CLINICAL IMAGING

CLINICAL IMAGING
AN INTRODUCTION TO THE ROLE OF IMAGING IN CLINICAL PRACTICE

Edited by

Matthew Freedman, M.D.

Associate Professor of Diagnostic Radiology
Georgetown University School of Medicine

Associate Professor of Diagnostic Radiology
The Russell H. Morgan Department of Radiology
The Johns Hopkins University School of Medicine

Associate Professor of Diagnostic Radiology
Assistant Professor of Orthopedic Surgery
The University of Maryland School of Medicine
Baltimore, Maryland

Churchill Livingstone
New York, Edinburgh, London, Melbourne
1988

Library of Congress Cataloging-in-Publication Data

Clinical imaging.

    Includes index.
    1. Diagnostic imaging.   I. Freedman, Matthew.
RC78.7.D53C565   1988   616.07'57   87-22986
ISBN 0-443-08623-0

Distributed in the United Kingdom by Churchill Livingstone, Robert Stevenson House, 1-3 Baxter's Place, Leith Walk, Edinburgh EH1 3AF, and by associated companies, branches, and representatives throughout the world.

Accurate indications, adverse reactions, and dosage schedules for drugs are provided in this book, but it is possible that they may change. The reader is urged to review the package information data of the manufacturers of the medications mentioned.

The Publishers have made every effort to trace the copyright holders for borrowed material. If they have inadvertently overlooked any, they will be pleased to make the necessary arrangements at the first opportunity.

Printed in the United States of America

First published in 1988

CONTRIBUTORS

J. Wolfe Blotzer, M.D.
Division of Rheumatology
York Hospital
York, Pennsylvania

Morgan G. Dunne, M.A., M.B., B.Ch., B.A.O.
Chief, Radiology Service
Baltimore Veterans Administration Medical Center
Baltimore, Maryland

David Graham, M.D.
Associate Professor
Obstetrics and Gynecology
University of Rochester Medical Center
Rochester, New York

Phillip J. Haney, M.D.
Associate Professor of Radiology
Department of Radiology
University of Maryland School of Medicine
Baltimore, Maryland

Peter M. Joseph, Ph.D.
Associate Professor of Radiologic Physics in Radiology
Department of Radiology
University of Pennsylvania
Philadelphia, Pennsylvania

Harry C. Knipp, M.D.
Department of Radiology
Carroll County General Hospital
Westminster, Maryland

Yu-Chen Lee, M.D.
Associate Professor of Medicine
Division of Cardiology
University of Maryland School of Medicine
Baltimore, Maryland

Erlinda McCrea, M.D.
Associate Professor of Radiology
Department of Radiology
University of Maryland School of Medicine
Baltimore, Maryland

John Meyerhoff, M.D.
Assistant Professor
Department of Medicine
University of Maryland School of Medicine
Baltimore, Maryland

CASE CONTRIBUTORS

Eric J. Blum, M.D.
Attending Radiologist
Chesapeake Imaging Specialists
Baltimore, Maryland

Janet Brown, M.D.
Radiologist
North Arundel Hospital
Pasadena, Maryland

Stephan J. Cisternino, M.D.
Associate Attending Physician
Department of Radiology
Suburban Hospital
Bethesda, Maryland

Charles M. Citrin, M.D.
Director of Radiology
The Neurology Center, P.A.
Chevy Chase, Maryland

Barry H. Friedman, M.D.
President
Chesapeake Imaging Specialists
Baltimore, Maryland

Rosemarie Greyson-Fleg, M.D.
Radiologist
North Charles General Hospital
Baltimore, Maryland

David Moses, M.D.
Director, Division of Nuclear Medicine
Acting Radiologist-in-Chief
Sinai Hospital of Baltimore
Baltimore, Maryland

Jerry Patt, M.D.
Attending Radiologist
Shultze, Snider, and Associates, P.A.
Baltimore, Maryland

Roger Sanders, M.D.
Professor of Radiology
Associate Professor of Urology
The Johns Hopkins Medical Institutions
Baltimore, Maryland

Margaret E. Toxopeus, M.D.
Attending Radiologist
Winchester Memorial Hospital
Winchester, Virginia

Mark Vaccaro, M.D.
Radiologist
Rouseau, Dominica
Windward Islands, West Indies

Nancy O. Whitley, M.D.
Professor of Radiology
Department of Radiology
University of Maryland School of Medicine
Baltimore, Maryland

PREFACE

As a child, I was fascinated by Superman's ability to see through walls and to spy on criminals. Perhaps this sparked the interest that eventually led me to study radiology. To the student coming to the radiologist with a radiograph, the diagnoses generated by the radiologist often seem as amazing as did Superman's feats, and the aid that the radiograph gives in solving clinical problems is often as dramatic as Superman's capture of the elusive criminal.

In modern medicine, the imaging techniques play an important role in solving patients' problems. In the past 15 years the ability of radiology to diagnose patients' problems has increased greatly because of the development of new modalities of imaging and the improvement of the older methods. At the same time, the growing complexity of the field has made it increasingly difficult for the student trying to learn the field.

With the increase in the number of techniques available for imaging the body, students have faced the prospect of learning each technique separately, attempting their own integration of the methods of interpretation and clinical use of these different modalities.

This text integrates the different imaging modalities and, as appropriate, discusses the common methods of imaging-guided surgical treatment. To simplify the process of learning, it looks at those features common among the imaging techniques and their method of interpretation. It makes recommendations for the evaluation of common clinical problems. Chapter 1 discusses the methods of analysis of imaging studies. Chapters 2 through 6 discuss the methods used for imaging the body. Chapters 7 through 62 discuss the clinical applications of the imaging methods, divided by anatomic region. Chapter 63 discusses medical economics and the impact of diagnostic imaging on the cost of health care.

Each chapter consists of several distinct parts:

1. Key concepts and objectives: a section that gives an overview of the most important information contained in the chapter.
2. Keynotes: comments within the text page that emphasize key points and define words or concepts.
3. Review questions: questions to help guide you back to the key points in each chapter and sometimes to guide you to questions that go beyond the text.
4. A vocabulary list: a list of key words in the chapter that you should know.
5. The chapter text: the text is designed to assist the resident in radiology and the medical student in learning an appropriate clinical approach to diagnostic imaging. It is intended to serve as a guide to the imaging studies seen on each clinical clerkship, as the text for a 3- to 5-week radiology course, and as a reference for first-year residents.

SUGGESTED METHODS OF USE DURING CLINICAL CLERKSHIPS

The book is divided into sections based on clinical anatomic groupings. There are sections on the imaging of lung disease, heart disease, abdominal disease, gastrointestinal disease, and so on. These sections can be used by students to gain a better understanding of the imaging component of the care of patients with these diseases. In some cases, the director of a clinical clerkship may specifically advise students to read selected chapters. In other cases, the chapters can be chosen by students to help them understand their own patients.

SUGGESTED METHOD OF USE DURING A RADIOLOGY COURSE

When used as the text for a 3- to 5-week radiology course, chapters can be selected to coordinate with the course your instructor has designed.

The contributors join me in hoping that this book will enrich your education and guide you to being a better physician and diagnostician.

MATTHEW FREEDMAN

ACKNOWLEDGMENTS

This book is the result of the influence and assistance of the many fine radiologists, physicians, residents, fellows, and students with whom I have had the privilege of working and from whom I have learned so much.

In addition to those contributors specifically acknowledged in the text as contributors, I would like especially to thank the following for their direct or indirect assistance in the preparation of this book and the teaching material that forms its core: From the University of Rochester: Stanley Rogoff, M.D.; Paul Ross, M.D.; Lionel Young, M.D.; Wendy Logan, M.D.; and Harry Fischer, M.D. From Rochester General Hospital: Ted Van Zandt, M.D. From the Johns Hopkins Medical Institutions: Martin Donner, M.D.; Stanley Siegelman, M.D.; and John Dorst, M.D. From the University of Maryland: Joseph Whitley, M.D., and Charles Edwards, M.D. From the Sinai Hospital of Baltimore: Spencer Foreman, M.D.; Robert Conaty; and the advisor and donor who wishes to remain anonymous.

Several cases came from the Pediatric Radiology Teaching File at Johns Hopkins, John Dorst, M.D., Director.

Thanks also go to General Electric Medical Systems and Philips Medical Systems for their contributions of illustrations.

I should like to thank the following for their photographic contributions: Henri Hessels, Willie Ragsdale, David Crandall, Donald Yeager, Harriett Sherr, and Bernard Bowers.

I should like to thank the following for their secretarial assistance: Dee Baer, Trisha Mead, Mary Baladarch, Millie Glass, and Margo Chisnell. Special thanks go to Debbie Trust for her work on Chapter 21.

I should like to thank Cass Schmidt for her artistic assistance.

I should especially like to thank my editors Robert Hurley, Linda Turner, Ray Moloney, Amarjit Chawla, and Sidney Landau, who kept me on track and working toward the distant goal of completing this book.

MATTHEW FREEDMAN

CONTENTS

1

HOW THE RADIOLOGIST WORKS

KEY CONCEPTS

This chapter discusses the process that a radiologist uses to arrive at a diagnosis.

1. There are five stages of the diagnostic process:
   a. Careful observation
   b. Comparison with mental images of normal and abnormal
   c. Tentative diagnosis
   d. Testing the tentative diagnosis
   e. Final diagnosis
2. In difficult cases, the radiologist uses a list of the categories of disease, dividing diseases into those that are

   Congenital
   Inflammatory-infectious
   Neoplastic
   Traumatic or surgical
   Metabolic
   Vascular
   Allergic
3. Three sequential stages of careful observation are used:
   a. The initial complete search
   b. A review of those places where findings are often missed—the check areas
   c. A survey of those places where that radiologist has missed findings—the psychological blind spots

OBJECTIVES

When you complete this chapter you will be able to

1. List the five stages of the diagnostic process.

2. List the categories of disease.
3. Generate a list of potential diagnoses using a list of the categories of disease.
4. List the three sequential stages of careful observation.

As you learn to practice medicine you will spend many hours looking at radiographs of your patients. You are likely to find the interpretation of radiographs difficult, but this should not discourage you from looking and learning. You may also frequently be startled by what the radiologist can tell you about your patient from a few images, and you may wonder how he does this.

How does the radiologist work? William James Morton was the first American radiologist and his method is the method we still use. Morton, a physician and a son of William Morton, a dentist and probable codiscoverer of ether anesthesia, had spent many years studying the application of electrical devices to the treatment of human illness. In 1898, on hearing of Roentgen's discovery, he realized that one of his experimental devices had probably been producing (unbeknownst to him) x-rays. He modified this device and started to make radiographs of all parts of the body. He was able in this way to assemble a large number of plates showing both normal and diseased people. When a patient was sent to him for a radiograph, he would compare the image he obtained with those in his file and would make his diagnosis by comparison.

How does a radiologist work? There are five stages:

1. Careful observation
2. Comparison with mental images of normal and abnormal

3. Tentative diagnosis (hypothesis)
4. Testing the tentative diagnosis (testing the hypothesis)
5. Final diagnosis

Each of these stages is important and each must be used.

CAREFUL OBSERVATION

Careful visual observation is probably the hardest skill for the student in medicine to master; examining the skin and external structure of the body, learning histopathology, examining the body's image on the radiograph—these cause the student of medicine great problems. Why should this be so? Visual skills are not often called upon in high school and college, where most of the learning depends on verbal memory and verbal analysis. Since they have not been needed, they often have not been learned. To succeed in radiology, a new skill must be learned, the skill of observing.

Some students bridge this gap quickly, but many struggle with it. Fortunately, only a few give up before they master the skill. What is the method of improving this skill? The prime method is to have a search pattern, a system of looking at everything; such search patterns are important but not sufficient. The search must be an active looking, both for abnormalities and always to test the hypotheses that each found abnormality generates.

For example, look at the chest radiograph in Figure 1-1. This is a chest film on a 35-year-old man. What do you see?

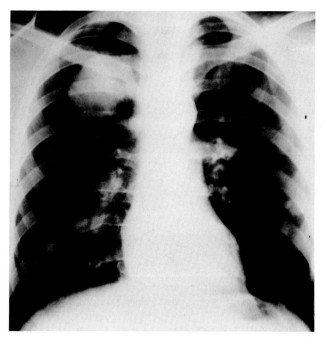

Figure 1-1. A patient with a large lung mass. In addition to the mass in the right upper lobe, there are smaller masses in the left hilum and in the left lower lung. This patient had metastatic testicular cancer.

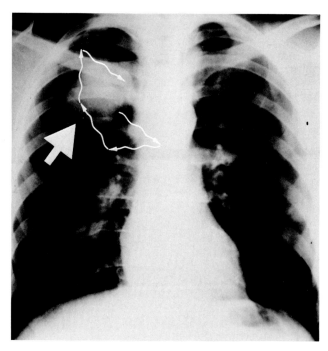

Figure 1-2. A search pattern typical of an inexperienced viewer. The viewer keeps looking at the big mass, entranced by having found an abnormality, and misses the smaller masses.

Most students will quickly see the large mass in the right upper lung; fascinated with having found an abnormality, they will cease to look more. Their search pattern, if recorded, might look like that in Figure 1-2.

What else do you see if you keep looking? There is a mass in the left hilum and another in the lower left lung (Fig. 1-3). With one mass, you might think of lung cancer. If you did, your hypothesis should lead you to search for metastases, helping you to find the other masses; if you found all the masses, then you would suspect metastatic cancer and could suggest a search for the primary tumor.

Each finding should lead you to search for more findings. The best visual search cannot find everything. The best search starts with an organized view of everything once; then the search is directed to look for specific, predictable abnormalities based on your hypothesis about the findings you have made.

Types of Search Patterns

On any radiograph, three consecutive search patterns are used:

1. *Initial complete search*
2. A search of the regions where lesions are most likely to be missed, the *check areas.*
3. A search in those areas in which you yourself have missed lesions before, your *psychological blind spots*

Initial Complete Search. There are two types of search patterns: the geographic and the anatomic. The first is a

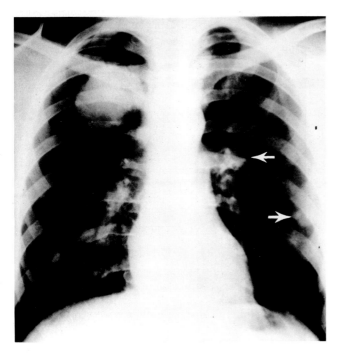

Figure 1-3. Additional masses marked.

search of the film by location, the second by organ and organ groups. The search patterns can start, respectively, with the region or organ most likely or least likely to be abnormal. In different parts of this book, different types of search patterns are suggested, not as absolute rules but as guides so that you can eventually choose your own patterns of systematic observation.

Check Areas. Even with careful, systematic search, lesions are missed on the radiograph, perhaps 20% on the initial survey. Because of this, additional observation is essential. Radiographs of each part of the body have their own areas of difficulty. Lists of these areas to check are given throughout this book. It is useful to memorize them because these are the places where lesions are most often missed.

Psychological Blind Spots. "Psychological" is overstating it, but many students who look at radiographs seem to have the same type of observational problem over and over. In a sense, these observation misses are built into the viewer, and it is only by conscious effort that the student's skill at observation improves. When you miss a finding on the radiograph, you should try to figure out why you missed the finding so that, by special attention, the same type of miss will not occur again.

Keynotes

• *The sequential search consists of*
  An initial complete search

The check areas
Your psychological blind spots
• *There are two types of search patterns:*
  Anatomic
  Geographic
• *Each time you miss an abnormality, try to figure out why you missed it so you will not miss it the next time.*

COMPARISON WITH MENTAL IMAGES OF NORMAL AND ABNORMAL

As William Morton did, we must develop our own memory sets of what normal and abnormal radiographs look like. The only way to do this is to look carefully at all the radiographs on your own patients. Athough books with patterns seen in normal and ill patients are available, these are cumbersome to use. The mental image is best.

What do you do when you see a pattern you have never seen before? You have to analyze the image. The technique of this analysis is discussed in Chapters 2–6 as part of the discussion of the individual types of imaging techniques.

TENTATIVE DIAGNOSIS (HYPOTHESIS)

Based on your observations and your comparisons of what you've seen with your mental images of normal and abnormal, you should make a hypothesis about what disease the patient may have. For each finding or group of findings, you should consider what kinds of diseases might result in the finding or findings. One of the useful ways of doing this is to have a list of categories of diseases. Thus an abnormality may be congenital, inflammatory-infectious, neoplastic, traumatic or surgical, metabolic, vascular, or allergic. For example, a patient with an interstitial lung process could have

Congenital lymphangiectasis
A viral infection
Lymphangitic spread of tumor
A lung contusion
Heart failure
Asthma

Using a category list of the types of disease helps in deriving hypothetical diagnoses, but then each of these hypotheses must be tested against the film, looking for other findings that might support or refute the hypothesis. Once the diagnosis or diagnoses are consistent with all the findings on the film, it is then helpful to consider the clinical information. Does the clinical information support your diagnosis? Does the clinical information suggest other possible diagnoses for the same findings? The clinical information should lead you back to the film to search again for those findings that could be present were the clinical diagnosis correct.

Radiologists often seem not to be interested in what you are telling them. When you talk to them, they tend not to look at you but at the film. Indeed, it is hard to get a radiologist to look you in the eye. Why? Because the good radiologist is always searching the film. Listening and searching. Even the skilled radiologist knows that he never sees all the findings on the film, and using what you say to guide his search may help him to make new observations, guiding you and helping your patient.

Active search based on continuous generation of hypotheses is the basis of the radiologist's skill, and it is something you can learn and should learn, because the same technique is also at the heart of the skill of the great clinical diagnosticians: listening to what the patient says, making hypotheses, probing with questions, examining the patient, making hypotheses based on the findings, and questioning and searching again.

Keynotes

- *Classification of diseases, method 1: Congenital, inflammatory, neoplastic, traumatic or surgical, metabolic, vascular, allergic.*
- *Classification of diseases, method 2: VICTIM, where V = Vascular; I = Inflammatory; C = Congenital, Cancer, Collagen-vascular; T = Traumatic; I = Idiopathic; and M = Metabolic.*
- *An active search based on the continous generation of hypotheses is the basis of the radiologist's skill.*

TESTING HYPOTHESES

Each hypothesis made is tested against the findings on the film and then against the patient's clinical history and physical examination. Initially, during learning, the generation of hypotheses comes first, followed by their testing. With experience, the two acts occur almost together; generation and critique are almost simultaneous. It is important to learn to do both.

FINAL DIAGNOSIS

It would appear obvious: the final diagnosis after all of the above *is* final! Unfortunately, it is not. People are complex and variable. The final radiographic diagnosis is a hypothesis to be tested against all the other information you have about *your* patient. The radiologist has the radiograph, but you have the complete clinical history, the results of the physical examination, the laboratory tests, the results of the radiography, and your own clinical skill. The clinician should use the radiological information, not be used by it.

SUMMARY

The evaluation of an image of the body is based on a directed search. Systematic observation based on either an anatomic or a geographic approach is followed by the generation and testing of hypotheses. Each search is really a sequence of searches: a directed complete search, a survey of check areas where people are likely to miss lesions, a recheck of places where you yourself have missed lesions in the past, and then a search based on hypotheses you have generated based on what you have found on your earlier searches.

The generation of the hypothetical diagnoses can be made more complete by using a list of disease categories. Although there are several that can be used, the following list is particularly helpful: congenital, inflammatory, neoplastic, traumatic or surgical, metabolic, vascular, allergic.

REVIEW QUESTIONS

1. What are the stages of the diagnostic process?
2. List the categories of disease.
3. A careful survey of an image can be made using two different approaches. They are . . . ?
4. What are check areas?
5. How do you discover your own psychological blind spots?
6. What should you do to overcome your psychological blind spots?

SUGGESTIONS FOR FURTHER READING

William J. Tuddenham, Ed. Perception of the roentgen image. *Radiologic Clinics of North America,* **7**(3), 1969.

Harold L. Kundel, Calvin F. Nodine, Dennis Carmody. Visual scanning: Pattern recognition and decision-making in pulmonary nodule detection. *Investigative Radiology,* **13**:175–181, 1978.

Harold L. Kundel, Paul S. LaFollett, Jr. Visual search patterns and experience with radiological images. *Radiology,* **103**:523–528, 1972.

Harold L. Kundel, D. John Wright. The influence of prior knowledge on visual search strategies during the viewing of chest radiographs. *Radiology,* **93**:315–320, 1969.

2

RADIOGRAPHIC TECHNIQUES

KEY CONCEPTS

This chapter discusses conventional radiographic techniques, that is, those techniques of imaging based on the transmission of a beam of x-ray photons through a patient. Computed tomography (CT), while based on these same principles of x-ray photon transmission, is discussed separately in Chapter 4.

Images can be produced by x-ray photons because the body selectively limits the amount of x-ray photons that pass through it, and this limitation is based on the electron density of different tissues. There are two different types of "density" in radiography: electron (or radio) density and optical density. *Electron density* is the number of electrons per unit of tissue thickness and so is based on the inherent structure of the substance radiographed. *Optical density* is the degree of blackness recorded on the film. It is based on the electron density of the substance radiographed, the x-ray techniques used, the film used to record the image, and how that film is developed. Five different substances have sufficient differences in *radiodensity* to be easily distinguished on radiographs: air, fat, water, bone, and metal. The transmission of x-ray photons is dependent on the type and amount of such substances the photons must pass through.

Radiographic images can be recorded in different ways: directly on film, transformed into light that exposes film, transformed into light that is viewed directly or with television amplification (*fluoroscopy*), or recorded on a xerographic plate.

This chapter also discusses the applications of these techniques to the visualization of blood vessels (*angiography*) and to the visualization of thin sections of the body (*tomography*).

OBJECTIVES

When you complete this chapter you will be able to

1. Describe the interaction of x-ray photons with atomic electrons.

2. Define electron density.

3. Describe the contributions of atomic number, physical state, and object thickness to the total electron density of an object.

4. List the five radiographic densities.

5. Describe the difference between the radiodensity of an object and its optical density as seen on a film.

6. Describe the different methods of viewing the image.

7. Describe the role of phosphor screens in converting x-ray photons into light photons.

8. Describe how tomography enables one to visualize thin layers of the body.

MAKING THE IMAGE: THE INTERACTION OF RADIATION AND MATTER

Radiography was the first method used for imaging of the interior of the body. X-ray photons of high energy are directed to pass through the portion of the body to be studied. A few of the photons are absorbed; others are deflected from their straight course by electrons in their paths. These deflected photons either miss the image recorder or strike it in the wrong place, resulting in a gray cast to the image, called noise. The x-ray image itself is made by those photons that pass through the patient without interacting with electrons and then interact with the image recorder to produce an image. In the abdomen only about 1% of the initial x-ray photons reach the image recorder to make the image; the rest are either absorbed or deflected.

The image produced, therefore, is dependent on the probability that an x-ray photon will not interact with an electron in its path, and that in turn is dependent on the

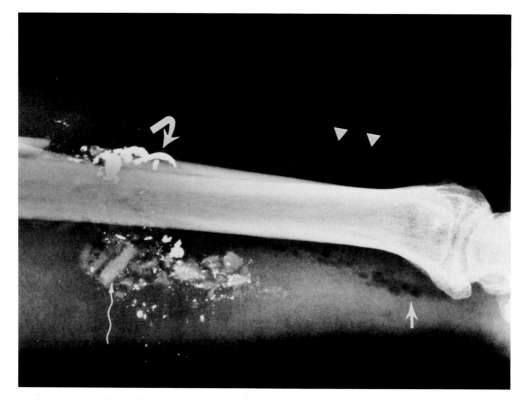

Figure 2-1. Radiograph of the forearm with a gunshot wound and fracture. The air outside the arm is black. Air within the soft tissues (straight arrow) is dark gray because it is radiolucent with water radiodensity material added to it. The subcutaneous fat (arrowheads) is dark gray. The bone of the radius, ulna, and fracture fragments (wavy arrow) is almost white, and the metal fragments from the bullet are white (curved arrow).

number of electrons in its path. The greater the electron density, the greater the likelihood of an interaction and, therefore, the less the likelihood that the photon will reach the image recorder. The greater the electron density, the less the exposure of the image recorder and the less the blackening or whitening seen on the image recorder.

The radiographic image, therefore, is a shadow reflecting areas of differing electron density. If the image is recorded on film, the greater the electron density, the less the exposure and blackening of the film; the lower the electron density, the greater the exposure of the film and the greater the blackening.

Two factors affect the electron density in the path of the x-ray photon: the thickness of the object and the number of electrons per unit thickness. The number of electrons per unit thickness depends on the atomic number and the physical state (gas, liquid, solid) of the substance. Air, composed of gases with low atomic numbers, has a low electron density and usually appears black on a radiograph. Bone, a solid composed of atoms with higher atomic numbers, has a high electron density and usually appears white on radiographs.

Using standard radiographic techniques, the eye can be expected to distinguish five different radiodensities, one from another, if they are placed side by side. These five basic radiographic densities are air, fat, water, bone, and metal. If the exposure is set properly, air can appear black, and metal white, with fat, water, and bone represented as shades of gray in between (Fig. 2-1). These densities are, however, relative. If a careless technologist were to turn up the output of the machine, eventually enough x-ray photons could traverse a piece of metal to blacken the film. But if this happened, all the other substances would also appear black. If the technologist turned the output of the machine low enough, even air might appear white because so few x-ray photons were being produced. But then everything on the film would be white. Although the radiodensity (based on the electron density) of an object cannot be changed in this matter, the film (or optical) density can be easily changed by changing the settings of the x-ray machine.

Changing the Radiodensity of Tissues

It is sometimes desirable to change the radiodensity of the body tissues. This can be done by the injection of a drug containing iodine. Such drugs, called contrast media, can increase the radiodensity in three ways: they can increase the radiodensity of blood vessels and organs with blood flow; they can be designed to be excreted and concentrated by the kidneys, permitting better visualization of the urinary system; they can be designed to be excreted by the biliary system, permitting visualization of the larger bile ducts and gallbladder.

Keynotes

- *The radiographic image is a shadow reflecting areas of differing electron density.*
- *The electron density in the path of a beam of x-ray photons is based on*
  The atomic number of the object
  Its thickness
  Its physical state (gas, liquid, solid)
- *The five basic radiodensities are air, fat, water, bone, and metal.*
- *Radiodensity is due to the number of electrons in the path of the x-ray beam and the energy of that x-ray beam.*
- *Optical density is the amount of blackening on the film.*

RECORDING THE IMAGE

There are several methods for transforming the x-ray photons that have been encoded, by their passage through the body, into an image. The x-ray photons can be used to expose photographic film directly, or directed onto a phosphor screen that will transform them into flashes of light. These flashes of light can then be used to expose film or amplified to produce an image that can be viewed as it is produced.

Direct Exposure Imaging

Films can be placed in the x-ray photon beam. This allows the x-ray photon to strike the film directly, deionizing the silver halide emulsion making the image. This technique gives an image with very high detail but requires relatively high doses of radiation because film is not very sensitive to x-rays. Most radiography no longer uses the direct imaging onto radiographic film because the excellent detail obtained is usually not necessary to diagnose the patient's problem. This technique is now usually limited to the study of the breast for cancer (mammography) and to the study of the hands for metabolic bone disease (hyperparathyroidism).

X-ray photons can also be directed onto a Polaroid radio-

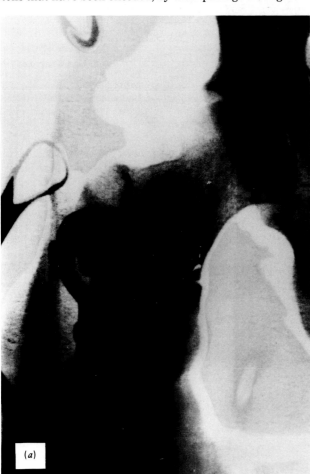

(a)

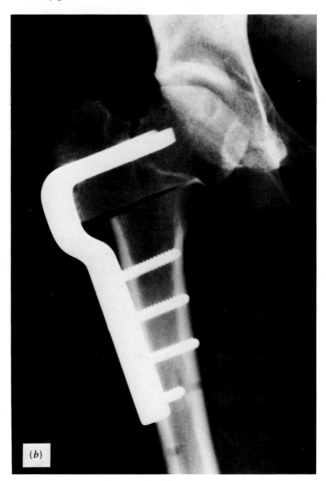

(b)

Figure 2-2. Right hip with metal plate holding position of fragments. Two different patients. (a) Polaroid image. (b) Conventional film image. The Polaroid image has less contrast. Black and white are reversed in the two images.

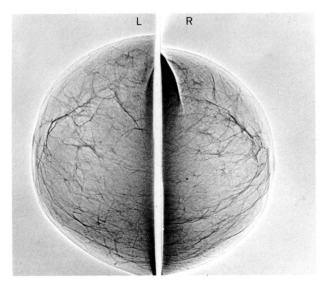

Figure 2-3. Xeromammogram of the breast. Normal fatty breast. L = left breast. R = right breast.

graphic film or onto a xerographic plate. Polaroid film permits the rapid development of the image without the need for developing tanks or machines but uses a relatively high radiation dose to give an image of low contrast (Fig. 2-2). Xerography has, in its response to x-ray photons, a special characteristic: edge enhancement. Minor changes in tissue structure are exaggerated by the electrostatic exaggeration of the images. This technique is usually limited to the study of the breasts (Fig. 2-3). It is occasionally useful in the study of the extremities and the neck (Fig. 2-4).

Phosphor Screen Exposure

X-ray photons when they strike an appropriate *phosphor screen* will generate a flash of light. Because the phosphor screen is more sensitive to x-ray photons than is film, and because film is more sensitive to light exposure than to x-ray photon exposure, the amount of radiation needed to make the image is less. Film can be placed next to the phosphor, to be exposed to flashes of light, and record an image. This technique gives an image with good detail (but not as good as direct exposure of the film to the x-ray photons) with much lower radiation dose.

By changing the crystal size, thickness, and phosphor chemistry in the screen, the phosphor can be made more or less sensitive to x-ray photons. For any particular phosphor structure, increasing the thickness of the phosphor layer decreases the amount of radiation needed to make an image, but it also decreases the detail resolution of the image. The radiologist can choose the appropriate phosphors for the part of the body being studied and thereby limit the radiation the patient receives to the minimal amount necessary to obtain adequate diagnostic detail.

Fluoroscopy

The light generated in the phosphor screen can be viewed in additional ways. If viewed as it is generated, the technique is called *fluoroscopy*. The phosphor screen can be viewed directly, via electronic magnification, or via electronic magnification and television enlargement. Viewing the movement of portions of the esophagus, stomach or heart and using fluoroscopy to position the patient for accurate filming is of great help in evaluating the patient's disease. The use of fluoroscopy is limited by the relatively high radiation dose and by the lack of a permanent record of what was seen. For this reason, fluoroscopy is often combined with the taking of radiographs. These radiographs can be taken by the conventional method or photographed from the electronically amplified image.

Keynotes

- *Direct film exposure is usually limited to*
  Mammography (the study of the breast for cancer)
  The study of the hands for hyperparathyroidism
- *The x-ray photon beam can directly expose film, xerographic plates, Polaroid film.*
- *Xerography has the special characteristic of edge enhancement.*
- *Phosphor screens transform x-ray photons into flashes of light.*
- *Fluoroscopy permits the immediate and continuous viewing of the x-ray image.*

TYPES OF RADIOGRAPHIC STUDIES

Radiography

Radiography is the recording of x-ray–produced images on film.

Advantages

1. High resolution.
2. Screening method: the same radiograph screens for many types of abnormalities.
3. Intermediate cost.
4. General physician familiarity with interpretation, indications, and reliability.

Disadvantages

1. Low-dose radiation hazard.
2. Ready availability leads to potential overuse.

Main Uses

1. Screening for chest, cardiac, renal, abdominal, gastrointestinal, and skeletal diseases
2. Evaluating the progression of pulmonary, gastrointestinal, skeletal, and occasionally renal disease

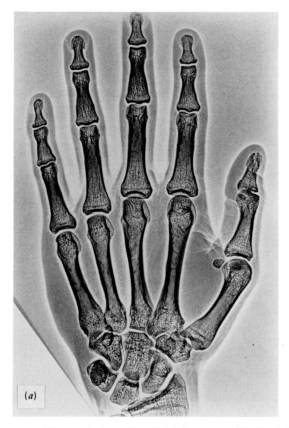 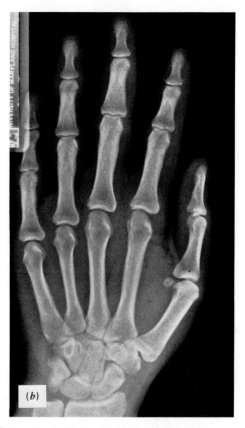

Figure 2-4. Normal hand. (*a*). Xerogram of the hand. (*b*) Conventional radiograph of the hand. Note the increased definition (edge enhancement) of the trabeculae of the bone on the xerogram.

Main Abuses

1. Search for pulmonary emboli (lung scan is preferred)
2. Evaluation of the bladder (if hematuria is present, cystoscopy is necessary).
3. Overused in screening patients with head injuries.

Fluoroscopy

Fluoroscopy is the continuous viewing of the image made as x-rays pass through the patient.

Advantages

1. Ability to see motion.
2. Permits accurate positioning for radiography.
3. Ability to see small amounts of calcification in moving structures (heart).

Disadvantages

1. Moderately high radiation dose
2. Lack of record of what is seen

Main Uses

1. Evaluation of physiological motion of the gastrointestinal tract

2. Evaluation of cardiac motion
3. Evaluation for cardiac calcification
4. Evaluation for diaphragmatic fixation and phrenic nerve paralysis
5. Localization of pulmonary abnormalities
6. Positioning for radiography of the gastrointestinal tract

Keynotes

- *Radiography: the recording of x-ray–produced images on film.*
- *Fluoroscopy: the continuous viewing of images made as x-rays pass through a patient.*

SPECIAL TECHNIQUES

The Angiogram

An *angiogram* is a method of radiographing blood vessels. A medicine containing iodine (called contrast medium or material) is injected into a vessel, filling its lumen. Multiple radiographs are taken to demonstrate the anatomy of the blood vessels (Figs. 2-5 and 2-6). The contrast material can be placed in the vessel by direct needle placement or by

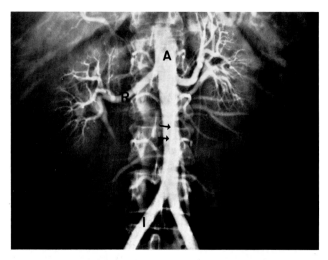

Figure 2-5. An angiogram of a normal abdominal aorta. A = aorta, R = right renal artery, I = iliac artery. The catheter can be faintly seen within the lumen of the aorta (arrows). The catheter was placed percutaneously into the right femoral artery and passed upward until the catheter tip was in the aorta. This procedure is called a transfemoral aortogram.

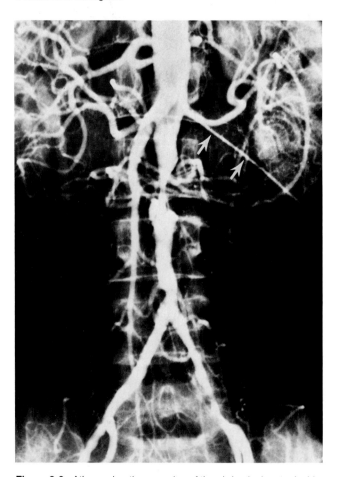

Figure 2-6. Atherosclerotic narrowing of the abdominal aorta. In this patient, a needle (arrows) was placed through the back into the aorta; the contrast was injected through this needle. This is called a translumbar aortogram.

positioning a tube called a catheter in the vessel of interest. These catheters are usually passed percutaneously into the femoral or axillary artery using the *Seldinger Technique.* By using long catheters, almost any vessel in the body can be imaged.

Advantages

1. Ability to see the anatomy of blood vessels:
   Contour
   Smoothness
   Luminal size
   Location
2. Placement of a catheter in a vessel permits therapy to be done in that vessel by passing instruments through the catheter. Vessels can be dilated or occluded, and medicines can be precisely administered.

Disadvantages

1. Risk of injury or death (1:100) from the procedure. Risk of injury is increased in children; risk of death is higher in the elderly. Both vary with procedure.

Arterial Studies

Main Uses

1. Evaluation of vascular luminal narrowing or occlusion (Fig. 2-6)
2. Operative planning for removal of vascular tumors

Secondary Uses

1. Evaluation of renal, hepatic, and pancreatic masses, if CT and ultrasound studies are unavailable or nondiagnostic (Fig. 2-7)

Venous Studies

Main Uses

1. Evaluation of thrombotic or thromboembolic disease (Fig. 2-8)
2. Evaluation of venous stasis preoperatively
3. Sampling of renal vein blood for renin (in patients with suspected renovascular hypertension)

Lymphatic Studies

Main Uses

1. Evaluation for nodal metastases from lymphoma or testicular tumors. Used to detect small metastases when CT is equivocal or normal.
2. Evaluation of lymphedema.

Interventional Techniques

Many organs in the body can be reached through the arterial or venous systems permitting:

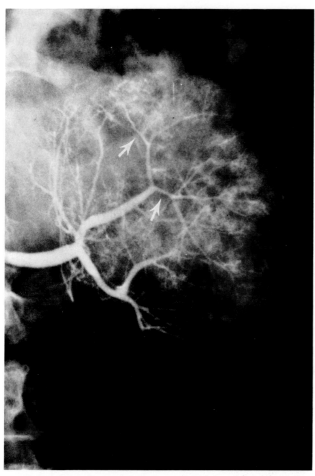

Figure 2-7. Left renal arteriogram. Vessels in the lower portion of the kidney are near normal (compare them with the renal vessels in Fig. 2-5). Those in the mid and upper portions of the kidney are in an area of renal cell carcinoma. Note the many additional fine vessels that are opacified. There is encasement (focal narrowing) of several vessels (arrows) caused by tumor compressing them. The small irregular vessels that form in tumor masses or in response to infection are called neovascularity.

1. Occlusion of bleeding vessels
2. Occlusion of vessels to vascular tumors to simplify surgery
3. Venous sampling for enzymes
4. Dilation of stenotic vessels
5. Administration of medicines

The Tomogram

The standard radiograph superimposes many layers of the body, each on top of the next. The image that results is difficult to evaluate because of the need to separate out these layers. *Tomography* is a technique that permits the imaging of a layer or section of the body while blurring out other layers. A tomogram is made on a special machine in which the x-ray tube and film move in opposite directions

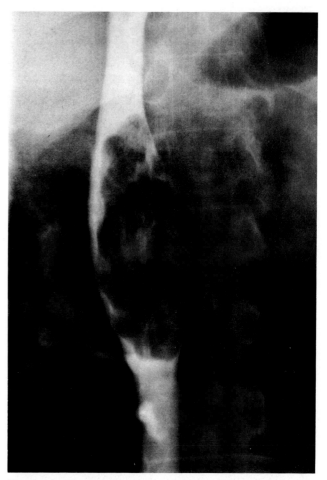

Figure 2-8. Inferior venacavagram. Normal opacification of the inferior vena cava is seen above and below a large mass of tumor that has extended from the tumor seen in Figure 2-7 into the inferior vena cava.

through an arc. From the viewpoint of the film, only a portion of the body at the center of rotation of this arc is still. This layer is in focus. All other layers are moving and are blurred. The tomogram can be helpful in selected cases in simplifying the analysis of complex regions of the body when standard radiography cannot adequately image this area (Fig. 2-9).

Tomography

Advantages

1. Blurring of overlying structures permits better visualization of the layer of interest.

Disadvantages

1. Moderate-to-high cost
2. Moderate radiation dose
3. Potential for sampling error
4. Ease of misinterpretation

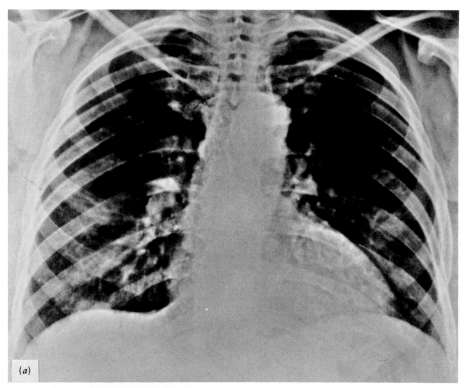

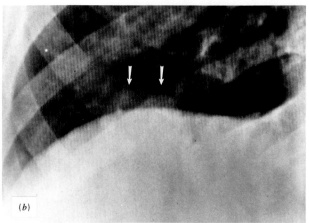

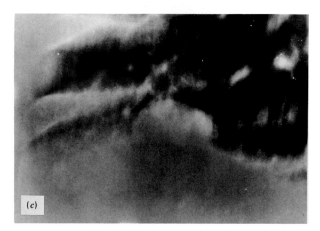

Figure 2-9. Conventional tomography used to evaluate a mass in the lower right side of the chest. (*a*) Conventional posteroanterior (PA) chest radiograph. The mass overlying the right hemidiaphragm is just visible. (*b*) Focal view demonstrates the mass (arrows) partially hidden behind the right hemidiaphragm. (*c*) Tomogram of the right lower lung demonstrates the mass. No calcium is demonstrated. Note that the mass itself is sharply seen, while the ribs that overlie it in *b* are not visible. They have been blurred out by the tomographic motion. A biopsy of this mass proved it to be a noncalcified tuberculoma.

Main Uses

1. Evaluation of location and of possible calcification in lung nodules 0.75 to 3 cm.

2. Evaluation of possibly abnormal hilum if oblique and lateral views cannot show it to be normal.

3. Evaluation for possible lung metastases in a patient with normal chest radiograph results before major ablative surgery, which would not be done if metastases were present.

    Bladder cancer
    Osteogenic sarcoma

4. As part of intravenous urographic studies of the kidney.

Caution

1. Always view a plain radiograph of the same area because sampling error may permit a lesion to be missed that can be seen on a standard radiograph.

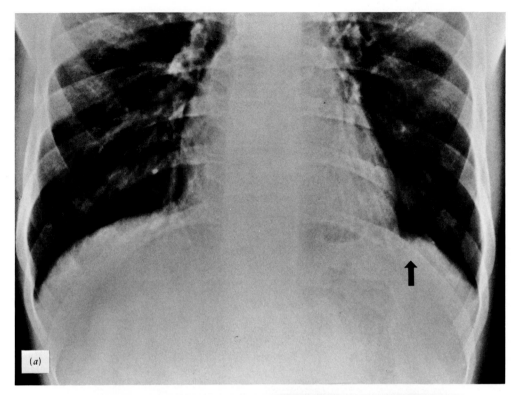

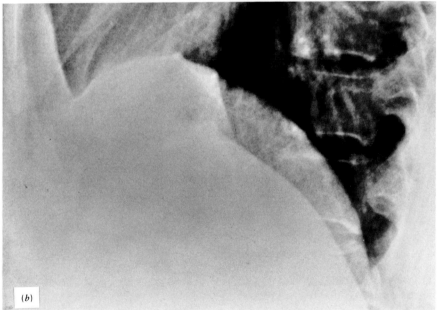

Figure 2-10. (*a*) Lower portion of the chest, PA view. A portion (arrow) of the left hemidiaphragm in this young, healthy patient cannot be seen because it is not tangential to the x-ray beam. The slope of the hemidiaphragm (as shown in *b*) is such that its margin is not tangential. The right hemidiaphragm in *a* has a different slope and its margin is distinct. (*b*) Lower portion of the chest, lateral view. The lower hemidiaphragm is the left hemidiaphragm; its anterior portion blends with the heart shadow. Its more posterior portion is not tangential to the x-ray beam on the PA view.

2. An edge not tangential to the beam in its arc of swing will disappear, suggesting that it is destroyed.

Keynotes

- *Angiography: the radiology of blood vessels.*
- *Angiographic catheters are placed through the skin, usually into the femoral or axillary artery. The method of placement is called the Seldinger technique.*
- *The Seldinger technique:*
  A needle is placed through the skin into a vessel.
  A wire is placed through the needle into the vessel.
  The needle is removed.
  A catheter is placed over the wire.
  When the catheter is within the vessel, the wire guide is removed.
- *Tomography: a technique of visualize one layer of tissue in the body by blurring out all other layers.*

INTERPRETING THE X-RAY IMAGE

What the Eye Can See

While there are a large number of potential densities that could be produced on a radiograph, the eye can only distinguish five of these, one from another: air, fat, water, bone, and metal. One of the great advantages that occurs from applying the computer to radiographic imaging is that the computer can separate additional levels of density, permitting us to see structures previously unseen on radiographs.

Evaluating an Unknown Image

The density on the film depends on the electron density of the substance radiographed, its thickness, and the exposure settings on the x-ray machine. If you can determine the thickness of an object, you can determine the type of substance it is made of; if you known what it is made of, you can determine its thickness.

The edge of an object can be seen easily only if it borders on a structure of different radiographic density and if the border is parallel to the direction of the x-ray beam. The heart margin on a chest radiograph (Fig. 2-9*a*) can be seen because the water-density heart is adjacent to the air-density lung and because the beam is in part parallel to the curved heart margin.

> *If two objects of the same radiodensity touch, the margin between them will not be seen.* Where the heart touches the diaphragm inferiorly, the border between them is invisible.

> *If the edge of an object is not parallel to the x-ray beam, it will not be seen.* The left hemidiaphragm in Figure 2-10 is of increased slope, and no portion of it is tangential to the beam, so its margin is indistinct.

> *If you know the density of an object and its shape, it will often be possible to determine what it is, based on a knowledge of normal and pathological anatomy.*

Keynotes

- *The edge of an object can be seen only if*
  1. *It borders on a structure of different radiographic density, and*
  2. *If the x-ray beam is tangential to the border of the object.*
- *When two objects of the same radiodensity touch, the margin between them will not be seen.*
- *If the x-ray beam is not tangential to the edge of an object, the edge of that object will not be sharp.*

SUMMARY

Radiography is the use of x-ray photons to create an image on film directly or by the generation of light from the exposure of a phosphor screen. Fluoroscopy is the direct viewing of the image created by the x-ray photons as it is being made. Fluoroscopy permits the motion of organs within the body to be seen.

The vessels within the body can be visualized by taking radiographs after injecting radiopaque medicine into them. Tomography is the radiography of thin layers of the body. The use of each of these techniques is summarized within this chapter; the important uses will be discussed more fully in subsequent chapters.

REVIEW QUESTIONS

1. List the different methods for recording radiographic images.
2. What does the phosphor screen used in radiography do?
3. What special property does xeroradiography offer?
4. In catheter angiography, the catheter is usually placed into one of two vessels and is then guided to the vessel of interest. What vessels commonly serve as the entry point for the catheter?
5. Tomography is used to evaluate the lung in what conditions?
6. What is the difference between optical density and radiodensity?
7. What are the five radiodensities distinguishable on a radiograph?

TRUE-FALSE

1. Two water-density objects that touch can be visually separated if their edges are parallel to the x-ray beam.
2. Two water-density objects that touch can be visually separated if their edges are not parallel to the x-ray beam.
3. If bone lies within fat, the two substances can be visually separated on a radiograph.
4. Tomograms should always be interpreted with a standard radiograph of the same portion of the body.

VOCABULARY

angiography   radiodensity
fluoroscopy   Seldinger technique
optical density   tomography
phosphor screen

SUGGESTIONS FOR FURTHER READING

The Fundamentals of Radiology, 12th Ed. Health Sciences Division, Eastman Kodak: Rochester, N.Y. 1980.

3

NUCLEAR MEDICINE: TRACER IMAGING TECHNIQUES

KEY CONCEPTS

This chapter discusses the methods by which the radiologist uses small amounts of gamma ray–emitting radioactive drugs to make images of the body. The names applied to this group of techniques are "nuclear medicine," "nuclear radiology," and "nuclear imaging." The images result from the preferential accumulation or exclusion of the radioactive *tracer* from the organ or tissue of interest. Nuclear medicine techniques are most often used to image the lungs, heart, liver, biliary tract, bone, thyroid, and kidneys.

OBJECTIVES

When you complete this chapter you will be able to

1. Give an example of a nuclear medicine–imaging method that depends on each of the following imaging methods:

   Radiotracer exclusion

   Metabolic accumulation

   Biologic mimicry

   Capillary occlusion

   Cellular or intracellular binding

   Excretion or secretion

2. List and describe the two main types of instruments used to produce nuclear medicine images.

3. Give at least three reasons why technetium 99m and its compounds are used for so many of the nuclear medicine–imaging techniques.

Nuclear medicine imaging techniques use small amounts of radioactive materials to image the body. The radioactive material can be used in its elemental form

(such as xenon 133, which is used in lung imaging), as an ion (such as gallium 67^{++}, which is used in imaging abscesses), or as one of the elements in a compound (such as technetium Tc 99m diphosphonate, which is used in bone scanning). Most of the isotopes used are gamma emitters, and it is the ability of gamma rays to penetrate through the body to a detector outside the body that permits these isotopes to be used for imaging. Less commonly, positron emitters are used for imaging. Positrons rapidly interact with electrons and decompose to form gamma rays that can then be detected and converted into an image.

Tracer images result either from the accumulation of the tracer in a region of interest or from its selective exclusion from a region of interest. The images can be clinically useful only if the disease being studied affects the localization of the tracer differently than the normal organ. For example, the ion pertechnetate Tc 99m is selectively excluded from brain tissue, but not excluded from most brain tumors. It is easy to see the region of activity within the nonradioactive brain tissue (Fig. 3-1). Conversely, technetium Tc 99m sulfur colloid particles are ingested by cells of the reticuloendothelial system of liver. Regions of tumor do not contain reticuloendothelial cells and will have less radioactivity than the normal portions of the liver (Fig. 3-2).

Keynotes

- *Nuclear medicine–imaging uses radioactive isotopes in small (tracer) quantities to image the interior of the body.*

- *Imaging results from the preferential accumulation or exclusion of the tracer from the organ or tissue of interest.*

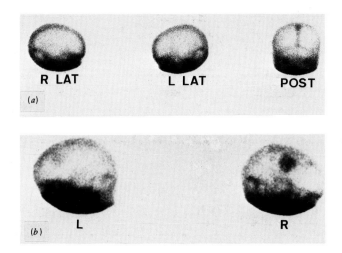

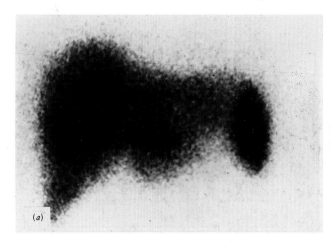

Figure 3-1. (a) A scan of a normal brain performed with sodium pertechnetate Tc 99m. The blacker areas represent areas of tracer activity in the blood. The ^{99m}Tc does not cross the blood-brain barrier. R Lat = right lateral, L LAT = left lateral, POST = posterior. (Courtesy of M. Vaccaro, M.D.) (b) A scan demonstrating metastasis in the right parietal lobe of the brain. While the ^{99m}Tc does not cross the blood-brain barrier, it does pass into the tumor, enabling us to see it. L = left lateral, R = right lateral. (Courtesy of M. Vaccaro, M.D.)

METHODS OF RECORDING THE TRACER IMAGES

The location of the isotope tracer within the body is detected by a sodium iodide crystal placed close to the body. The sodium iodide detector can measure the total accumulation of tracer in the region; the rate of accumulation or disappearance can also be measured. To make an image, it is necessary to limit the recording by the detector to one localized region within the pool of generalized activity. This is done by using a lead *collimator*. Multiple holes within the thick piece of lead limit the recording of gamma rays to those traveling along the longitudinal axis of these holes. Gamma rays traveling obliquely will be absorbed by the lead in the collimator.

Rectilinear Scanner

In the *rectilinear scanner,* the sodium iodide detector and the collimator move back and forth across the patient, recording the activity from multiple locations in the body, one at a time. As each gamma ray strikes the sodium iodide crystal, a flash of light is produced. In the rectilinear scanner, all light flashes are amplified by a single electronic photomultiplier tube, blending together all of the spatial information. The collimator used with rectilinear scanners has a predetermined focal depth at which maximum resolution is obtained. Activity in structures outside the focal plane is still imaged, but with lesser intensity and resolution.

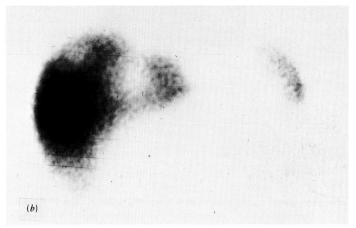

Figure 3-2. (a) A scan of a normal liver performed with technetium Tc 99m sulfur colloid. The tracer is taken up by the reticuloendothelial phagocytic cells of the liver and spleen, which are seen as the blacker areas of the image. (Courtesy M. Vaccaro, M.D.) (b) A liver scan from a patient with metastatic carcinoma of the colon. The rounded white areas within the liver are areas where tumor has replaced the normal liver. Since the tumor does not have reticuloendothelial cells, no tracer is phagocytosed in the regions of tumor, leaving them as white areas within the surrounding blackness of the activity in the liver. (Courtesy M. Vaccaro, M.D.)

Gamma Camera

The second type of imaging device is called the *gamma camera* (Fig. 3-3). In this device, a large sodium iodide crystal is used as a detector. Multiple (usually 19 or 37) photomultiplier tubes are used, each recording from its own and adjacent segments of the sodium iodide crystal. A computer can then use this data to produce a two-dimensional image. This spatial resolution is achieved by recording the difference in intensity of the flash of light as recorded by adjacent detectors. Because the flash of light is attenuated by a constant rate as it passes through the sodium iodide crystal to the photomultiplier tubes, the distance of the flash from each photomultiplier tube can be calculated. As multiple flashes of light are localized, an image is made. Usually, more than 100,000 flashes are recorded to make an image.

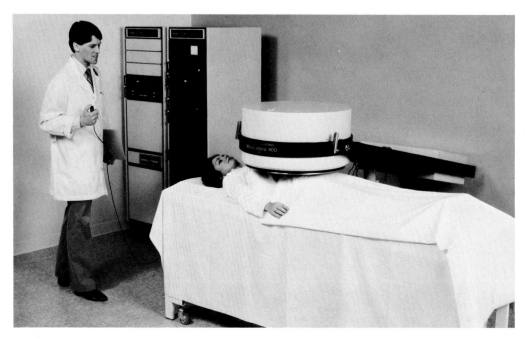

Figure 3-3. A photograph of a gamma camera. (Courtesy of the General Electric Company.)

Emission Computed Tomography

In addition to the standard rectilinear scanner and gamma camera, there are newer devices that permit the imaging of the radioactivity within a thin layer in the body. These machines are of two types, those that use gamma ray—emitting agents and record the activity of single gamma photons (called SPECT) and those that use positron-emitting agents using the paired gamma rays that result from the collision of a positron with an electron (called PET). These devices are not in wide clinical use and will not be discussed further.

Keynotes

- *Sodium iodide crystals are used to detect the tracer activity.*
- *A collimator limits the gamma rays reaching the detector to those coming from a single direction.*
- *Tracer images can be made with rectilinear scanners or with cameras.*

TRACER CHEMISTRY

Only five radioactive tracers are in common clinical use: technetium 99m, iodine 131, xenon 133, thallium 201, and gallium 67 (Table 3-1). Of these the most versatile is ^{99m}Tc. It serves as the *radiotracer* in many *radiopharmaceuticals* because of several important properties:

1. Its gamma ray energy of 140 keV is suited for imaging by the sodium iodide crystals used in the imaging devices.

TABLE 3-1 RADIOACTIVE TRACERS IN COMMON CLINICAL USE

	Physical Half-life	Main Energy
^{99m}Tc	6 hours	140 keV
^{131}I	8 days	364 keV
^{133}Xe	5.3 days	81 keV
^{201}Tl	73 hours	135 keV
		167 keV
^{67}Ga	79 hours	94 keV
		184 keV
		296 keV

2. It is produced from a more stable source, from which it can be eluted (washed out) as needed. This process of *elution* is called "milking the cow."

3. Its physical half-life of 6 hours is long enough to permit imaging but short enough to limit the radiation dose to the patient.

Because of these desirable properties, many compounds incorporating ^{99m}Tc have been tried as biologic markers: technetium 99m can be bound to phosphate complexes to image bone, to colloidal sulfur to image the liver, to iminodiacidic acid derivatives to image the biliary tree, to albumen aggregates to image the location of pulmonary blood flow, to several compounds to image the kidney, or used in its ionic form (sodium pertechnetate Tc 99m) to image the heart, the brain, the thyroid, and the urinary system.

TRACER LOCALIZATION

Six different mechanisms are employed to achieve tracer localization.

Exclusion

A drug may be selectively excluded from an organ except in the presence of disease.

1. Sodium pertechnetate Tc 99m placed in the urinary bladder normally will not pass into the ureters. Its passage into the ureters is a sign of vesicoureteral reflux, a process often associated with renal infection and renal damage.
2. Sodium pertechnetate Tc 99m swallowed should not reflux into the esophagus. Gastroesophageal reflux, if frequent, can be associated with peptic esophagitis.
3. Sodium pertechnetate Tc 99m is excluded from the brain substance by the blood-brain barrier. Many brain diseases interfere with the blood-brain barrier, permitting the technetium to be imaged within the brain (Fig. 3-1).

Metabolic Accumulation

A drug may be metabolically active within an organ, thus accumulating there. Iodine is concentrated in the thyroid gland. Tracer doses of radioactive iodine will also accumulate within the gland, and the amount of iodine uptake can be measured. Once in the gland, radioactive iodine can be used to image the thyroid gland. Its size can be estimated and the homogeneity of its activity judged. Masses within it can be seen to function or not function. Some nonfunctioning solitary nodules are cancer.

Drug Mimicry

A drug may resemble a substance that is normally metabolically active in an organ, be taken up by that organ, and used to image it.

1. Sodium pertechnetate Tc 99m is taken up by the thyroid gland in the same manner as iodine. It can be used to image the thyroid (Fig. 3-4).

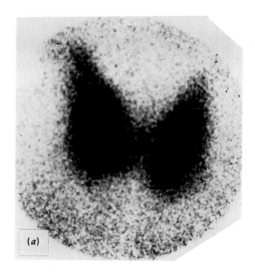

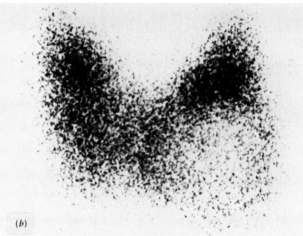

Figure 3-4. (*a*) An image of a normal thyroid gland made with sodium pertechnetate Tc 99m. (Courtesy of M. Vaccaro, M.D.) (*b*) An image of a thyroid gland with a cold nodule within the lower portion of the left lobe. Some cold nodules are cancerous; this was an adenoma. (Courtesy of M. Vaccaro, M.D.)

2. Technetium Tc 99m polyphosphate, technetium Tc 99m pyrophosphate, and technetium Tc 99m methylene diphosphonate are adsorbed onto the surface of newly formed bone and reflect the bone's metabolic activity (Fig. 3-5).
3. Technetium Tc 99m sulfur colloid particles mimic bacteria in size and are phagocytosed by the liver, spleen, and bone marrow, permitting these organs to be imaged (Fig. 3-2).
4. Xenon 133 gas when breathed distributes in the lung similarly to nitrogen and can be used to image the local respiratory function of the lung. It is used to find areas of the lung that are poorly ventilated (Fig. 3-6).
5. Thallium 201 is concentrated in muscle tissue in the same manner as potassium and can be used to image the myocardium (Fig. 3-7).

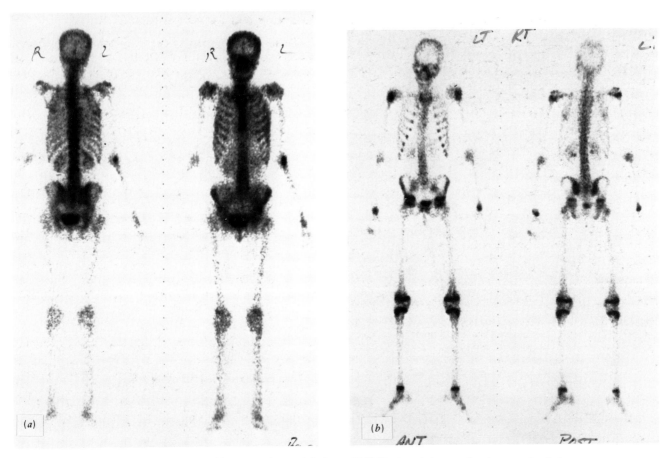

Figure 3-5. (a) A normal bone scan in an adult, done with ^{99m}Tc phosphate complex. Increased activity is seen at the left elbow at the site of injection, a common normal finding. (Courtesy of M. Vaccaro, M.D.) (b) A normal bone scan in a child. Increased tracer activity is present at the sites of rapid bone growth: the wrists, shoulders, knees, and ankles. (Courtesy of M. Vaccaro M.D.)

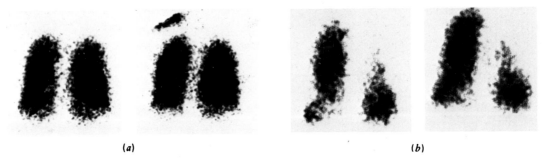

Figure 3-6. (a) Selected views of a lung scan showing normal ventilation, done with xenon 133 gas. These posterior views demonstrate equal activity throughout the lungs. (Courtesy of M. Vaccaro M.D.) (b) Limited views of the lungs in a patient with severe emphysema, demonstrating several focal areas of lack of ventilation. (Courtesy of M. Vaccaro, M.D.)

Capillary Occlusion

A tracer may be bound to particles large enough to occlude a capillary bed partially and, once lodged there, be used to image the organ. Iodine 131 or technetium Tc 99m albumen aggregates injected intravenously will lodge in the capillary bed of the lung, permitting that organ to have its own vascular bed mapped (Fig. 3-8).

Cellular Binding

Certain toxins, drugs, and antibodies adhere or bind to particular cells or particular enzyme systems. If these substances are radiolabeled, they can be used to image the cells adhered to.

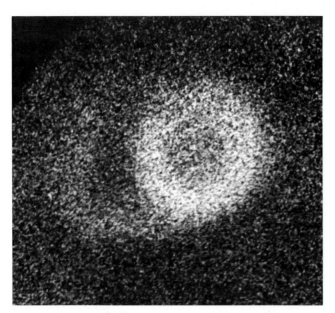

Figure 3-7. A Thalium 201 scan of the myocardium. In this view, the left ventricular myocardium appears like a doughnut. The right ventricular myocardium is a faint "U". (Courtesy of M. Vaccaro, M.D.)

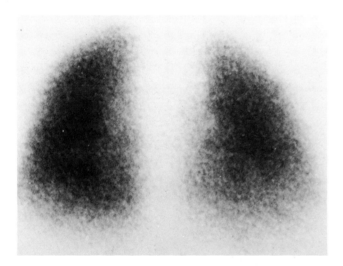

Figure 3-8. Single view from a scan of the capillary bed of normal lungs, done with technetium Tc 99m albumen aggregates. Uniform activity is seen throughout the lungs. (Courtesy David Moses, M.D.)

1. Certain diuretics bind to renal tubular cells. Chlormerodrin Hg 197 can be used to image the location of renal tubular cells.
2. Antibodies to particular cells can be radiolabeled and used to image their locations. This procedure is being used experimentally to determine the sites of tumors within the body.
3. Gallium 67 is bound both to white blood cells and to bacteria and can be used to locate abscesses and enlarged lymph nodes (Fig. 3-9).

Excretion and Secretion

Radiolabeled drugs can be excreted by the normal pathways of urinary and biliary excretion or of gastric or pancreatic secretion. These properties can be used to image the organs involved.

1. Many small molecular weight drugs, when injected into the body, can be excreted by the kidney and be used to image it. ^{99m}Tc diethylene triamine pentaacetic acid (DTPA) is the drug most often used for this function.
2. Sodium pertechnetate Tc 99m is secreted by gastric mucosa. This technique is used to image aberrant gastric mucosa in a Meckel's diverticulum of the distal ilium; clinically, this technique is used to identify the site of occult bleeding and ulceration.
3. Iminodiacetic acid derivatives labeled with ^{99m}Tc (IDA compounds) are excreted by the biliary tract and can be used to evaluate the rate of excretion and the anatomy of the organ (Fig. 3-10).

Keynote

- *The six methods of tracer localization are*
  Exclusion
  Metabolic accumulation
  Mimicry
  Capillary occlusion
  Cellular binding
  Excretion and secretion

NUCLEAR MEDICINE IMAGING

Nuclear medicine techniques can be used to image many organs in the body.

Advantages

1. Relatively low radiation dose
2. Ability to image organs not visible by routine radiography
3. Ability to measure metabolic and physiological activity coincident with obtaining the image
4. High sensitivity for detecting bone, liver, and lung disease

Disadvantages

1. Low resolution: lesions smaller than 2 cm may be missed.
2. Low specificity: imaging techniques are sensitive for finding whether disease is present, but abnormalities found by tracer imaging are often not specific for only one diagnosis.

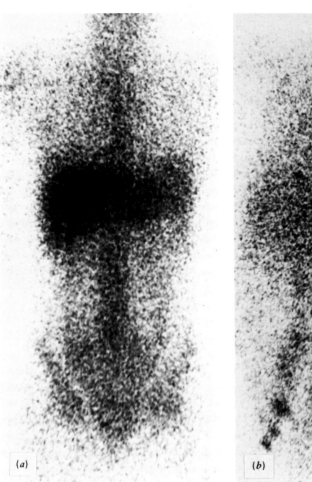

(a)

(b)

Figure 3-9. (a) A scan done with gallium citrate Ga 67 in a normal person. Activity is seen in the liver. (b) A scan done with gallium citrate Ga 67 in a patient with lymphoma. Abnormally increased activity is seen in iliac lymph nodes that contain lymphoma. (Both courtesy of M. Vaccaro, M.D.)

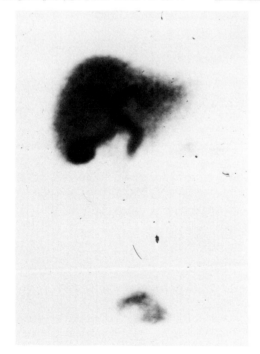

Figure 3-10. A biliary tract scan done with a technetium 99m IDA compound demonstrating a normal gallbladder and major biliary ducts.

3. Expense: Certain of the abnormalities detectable by nuclear medicine imaging techniques are found more cheaply by laboratory tests (e.g., 80% of liver metastases will result in an abnormal alkaline phosphatase level. A liver scan detects only 80% of metastases). A clinical decision must be made as to when the specific imaging technique is necessary.

Main Uses

1. Evaluation of pulmonary emboli.
2. Screening for hepatic metastases.
3. Evaluation of thyroid disease:
   Masses
   Hyperthyroidism.
4. Screening for bone metastases.
5. Screening for brain metastases and tumors. (CT is preferred if available.)
6. Diagnosis of acute cholecystitis.
7. Evaluation of cardiac function:
   Cardiac output
   Myocardial contractility

Segmental
Generalized
Myocardial ischemia.

Secondary Uses

1. Evaluation for vesicoureteral reflux
2. Evaluation of renal function
3. Evaluation of cerebral blood flow
4. Evaluation of gastroesophageal reflux

SUMMARY

Nuclear medicine imaging techniques use a small quantity of a gamma emitting–radioisotope to image the body. This administered internal emitter can be detected by sodium iodide crystals placed outside the body. Two types of detection systems are in common use: the rectilinear scanner, in which a single sodium iodide crystal is mechanically passed multiple times across the body, and the gamma camera, in which data manipulation is used to create spatial images.

Five radiotracers are in common clinical use (Table 3-1). Technetium 99m is the most versatile, and compounds to image bone, liver, lung, biliary tree, kidney, heart, brain, and thyroid have been developed incorporating it.

The main advantages of tracer imaging are its ability to provide metabolic, physiological, and anatomic information from the same study; its relatively low radiation dose; its safety; and its ability to visualize organs not adequately seen by other methods.

REVIEW QUESTIONS

1. What is a radiotracer?
2. What physical property permits a radiotracer to make an image?
3. What are the methods by which a tracer can accumulate in or be excluded from an organ or tissue?
4. Which five radiotracers are in common clinical use?
5. What is a "cow"?
6. Why is ^{99m}Tc the tracer used for imaging so many different organs in the body?
7. How does a rectilinear scanner work?
8. How does a gamma camera work?
9. What is the function of the sodium iodide crystal?
10. What are the main uses for tracer imaging?
11. Nuclear medicine imaging is one of several names applied to this type of imaging. What are the others?

VOCABULARY

collimator	rectilinear scanner
gamma camera	radiotracer
radiopharmaceutical	tracer

SUGGESTIONS FOR FURTHER READING

Leonard M. Freeman. *Freeman and Johnson's Clinical Radionuclide Imaging,* 3rd Ed. Grune & Stratton: Orlando. 1984.

Henry N. Wagner, Jr., Julia W. Buchanan, Danilo Espinola-Vassallo. *Diagnostic Nuclear Medicine Patient Studies,* Year Book Medical Publishers: Chicago. 1986.

4

TRANSMISSION COMPUTED TOMOGRAPHY

PETER M. JOSEPH
MATTHEW FREEDMAN

KEY CONCEPTS

This chapter discusses transmission computed tomography. This technique, which is also known as "computed tomography," "CT," and "CAT scanning," produces an image by directing many beams of x-rays through the body, recording their magnitude and energy levels as the beams exit from the body, and then computer processing the encoded information to produce an image.

The image that is produced is composed of small units called *pixels*, or picture elements, each of which reflects the radiodensity of a small unit of tissue in the body, called a *voxel*. Because the radiodensity of the voxel is recorded in the computer, the computer can be used to accentuate voxels of specific radiodensities by adjusting controls called "window level" and "window width." The computer can also display the relative radiodensity of each voxel compared with the radiodensity of water. The unit of relative radiodensity used is called the "CT unit," or *Hounsfield unit*. CT units are not standardized and are machine dependant.

The simplest method of image analysis for the CT image consists of two parts. First, identify all normal structures. Structures not identified as representing normal anatomy should be further evaluated because they often represent disease. Second, evaluate the internal pattern of radiodensity seen in each organ. Distortions of the patterns within an organ indicate disease.

OBJECTIVES

When you complete this chapter you will be able to

1. Describe the method by which a CT scanner produces an image.
2. Identify normal anatomy on selected CT sections through the brain, chest, and abdomen.
3. Describe the difference between window level and window width.

4. Define and describe the differences between a pixel and a voxel.

A computed tomogram is an image produced by computer processing of data obtained by directing multiple narrow beams of x-ray photons through the patient into detectors. The detectors, which can be solid phosphorescent crystals or gaseous ionization detectors, measure the intensity of each narrow beam as it emerges from the patient. Each single beam, therefore, represents a measurement of the x-ray attenuation of the tissues in its path (Fig. 4-1); the value obtained will depend on the length of the path as well as on the radiodensity and chemical composition of the tissues. Many such paths are recorded as the x-ray tube and detectors rotate around the body.

The computer then processes the data and mathematically superimposes all the path attenuation measurements to create an image in which the intensity at each location in the image reflects the radiodensity of that place within the body (Fig. 4-2). It must be understood that this CT process gives a true image of those tissues lying within the selected slice, with no contribution from tissues outside of the slices. This is in contrast to conventional tomography, where many objects lying outside of the desired slice will nevertheless cause "phantom" or "ghost" shadows that appear as though they were objects in the slice. Thus, CT sections have greater geometric selectivity than the conventional tomographic sections.

Keynote

- *The intensity (whiteness) of each point on a CT scan is related to the radiodensity of the place within the body.*

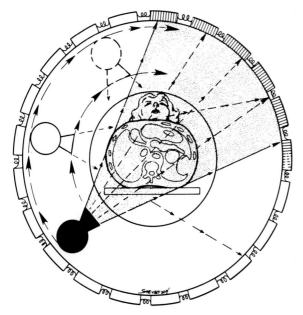

Figure 4-1. Drawing of a CT scanner. The x-ray tube rotates around the patient, directing multiple beams of x-rays through the patient to a ring of detectors. The computer analyzes the amount of transmission of x-ray photons in these multiple beams and calculates the radiodensity of separate points within the body. (Illustrative Services, Art Department, University of Maryland Medical School.)

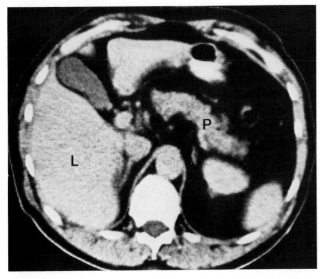

Figure 4-2. A CT scan section corresponding to the drawing and containing the liver (L) and the body and tail of the pancreas (P).

PIXELS AND VOXELS

The slice of tissue that is imaged with CT is a slice with thickness. The radiodensities ascribed to a specific location within the body are being ascribed to a volume of tissue called a voxel, rather than to a point within the body. Within each of these voxels, the tissue radiodensities are averaged. If the radiodensities within a voxel differ greatly, the image made will give a false impression

of the radiodensity of an object. This distortion of the radiodensity recording is called the *partial volume effect*. For example, if voxel contains an area of calcium and also contains soft tissue, the image may, because of tissue radiodensity averaging, be misinterpreted as not showing the presence of calcium.

The amount of detail available within the image is limited by the size of the voxel. The size of the voxel is determined by the product of the smallest unit of surface area (the pixel) that the computer is programmed to analyze and the thickness of the beam. The size of the pixel can be varied with computer software, and the thickness of the beam can be varied by the collimator (Fig. 4-3). A thick beam increases the number of x-ray photons used and therefore results in a less grainy picture. A thin section permits smaller anatomic structures to be seen but usually uses a higher total radiation dose for the entire CT study.

Keynotes

- *The voxel is the smallest unit of tissue volume imaged by the CT scan.*
- *The partial volume effect is the distortion of the measurement of tissue radiodensity that occurs because the CT scan is measuring a volume of tissue. If the same voxel contains tissues of different radiodensities, the radiodensity recorded for that voxel will be between the two true radiodensities.*
- *The pixel is the smallest unit of surface area that the computer is programmed to analyze.*

CT IMAGE ORIENTATION

The images made by a CT scanner are usually thin (2–10 mm) transverse (axial) sections across the head or body (Fig. 4-4*a*). The computer can, however, recombine the voxels in its memory to create coronal or sagittal images (Fig. 4-4*b*). Because the thickness of a voxel is always greater than the size of the pixel, these reconstructed images always have less detail than the original image.

CONTRAST

Once the data for the image is stored in the computer, the computer can be used to exaggerate differences in radiodensity, permitting the visualization of structures whose intrinsic radiodensities are too similar to be detected by radiography but which, once processed, can be seen (Fig. 4-5). This computation is made by having the operator direct the machine to make an image of all points within a specific range of radiodensities. Because of the freedom to adjust the "viewing window," the operator can select a specific range of radiodensities to be imaged as shades of gray in the picture. This is done by adjusting two controls known as the "window level" and "window width" (Fig. 4-6).

The *window level* represents the average or central radiodensity of the particular tissue to be seen. The *window*

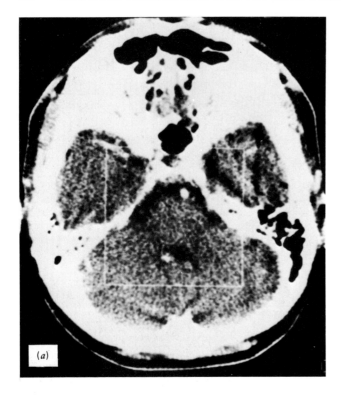

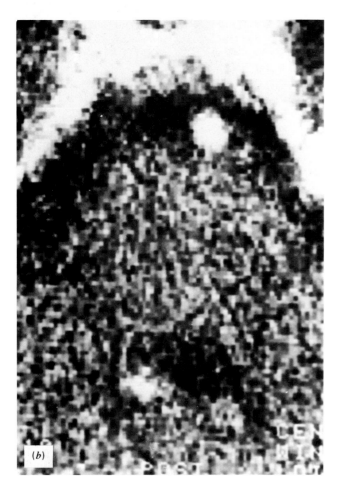

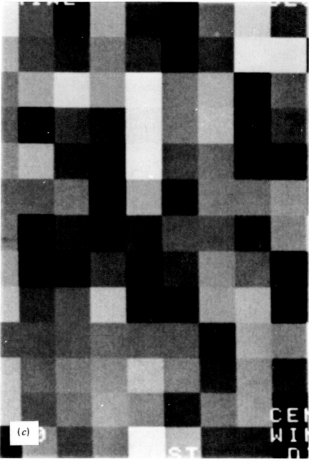

Figure 4-3. Demonstration of pixels by progressive magnification of a CT image. (*a*) CT image through the posterior fossa of the brain. The white box indicates the portion to be magnified. (*b*) Magnification of the area within the box in *a* demonstrating the pixels. (*c*) Further magnification of *b* demonstrates the individual pixels, each one with its own shade of gray.

width determines the range of radiodensities, both greater or smaller than the window level, that will result in distinguishable gray shades on the image. All tissues whose radiodensities are greater than the window level *plus* one-half of the window width will appear uniformly white, while all those with radiodensities less than the window level *minus* one-half window width will appear uniformly black. Only those radiodensities within the "window" will be distinguishable as shades of gray. It is imperative that the viewing window controls be properly adjusted so that the desired tissues will be well visualized. As an example, in Figure 4-7, two different window settings of the same image demonstrate the patient's lungs (*a*) and bones and mediastinum (*b*).

THE LIMIT TO DATA MANIPULATION

There is, however, a limit to the degree of such contrast enhancement. It is determined by the appearance of

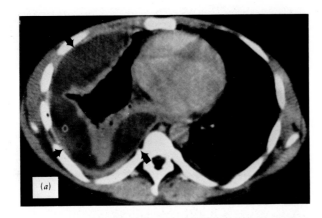

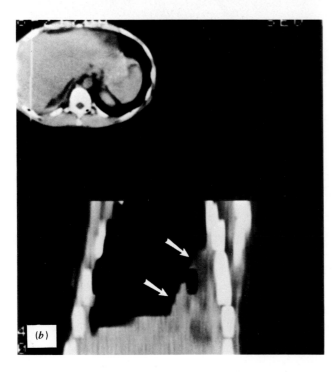

Figure 4-4. Demonstration of the reformation of a nonaxial image from a series of axial images. (*a*) A transverse image through the lower chest demonstrates multiple areas of empyema (arrows). To aid the radiologist in his insertions of drainage catheters, images were reconstructed in different planes. (Courtesy E. Blum, M.D.) (*b*) Demonstration of one of the sagittal planes of reconstruction used to guide the insertion of a drainage catheter into the empyema (arrows). (Courtesy E. Blum, M.D.).

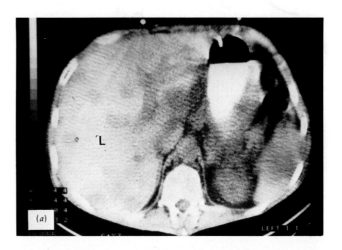

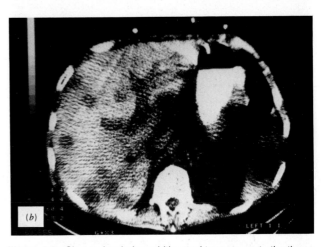

Figure 4-5. Change in window width, used to exaggerate the tissue radiodensity differences in hepatic metastases (liver = L). (*a*) Wide window width. The hepatic radiolucencies are poorly seen. (Courtesy M. Dunne, M.D.) (*b*) Narrow window width. The radiolucent hepatic metastases are easier to see. (Courtesy M. Dunne, M.D.)

Keynotes

- *Voxels are usually assembled to form a transverse (axial) image, but they can be assembled by the computer to form coronal or saggital sections.*
- *The window level is the median point of radiodensities chosen to be shown as shades of gray in the image.*
- *The window width determines the range of radiodensities shown as shades of gray.*

RADIATION EXPOSURE IN COMPUTED TOMOGRAPHY

In CT, only the imaged slice is (in principle) irradiated by the direct beam; thus imaging additional slices does not increase the direct radiation exposure of any given element of tissue but merely increases the volume of tissue that is irradiated. This can be contrasted with conven-

"grain," or "noise," which appears superimposed on the image (see Fig. 4-5). This grain is due to the inevitable statistical fluctuations in the number of x-ray photons in each narrow beam measured. It can be reduced only by increasing the number of photons used, which means, of course, that the patient would receive more radiation. Thus, there is a direct relationship between the radiation exposure used and the ability of the scan to differentiate between tissues of similar density.

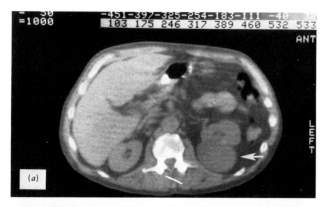

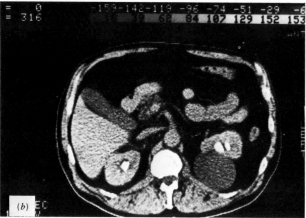

Figure 4-6. Images through the abdomen demonstrating a left renal cyst (arrow) shown at two different window widths. The band of numbers at the top of the images indicates the degrees of gray assigned to different CT numbers. (a) Image made with a window level of 50 and a window width of 1,000. (b) Image made with a window level of 0 and a window width of 316. Intravenously administered contrast medium has increased the radiodensity of the kidneys and liver and is being excreted into the collecting system of the kidneys.

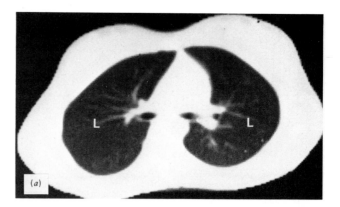

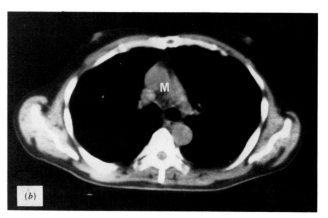

Figure 4-7. Chest CT sections done at two different window settings. (a) Image obtained with a wide window setting demonstrates the lungs (L) and their vessels. (b) Image done with a narrower window width demonstrates the mediastinum (M) and the bones of the chest.

tional tomography, in which a region of the body much larger than the imaged plane must be irradiated; each additional conventional tomographic section increases the radiation exposure to all tissues in the region. A typical CT slice through the head exposes the tissue in that slice to 1–2 R; one through the abdomen 2–3 R.

THE INTERPRETATION OF THE CT IMAGE

The CT image can contain both normal and abnormal structures. The easiest way for the novice to interpret this image is to identify all the normal structures seen on the image and then to attempt to determine what the other structures are. For example, in the slice through the mid-abdomen shown in Fig. 4-8a, it is possible to identify the kidneys (K), the aorta (A), the inferior vena cava (C), the tip of the liver (L), and the bowel (B). In Figure 4-8b, there is an added structure (arrow), which should not be there. Each visualized organ must have a normal size and shape

and a normal radiodensity. This ls learned by viewing the images of many patients.

METHODS OF EVALUATING AN UNKNOWN OBJECT

An unknown object in the body can be separated from its surroundings only if it has a different radiodensity. The conventional radiograph is limited in its ability to record differential radiodensities to the differentiation of air-fat-water-bone-metal interfaces. CT, because of its computer processing of the image and its tomographic effect, can permit the differentiation of even smaller differences of radiodensity, such as water-radiodensity differences between the brain and the cerebrospinal fluid that fills its ventricles and sulci. The image of these radiodensity differences can be intensified by the proper adjustment of the window width and level.

Individual organs can be imaged if they are surrounded by a structure of different radiodensity. Air and fat are the major structures separating organs within the body. In the abdomen and retroperitoneum, CT works best in patients

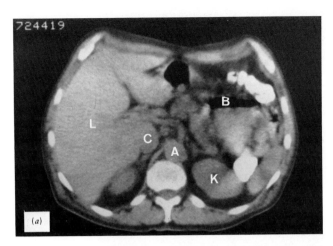 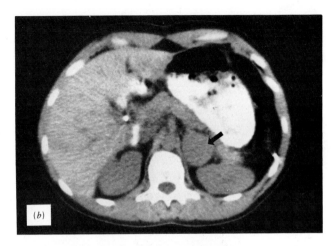

Figure 4-8. (*a*) Midabdominal CT in a normal person. K = kidney, A = aorta, C = inferior vena cava, L = liver, B = bowel. (*b*) Midabdominal CT revealing an abnormality. The arrow points to a structure that should not be present, a left adrenal mass that turned out to be a pheochromocytoma. This type of tumor can be associated with intermittent high blood pressure.

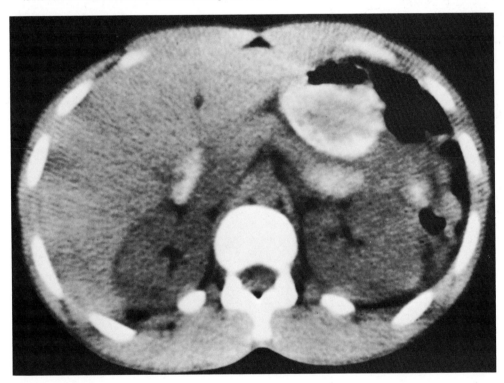

Figure 4-9. CT in an emaciated patient. This patient had a chronic liver abcess and had catabolized body fat. The organs are poorly delineated from adjacent organs. Compare this section with the CT of a normal abdomen shown in Figure 4-8*a*.

with an ample amount of nonedematous fat. Therefore, normal children and emaciated patients are less well imaged (Fig. 4-9). If infection or tumor has invaded the fat, the edges of organs may be difficult to define.

When the edge of an organ is poorly defined or there is an unidentified structure, several additional methods may aid in evaluating the image. In some cases, turning the patient on his or her side may shift structures, permitting

an unknown structure to be identified. In other cases, contrast media can be given to the patient to outline an unknown strucure, perhaps permitting it to be identified.

The intravenous injection of an iodinated water-soluble contrast medium increases the radiodensity of large vessels (Fig. 4-10) structures with extensive capillary blood flow, the kidneys, ureters, and bladder (Fig. 4-11). Swallowed water-soluble contrast material increases the radio-

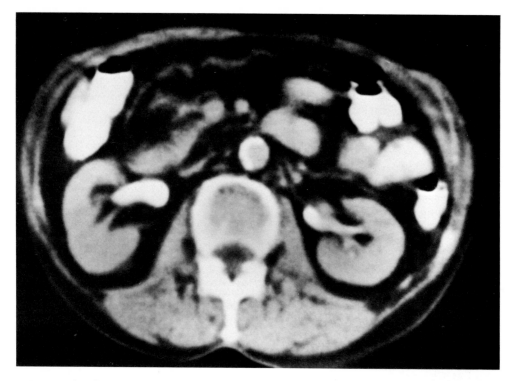

Figure 4-10. CT through the midabdomen with opacification of the bowel, kidneys, and aorta. Swallowed contrast medium has been used to opacify the bowel. Intravenously injected contrast medium has been used to opacify the aorta and the kidneys. The aorta is almost as radiopaque as the bowel (compare with figs. 4-8 and 4-9). Contrast is also seen in the renal pelves.

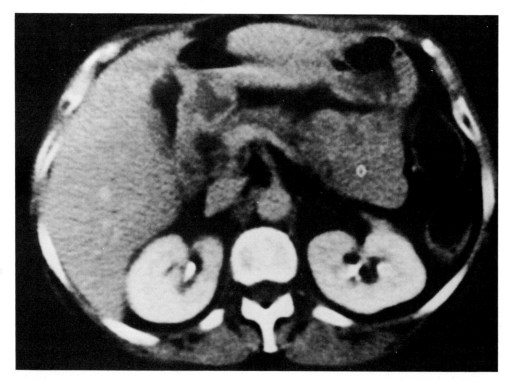

Figure 4-11. CT with intense opacification of the kidneys. In this section, the kidneys have concentrated the contrast, while the blood level of contrast has decreased. In this study, the bowel has not been opacified.

density of the esophagus, stomach, duodenum, and small bowel (Fig. 4-10). Water-soluble contrast media can be placed in the rectum or sigmoid colon as an enema. Air can be placed in the bladder or rectum with a catheter to outline these structures.

A disadvantage of using iodinated contrast agents is their tendency to produce streak or band artifacts adjacent to the organ containing the contrast. Streak artifacts also occur when there is metal in the field of view (Fig. 4-12).

The measurement of the CT number can also aid in the evaluation of an unknown object. The *CT number* is a number measuring the radiodensity of an object seen on the CT scan. The machine can be directed to calculate it for any group of voxels within the image. In general, water has a CT number of 0 Hounsfield units, air minus 1,000 units, fat minus 75 units, and blood plus 40 units. Calcifi-

cation in a mass usually has a radiodensity of greater than 150 Hounsfield units.

At appropriate places in this text, examples of CT images of normal and abnormal conditions will be presented to help you learn to interpret them.

Keynotes

- *Tissue or organ radiodensity can be altered by administering contrast media into vessels or into the lumen of the gut.*
- *The CT number is a measure of the radiodensity of an object imaged by the CT scan. It is measured in Hounsfield units.*

COMPUTED TOMOGRAPHY IMAGING

Advantages

1. Transverse image
2. Exaggeration of tissue radiodensity difference
3. Tomographic (thin-layer) visualization

Disadvantages

1. High cost of equipment
2. High physician time input

Main Uses

1. Visualization of the brain and ventricular system (Fig. 4-13)
2. Visualization of the pancreas
3. Evaluation of retroperitoneal tumors
4. Detection of calcium in pulmonary nodules

Secondary Uses

1. Differentiating a renal cyst from a renal tumor
2. Staging of cancers: evaluating local extent and distant metastases of ovary, lung, kidney, bladder, and cervix cancer

SUMMARY

Transmission computed tomography derives an image of the body by the mathematical analysis of multiple recordings of bands of tissue radiodensity. The computer analysis calculates the radiodensities of small volumes of tissues called voxels, which the computer can then combine to make images in different planes of the body. The window level and width determine the range of radiodensities imaged as varying shades of gray within the image. These adjustments, made by the operator, greatly contribute to the analysis of the image of the body.

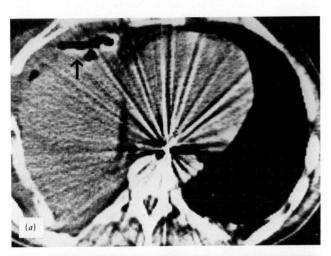

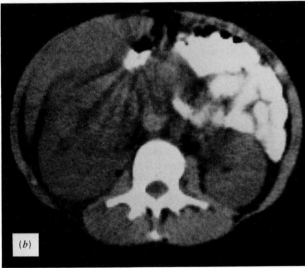

Figure 4-12. CT streak artifacts. (a) Streak artifacts caused by metallic surgical clips. The air anterior to the liver (arrow) was a subphrenic abscess. (b) Streak artifacts caused by an iodinated contrast medium in the bowel. Thr right renal mass proved to be a renal cell cancer.

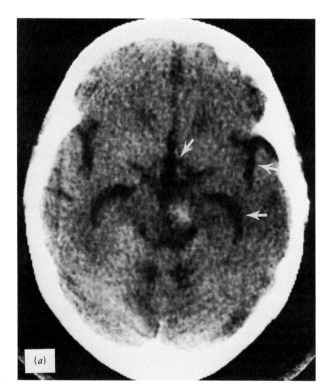 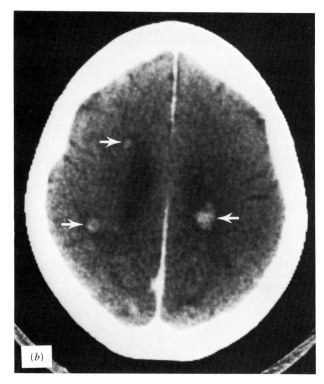

Figure 4-13. CT sections through the brain. (*a*) Section through the base of the brain. The darker areas (arrows) are the cerebrospinal fluid–containing cisterns. (*b*) Section through the ventricular system. The ventricular system appears less radiodense (blacker) than the surrounding brain. The few focal white areas (arrows) seen in the cortex represent metastases to the brain from breast cancer. CT is often used to detect cancer metastatic to the brain.

REVIEW QUESTIONS

1. How does the CT scanner measure tissue radiodensities?
2. How does the computer create an image from the stored data?
3. What is a voxel?
4. What is the partial volume effect?
5. What is meant by the term *window level?*
6. What is meant by the term *window width?*
7. What effect does changing the window level and window width have on the image?
8. What are the methods of changing tissue or organ radiodensities to aid in the interpretation of CT images?
9. What is the CT number?

VOCABULARY

CT number

Hounsfield units

partial volume effect

pixel

voxel

window level

window width

SUGGESTIONS FOR FURTHER READING

John R. Haaga, Ralph J. Alfidi. *Computed Tomography of the Whole Body.* C. V. Mosby: St. Louis. 1983.

Joseph K.T. Lee, Stuart S. Sagel, Robert J. Stanley. *Computed Body Tomography.* Raven Press: New York. 1983.

5

MAGNETIC RESONANCE IMAGING

KEY CONCEPTS

Magnetic resonance imaging (MRI) is based on the interaction between atoms that have been aligned in a strong magnetic field and radiofrequency electromagnetic radiation. Hydrogen atoms (usually referred to as "protons") are the atoms most easily imaged by this process. Because most of the hydrogen in the body is in water, water is the main substance imaged by this technique.

Images are produced by first aligning some of the atoms in the body by placing the body in a strong magnetic field. *Radiofrequency electromagnetic waves* are then used both to deflect this alignment and to cause the deflected atoms to spin in phase with each other. The radiofrequency electromagnetic waves are then stopped. The atoms then realign themselves in the strong magnetic field, releasing electromagnetic energy as they are realigned. This energy can be measured and localized and used to form an image: the magnetic resonance image. Different tissues appear different from each other because the "decay" of this angular and spin alignment differs among tissues.

Magnetic resonance imaging:

1. Provides excellent anatomic definition of the brain and spinal cord and can demonstrate areas of demyelination.
2. Can demonstrate disc hernations in some patients.
3. Can demonstrate the muscles of the heart and the heart chambers.
4. When the technique is correctly chosen, can create the *flow-void phenomenon* whereby flowing blood produces no signal. Thus the lumen of blood vessels and the chambers of the heart can be visualized as though free of blood.

OBJECTIVES

When you complete this chapter you will be able to

1. Describe how the strong magnet aligns atoms and how the electromagnetic field deflects them.

2. Describe the flow-void phenomenon and how it is used in imaging the body.
3. Identify major anatomic structures in the brain, heart, abdomen, and pelvis on MR images.

The application of the magnetic resonance of atomic nuclei to medical imaging represents its newest development. This chapter discusses briefly the basic principles of MRI and some of its current applications and suggests its probable future applications. Because of government-enforced restrictions on the introduction of MRI machines, not enough have been available for clinical research; therefore, the appropriate clinical role of MRI is uncertain. The clinical applications suggested in this book are therefore tentative, and some will need to be revised as greater experience is gained.

Keynotes

- *Magnetic resonance imaging (MRI) is also known as nuclear magnetic resonance (NMR) imaging.*
- *At the time this book is being written, the potential clinical applications of MRI are still being investigated and critically evaluated. Only a limited number of studies comparing its clinical utility with other diagnostic techniques have been reported.*

BASIC PRINCIPLES

Magnetic resonance imaging is based on the interrelation of magnetism, electricity, and *electromagnetic radiation.*

All atomic nuclei have an inherent *nuclear spin,* and in those with an odd number of protons, this spin results in a magnetic field. In the normal state, the electromagnetic field from each atomic nucleus is too small to be detected, in part because of its low magnitude and in part because its small magnetic force is canceled by the small magnetic forces of other nuclei that are aligned in other directions.

In MRI, the patient is placed in a very strong magnetic field. This magnetic field will align some of the nuclei in the body. Those nuclei most subject to being aligned by the strong magnetic field are those with an unbalanced (odd) number of protons in the nucleus. After the machine is tuned, a short burst of radiofrequency electromagnetic radiation is used to induce a magnetic field in a direction different from that of the strong magnetic field. A radiofrequency field is chosen to have an orientation that will change the angular alignment to a new direction and cause nuclei of similar types to spin in phase.

When this radiofrequency electromagnetic pulse stops, the nuclei will begin to realign themselves with the strong magnetic field, and the spins of the phase-aligned atomic nuclei will start to shift out of phase. At this point, a second radiofrequency electromagnetic wave is often used to realign the angular and spin alignment of the nuclei because this second pulse seems to exaggerate the differences between tissues.

When this second pulse stops, realignment with the strong magnetic field again begins. The change in the angular alignment and the spin dephasing both produce electromagnetic signals that can be detected by a radiofrequency antenna, processed by a computer, and used to create the MR image.

The signal usually recorded to make the magnetic resonance image is an image of the loss (decay) of angular and spin alignment that occurs as the atomic nuclei realign in the strong magnetic field. These decay signals have proved useful because different tissues have different interatomic forces, and these differing interatomic forces result in differing patterns of loss of angular and spin alignment.

Keynotes

- *Magnetic resonance imaging is based on the interrelation of magnetism, electricity, and electromagnetic radiation.*
- *The spin of atomic nuclei with an odd number of protons results in an electromagnetic field.*
- *The radiofrequency electromagnetic waves produced by the machine are used to cause angular and spin alignment.*
- *The electromagnetic waves produced by the decay of the angular and spin alignment are used to create the MR image.*
- *Different interatomic forces in different tissues are thought to be part of the cause for differing patterns of the decay of angular and spin alignment in different tissues.*

HYDROGEN OR PROTON IMAGING

Because the electromagnetic waves produced by each atomic nucleus are of low magnitude, it is desirable to image common atomic nuclei so that their individual forces can be additive. The most common atomic nucleus with an unbalanced (odd) number of protons is hydrogen; because of their abundance, hydrogen protons, usually in water molecules, are the protons most strongly and commonly imaged. Variations in the image are seen in different tissues because of their different water contents and probably because of different interatomic and intermolecular forces affecting the hydrogen nuclei in different tissues. Other atoms with odd numbers of protons in their nuclei, for example, sodium and phosphorus, can also be imaged, though the image quality is poorer.

Keynote

- *Most MR imaging is of hydrogen atoms because they are the most abundant atoms containing an odd number of protons in their nuclei. Most hydrogen atoms are in water, and thus MR mainly images the location of water in the body.*

SPECTRAL ANALYSIS AND IMAGES

In addition to forming an image of the magnetic resonance of nuclei, it is also possible to use the same detected electromagnetic information with a *spectral analysis* to gain biochemical information about tissues. Because the pattern of the decay of angular and spin alignment is affected by interatomic and intermolecular forces, it is possible to determine the decay pattern of specific molecules and then to quantify the amount of each of these molecules in the tissue under study. This type of investigation is still experimental, the major work having been done in quantifying adenosine triphosphate (ATP) and related compounds.

Keynote

- *MR spectroscopy is possible because there are different interatomic forces affecting the nucleus of an element in different molecules. These different interatomic forces result in different patterns of decay for angular and spin alignment.*

IMAGE SEQUENCES

Depending on the sequence of the electromagnetic radiation used to magnetically deflect the angular alignment and phase-align the spinning protons (or other nuclei), different types of images are produced. The names for these include "saturation recovery," "partial saturation," "inversion recovery," "spin echo," "T-1–weighted images," and "T-2–weighted images." Because these different patterns change the relative amounts of signal received from different tissues, there can be a particular imaging sequence pattern in which an abnormality is not seen, whereas another imaging sequence pattern could demonstrate it. The correct selection of the imaging pattern is necessary to be

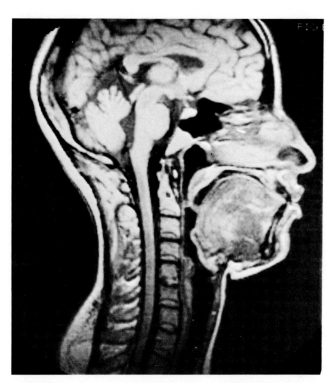

Figure 5-1. Sagittal image of the brain and cervical spinal cord. The gyri and sulci of the brain are well seen, as are the pons, medulla, and spinal cord. (Courtesy C. Citrin, M.D.)

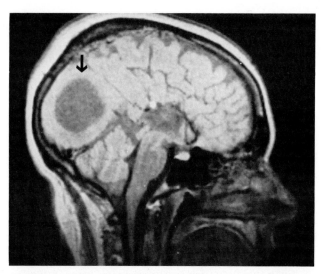

Figure 5-2. Sagittal MR midline image, demonstrating a tumor and its surrounded edema (arrow) in the occipital lobe of the brain. (Courtesy C. Citrin, M.D.)

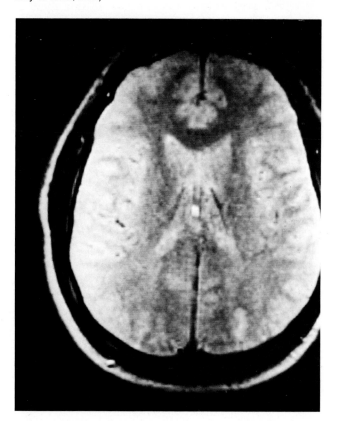

Figure 5-3. Axial MR image of the brain, demonstrating white matter–gray matter differentiation. (Courtesy C. Citrin, M.D.)

certain that the disease looked for can be seen, and this selection is dependant upon the skill of the radiologist operating the machine.

APPLICATIONS OF MRI

Images of the Brain

MRI gives exquisitely detailed images of the brain and spinal cord. In Figure 5-1, a normal sagittal image of the brain and spinal cord is shown. The brain portion demonstrates the gyri and sulci as well as the brainstem and spinal cord clearly demarcated by the cerebrospinal fluid that surrounds them. In Figure 5-2, a mass can be seen posteriorly in the occipital lobe of the brain as a rounded area of decreased whiteness. The sulci in this area are not visible because the swelling of the brain has compressed them. Figure 5-3 demonstrates a normal axial section of the brain and demonstrates differentiation between the *white* and *gray matter*. At least part of the image difference between white and gray matter is the result of more fat in the white matter.

Magnetic resonance imaging appears to have a greater sensitivity for brain lesions than CT. It is particularly useful in finding areas of *demyelination* of brain, as in multiple sclerosis. Because of the absence of bone artifacts, it will probably be most useful in the evaluation of the structures of the *posterior fossa of the cranium,* an area

often suboptimally seen on CT because of the adjacent bone.

The clinical role of MRI in the supratentorial portions of the brain (i.e., the cerebrum) and adjacent structures is less certain. Although its sensitivity for the detection of cerebral lesions is greater than that of CT, it is not clear

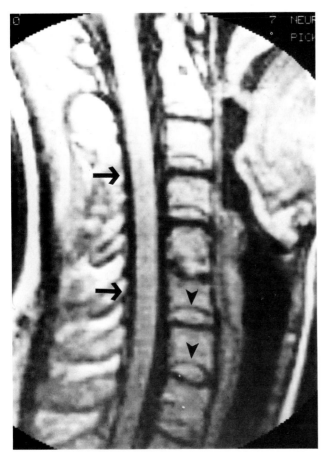

Figure 5-4. Sagittal MR image through the cervical spine and spinal cord. The spinal cord (arrows) is well seen. The nuclei pulposi (arrowheads) of the intervertebral discs appear white on this normal image. On this T-1–weighted image the cerbrospinal fluid appears black. Compare this appearance to that in Figure 5-5, where a T-2–weighted image results in white cerebrospinal fluid. (Courtesy C. Citrin, M.D.)

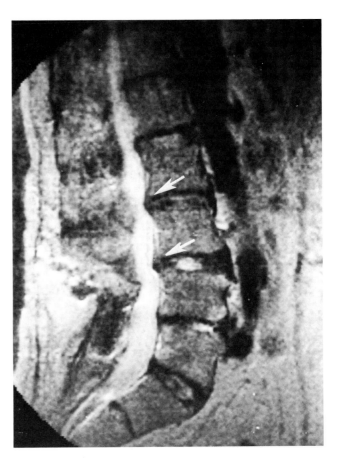

Figure 5-5. Lumbar spine and spinal canal. This T-2–weighted image demonstrates that the spinal fluid in the subarachnoid space is white. This MRI technique permits direct visualization of the subarachnoid space without the injection of a myelographic contrast medium and permits the identification of subarachnoid space impingement. In this patient, bulging, but not herniated, intervertebral discs (arrows) indent the subarachnoid space. (Courtesy C. Citrin M.D.)

whether this increased sensitivity is sufficient to justify the increased cost of MRI.

Images of the Spine

Magnetic resonance imaging is likely to find its most important application in the evaluation of spinal canal and nerve root disease. By varying the image sequence, images of the spinal cord and discs (Fig. 5-4) as well as images of the fluid in the *subarachnoid space* (Fig. 5-5) can be easily obtained. This permits an evaluation for spinal cord tumors, *syringomyelia,* herniated discs, and other spinal processes without injecting contrast into the spinal canal. Though only preliminary data are available, it seems likely that MRI will become the procedure of choice in the evaluation of *sciatica* and related back-pain syndromes.

Images of the Cardiovascular System

Figure 5-6 demonstrates MR images of a normal heart and aorta. These are cardiac-gated images. *Cardiac gating* is a process by which the imaging information is acquired only during a selected portion of the cardiac cycle. This permits cardiac images to be obtained during systole, diastole, or anywhere in between.

In addition to gating these images to the cardiac cycle, the imaging sequence was also selected to use the flow-void phenomenon. This phenomenon occurs because the imaging parameters selected permit the blood that has been excited by the radiofrequency electromagnetic pulse of the machine to flow out of the imaging field and new, unexcited blood to flow into the field before the excited blood transmits its decay signal back to the antennae of the machine. This means that structures filled with flowing blood will appear black on the image because they produce no signal.

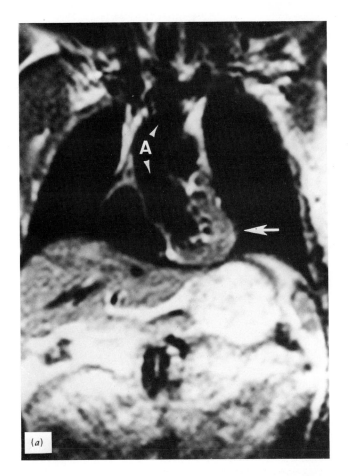

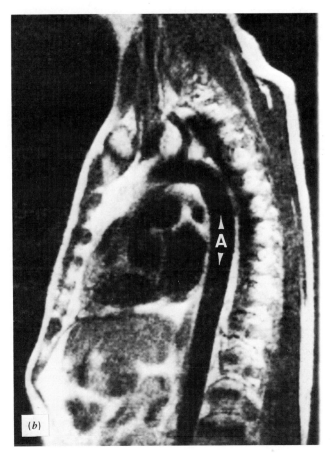

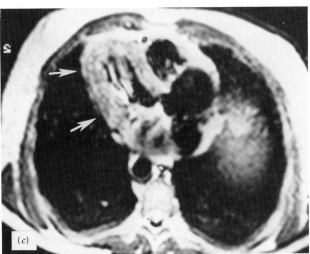

Figure 5-6. MR images of the normal heart and aorta: (*a*) coronal view, (*b*) sagittal view, and (*c*) axial (transverse) view. These views demonstrate the heart and great vessels. The left ventricular myocardium is particularly well seen (arrows). The flow-void effect permits clear differentiation of the myocardial wall from the cardiac lumen and also allows clear demonstration of the lumen of the aorta (A and arrowheads). (Images provided courtesy Philips Medical Systems, Inc.)

If different imaging parameters were selected, the flow-void phenomenon might not be produced and the blood-filled lumen could produce a signal. Because the imaging parameters can be varied to produce or fail to produce the flow-void effect, investigators are studying this phenomenon to see if it can be used to calculate accurately blood flow velocity and possibly blood flow volume.

The flow-void phenomenon currently permits the clinical evaluation of cardiac chamber size, myocardial thickness, and cardiac structure in patients with congenital heart disease. It is also used in evaluating major vessels and may in the future be used to substitute for certain types of diagnostic angiography.

Images of the Abdomen

Magnetic resonance can be used to image the abdomen but currently does not appear to offer any advantage over CT and is being used in this capacity only as a clinical research tool. Although MR can image abdominal structures such as the liver and kidney, as shown in Figure 5-7, the images of the upper abdomen are degraded in quality by respiratory motion. Respiratory gating is being used on some machines; however, the image quality still does not equal that of CT.

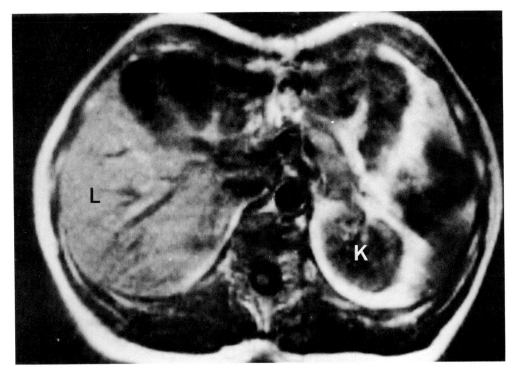

Figure 5-7. MR image through the upper abdomen. The liver (L) and left kidney (K) are identified.

In the pelvis, MRI may have greater promise. Because it can visualize the body in multiple planes, it may prove of value in complex anatomic regions. Figure 5-8 demonstrates MR images through a man's pelvis showing the bladder and prostate.

Keynotes

• *Magnetic resonance images of the brain demonstrate excellent anatomic detail.*

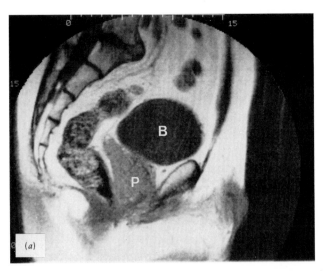

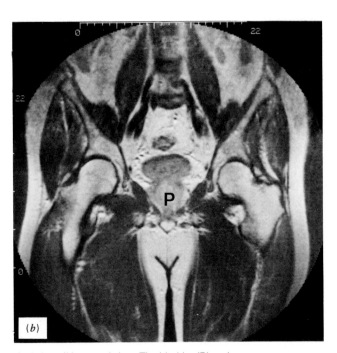

Figure 5-8. MR images through the male pelvis: (*a*) sagittal view: (*b*) coronal view. The bladder (B) and prostate (P) are identified. (Courtey C. Citrin M.D.)

- *Magnetic resonance images of the brain allow discrimination of the gray and white matter.*
- *Magnetic resonance imaging is the most sensitive method for demonstrating brain myelination and demyelination.*
- *Magnetic resonance imaging is better than CT at demonstrating disease in the posterior fossa of the skull.*
- *Magnetic resonance imaging of the spine can demonstrate the spinal cord, discs, and subarachnoid space.*
- *Gated cardiac MR images permit the imaging of the heart in systole, diastole, or anywhere in between.*
- *The flow-void phenomenon results in flowing blood having no MR signal, permitting the chambers of the heart and the lumina of vessels to be sharply delineated from the structures that surround them.*
- *At the current time, MR appears to offer no advantages over CT for imaging of the abdomen.*

SUMMARY

Magnetic resonance imaging is the newest major development in medical imaging. The precise clinical role of this modality still needs to be defined; however, based on current information it seems likely that MR imaging is now the imaging procedure of choice for suspected spinal cord disease and multiple sclerosis. It is also probably the procedure of choice in the posterior fossa of the brain and in patients with spinal nerve compression syndromes (such as cervical radiculopathy and sciatica).

In the future, MRI is likely to play a major role in the evaluation of patients with congenital heart disease and diseases of major vessels. Other future applications are less certain, but as with any new technique additional applications are likely to be found as clinical investigation proceeds.

REVIEW QUESTIONS

1. What is the function of the strong magnetic field in MR imaging?
2. What is the function of the radiofrequency electromagnetic pulse in MR imaging?
3. What part of the magnetization, radiofrequency cycle of MR imaging produces the data used to construct the MR image?
4. What types of nuclei are best for MR imaging? Why are those nuclei preferred?
5. What is the advantage of MR imaging of the brain and posterior fossa structures?
6. What structures in the spinal column can MR image?
7. What is the clinical application of MR imaging of the brain? Of the spinal column? Of the cardiovascular system?
8. What is the flow-void phenomenon? What does it look like on MR images?

VOCABULARY

cardiac gating	posterior fossa of the cranium
demyelination	radiofrequency electromagnetic waves
electromagnetic radiation	
flow-void phenomenon	sciatica
gray matter of the brain	spectral analysis
nuclear magnetic resonance (NMR)	subarachnoid space
	syringomyelia
nuclear spin	white matter of the brain

SUGGESTIONS FOR FURTHER READING

Steven E. Harms, David M. Kramer. Fundamentals of magnetic resonance imaging. *CRC Critical Reviews in Diagnostic Imaging,* **25:**79–111. 1985.

6

ULTRASONOGRAPHY: IMAGING WITH SOUND

KEY CONCEPTS

This chapter discusses ultrasonography, a technique of imaging that uses high-frequency sound waves to create an image of the interior of the body. Images can be produced because there are acoustic interfaces in the body that reflect some of the high-frequency sound waves. This reflected sound is then converted into an image.

The images consist of outlines of organs or masses and their internal echo texture. The echo texture is classified by whether or not there are internal echoes. Those structures without internal echoes are called *anechoic* or *sonolucent* structures. Those with internal echoes are called *echogenic* structures. The amount of echogenicity of a structure is compared with structures of known echogenicity to grade the quantity of internal echoes.

Evaluation of a sonographic image begins by determining what part of the body is being imaged. This is done by looking for easily recognized organs such as the liver, kidney, gallbladder, urinary bladder, uterus, vagina, and major vessels. Once oriented, evaluation consists of determining whether these organs are of normal shape and echogenicity and whether there are masses that are not part of normal organs.

OBJECTIVES

When you complete this chapter, you will be able to

1. Identify the liver, kidney, gallbladder, gallstones, and normal uterus on selected sonographic images.
2. Differentiate echogenic and anechoic structures.
3. Identify what part of the body is being imaged by
   a. Translating the shorthand labeling of images.
   b. Orienting the image by identifying major abdominal organs.

The *sonogram* uses high-frequency sound waves to image the body. Sound waves propagate through the body in relatively straight lines. For any specific tissue the speed of movement is constant. When tissues change and the change in speed of sound movement is great enough, part of the sound will be reflected back from the tissue interface. When this interface is perpendicular to the path of the sound waves, the reflected sound will be reflected back at the crystal transducer, which can record its return. The time taken for it to return can be electronically converted into the distance traveled by the sound, permitting an image in depth to be made. Multiple images can be arrayed to create a two-dimensional image of the location of echo surfaces within the body(Fig. 6-1).

High-frequency sound waves propagate well through soft tissues and fluid spaces. They are stopped by air or bone. Thus the technique is most useful in the eye, heart, abdomen, pelvis, and retroperitoneum. It has been used to a lesser degree in imaging the thyroid, carotid arteries, and extremities.

Some structures, such as the gallbladder (GB) in Figure 6-2, produce few or no echoes and are called anechoic or sonolucent structures. Others, such as the liver (L) in Figures 6-1 and 6-2, produce many echoes and are called echogenic structures. Fluid filled structures, large vessels, masses of lymphoma, and some neurogenic tumors are usually anechoic. Air and calcium are markedly echogenic and stop the transmission of sound. Large amounts of air or calcium prevent imaging. Small amounts of calcium (as seen in biliary and renal calculi) and small amounts of air (as might be seen in an abscess) will result in small acoustic "shadows," permitting the diagnosis of these entities (Fig. 6-3).

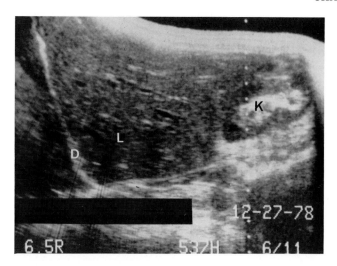

Figure 6-1. This parasagittal sonographic image of the right upper quadrant of the abdomen demonstrates the liver (L), right hemidiaphragm (D), and right kidney (K). (Courtesy of Morgan Dunne, M.D.)

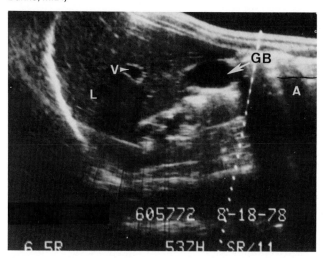

Figure 6-2. This parasagittal sonographic section through the right upper quadrant of the abdomen demonstrates the gallbladder (GB arrow), a structure that when normal is sonolucent; a portal venous branch (V arrowhead), with a sonolucent center and an echogenic rim; and the liver (L), which has an intermediate degree of echogenicity. Air in the bowel (A) is markedly echogenic and prevents the imaging of the structures beneath it. (Courtesy of Morgan Dunne, M.D.)

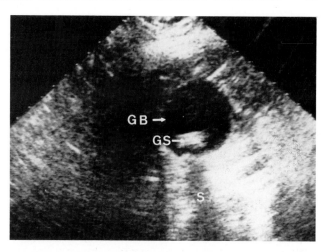

Figure 6-3. This sonographic section through the gallbladder (GB) demonstrates the sonolucent gallbladder with an echogenic focus, representing a gallstone (GS), within it. Behind this gallstone there is a band of nonecho (S) representing an area of sonic shadowing. Because the gallstone has stopped all the sound, no echos are produced distal to it. (Courtesy of Eric Blum, M.D.)

depth below the skin surface is proportional to the depth of the point imaged within the body. The horizontal axis reflects the movement of the transducer along the skin surface as the image is made.

There are several different formats for displaying the B-mode image. Black-white inversion of the image is possible. In the white-on-black format (Fig. 6-5a), the intensity of echogenicity is proportional to the amount of whitening on the film. Echogenic areas are white; anechoic areas are black. In the black-on-white format (Fig. 6-5b), echogenic areas are black, and anechoic areas are white. Both formats are in common use.

Some newer B-mode machines, the real-time machines, have special transducers and electronics that permit the making of rapid sequential images. These machines permit rapid viewing of multiple images as in a movie, allowing a greater choice in the final image. They also permit the motion of an organ to be viewed.

The M-mode image's main use is in echocardiography; it is explained in Chapter 21. The M-mode image demonstrates the motion of a structure in the body (such as a heart valve) as it rapidly changes position over time.

Three different methods are used for recording the image, the A, B, and M modes. The A-mode image (Fig. 6-4) is like a line graph. The height of the line represents the intensity of echogenicity; the length along the graph represents the depth of that echo source within the body.

In the B-mode image (see Figs. 6-1, 6-2, and 6-3), the intensity of echoes from a point in the body is related to the intensity of the light exposing the film and making the image. A two-dimensional image is constructed in which the top of the image represents the skin surface and the

---

Keynotes

- *The sonogram uses high-frequency sound waves to image the body.*

- *The high frequency sound waves are stopped by air or bone.*

- *Tissues without internal echoes are described as sonolucent or anechoic.*

- *An echogenic structure is one with many internal echoes.*

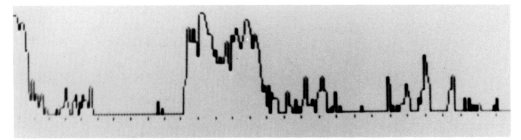

Figure 6-4. A-mode ultrasound. The line represents the amount of echo at increasing depths within the body.

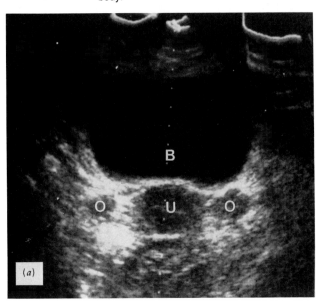

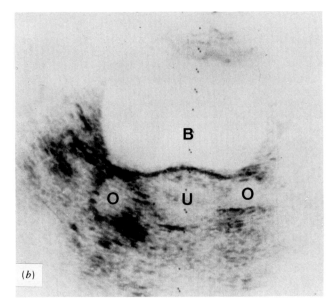

Figure 6-5. These transverse sections through a woman's pelvis demonstrate the two formats for the sonographic image: (a) white on black; (b) black on white. The sonolucent bladder (B), the echogenic uterus (U), and the ovaries (O) are labeled. (Courtesy of Roger Sanders, M.D.)

INTERPRETATION OF THE SONOGRAPHIC IMAGE

Sonographic images can be made in any plane of the body. There are two methods of determining the location of the section: by reading the label and by looking for certain organs to use as landmarks to determine where you are.

The Label System

Vertical axis:

X = Xyphoid
U = Umbilicus
S or P = Symphysis pubis

Measurements are given in centimeters above or below these landmarks:

X − 2 = 2 cm below the xyphoid
U + 4 = 4 cm above the umbilicus

Horizontal axis:

M = Midline
R = Right
L = Left
L + 2 = 2 cm to left of midline
R + 4 = 4 cm to right of midline

Scans not in the vertical or horizontal axes are usually labeled "free" scans.

The Organ Identification System

Any organ you identify can be used to help you determine where you are in the abdomen; however, the liver, kidneys, aorta, inferior vena cava, bladder, and vagina are the organs that are most often helpful:

The liver is a triangular organ, moderately echogenic, in the right upper quadrant of the abdomen. Its typical appearance is shown in Figures 6-1, 6-2, and 6-6.

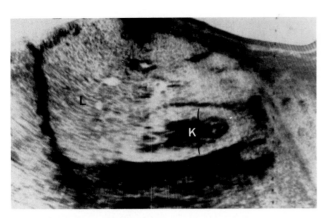

Figure 6-6. This parasagittal section through the right upper quadrant of the abdomen demonstrates, in the black-on-white format, the liver (L) and kidney (K). Compare these images with the similar images done in the white-on-black format in Figures 6-1 and 6-2. (Courtesy of Roger Sanders, M.D.)

The kidney appears as an oval organ, with sonolucent parenchyma and an echogenic core of central structures (Figs. 6-1, 6-6, and 6-7).

In Figure 6-8, the aorta and the superior mesenteric artery are sonolucent.

The bladder is a sonolucent structure in the pelvis (Figs. 6-5 and 6-9).

On longitudinal scans, the vagina consists of two moderately sonolucent lines with a central echogenic core (Fig. 6-9). Identification of the splenic vein can aid in identification of the pancreas, and identification of the portal vein can aid in the identification of the common bile duct.

SONOGRAPHIC IMAGING

Advantages

1. Uses no x-radiation; safe for use in children and pregnant women.
2. Is relatively inexpensive.
3. Has high sensitivity and specificity in retroperitoneal disease, pelvic disease, and structural cardiac disease.

Disadvantages

1. Image is blocked by air.
2. Image quality deteriorates in a very fat person.
3. Frequent inability to image the upper pole of the left kidney.
4. Possibility of confusion of fluid-filled colon with mass or abscess.
5. Poor screening technique because of sampling error. Technique is best when site of abnormality is known.

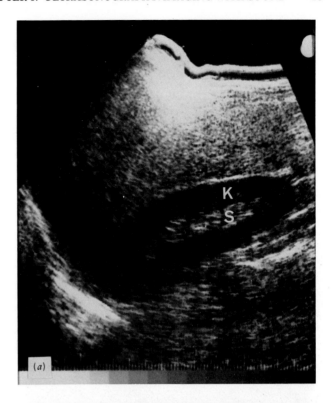

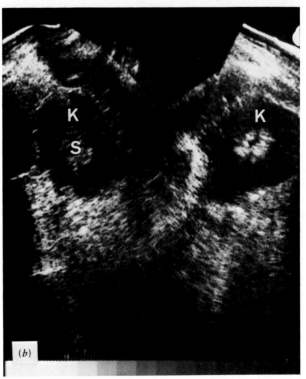

Figure 6-7. These parasagittal (*a*) and transverse (*b*) sonographic sections demonstrate the parenchyma of the kidney (K) as a minimally echogenic oval structure with a central area of increased echogenicity containing the fat of the renal sinus (S) and the renal collecting system. (Courtesy of Morgan Dunne, M.D.)

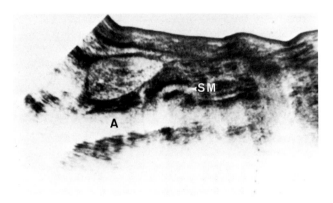

Figure 6-8. This parasagittal section through the midabdomen demonstrates the sonolucent aorta (A) and the superior mesenteric artery (SM) arising from it. The patient's head is to the left, the feet to the right. (Courtesy of Roger Sanders, M.D.)

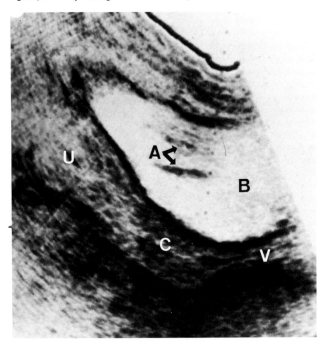

Figure 6-9. This midline sagittal section through the pelvis of a woman demonstrates the uterus (U), the cervix (C), the vagina (V), and the bladder (B). The vagina appears as two bands of low echogenicity with a central echogenic core resulting from the vaginal lumen. The bladder in this patient appears different from those in the preceeding images, for it appears to contain some echoes. The horizontal bands of apparent echogenicity within the bladder are a common artifact (A) caused by reverberation. They result from having the machine settings too high, and can be recognized because they are always parallel to each other. (Courtesy of Roger Sanders, M.D.)

6. More than in other imaging techniques, the image obtained on the sonogram depends on the skill of the person moving and positioning the transducer and adjusting the intensity controls of the machine. Echoes can be amplified or dampened by the machine, and thus the operator can markedly affect the appearance of the final image. By changing the setting on

the controls, echogenic structures can become anechoic, and anechoic structures near the skin surface can appear echogenic. It is necessary to compare an object under investigation to a structure of known echogenicity. Most useful comparison structures are the bladder, aorta, inferior vena cava, kidney parenchyma, and liver parenchyma.

Main Uses

1. Evaluation of the fetus and pregnant uterus (Fig. 6-10)
2. Evaluation of kidneys in renal failure
3. Evaluation of renal masses, cysts versus tumors (Fig. 6-11)

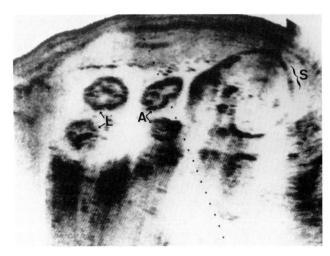

Figure 6-10. Normal fetus, third trimester. This coronal view of the fetus demonstrates the skull (S), the arms (A), and the legs (L).

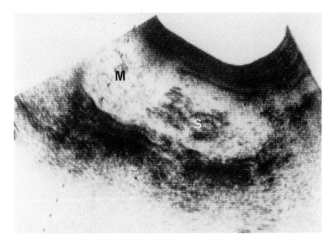

Figure 6-11. This parasagittal image through the left kidney demonstrates additional tissue at the upper pole (to the left of the image) that extends well above the normal central echo pattern of the renal sinus (S). This mass (M) contains echoes and represents a renal cell cancer.

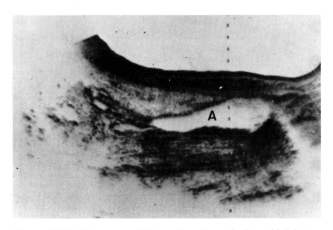

Figure 6-12. This parasagittal section through the midabdomen demonstrates the sonolucent aorta (A). The head is to the left of the image, the feet to the right. In the more distal aorta (to the right of the image), the lumen of the aorta widens, indicating the presence of an aneurysm.

4. Evaluation of suspected abdominal aortic aneurysm (Fig. 6-12)
5. Evaluation of the biliary system in acute biliary tract disease or in the presence of jaundice
6. Detection of pancreatic pseudocyst
7. Detection of ascites (small or large amount)
8. Evaluation of cardiac valvular disease
9. Detection of pericardial effusion
10. The evaluation of masses in the female pelvis

Secondary Uses

1. Evaluation of hepatic masses found by tracer-imaging methods
2. Localization of loculated pleural effusions before thoracentesis

SUMMARY

Imaging by sound is possible because tissue interfaces are often echogenic. Changes in the shape of organs or of the structure of their internal architecture are the basis for diagnosing the presence of abnormalities. An abnormality detected by sonography may be without internal echoes (anechoic or sonolucent) or with internal echoes (echogenic). There are three image formats: the A, B, and M modes. Most organs in the body are displayed in B mode because this best shows the anatomic shape of the organs. M-mode sonography is used primarily in studying the heart.

REVIEW QUESTIONS

1. What causes sonographic echoes?
2. What tissues prevent the passage of the sonographic beam?
3. What structures are usually anechoic?
4. What are A-, B-, and M-mode sonographic formats?
5. The following are typical labels from a sonogram. What does each mean?

   X − 4
   U + 6
   P + 2
   M
   R + 4
   L + 5
   Free

VOCABULARY

anechoic   sonogram

echogenic   sonolucent

SUGGESTIONS FOR FURTHER READING

Roger C. Sanders, the Ultrasound Technologists at Johns Hopkins. *Clinical Sonography: A Practical Guide.* Little, Brown: Boston. 1984.

Kenneth J.W. Taylor. *Atlas of Ultrasonography.* 2nd Ed. Churchill Livingstone: New York. 1985.

PART 1

THE THORAX

The discussion of imaging in the evaluation of diseases of the thorax is divided into

Section A: The Lungs
Section B: The Pleura
Section C: The Hilum
Section D: The Heart
Section E: The Breast

Within each section, the common patterns of abnormality are demonstrated, and common diseases and their diagnosis are discussed.

SECTION A

THE LUNGS

The major processes that can affect the lungs are discussed sequentially: lung masses, alveolar and interstitial lung processes, and decreased lung volume. These chapters are followed by discussions of respiratory disease in the child and the evaluation of lung disease in the patient with a normal chest radiograph.

7

INTRODUCTION TO LUNG IMAGING

KEY CONCEPTS

This chapter discusses the main methods used to evaluate lung disease. The chest radiograph is the main method of evaluating the lungs for pneumonia, cancer, metastases, and heart failure. The *perfusion lung scan* demonstrates areas of lung without blood supply; combined with the *ventilation lung scan,* it is used mainly to demonstrate the presence of pulmonary emboli. The pulmonary arteriogram is occasionally used to confirm the presence of pulmonary emboli. Tomography and computed tomography are used to evaluate solitary pulmonary masses and to look for metastatic disease in patients with a normal chest radiograph.

OBJECTIVES

When you complete this chapter you will be able to

1. List the major indications for obtaining a chest radiograph.
2. Describe the differences between the two types of lung scans.
3. Give the probable clinical diagnosis when the perfusion lung scan is abnormal and the ventilation scan is normal.
4. Give the probable clinical diagnosis when the perfusion lung scan and ventilation lung scan are both abnormal in the same region of the lungs yet the chest radiograph is normal.
5. Give the probable clinical diagnosis when the perfusion and ventilation lung scans and chest radiograph are all abnormal in the same region of the lungs.
6. List the indications for traditional and computed tomography of the lungs.

THE CHEST RADIOGRAPH

The chest radiograph is the initial imaging method for evaluating the lung. Two views are usually obtained: a frontal view, usually taken with a postero-anteriorly directed beam (the PA view), and a lateral view (Fig. 7-1). In sicker patients, the only obtainable view may be the frontal view, usually taken with an anterioposteriorly directed beam (the AP view). This view is usually taken with the x-ray tube closer to the patient, and this magnifies structures in the anterior portion of the chest (the anterior mediastinum and the heart).

The chest radiograph is best for the initial evaluation of the lungs for possible

> Pneumonia
> Cancer
> Metastases
> Heart failure

It can also detect moderate-to-severe chronic obstructive pulmonary disease (COPD). Pulmonary function tests, which measure the vital capacity and the timed forced expiratory volume at one second (FEV_1), are, however, much more sensitive and accurate.

Keynotes

- *The chest radiograph evaluates the lung for*
  Pneumonia
  Cancer
  Metastases
  Heart failure
- *Chronic obstructive pulmonary disease is best detected by pulmonary function tests.*

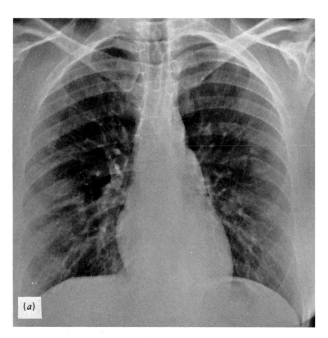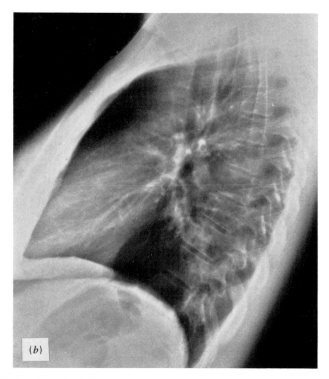

Figure 7-1. Chest radiograph of normal lungs. (*a*) PA view. (*b*) Lateral view.

NUCLEAR MEDICINE TRACER IMAGING TECHNIQUES

Two types of tracer imaging techniques are used for evaluation of the lung: the perfusion scan and the ventilation scan.

The Perfusion Scan

The perfusion scan images the capillary bed of the lung (Fig. 7-2). Small radiolabeled particles of albumen, each slightly larger than a pulmonary capillary, are injected intravenously, circulate to the lung, and lodge in the pulmonary capillaries. The gamma rays they emit can then be used to map the locations of lung perfusion.

The Ventilation Scan

The ventilation scan uses xenon 133, a gamma-emitting inert gas, which functions in the respiratory system in a manner similar to nitrogen. With repetitive breathing, it mixes with the nitrogen and is distributed to the pulmonary airspaces. Images obtained after equilibrium demonstrate regions that are ventilated (Fig. 7-3*a*). After equilibrium, the rate of regional ventilation can be evaluated on serial images obtained as the patient breathes room air (Fig. 7-3*b*) These images can be used to show regions of *airtrapping* (Fig. 7-4).

The perfusion lung scan is best for the evaluation of suspected pulmonary emboli. When perfusion defects are found on the perfusion scan, the ventilation scan is then compared with it to demonstrate whether the regions of perfusion deficit are ventilated. Regions with absent perfusion but normal ventilation have embolic vascular occlusion (Fig. 7-5).

Regions with absent perfusion but with absent or diminished ventilation are indeterminate and must be evaluated further by comparison with a chest radiograph. If the lung is whitened by *infiltrate* at the same site at which the scan shows decreased perfusion and ventilation, the diagnosis is likely to be either pneumonia or embolus, each of which will show matched abnormalities on chest radiograph, perfusion scan, and ventilation scan (Fig. 7-6). If the radiograph shows no infiltrate at the site of absent perfusion and absent ventilation, the likely diagnosis is obstructive pulmonary disease. Less commonly, the lung scan is used to determine the relative function of different portions of the lung to evaluate the consequences of resection of a portion of diseased lung. These changes are summarized in Table 7-1.

Keynote

• *The perfusion and ventilation lung scans are most useful in diagnosing pulmonary emboli.*

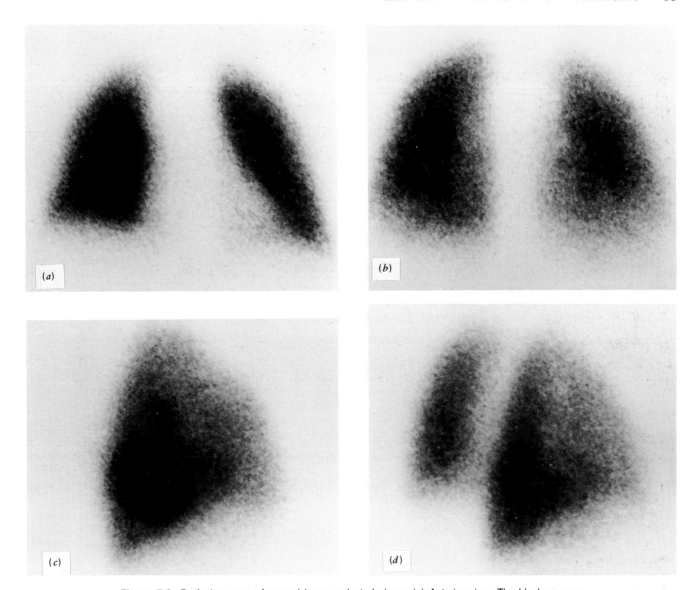

Figure 7-2. Perfusion scan of normal lungs, selected views. (*a*) Anterior view. The blacker areas demonstrates areas of perfused lung. The whiter area in the middle is the location of the heart. (*b*) Posterior view. (*c*) Lateral view. (*d*) Oblique view.

ANGIOGRAPHY

Angiography is not commonly used for the evaluation of the lung; however, it can be used in the patient with a matched defect on lung perfusion scan and chest radiograph to determine the presence or absence of emboli. It can also be used for the confirmation of suspected vascular malformations of the lung (arteriovenous malformations, congenital pulmonary sequestrations).

TRADITIONAL TOMOGRAPHY

Lung tomography is used for the evaluation of solitary lung masses to determine the presence or absence of calci-

fications (Fig. 7-7) and for accurate localization. In most cases, the presence of calcification means that the mass is benign. It is also used in patients whose chest radiograph findings were normal to exclude small pulmonary metastases before major ablative surgery.

COMPUTED TOMOGRAPHY

Computed tomography is not used for the initial evaluation of the lungs; however, masses seen on chest radiography (0.5–3.5 cm in diameter) can be studied for the presence or absence of calcification by traditional or computed tomography (Fig. 7-8). Subpleural metastases may be better seen on computed than on regular tomography. The preferred

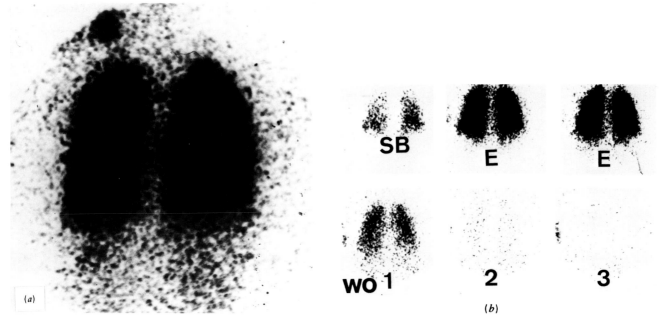

Figure 7-3. Ventilation scan of normal lungs. (*a*) Equilibrium view. (*b*)Single-breath (SB), equilibrium (E), and washout (WO) views at 1, 2, and 3 s.

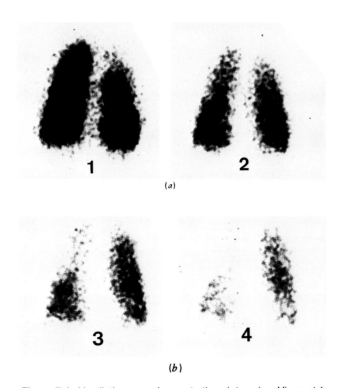

Figure 7-4. Ventilation scan demonstrating air trapping. Views at 1, 2, 3, and 4 s show retention of xenon 133 in the lung of a patient with chronic obstructive pulmonary disease.

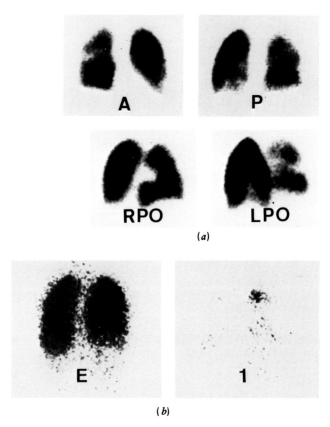

Figure 7-5. Multiple pulmonary emboli. (*a*) Perfusion scan demonstrates several lung segments with perfusion defects. These are represented as the whiter areas within the blacker regions of radioactivity. P = posterior view, A = anterior view, RPO = right posterior oblique view, LPO = left posterior oblique view. (*b*) Ventilation scan; the washout view at 1s demonstrates only one region of air trapping, in the right upper lobe. E = equilibrium.

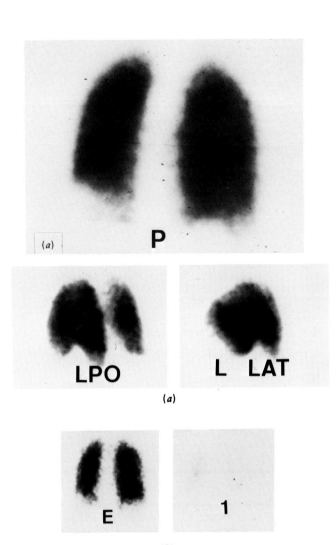

(a)

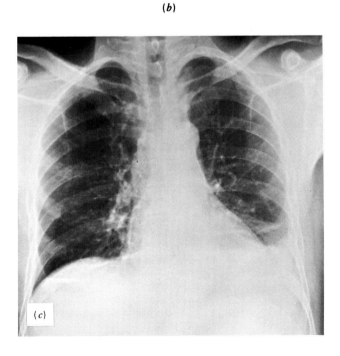

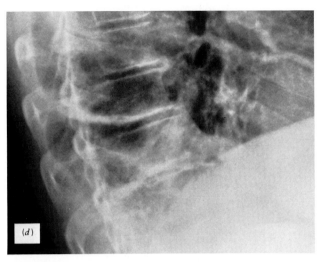

Figure 7-6. Perfusion and ventilation scans showing defects and matched to a chest radiograph to reveal an abnormality that angiography proved to be a pulmonary embolus. (a) Perfusion scan views demonstrating left basilar perfusion defect. P = posterior view, LPO = left posterior oblique view, L LAT = left lateral view. (b) Ventilation scan demonstrating decreased ventilation at the left lung base. E = equilibrium view, followed by 1-s washout view. (c) PA and (d) lateral radiographic views demonstrating focal atelectasis and small pleural effusion at left base.

method of screening for pulmonary metastases in patients whose lungs appear normal on chest radiographs taken before major ablative surgery is still undecided and is under active study. Currently CT seems to be more accurate, but these findings need additional confirmation.

Keynote

- *Conventional and computed tomography are used to evaluate for Calcification in lung nodules*
  Metastases not seen on standard chest radiographs when major ablative surgery is planned.

TYPES OF LUNG PROCESSES

Though there are many types of lung disease, there are only a few different patterns of imaging abnormalities. Lungs can be infiltrated with blood, pus, edema fluid, or fibrosis; lung volume can be decreased or increased; masses can be present; vessels can be occluded. These patterns make the images of disease that will be discussed in more detail in the following five chapters.

SUMMARY

Each of the imaging methods used with the lung has its own role. The radiograph is best in evaluating the lungs for pneumonia, cancer, metastases, and heart failure. The

TABLE 7-1.   LUNG SCAN AND RADIOGRAPH FINDINGS

Perfusion	Ventilation	Radiograph	Likely Diagnosis
Focal defect	Matched area normal	Normal	Embolus
Focal defect	Matched defect	Normal	COPD
Focal defect	Matched defect	Matched area is white	⅔ pneumonia or: ⅓ embolus, if history suggests embolus
Normal	+or −	+or −	No embolus
+or −	Unmatched defects	Normal or COPD	COPD

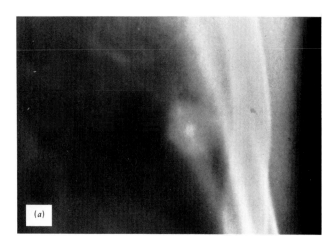 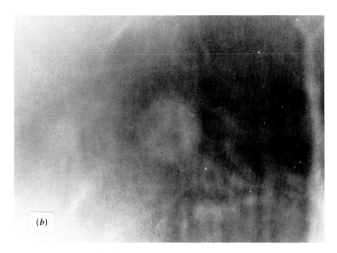

Figure 7-7. Lung granulomas shown on conventional tomography. (*a*) Calcified granuloma. Focus of increased radiodensity (whiteness) in center of mass due to calcium deposit. (Courtesy of E. McCrea, M.D.) (*b*) Noncalcified lung mass. Biopsy demonstrated this to be a tuberculoma.

perfusion lung scan is used to look for areas of decreased blood flow. Because there are several diseases that decrease pulmonary blood flow, ventilation lung scans and chest radiographs may be necessary to evaluate more completely the patient with an abnormality shown on a perfusion lung scan. Occasionally, angiography is necessary to evaluate embolic disease or vascular malformation of the lung.

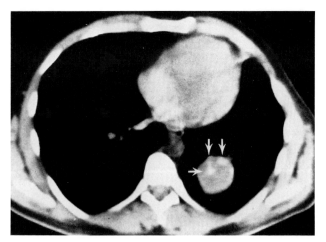

Figure 7-8. CT of a lung mass with focal calcifications; whiter areas (arrows) are calcifications. Diagnosis metastatic chondrosarcoma. (Courtesy of N. Whitley, M.D., University of Maryland Hospital.)

Traditional tomography and CT are both used to evaluate a solitary lung mass for calcification. They are also both used to evaluate possible metastatic disease when lungs appear normal on a chest radiograph and major ablative or deforming surgery is planned, if the surgery would not be done were metastases demonstrated. The choice between traditional tomography and CT for each of these uses is currently being studied. In each case, CT seems to be more accurate, but additional studies are necessary to confirm this apparent advantage.

REVIEW QUESTIONS

1. For which of the following is a chest radiograph preferred and for which is the lung scan preferred: possible pneumonia, pulmonary embolus, metastases, COPD, heart failure, lung cancer.

2. What is the most sensitive test for COPD?

3. If the perfusion lung scan, ventilation scan, and chest radiography each show an abnormality in the same location, what is the likely diagnosis?

4. If the perfusion lung scan shows a focal abnormality and the ventilation scan and chest radiograph show no abnormality, what is the likely diagnosis?

5. When should traditional or computed tomography of the lung be performed?

VOCABULARY

air trapping	infiltrate
COPD	perfusion lung scan
FEV_1	ventilation lung scan

SUGGESTIONS FOR FURTHER READING FOR CHAPTERS 7 TO 18

George Simon. *Principles of Chest X-ray Diagnosis,* 4th Ed. Butterworth: London. 1978. (Introductory text)

Robert G. Fraser, J.A. Peter Pare. *Diagnosis of Diseases of the Chest.* W.B. Saunders: Philadelphia. 1979. (Reference text)

Benjamin Felson. *Fundamentals of Chest Roentgenology.* W.B. Saunders: Philadelphia. 1960. (Classic introductory text)

Anthony V. Proto, Raymond C. Rost, Jr. CT of the thorax: Pitfalls in interpretation. *RadioGraphics,* **5**(5), 1985.

8

WHAT'S WRONG WITH THIS PATIENT? THE SOLITARY LUNG MASS

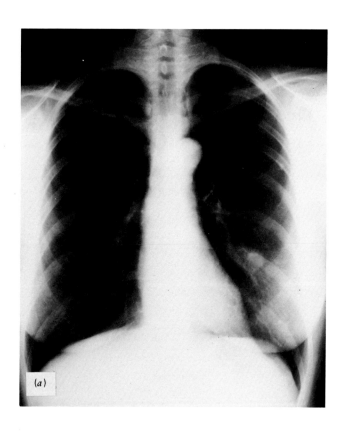

(a)

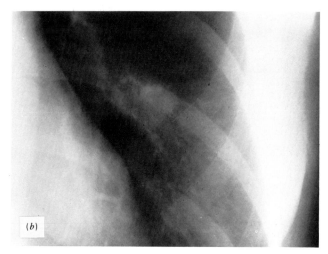

(b)

Figure 8-1. Look at *a*. Did you find the lung mass near the left border of the heart? If not, look at the limited view of the chest in *b*. What do you think the mass might be? How would you find out?

KEY CONCEPTS

This chapter discusses the evaluation of the patient with a single mass in the lung seen on a chest radiograph. If you can demonstrate that the mass is on the skin, was present on films more than 2 years old, or is calcified, additional work-up is usually not needed. If further evaluation is needed to show that the lesion is not cancer, tomography, CT, and biopsy may be needed. Because of the expense of each of these procedures, the search for an old film, even if difficult to locate, is of prime importance.

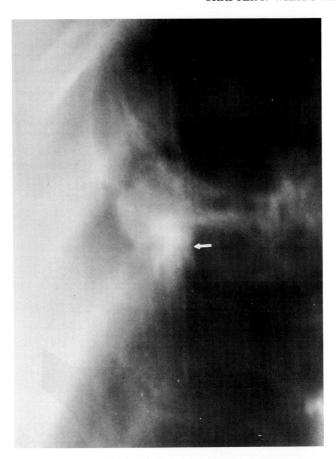

Figure 8-2. Scar carcinoma. This lung tomogram demonstrates calcium (arrow) in the lower portion of the lung mass. The region of calcium looks whiter because calcium is more radiodense than the cancer around it. *Scar carcinoma* is a cancer that arises in a scar.

OBJECTIVES

When you complete this chapter you will be able to

1. List the steps to follow in evaluating a solitary lung mass.
2. List five potential places to check for older comparison films.
3. Discuss the significance of calcium found in a solitary lung mass.

There is a mass-like density in the mid left portion of the chest. What could it be?

Cancer?
Granuloma?
Focal pleural fibrosis?
Something on the skin?

How would you evaluate it? Is there anything about the lesion that could tell you that your patient needn't worry about it?

What if the patient is 30 years old? Can you stop your work-up then? If the patient has no symptoms and has had no known primary tumor, the answer is usually yes—no work-up except a follow-up film 3 and 6 months later looking for change.

What if the lesion was on an old chest radiograph more than 2 years old? If the lesion is unchanged for 2 years, it is not a primary lung cancer.

What if the lesion is on the skin? A nipple, a sebaceous cyst, a skin tag? Then you can forget about it, but how do you know it's on skin? You look at the skin in the same position used for taking the radiograph (arms up), looking at both front and back skin (for the PA view) and at the right and left sides (for an abnormality seen on the lateral view). If you find a possible lesion, repeat the radiograph with a lead marker on the lesion.

What if the lesion has calcium in it? Calcified lesions are usually benign. What if the calcium looks like that in Figure 8-2? There the calcium is localized in the periphery of the lesion. In this case, a growing tumor could have engulfed a calcified granuloma. Only when the calcium occupies a major portion of the lesion can it be considered benign.

What if you can't see calcium in the lesion? What then? If the lesion is less than 0.5 cm, is solitary, and you can see it easily, it has to be calcified. A water-density solitary lesion less than 0.5 cm is only faintly visible. Lesions 0.5–1 cm can be easily seen only if they are superimposed on the ribs, spine, or heart. If you can see a 1-cm lesion easily and it is not superimposed on any of these structures, it is calcified.

If the mass is larger than 3.5 cm and is calcified enough to be definitely benign, clumps of calcium should be clearly visible on the standard film (Fig. 8-3). A lesion between 0.5 and 3.5 cm that is not obviously calcified should be studied with tomography. Conventional linear tomography is standard. Computed tomography is becoming more popular and may replace it once it has been shown to be cost effective and of equal value or better accuracy.

What if you find a lesion that it totally calcified? Is it benign? Usually yes, but can you think of any tumor whose metastases might be densely calcified? Osteogenic sarcoma and chondrosarcoma metastases may be densely calcified; but those tumors usually produce symptoms at the site of the primary tumor that should cause you to suspect their presence.

Case 8-1

Your patient (Fig. 8-1), whose radiograph introduces this chapter, is a 43-year-old man who came to you with symptoms of a morning cough. He smokes two packs of cigarettes a day and has occasionally hemoptysis. You obtain a chest radiograph that reveals a masslike density on the mid left side of the chest. What should you do first?

Old films?
Tomography?
Biopsy?

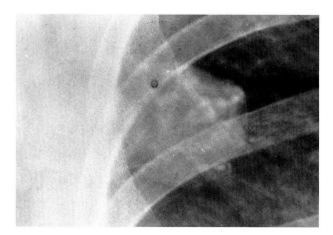

Figure 8-3. Lung mass containing many separate areas of increased radiodensity caused by calcium deposits. This mass was a hamartoma of the lung. Approximately 50% of lung hamartomas contain calcium.

No. First you work with the film you have. You've found a possible mass. Are there others? Are there bony, hilar or mediastinal metastases? Are there enlarged lymph nodes in the supraclavicular fossa? (Fig. 8-4 demonstrates each of these possibilities. Do they look like your patient?) Is the lesion calcified? It's larger than 1 cm and less than 3.5 cm with no definite clumps of calcium in it.

What do you do next?

Check the skin? No possible lesions. Then check for old films. You look in the patient's film jacket and find no old films. What next? Next find out whether the x-ray department you are using has a remote storage area (most radiology departments maintain a separate file of old inactive films away from the main hospital department). Ask them if your patient's old film might be there so you can check for the mass.

If that fails, what next?

Next ask the patient, "Have you ever had a chest radiograph before?" This will probably make him nervous. He'll want to know why you're asking, so tell him there's a suspicious shadow on the chest radiograph. Ask him if anyone ever told him about a problem with the chest radiograph or a spot on the lung. If your pa-

tient is like most patients, there is a good chance he won't remember his last chest radiograph; he'll tell you he's never had one before.

"Doc, is it cancer?" What do you do now?

You can tell him, "Maybe, but it may be an old scar," and that's why you need the old films.

But he can't remember any. So what do you do?

There are many situations in which people have chest

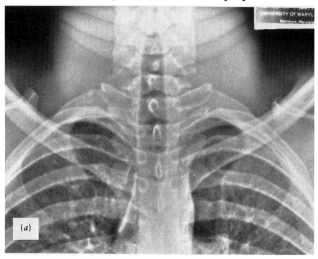

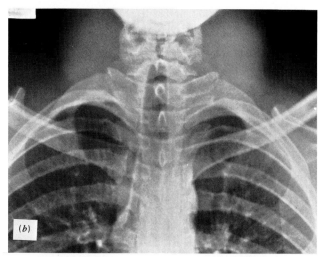

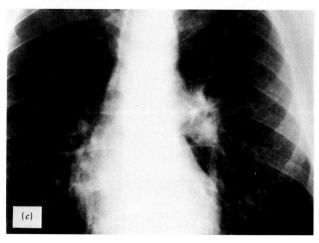

Figure 8-4. (*a*) Normal supraclavicular fossae. The tissue line (called a *companion shadow*) along the superior portion of the clavicles reflects the depressed supraclavicular fossa. In thin people, the supraclavicular fossae are depressions in the body surface. In obese people, the depression, and therefore the companion shadow, may be absent. (*b*) There is a lymph node mass in the left supraclavicular fossa. The companion shadow on the right is present; the companion shadow on the left is obliterated because the lymph node masses fill the supraclavicular depression. Diagnosis: metastatic cancer of the lung. (*c*) There is a left hilar mass in this 45-year-old man with squamous cell cancer of the lung. In this patient, the mass is the primary cancer, not a metastasis. The mass can be detected because the left hilum is larger and more radiodense than the right hilum.

radiographs but don't remember them. How many situations can you think of to ask him about? Review the list that follows.

The Forgotten Chest Radiograph

Insurance physicals
College physicals
Jail or imprisonment
Military service
Preemployment
  Food handlers
  Hospital workers
  Teachers
Heavy Industries
  Coal miners
  Chemical workers
  Shipyard workers
  Steelworkers
Prehospitalization
During chest illness
Tuberculosis screening
Mobile street units

List exhausted, you find a film from 1 year ago, but that's the only film. What next?

A lesion unchanged for 2 years is not a primary lung cancer, but some metastases may sit unchanged in the lung for many years and then start growing. Renal cancer may sit 3 years unchanged, breast cancer 5–10 years, and, rarely, thyroid cancer stays unchanged for 15–20 years. With only 1-year follow-up, what do you do next?

Next get tomograms or CT, first, to see that the lesion is really in the lung rather than in the pleura; second, to look for calcification; and third, to measure the size of the lesion accurately. The lesion is 2.2 cm and has no calcium in it. It is in the upper anterior segment of the left lung. What next?

Most people would do a biopsy of the lesion at this time. What is the easiest way to do a biopsy? With a needle passed from the skin, guided into the lesion by fluoroscopy or CT (Fig. 8-5). But that technique is available only at a limited number of institutions. If needle biopsy technique is unavailable, thoracotomy with an excisional biopsy can be done but is more hazardous. Some physicians confronted with a lesion unchanged for 1 year would follow it every 3 months, accurately measuring it with repeated tomography. Any evidence of enlargement mandates a biopsy. A newly discovered mass should not be followed in this manner, but a mass unchanged for 1 year can be followed safely in this manner.

In this case, you are able to have the lesion biopsy done percutaneously, and the mass is a granuloma. What should you do now?

Bronchoscopy is indicated to look for the possible cause of the patient's hemoptysis (this can be done be-

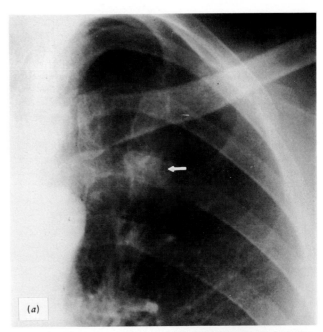

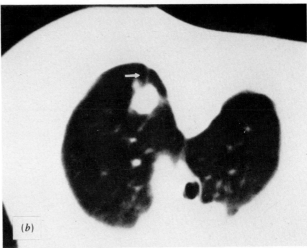

Figure 8-5. Left-upper-lobe squamous cancer. (*a*) Limited view demonstrates a small mass overlying the first rib (arrow). (*b*) CT demonstrates the mass. The arrow marks the needle that has been passed through the skin into the mass to biopsy it. Cytological examination of the specimen demonstrated squamous cell cancer.

fore or after the biopsy). The bronchoscopy results are normal. What now?

Now you should attempt to counsel and work with the patient to decrease the amount that he smokes and to urge him to change to a cigarette with a lower tar level. Occasionally, a patient can, with encouragement, stop smoking; more often, the goal must be only to reduce the amount of carcinogen he exposes himself to.

Keynotes

• *A lung mass unchanged on radiographs for two years is not primary lung cancer but could be a metastasis.*

- *Always check the skin when you think a mass may be in the lung.*
- *Cancer can originate in a scar. Peripheral calcification does not indicate that a mass is benign. A mass unchanged for years that starts to enlarge can be a cancer.*
- *Lung masses easily seen but less than 0.5 cm are calcified. Lung masses larger than 3.5 cm, if calcified, should show the calcification on the conventional chest radiograph.*
- *Finding an old chest film for comparison is the cheapest method of evaluating a lung mass.*
- *Remember that patients don't always remember where they've had chest radiographs. Be prepared to suggest where they might have had them.*

SUMMARY

Work-up of a Mass Lesion

Take a clinical history.

Check for old films (local jacket, remote storage area).

Check skin with arms in position used for radiograph (arms up).

Film with lead marker on skin lesion.

Ask patient about known lung lesions.

Check for films taken elsewhere. remembering to jog patient's memory about situations listed in the case example.

Order tomography or CT for location, calcification.

Order biopsy, by percutaneous needle (controlled by fluoroscopy or CT), by bronchoscopy, or by open thoracotomy.

Order bronchoscopy (sometimes done before a biopsy to exclude other lesions).

REVIEW QUESTIONS

1. When the radiograph on your patient shows a single lung mass, what else should you look for on the film to help you?
2. List the places where an old chest film might be found, if needed for comparison.
3. What is the significance of calcification in a solitary lung mass?
4. List the work-up of a newly found solitary lung mass in a man over the age of 40.

VOCABULARY

granuloma

hamartoma

scar carcinoma

sebaceous cyst

skin tag

SUGGESTIONS FOR FURTHER READING

R. Konig et al. Computed tomography for staging bronchogenic carcinoma. *European Journal of Radiology,* **5**:91-93, 1983.

Benjamin Felson, Ed. Solitary lung lesions. *Seminars in Roentgenology,* **19**(3), 1984.

Benjamin Felson, Ed. Pulmonary neoplasms. *Seminars in Roentgenology,* **12**(3), 1977.

For additional suggested reading see Chapter 7.

9

LUNG INFILTRATES: INTRODUCTION

KEY CONCEPTS

When you look at a chest radiograph, there are often areas of increased radiodensity that might represent disease. Some of these are in the lungs and are classified into *alveolar processes,* in which the alveoli are filled with fluid, and *interstitial processes,* in which the interstitial support structures of the lungs are thickened. Often, the radiodensity seen on the radiograph does not represent lung disease but is the result of a process or structure that is outside the lung but superimposed on it. Structures and processes such as breast tissue, skin bumps, or pleural disease can result in pseudopulmonary radiodensities. The best way to distinguish the true pulmonary processes from the pseudopulmonary is by the identification of the signs of true pulmonary processes, signs discussed in the two chapters that follow this one.

OBJECTIVES

When you complete this chapter you will be able to

1. Describe what an alveolar process is.
2. Describe what an interstitial process is.
3. List five pseudopulmonary radiodensities.

The chest radiograph frequently has radiodensities superimposed over the lungs. Some of these are in the lung, some in the pleura, some in the chest wall, and some outside the body. Those within the lung, *pulmonary radiodensities,* are often called *infiltrates,* a term that is acceptable but etymologically applies only to a subgroup of these processes. This text uses *pulmonary radiodensities* or *pulmonary processes* rather than the overly specific term *in-*filtrate whenever a general term is needed and uses *infiltrate* only when the process is due to fluid infiltration.

Pulmonary radiodensities result from two types of processes: Those in which the alveoli are filled with a material other than air and those in which the interstitial supporting structures are enlarged, thickened, or infiltrated. Most acute and most chronic lung diseases cause abnormal pulmonary radiodensities. Of the few that do not, the most common are pulmonary emboli and obstructive pulmonary disease, and these are discussed in more detail later. The classic division of pulmonary radiodensities is into alveolar (or airspace) and interstitial processes, although few processes are purely alveolar or purely interstitial. The predominant pattern is selected to aid in classification and to limit the differential diagnostic possibilities.

Many of you may already have had the experience of viewing a chest radiograph on one of your patients. Convinced that the patient has a pneumonia, you have taken the film to the radiologist for confirmation, only to be told that the radiograph results are normal. It is very common for the inexperienced to identify pulmonary radiodensities when none exist. Do you remember what it was that confused you? Often it is breast tissue, or a pleural effusion or fibrosis, or clothing, or just a poor inspiratory film. The radiodensity of each of these things, not in the lung but simulating lung disease, I like to call pseudopulmonary processes. As it is never fun to be wrong in public, my list of the types of lung processes is:

1. Pseudopulmonary processes
2. Alveolar (or airspace) processes
3. Interstitial processes
4. Mixed interstitial and alveolar processes

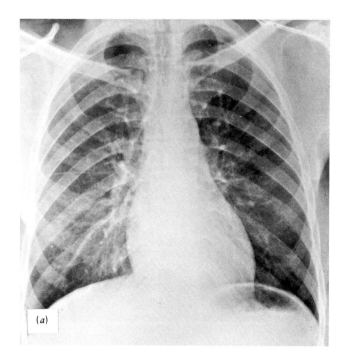

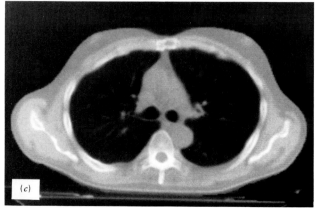

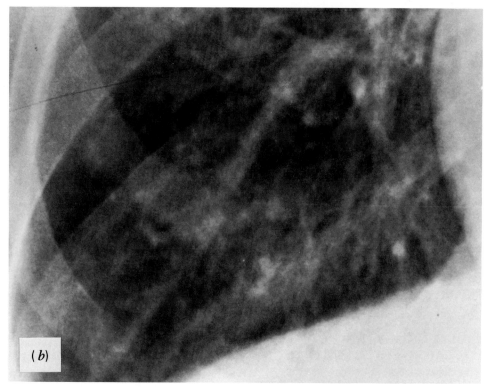

Figure 9-1. (*a*) Normal PA chest radiograph. Multiple layers of tissue overlie the lungs. The lungs themselves are seen only because the vessels in them are more radiopaque than the air in them. (*b*) A close-up view demonstrates the vessels coursing in the lower right lung. (*c*) A CT scan photographed at lung windows demonstrates the whiter vessels coursing through the blacker air-containing lung.

Often if you think of the possibility that something might be pseudopulmonary, it becomes obvious that it is. In much of medical practice, there are false signs, misinterpretations, confusing test results. Often the hardest decision is to realize that something may be a false sign, but when you do, then it quickly becomes obvious that it is. The second method of diagnosing a pseudopulmonary process is by looking for the specific signs of true pulmonary processes. There are specific signs of alveolar processes and specific signs of interstitial processes. Any radiodensity that does not show a specific sign is probably pseudopulmonary.

So what are the specific signs? The normal lung on a radiograph or CT consists of air and blood vessels (Fig. 9-1). All other markings are so thin that they cannot be seen. Alveolar air and bronchial air blend with no separation. Fibrous septa and lymphatics are invisibly thin. You find pulmonary radiodensities by looking for fluid where there should be air and for the thickening of structures normally too thin to see.

Keynotes

- *An alveolar (or airspace) process is one in which the alveoli of the lung are filled with fluid.*
- *An interstitial process is one in which the interstitial support structures are enlarged, thickened, or infiltrated.*
- *A pseudopulmonary process is any process that appears to add to the radiodensity of the lung by being superimposed on the lung.*
- *Any process not showing the specific signs of an alveolar or interstitial process should be evaluated as more likely lying outside than inside the lungs.*

SUMMARY

Three types of processes can add to the apparent radiodensity of the lung: the alveolar processes, in which alveoli are filled with fluid; the interstitial processes, in which the interstitial supporting structures of the lung are thickened; and pseudopulmonary processes, in which structures outside the lungs are superimposed on the lung and add to the lung's apparent radiodensity. The pseudopulmonary processes are those that most often confuse the student, and care is needed not to confuse breast tissue, clothing, hair, and pleural changes for true lung processes.

REVIEW QUESTIONS

1. What is an alveolar process?
2. What is an interstitial process?
3. Name five pseudopulmonary radiodensities.

VOCABULARY

alveolar processes

infiltrate

interstitial processes

pseudopulmonary process

pulmonary radiodensities

SUGGESTIONS FOR FURTHER READING

For suggested reading see Chapter 7.

10

ALVEOLAR PROCESSES

KEY CONCEPTS

Radiological

The main radiological signs of an alveolar pulmonary process are air bronchograms, a positive silhouette sign, lobar or segmental distribution, and certain patterns of inhomogeneous consolidation. *Air bronchograms* are air-filled bronchi seen as branching black lines because they are surrounded by water-density material in alveoli. A positive *silhouette sign* is the failure to seen the margin of an organ because a lung process of the same radiodensity lies immediately adjacent to it.

Clinical

Bacterial and mycoplasma pneumonias, cardiac pulmonary edema, and pulmonary emboli are the most common causes of processes with alveolar filling. It often takes bacterial pneumonias 1–3 days to produce enough alveolar filling to be seen on radiographs, and it may take up to 8 weeks for a pneumococcal pneumonia to clear up.

OBJECTIVES

When you complete this chapter you will be able to

1. List and describe the major radiological changes of alveolar infiltrates.
2. Discuss why air bronchograms are often not present in the patient with an alveolar infiltrate.
3. Describe the application of the silhouette sign to the identification of alveolar infiltrates.
4. Describe the advantages and disadvantages of the classic silhouette sign and the silhouette sign as applied to the intrapulmonary blood vessels.

5. Select an appropriate interval for obtaining chest radiographs in a patient with pneumonia and explain your choice.

The first major category of processes that increase the radiodensity of the lung are the *alveolar* or *air-space* processes. These processes result in increased lung radiodensity by filling the alveoli and, in some cases, the smaller bronchi with material other than air. On the radiograph, the lung will have increased radiodensity in patterns that allow the classification of the process as alveolar. Some of the patterns are specific for alveolar processes, some nonspecific.

ALVEOLAR PROCESS

Specific Signs	Nonspecific Findings
Air bronchogram	Fluffy margin
Silhouette sign	Lobar distribution
Inhomogeneous alveolar	Segmental distribution
infiltrates	Central fluffy pattern
Emphysema	
Lung abscesses	
Pneumatoceles	

SPECIFIC SIGNS

Air Bronchogram

Air bronchograms are a specific but uncommon sign of alveolar processes. Normally the alveoli and the bronchi contain air, and the bronchial wall is too thin to be seen. If the alveoli are filled with fluid and the bronchi are not, it

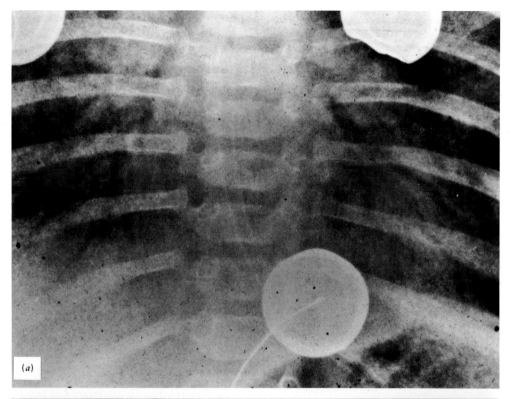

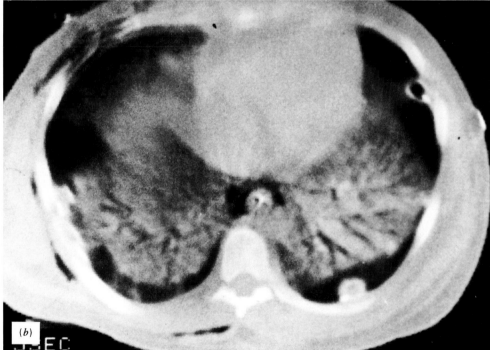

Figure 10-1. Alveolar processes with air bronchograms: (*a*) *Pneumocystis carinii* pneumonia. The branching black lines in the lung bases are air bronchograms. (*b*) Adult respiratory distress syndrome. The branching black lines on the CT examination of the chest are air bronchograms. (Courtesy of N. Whitley, M.D., University of Maryland Hospital.)

is then possible to see the bronchi as branching black lines surrounded by the radiodensity of fluid-filled alveoli (Fig. 10-1). This sign is amost specific for alveolar processes, but it is infrequent.

Why should it be uncommon? It is uncommon because the most common symptom associated with alveolar processes—for example, pneumonia, pulmonary edema, or hemorrhage—is . . . ? Sputum production. And how does the sputum get from the alveoli to the mouth? Through the bronchi. Air bronchograms are rare because secretions usually fill both the alveoli and the bronchi.

Silhouette Sign

The silhouette sign is a common sign that, when used properly, is specific for alveolar processes. Étienne de Silhouette, the French comptroller general for finances in 1759, was ridiculed for his unpopular economic policies by having his name applied to black paper cutouts of the profiles of people (the author's silhouette is shown in Fig. 10-2). In the same way that the black profile can be easily seen against the white background, the sharp outline of the water radiodensity heart, diaphragm, and aorta on a chest radiograph can be seen against the air radiodensity of the adjacent lung (Fig. 10-3). When the lung adjacent to

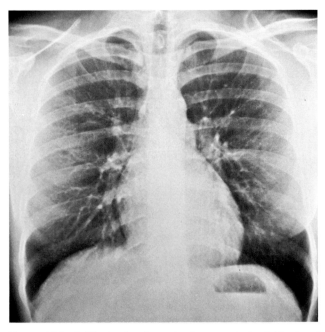

Figure 10-3. A PA chest radiograph of a normal chest. The heart and diaphragm are distinctly limited by the blacker appearing lung.

these water-density structures is replaced by fluid, the outline is lost. This loss of outline is called a *positive silhouette sign*.

The classic silhouette sign is used as follows: A radiodensity at the left of the midchest which "silhouettes out" the left heart border must be an alveolar process in the lingula (Fig. 10-4). A radiodensity in the right lower chest which silhouettes out the margin of the right hemidiaphragm must be an alveolar process in the right lower lobe. The aortic knob borders on the posterior segment of the left upper lobe (Fig. 10-5). The right heart border lies against the right middle lobe.

Unfortunately, there are two problems with the classic

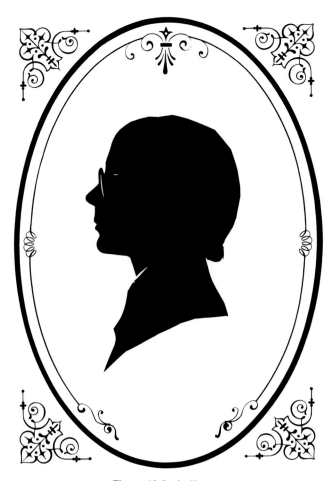

Figure 10-2. A silhouette.

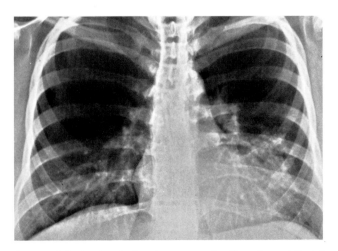

Figure 10-4. An alveolar lingular pneumonia silhouettes out the left side of the heart border, making its margin indistinct.

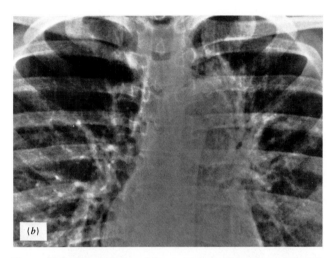

Figure 10-5. This left-upper-lobe pneumonia silhouettes out the left upper hilum and the aortic knob.

silhouette sign that markedly limit its usefulness. The first is that there are large regions of the lung not adjacent to a major water-density structure; if the alveolar process does not touch the margin, loss of its silhouette will not occur. The second problem is that the structures whose margins are to be affected lie outside the lung; it is possible, therefore, for processes not in the lung to obliterate their margins: a pericardial effusion obliterates the heart border; a pleural effusion silhouettes out the hemidiaphragm; a pericardial fat pad can simulate a lingular pneumonia by obscuring the lower portion of the left heart border; fat in the major fissures can silhouette out the hemidiaphragm.

Given these problems, how can you reconstruct the silhouette sign so that it becomes less trivial than its ridiculed namesake? How can you use it to show that a small radiopacity superimposed anywhere on the lung is in the lung? What water-density structure is available throughout the lung that can lose its margin when adjacent to or surrounded by an alveolar process?

If you realize that the pulmonary blood vessels are available, you are right. The silhouette sign is useful because there are blood vessels throughout the lung whose profile can disappear when surrounded by fluid-filled alveoli (Fig. 10-6). Care is necessary, however, because the blood vessels you trace on a normal radiograph also disappear—when they get close to the periphery of the lung, and throughout the lung when they change direction to run directly toward you or directly away from you.

Careful observation is the key. A vessel that turns is thicker as it courses toward you or away from you, and thus it is more radiodense; a white dot is seen at the end of these vessels (Fig. 10-6a, b, and c). A vessel disappearing into a focus of fluid-filled alveoli just disappears and does not change radiodensity.

Case 10-1

JB is a 28-year-old man with sickle cell disease who came to his physician with an acute onset of chest pain,

shaking chills, and fever to 105 °F (40.5 °C). The radiograph in Figure 10-7a was obtained about 6 hours after he started to feel sick. What do you see?

At this time, the radiograph was almost normal. There are a few linear radiodensities at the right lung base, which were on previous films and represent lung scars.

A smear of the sputum disclosed many bacteria grouped in twos or in chains, staining Gram-positive. Many of these had been ingested by polymorphonuclear leukocytes. What should you do now?

If your diagnosis is pneumococcal pneumonia, why does the chest radiograph look normal?

JB's physician started treatment with penicillin and hospitalized him.

Another chest film was taken the next day (Fig. 10-7b). What does it show?

There is minimal alveolar infiltrate in the right lower lobe. Several blood vessels fade as they enter the infiltrate (see close-up Fig. 10-7c). With the infiltrate getting worse while the patient is on penicillin, what should you do?

His fever is still high; but this is still only 1 day after the start of treatment, and neither the fever nor the radiograph will change that fast. Penicillin and supportive fluids given by intravenous infusion were continued.

The next day, a chest radiograph was obtained (Fig. 10-7d). What does it show?

There is marked right-lower-lobe infiltrate. The margin of the right hemidiaphragm is obliterated. The infiltrate is much larger. Is the therapy in error?

No, because the fever has decreased (in this case by lysis, rather than by crisis). Temperature is now 101 °F (38 °C), the patient feels weak, but the chills are gone and he's starting to feel hungry as well as thirsty.

How do you explain the radiograph results getting worse?

Two days later, the patient was sent home without further radiographs. Four weeks later, when the patient felt fine, a repeat radiograph was obtained and showed normal lungs. What should you do now?

Questions

This case of classical pneumococcal pneumonia in a patient with sickle cell disease poses several problems:

1. Why was the radiograph normal when the pneumonia was already causing severe symptoms?
2. Why did the radiograph finding continue to get worse while the patient was getting better?
3. Were all these chest radiographs really necessary? Could the patient have been managed with less expense?
4. Was the final film, showing normal lungs, needed?
5. What additional therapy should the patient have now that he has recovered from the pneumococcal pneumonia?

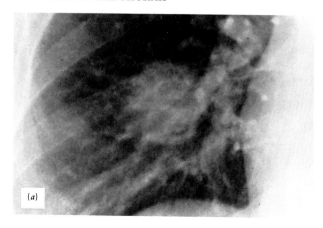

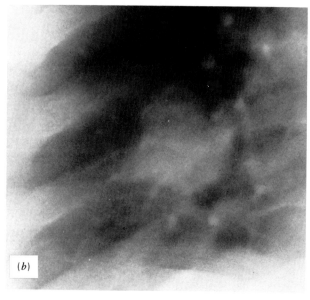

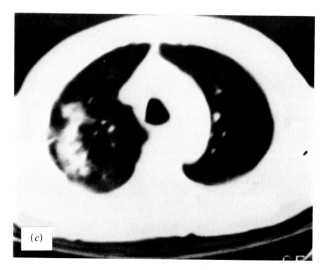

Figure 10-6. This masslike pneumonia does not touch any major water-density object, but it does silhouette out some of the vessels crossing it, indicating that it is alveolar. Some pneumonias are rounded and appear masslike. (*a*) Focal view of the pneumonia. (*b*) Tomogram of the infiltrate, demonstrating several vessels entering, and being silhouetted out by, the infiltrate. Other vessels end as white dots as they turn toward you or away from you. (*c*) CT of a peripheral alveolar infiltrate. Several vessels are silhouetted out by the infiltrate. Some vessels appear as white dots as they course in and out of the plane of the CT.

Answers

1. In diseases with an acute onset of severe symptoms, the patient will often turn to the physician for relief before there is enough change on the radiograph to be visible. This is particularly true for acute severe infections: bacterial pneumonias, osteomyelitis, abscesses. The lag between clinical symptoms and radiographic findings in pneumococcal pneumonia is 24–48 hours.

2. Because of the lag in response time of the radiograph, there is often a phase during the treatment of bacterial pneumonias when the patient is getting better, but the radiograph is getting worse. Clinical symptoms should be the guide, not the radiograph.

3. Were all these radiographs necessary? Probably not. Were I managing the case, I would have gotten a radiograph at the time of initial presentation, more to serve as a baseline of normal for the patient, though it might show some pneumonia. If the physical examination results were classic for a localized pneumonia, I probably would not have requested the next film until discharge at about 5 days. If the physical examination was equivocal for pneumonia, I would have obtained a film on day 2 to confirm the diagnosis. A film on discharge would still have been necessary to confirm the extent of the disease so that if the patient came back with a new fever, I would be able to tell whether there was a new infiltrate.

4. Was the final film, showing normal findings, needed? This depends on the age of the patient, but any patient in a cancer-risk age group does need a final film with a normal finding to avoid the problem in Figure 10-8. In this example, the later film (Fig. 10-8*b*) demonstrates a large mass in the hilum. The pneumonia is secondary to a partially obstructed bronchus. When should this final film be taken? It can take as long as 8 weeks for a pneumococcal pneumonia to clear.

5. What additional therapy should the patient have now? He should be vaccinated against pneumococcal infection. Any patient with increased risk of pneumococcal disease should receive the vaccine. A nonfunctional spleen increases the risk of pneumococcal disease. Sickle cell disease results in spleen infarction and atrophy.

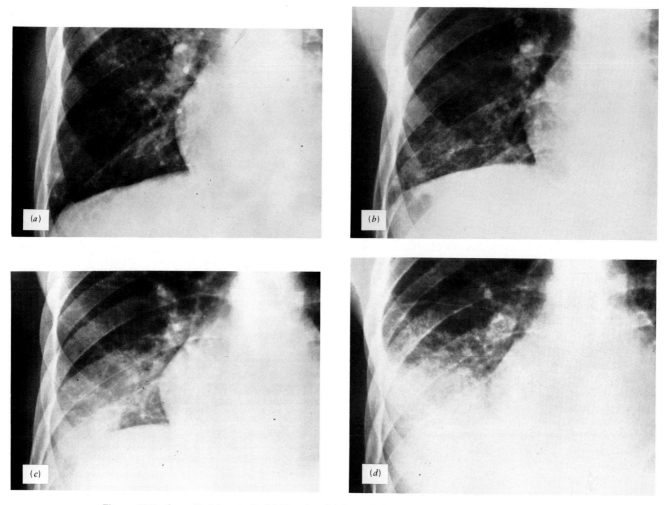

Figure 10-7. Case 10-1 (see text). (*a*) First day. (*b*) Second day. (*c*) Third day. (*d*) Fifth day.

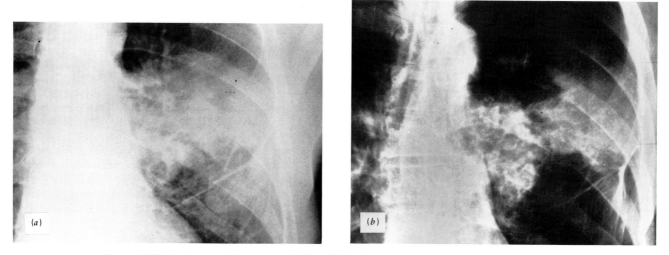

Figure 10-8. Squamous cell lung cancer in hilum hidden by alveolar infiltrate. (*a*) Hilar mass hidden by infiltrate. (*b*) Hilar mass visible through infiltrate.

Inhomogeneous Alveolar Infiltrates

Most alveolar processes are moderately homogeneous. Occasionally radiolucencies other than air bronchograms can be seen within them. Sometimes these inhomogeneous patterns are specific for alveolar processes, permitting accurate differentiation from pseudopulmonary processes. Often they point to other underlying or coexistent lung disease. Four patterns are seen:

1. Acinograms
2. Emphysematous blebs within areas of alveolar infiltrate
3. Lung abscesses surrounded by alveolar infiltrates
4. Pneumatoceles

Air acinograms are focal regions of air radiolucency occurring within a larger region of homogeneous water radiodensity. The *acinus* is a substructure of lung defined as being those alveoli ventilated by one terminal bronchiole. The acinus measures approximately 1 cm in diameter, and the identification of multiple 1-cm radiolucencies within a region of suspected lung infiltrate is usually sufficient to place the process within the lung and to identify it as being alveolar in nature. Less commonly, the alveolar process may fill scattered acini with fluid, resulting in multiple ill-defined lung nodules (Fig. 10-9).

Emphysematous blebs and foci of centrilobular emphysema frequently do not fill with exudate when surrounded by pneumonia. These focal radiolucencies of differing size demonstrate both that the process is in the lung and that the lung is emphysematous (Fig. 10-10).

Lung abscesses are regions of necrosis within the lung. Large radiolucencies within the region of radiodensity often permit the localization of the process to the lung (Fig. 10-11). Occasionally, subcutaneous or pleural abscesses may have similar appearances.

Pneumatoceles are air-containing spaces that develop

within certain pneumonias, as they clear, because of bronchial obstruction with air trapping (Fig. 10-12). Their appearance can be mimicked by pleural and subcutaneous abscesses.

Keynotes

- *Air bronchograms are air-filled bronchi that can be seen because the bronchi are surrounded by fluid-filled lung alveoli.*
- *The silhouette sign is present when the margin of a water-density organ cannot be seen because fluid replaces the air in the lung adjacent to it.*
- *In acute bacterial infections, the radiographic appearance often lags behind the clinical features of the disease.*
- *Any patient with pneumonia in the lung cancer–risk age group should be followed with radiographs to confirm clearing of the pneumonia. Lack of clearing in an appropriate interval suggests the possibility that cancer is partially blocking the bronchus.*

NONSPECIFIC (BUT COMMON) FINDINGS

Fluffy Margin

The margin of most alveolar-filling processes is fluffy or irregular (Fig. 10-9). This is due to the anatomy of the alveoli. Can you figure it out?

Alveoli are grouped into acini. These acini are arranged like a bunch of grapes. The margin of a clump of grapes will appear fluffy or irregular in contour. Alveolar processes are also fluffy because of the ways in which alveolar processes are spread. Alveolar processes spread through the bronchial tree (from acinus to acinus) and through the *pores of Kohn*—interalveolar channels—which permits a fairly random spread of the fluid material through the lung. A randomly spreading process will appear fluffy or irregular. Although the fluffy margin is common, it is not specific for alveolar fluid, since many pseudopulmonary processes also appear fluffy.

Lobar Distribution

Many alveolar processes assume a lobar distribution: they spread until they reach a margin they cannot cross. The pleura is such a boundary. The alveolar processes spread until they reach the pleural boundaries of the lobe filling it.

Processes partially filling a lobe of the lung can be alveolar or interstitial, and an occasional pseudopulmonary process will appear to be lobar in distribution. Processes extending to a fissure and stopping, and obscuring one margin of a fissure, are usually alveolar; but fluid in the pleural space filling the fissure can have a similar appearance.

Case 10-2

The radiographs in Figure 10-13 are those of a 47-year-old man taken to the emergency room. What do you think is going on?

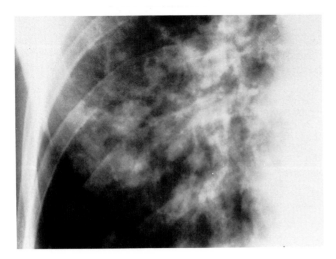

Figure 10-9. Bronchopneumonia. Multiple ill-defined acinar nodules are one of the patterns of alveolar infiltrates.

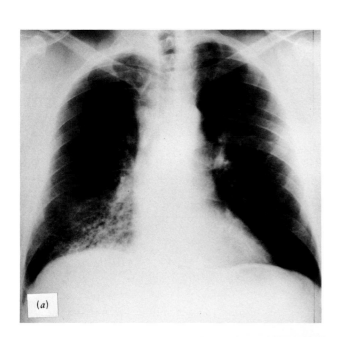

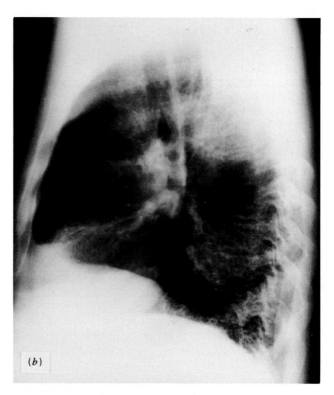

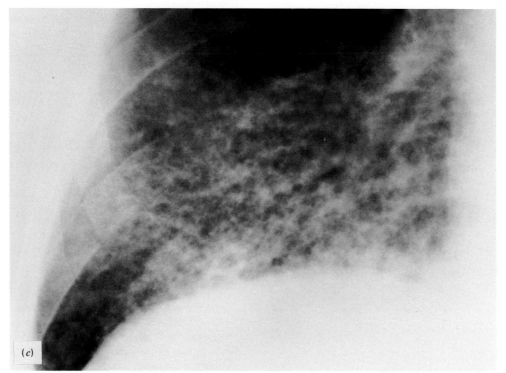

Figure 10-10. Inhomogeneous right-lower-lobe infiltrate caused by pneumococcal pneumonia in a patient with centrilobular emphysema. (*a*) PA view. (*b*) Lateral view. (*c*) Focal view of right lower lung.

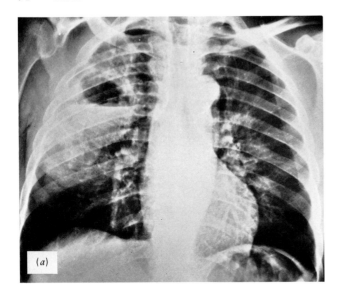

(a)

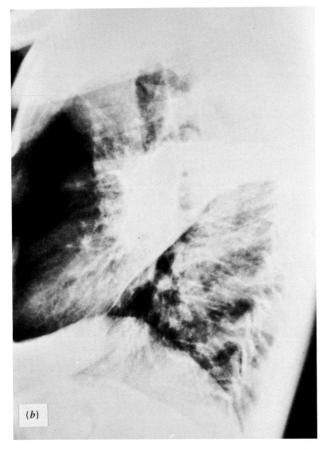

(b)

Figure 10-11. Right-upper-lobe lung abscess. Mixed-flora aspiration lung abscess in an alcoholic patient. (a) PA view. (b) Lateral view.

There is an alveolar process filling the right lower lobe. The right hemidiaphragm margin is obliterated. The process extends to the major fissure on the lateral view.

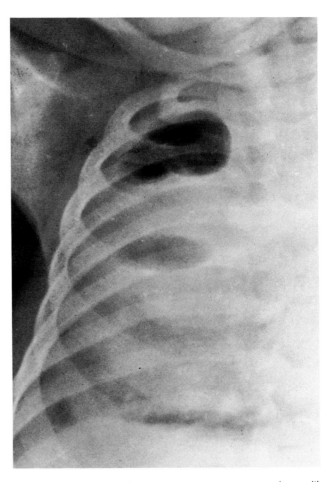

Figure   10-12. *Staphylococcus   aureus*   pneumonia   with pneumatoceles.

The patient says he "feels awful" and has been sweating and shivering. His temperature is 105 °F (40 °C). What do you do?

Look at his sputum. It is loaded with diplocci in chains. What is your diagnosis?

Pneumococcal pneumonia.

What is unusual about the presentation of this case? Compare it with the other case in this chapter.

Patients with pneumococcal pneumonia get sick very fast. Their temperatures rise quickly, and they have severe chills and rigors. Normally they come for medical care quickly, usually while their radiograph findings are normal or near normal. In this case, the right lower lobe is filled with infiltrate when the patient comes for treatment. What does this mean?

It means either that the patient has an underlying process—a pre-existing viral or mycoplasma pneumonia or an obstructing cancer—or that there is a social reason why he did not seek care sooner. He could have been an institutionalized patient, a bedridden patient, an addict who did not want his addiction discovered, or an alcoholic. This patient was an alcoholic who thought that if he drank more, he would feel better. It took him several days to run out of whiskey and come to the hospital.

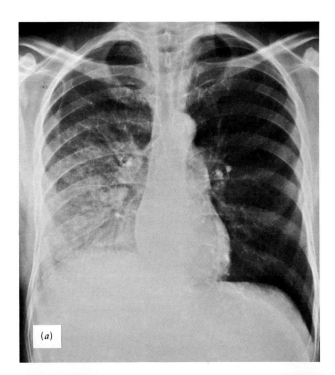

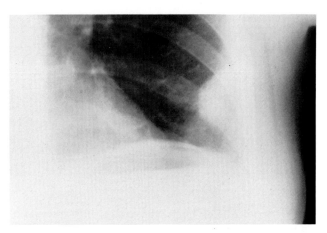

Figure 10-14. Pulmonary embolus in the lateral segment of the left lower lobe. The rounding of the medial portion of the infiltrate, called *Hampton's hump,* is a sign that the infiltrate is due to an embolus

areas of pulmonary hemorrhage from infarction will follow the same pattern (Fig. 10-14).

Perfusion lung scans often show segmental defects in patients with pulmonary emboli. A segmental defect on the perfusion scan associated with normal ventilation in the same region is diagnostic of a pulmonary embolus.

Pneumonias can also follow a segmental pattern, probably because some pneumonias have such viscous secretions that they cannot easily pass through the pores of Kohn and, therefore, can spread more easily through the bronchial tree.

Central Fluffy Pattern. Alveolar infiltrates caused by heart failure or heart failure associated with uremia may show a central fluffy pattern (Fig. 10-15). The pathophysiology

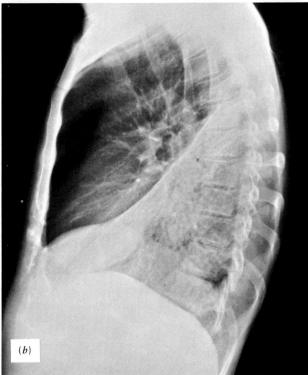

Figure 10-13. Case 10-2 (see text). (*a*) PA view. (*b*) Lateral view.

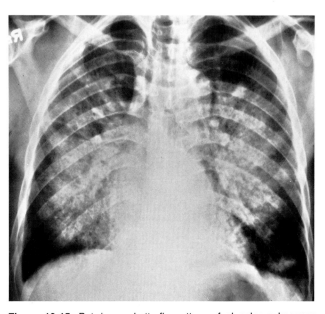

Figure 10-15. Batwing or butterfly pattern of alveolar pulmonary edema in a patient with uremia and congestive heart failure.

Segmental Distribution

Less commonly, alveolar processes follow a segmental pattern. This can occur with pulmonary emboli with hemorrhage. Since the vessels follow a segmental pattern, the

TABLE 10-1. PROCESSES RESULTING IN FLUID-FILLED ALVEOLI

Common Processes	Less Common Processes
Bacterial and mycoplasmal pneumonias	Viral and fungal pneumonias
Pulmonary edema from heart failure	Transfusion reaction
Bleeding and exudation from pulmonary embolus	Tuberculosis
Adult respiratory distress syndrome	Toxic exposure (including inhaled toxic gases)
	Cancer with secretions or bleeding (esp. bronchoalveolar carcinoma)
	Goodpasture's syndrome (autoimmune renal and pulmonary disease)
	Pulmonary hemosiderosis
	Many other diseases

for this pattern is easier to understand after interstitial infiltrates have been discussed, so its explanation is postponed.

TYPES OF PROCESSES CAUSING FLUID TO FILL ALVEOLI

The major processes resulting in fluid-filled alveoli are listed in Table 10-1.

SUMMARY

The filling of alveoli with fluid is a common manifestation of pulmonary disease. The identification of air bronchograms or positive silhouette sign can indicate that these processes are alveolar. Less often, specific inhomogenous radiodensity patterns can indicate that the disease is probably alveolar. Bacterial and mycoplasmic pneumonias, cardiac pulmonary edema, and pulmonary embolus are the most common causes of processes with alveolar filling.

REVIEW QUESTIONS

1. What is an air bronchogram?
2. Describe the silhouette sign and give several examples of how it is used.
3. What are the four reasons that inhomogeneous alveolar infiltrates occur?
4. Describe the clinical and radiological courses of a typical patient with pneumococcal pneumonia.
5. What can predispose a patient to pneumococcal pneumonia?
6. What can cause a segmental alveolar process?
7. What are the common causes of alveolar pulmonary processes?

VOCABULARY

acinograms
acinus
air bronchograms
airspace process
emphysema
Hampton's hump

pneumatoceles
Pneumocystis carinii
pores of Kohn
sickle cell disease
silhouette sign

SUGGESTIONS FOR FURTHER READING

George Genereux. CT of acute and chronic distal air space (alveolar) disease. *Seminars in Roentgenology,* **19**(3): 211-221, 1984.

For additional suggested reading see Chapter 7.

11

INTERSTITIAL PROCESSES

KEY CONCEPTS

Radiological

Interstitial processes are those that add to the radiodensity of structures in the lung interstitium. Thickened bronchial walls, thickened interlobular septa, engorged lymphatic channels, nodules, and thick bands of fibrosis are the abnormal structures sought, and they appear as lines, nodules, and ring shadows.

Kerley's A lines occur in the upper lobes; *Kerley's B lines* occur in the lower lobes. Both represent thickened interlobular septa and are often called "septal lines."

Clinical

Thickened bronchial walls can be seen in cystic fibrosis, bronciectasis, asthma, chronic bronchitis, heart failure, and with tumor engorgement of lymphatic channels.

Linear interstitial patterns can be seen with interstitial pulmonary edema, fibrosis, granulomatous diseases, viral pneumonia, metastatic tumor, connective tissue diseases, and interstitial pneumonitis. Thick bands of fibrosis are scars from prior disease.

Nodular interstitial patterns can be seen in granulomatous diseases, metastatic disease, and pneumoconiosis.

OBJECTIVES

When you complete this chapter you will be able to

1. List the major radiological patterns of interstitial disease.
2. List at least four diseases that result in each of the radiological patterns.
3. Identify on a radiograph Kerley's A and Kerley's B lines.
4. List three symptoms and three signs seen in a patient with miliary tuberculosis.
5. List three patterns of secondary or reactivation tuberculosis.

The second major category of processes that increase the radiodensity of the lung are the interstitial processes. These processes result in thickening of the interstitial supporting structures of the lung: the bronchi and the septa. Because the bronchi and the septa have characteristic shapes, it is usually possible on a radiograph to determine that the bronchi or the septa are thickened and thereby ascribe a pulmonary process to the interstitium. Some of the signs of interstitial processes are specific for the interstitium, some nonspecific.

INTERSTITIAL PROCESSES

Specific Signs	Nonspecific Findings
Bronchial patterns	Pseudonodules
Ring shadows	Increased lung markings
Parallel lines	
1- to 3-cm circular shadows (some with air-fluid levels)	
Linear patterns	
Septal	
Lymphatic	
Thick, fibrotic lines and fissures	
Honeycombing	
Nodular pattern	

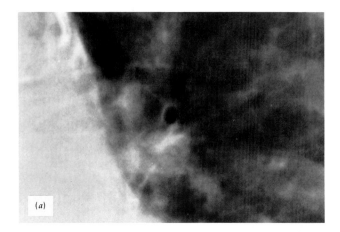

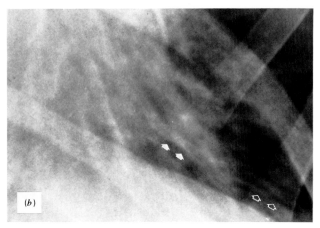

Figure 11-1. Thickened bronchial walls. (*a*) Ring shadow of bronchus, from increased lymphatic flow in a patient with interstitial pulmonary edema. (*b*) Thickened bronchial walls (arrows) in a patient with bronchiectasis.

SPECIFIC SIGNS

Bronchial Patterns

The normal bronchial wall is too thin to be seen on the radiograph. With air within it and air surrounding it, it is invisible. When the bronchial wall is thickened, it becomes visible. Seen end on, it is circular (Fig. 11-1*a*); seen en-face, the parallel lines of its wall can be seen (Fig. 11-1*b*). Less commonly, its walls may be thickened, but not parallel. Thickened walls of fusiform dilated bronchi may be seen. Rarely, sacules arising from the bronchi can result in inferiorly rounded shadows with air-fluid levels in them (Fig. 11-2).

In the mediastinum on a normal radiograph or CT, the air within the trachea and right and left main bronchi can be seen surrounded by a shadow composed of tracheal wall and mediastinal fat. Only the right wall of the trachea can be delineated on a radiograph or CT of the normal chest (Fig. 11-3). (The CT appearance of the right paratracheal region is shown in Fig. 11-4). Visibility of the air within the lumen of the smaller bronchi within the lung indicates

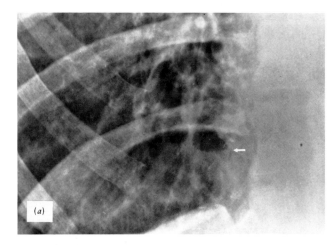

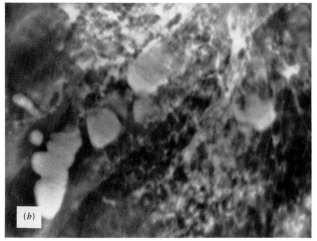

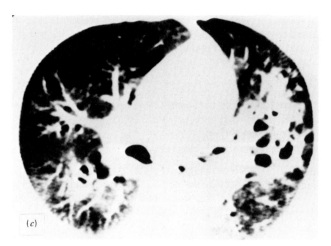

Figure 11-2. Cystic bronchiectasis. (*a*) Focal view of the right lower lung demonstrating focal radiolucencies with air-fluid levels (arrow) (*b*) A bronchogram demonstrates cystic areas of bronchial dilation. (A bronchogram is a study in which a radiopaque contrast medium is placed within the bronchi.) (*c*) CT scan of another patient with cystic bronchiectasis. Arrows point to the cystic areas.

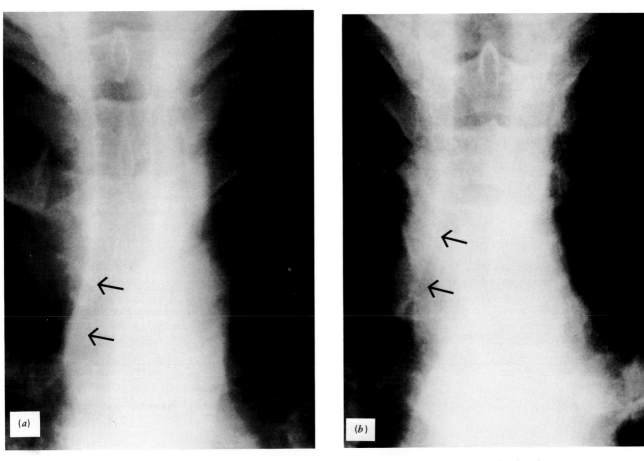

Figure 11-3. Right tracheal wall and right paratracheal region. (*a*) Normal right paratracheal region. The right wall of the trachea (arrows) is less than 4 mm thick. (*b*) Right paratracheal lymph node mass in a patient with sarcoid. The thickness of the right tracheal wall and paratracheal tissues (arrows) exceeds 4 mm.

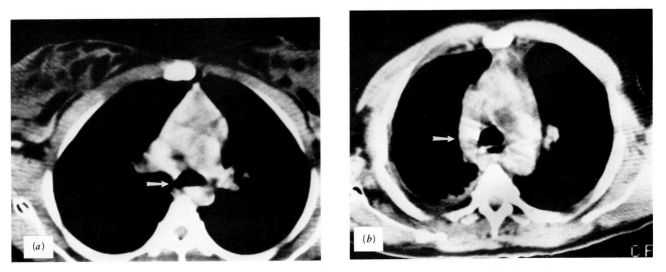

Figure 11-4. The right paratracheal region on CT. (*a*) Normal appearance (arrow). (*b*) Adenopathy (arrow) in a patient with oat cell cancer of the lung.

the presence of fluid-filled alveoli surrounding the bronchi (the air bronchogram, previously described). This pattern is an alveolar pattern and is different from bronchial wall thickening.

In an older person, an occasional ringlike shadow near the hilum can be seen, unrelated to current symptoms: the result of fibrosis from prior disease, air pollution, etc. Calcification of the trachea and bronchi (Fig. 11-5) is uncommon. It usually occurs in the elderly and is of no clinical significance. In the young, it is uncommon, usually is of clinical significance and should be investigated.

Bronchial-wall thickening can be seen in several diseases. What disease would you predict would cause it? Some are shown in Table 11-1, page 89.

Linear Patterns

The supporting structures of the lungs, the septa and lymphatic channels, are normally too thin to be seen. When thickened, these surfaces can be seen only when their edges are tangential to the x-ray beam—they project as lines. These lines were originally described by Peter Kerley, who described three patterns of lines, which he named A, B, and C lines.

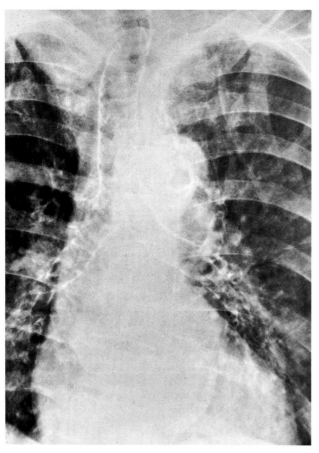

Figure 11-5. Tracheal- and bronchial-wall calcification in an elderly patient.

The A lines are in the upper lungs and are 1.5–2.5 cm long (Fig. 11-6a and b). Sometimes an angular bend is present. They can radiate from the upper portion of the hilum or from the periphery of the upper-lung pleural margin. The B lines are 1 cm long in the periphery of the lower lungs (Fig. 11-6c). They extend to a pleural margin, but because the lung is curved, some of them project more centrally in the lung. The C lines are the result of the superimposition of many B lines in the lower central portion of the lung and have the appearance of a crosshatch. An easy way to remember which line is which is that the A lines are near the apex, the B lines are near the lung base, and the C lines are central.

Kerley's lines can be caused by thickening of the interlobular septa or by distention of the lymphatics that run in the interlobular septa. They can be caused by chronic fibrosis, acute inflammation, or edema. Although it is not possible to tell acute inflammation from acute edema, it is often possible to tell chronic fibrosis from acute enlargement. In general, the lines caused by acute processes are thicker (1.5–2 mm), whereas those from fibrosis are usually hairline thick (0.5 mm) (compare Figs. 11-7 and 11-6c).

Other Lines

Sometimes lines are seen that are not Kerley's lines. These lines can represent engorged lymphatic channels (interconnecting lymphatics), thickened fissures or thick bands of lung fibrosis.

Honeycombing

Densely fibrotic lung can take on an appearance of a honeycomb: multiple, small, air-containing spaces surrounded by thick-walled septa (Fig. 11-8). Although honeycombing can occur in any interstitial disease, it is more common in Hamman-Rich disease, scleroderma, pneumoconiosis, and eosinophillic granuloma of the lung. The pattern of honeycombing can be confused with that of an alveolar infiltrate in a patient with emphysema. Fibrosis in breast tissue superimposed on the bases of the lung sometimes looks like the honeycomb pattern.

Case 11-1

The radiograph in Figure 11-9 is that of a 44-year-old man who felt as if someone were sitting on his chest and he was about to die. What do you see? What do you think is going on?

There are Kerley's B lines at the lung bases and a few A and C lines. Near the hili, the bronchial walls are thickened and can be seen. The minor fissure is thickened. What is causing all these findings?

The patient is in interstitial congestive heart failure (which is probably the most common cause of widespread interstitial infiltrates).

What do you think you would hear, were you to listen to his lungs?

If the process is completely interstitial with no alveo-

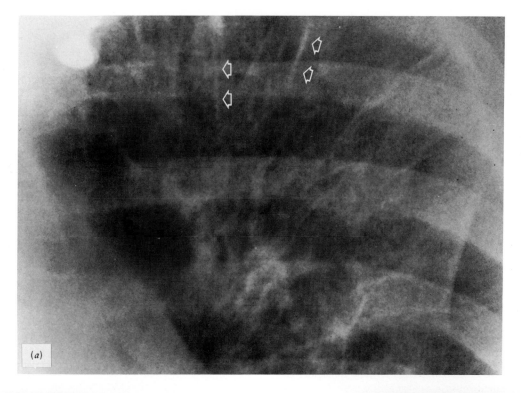

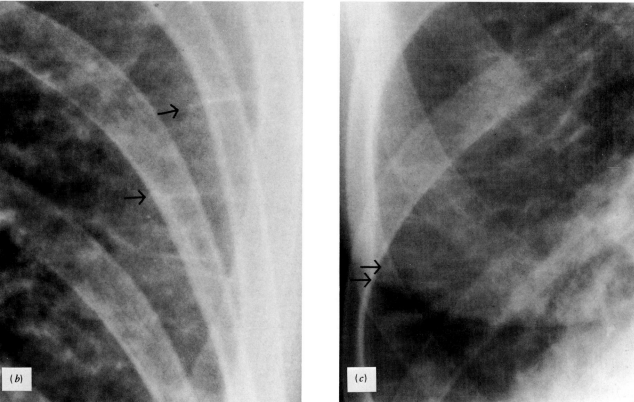

Figure 11-6. Kerley's lines. (*a*) Kerley's A lines (arrows) radiating toward the hilum, caused by interstitial pulmonary edema. (*b*) Kerley's A lines (arrows) radiating from the upper lung margin, also in interstitial pulmonary edema. (*c*) Kerley's B lines (arrows) in the periphery of the lower lung, caused by Interstitial edema and pulmonary hemosiderosis in a patient with mitral valve stenosis.

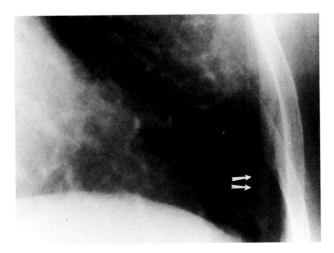

Figure 11-7. Interstitial fibrosis with Kerley's B lines (arrows).

lar component, the breath sounds would probably be normal; though if you were particularly skilled, you might detect that the tidal volume and vital capacity were decreased (because of a stiff lung) and that the respiratory rate was increased. You might hear a cardiac gallop.

Were you not to obtain a chest radiograph, how might you know that the patient had interstitial edema?

Pulmonary spirometry would give an abnormal result, and blood arterial oxygen level would be decreased because the edema would result in a mild diffusion impairment. Carbon dioxide level would be normal or decreased.

How would you treat this interstitial edema? Despite the limited findings on physical examination, it is important to treat this patient as having heart failure. If interstitial heart failure is not treated, alveolar pulmonary edema often will develop, increasing the chance of death.

The Etiology of Kerley's Lines in Interstitial Edema. The lymphatic lines (Kerley's A, B, and C lines) and the thickening of the fissures are both important signs of this patient's heart failure. Why do they occur? It has to do with the anatomy of the lung lymphatics. The lung is supplied with two lymphatic draining systems. The lymphatics in the inner two-thirds of the lung follow the septa and bronchial walls toward the hilum (resulting in the ringlike bronchial shadows in Fig. 11-1*a*). The lymphatics in the outer one-third of the lung follow the interlobular septa out toward the visceral pleura. Just beneath the visceral pleura, the lymphatics interconnect and then run in many channels along the fissures to the hili.

Thick Fissures. Thickening of the fissures is an important early sign of minimal interstitial edema (Fig. 11-10). It is often the only sign in the clinically confusing case of a patient who develops cardiac dyspnea, is brought to the hospital, but feels fine by the time she or he is seen by the

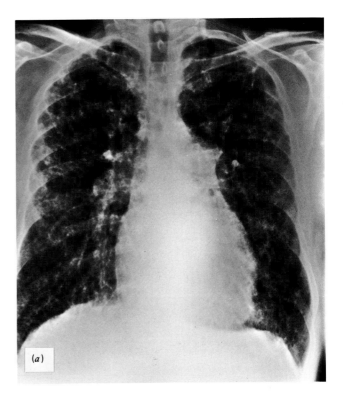

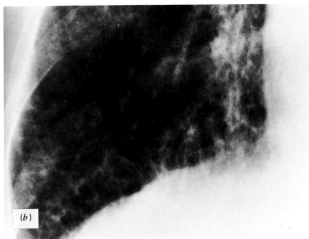

Figure 11-8. Honeycomb appearance of the lung in a patient with coal miner's pneumoconiosis (anthrosilicosis).

physician. This finding is most helpful and is one especially to watch for.

Does a thickened fissure mean that there is pleural fluid trapped in the fissure, between two layers of visceral pleura? Sometimes there is pleural fluid present in the patient with heart failure, in which case, the fissural thickening may be due to pleural effusion. More often, only minimal or no pleural fluid is present and the thickening of the fissure is due to distention of the subpleural lymphatics.

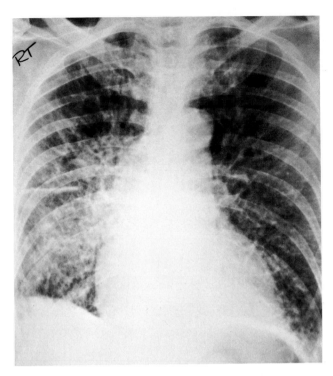

Figure 11-9. Case 11-1 (see text).

Why Should Heart Failure Result in Interstitial Edema?

The explanation is incorporated in Starling's law of fluid transport. Because many of the abnormalities seen on radiographs result from abnormal collections of fluids, a review of Starling's law is appropriate. What is this law? Starling's law states that if you have a membrane separating two regions of fluid, there are certain things that will push the fluid across the membrane and other things that will hold the fluid, limiting its passage. Hydrostatic pressure pushes fluid across a semipermeable membrane into a region of lower hydrostatic pressure. Colloid osmotic pressure tends to hold fluid on the same side of the membrane and to pull fluid to the site of higher colloid osmotic pressure. Certain processes can change the permeability of the membrane, permitting smaller or larger amounts of fluid (and colloid) to cross.

In a normal pulmonary capillary, the colloid pressure is fixed. Arterial pressure is sufficiently high on the arteriolar side of the capillary to push fluid into the interstitium. On the venule side, the hydrostatic pressure is lower, and much (but not all) of the fluid pushed out on the arteriolar side can be resorbed. The small portion that is left is transported by the pulmonary lymphatic vessels.

The patient with congestive heart failure has an elevated pulmonary venule pressure. This decreases the resorption of the interstitial fluid on the venule side of the capillary and increases the fluid load in the lymphatic channels. The increased fluid in the lymphatic channels and the perilymphatic fluid can be recognized as Kerley's lines.

Why Does Alveolar Edema Occur?

The alveolar wall is also a semipermeable membrane. As less and less fluid is resorbed on the venule side of the capillary, more and more is carried by the lymphatic channels. As these channels become overloaded, the pressure in the interstitium increases until it is sufficient to drive fluid across the alveolar-wall membrane, resulting in alveolar edema.

Case 11-2: The Batwing Pattern of Alveolar Pulmonary Edema

The patient whose radiograph is in Figure 11-11 is a 47-year-old woman with chronic renal failure. The pattern of perihilar alveolar infiltrate is described as a batwing or butterfly pattern of edema. How does it occur? Here are two clues:

1. The anatomy of the lymphatic system is important.
2. The force that drives fluid through lymphatic channels is important.

There are two pathways for interstitial fluid to return to the hili and circulation. The inner two-thirds of the lung has channels that run directly toward the hili; the outer one-third has lymphatic channels that run peripherally toward the pleural margins and then extend toward the hili.

Respiratory motion is the main driving force for movement of pulmonary lymph. Lymph channels have no muscle in their walls, but they do have valves. Motion increases the pressure sporatically in different portions of lymphatic channels, pushing the fluid past the valves, and thus clearing the lymph. Most of the motion of the lung takes place in the outer one-third of each lobe. These regions are less stiff (fewer bronchi and vessels) and expand more because there are more alveoli per unit volume. Thus lymph clears faster from the outer one-third of the lung.

Tachypnea will increase this lymphatic clearing, and most patients who develop the batwing pattern are tachypneic because of acidosis (in this case a metabolic acidosis from the renal failure).

Nodular Pattern

When the interstitial septa are diffusely infiltrated or thickened, lines are visible on the radiograph. When the thickening is nonuniform, it may be possible to recognize nodules on the radiograph (Fig. 11-12). The presence of small nodules is one of the interstitial patterns. Interstitial nodular patterns can be seen in:

Tuberculosis
Metastases (hematogeneous)
Sarcoid
Pneumoconiosis

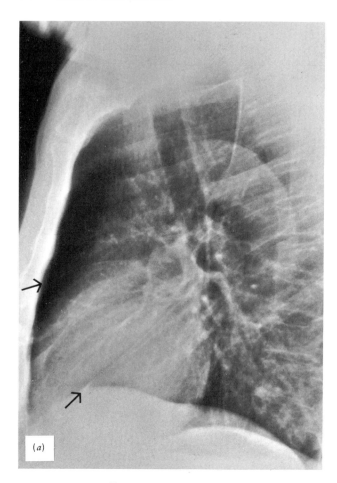

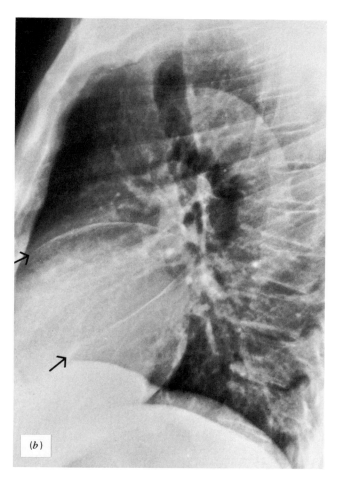

Figure 11-10. Thickening of the fissures from increased lymphatic flow. (*a*) Normal baseline appearance of the fissues (arrows) in a 61-year-old man. (*b*) Thickened fissures (arrows) are present when this man came to the emergency room with paroxysmal nocturnal dyspnea.

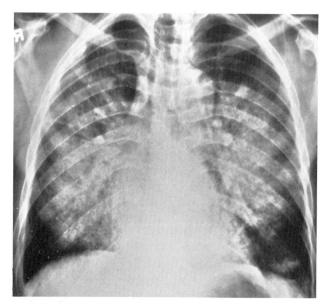

Figure 11-11. Batwing pattern of pulmonary edema in a uremic patient with heart failure.

Keynotes

- *The bronchial patterns are due to thickened bronchial walls. The bronchi may have their normal shape, or they may be dilated. Occasionally, large rounded sacules arise from bronchi.*

- *The right wall of the trachea should be outlined by air. Inability to see the outer wall may indicate the presence of a right paratracheal mass.*

- *Kerley's A lines are near the apices.*
  Kerley's B lines are at the lung bases.
  Kerley's C lines are central.

- *Untreated, interstitial edema often leads to alveolar edema.*

- *Thickening of the fissures may be the only remaining sign in the patient with paroxysmal nocturnal dyspnea who feels fine by the time he or she gets to the hospital.*

- *Minimal thickening of the fissures is often due to the distension of the subpleural lymphatic channels.*

- *Increased fluid in the lungs, pleural space, and peritoneal cavity can often be explained by using Starling's law of fluid transport.*

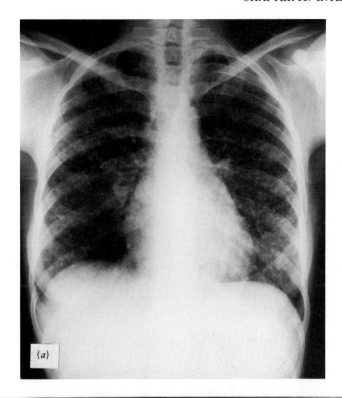

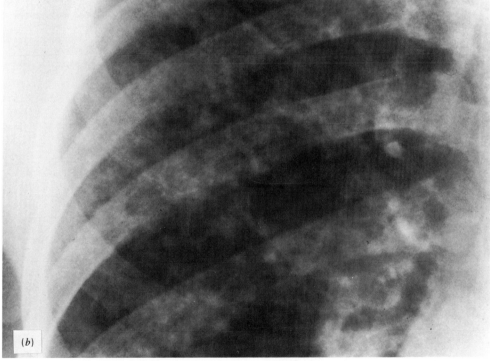

Figure 11-12. Interstitial nodular pattern in a patient with sarcoid.

Case 11-3

W.S., whose radiograph is in Figure 11-13, is a 72-year-old woman who has been losing weight for 3 weeks. What do you see?

There are many lung nodules, each quite small. Many calcified nodules are also present in the hilar lymph nodes. On the lateral view, the patient is strangely slanted because someone is helping her stay up by holding her arms.

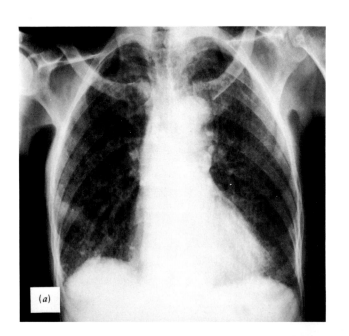

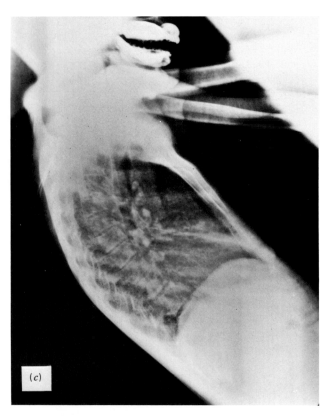

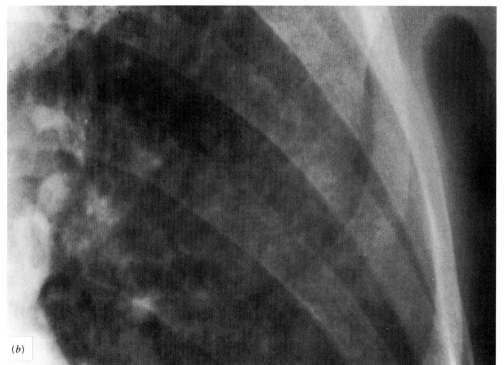

Figure 11-13. Radiographs of the chest of a 72-year-old woman with 3 weeks of weight loss.

What do you think is going on?

Nodular infiltrates can include blood-borne metastases, pneumoconiosis, granulomatous disease, and collagen vascular disease. This patient has miliary tuberculosis. She died 4 days after this study. Miliary tuberculosis has a high mortality rate because the disease is often not considered until the patient is moribund. It can have many different symptoms.

What sort of symptoms does the usual patient with miliary tuberculosis have?

There are two main forms: acute severe and subacute indolent. The acute severe form is more likely to occur in children than adults. Its victims are very sick with a high fever and often show no localizing symptoms. Death usually occurs in several days if not diagnosed.

The indolent form is more insidious in onset. The patient often has a low-grade fever but may not be aware of it. Weight loss is common. Any organ system may be involved, with localizing symptoms as follows:

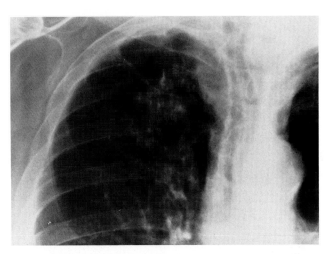

Figure 11-14. Right apical nodular pattern with some calcium deposits, a result of reactivation (or secondary) tuberculosis of unknown activity.

> Liver: hepatocellular jaundice, hypoalbuminemia
>
> Bone marrow: anemia
>
> Pleura: effusion
>
> Lung: diffusion block, hypoxemia
>
> Peritoneum: ascites
>
> Gut: diarrhea
>
> Uterus: amenorrhea
>
> Kidney: hematuria, renal failure
>
> Muscle: weakness, abnormal enzyme levels
>
> Brain: encephalitis, focal abscesses, meningitis (often with cranial nerve palsies and obstructive hydrocephalus)
>
> Heart: conduction defects
>
> Pericardium: effusion (with late fibrosis and calcification)

Essentially, any symptoms associated with fever may be caused by miliary tuberculosis.

How, then, do you make a diagnosis of miliary tuberculosis?

The best method is to order a liver biopsy. One biopsy has a yield of 50%. Multiple biopsies pick up 75%. Results of a bone marrow biopsy are abnormal in about 25% of patients.

The chest radiograph is usually normal in miliary tuberculosis until the disease is quite far advanced and the patient is moribund. Only rarely will the chest radiograph be any more than suggestive of miliary nodules.

How long does it usually take to make a diagnosis of miliary tuberculosis?

Three to six weeks from onset of illness to diagnosis is not uncommon. It is a difficult diagnosis to make and to be sure of.

Keynotes

- *Miliary tuberculosis has a high mortality rate because it is so difficult to diagnose and because its clinical symptoms are so varied.*
- *The liver biopsy (repeated if normal) is the best method for diagnosing miliary tuberculosis.*
- *The chest radiograph is usually normal until late in the course of miliary tuberculosis.*

Patterns of Pulmonary Tuberculosis

Pulmonary tuberculosis occurs in several different forms. *Primary tuberculosis* has an appearance often indistinguishable from other bacterial pneumonias, though hilar adenopathy is more common in primary tuberculosis than in infections caused by other bacteria. Uncommonly, primary tuberculosis presents with a massive unilateral effusion. This form usually occurs in previously healthy young adults who have a sudden onset of high fever and dyspnea.

Secondary or *reactivation tuberculosis* usually occurs in the apical or posterior segment of an upper lobe or in the superior segment of a lower lobe. A coarse, irregular nodular pattern is most common (Fig. 11-14), but any infiltrate in these segments could be due to secondary tuberculosis.

Secondary tuberculosis can also result in cavitation (Fig. 11-15a), and those patients with cavitary tuberculosis can develop a spreading form of tuberculosis that spreads through the bronchial tree into one or both lower lobes (Fig. 11-15b). The CT appearance of tuberculous cavities is shown in Figure 11-15c.

It can be quite difficult to tell by radiography whether the tuberculous infection is active. A progressive increase in the amount of infiltrate on serial films indicates activity. Cavities often indicate that the process is active, but with modern chemotherapy cavities can be made inactive.

When tuberculosis heals, it often calcifies. Calcium in

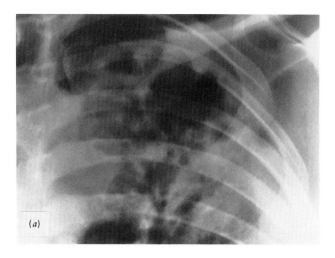

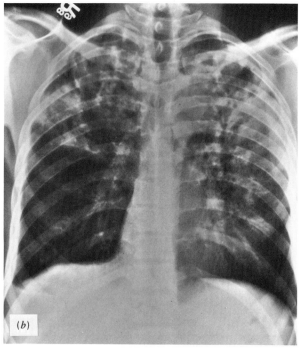

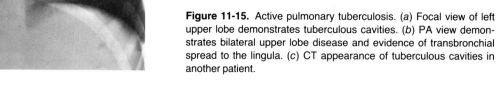

Figure 11-15. Active pulmonary tuberculosis. (a) Focal view of left upper lobe demonstrates tuberculous cavities. (b) PA view demonstrates bilateral upper lobe disease and evidence of transbronchial spread to the lingula. (c) CT appearance of tuberculous cavities in another patient.

a lesion does not mean, however, that the tuberculosis is inactive. While the calcified lesion is inactive, other foci of active infection can be present, but they may be so small that they cannot be seen on the radiograph. If the patient has symptoms, culture of sputum or gastric washings is the only way to be certain of the status of activity of tuberculosis.

NONSPECIFIC FINDINGS

Pseudonodules

Nodules must be distinguised from pseudonodules to differentiate accurately interstitial from alveolar processes. True nodules are moderately well defined and distinct foci of in-

creased radiodensity. Pseudonodules fall into two categories: confluent punctate radiodensities and acinar nodules.

Confluent punctate radiodensities are similar to those shown in Figure 11-16. These radiodensities are not distinct each from the other, and this kind of confluent radiodensity can occur in both interstitial and alveolar disease and cannot be used to distinguish one type from the other.

Acinar nodules are ill defined radiodensities approximately 1 cm in diameter resulting from alveolar filling of acini (Fig. 10-9). They are alveolar in nature and occur in the processes listed in the alveolar disease table, Table 10-1.

Increased Lung Markings

Increased lung markings are a nonspecific finding on chest radiographs. Sometimes they are caused by interstitial in-

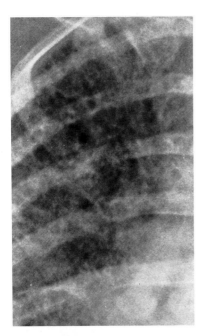

Figure 11-16. Confluent punctate radiodensities in a patient with *Pneumocystis carinii* pneumonia.

filtrates or fibrosis; the markings, however, can appear increased when the vessels are crowded together by lung hypoinflation or by an elevated hemidiaphragm. In women, mainly older women, fibrotic strands in the breast can be superimposed on the bases of the lungs simulating increased lung markings.

Mixed Alveolar and Interstitial Processes

Based on what you already know about alveolar and interstitial pulmonary processes, under what circumstances might you see both together? Make a list.

Mixed alveolar and interstitial patterns can be seen when the same disease can appear with either pattern. Which diseases appear in Table 10-1 and in either Table 11-1 or 11-2? Pulmonary edema can be interstitial *or* alveolar; so it can be both at the same time. Mycoplasmal pneumonia is in both Tables 10-1 and 11-2.

Many of the conditions in the interstitial lists are chronic. It is possible to have an acute process superimposed on a chronic process: pneumococcal pneumonia superimposed on sarcoid, for example. Sometimes viral (interstitial) pneumonia becomes secondarily infected with bacteria, resulting in a mixed pattern of infiltrate.

Many alveolar processes clear partially through the bronchial tree and partially via the lymphatic system. It is possible to see Kerley's lines developing in a region of bacterial pneumonia as the process is clearing.

TABLE 11-1. PROCESSES RESULTING IN BRONCHIAL-WALL THICKENING

Cystic fibrosis
Bronchiectasis
Asthma
Chronic Bronchitis
Increased lymphatic flow (congestive heart failure)
Tumor in lymphatic system

There are lymphatics in the walls of bronchi.

TABLE 11-2. PROCESSES RESULTING IN THE LINEAR PATTERN OF INTERSTITIAL INFILTRATES

Interstitial edema
Interstitial fibrosis
Sarcoid
Viral pneumonia
Mycoplasmal pneumonia
Lymphangitic spread of tumor
Lymphatic obstruction
Pneumonconiosis
Connective tissue diseases
Scleroderma
Rheumatoid arthritis

Keynote

- *Mixed processes can occur in three settings:*
  Different manifestations of the same disease
  Two different diseases superimposed
  During resolution of an acute alveolar process

IMAGING THE LUNG

When you see a region of increased density on a chest radiograph, it is first necessary to show that it is in the lung. Once shown to be in the lung, it should be classified as alveolar, interstitial, or mixed pattern. The pattern should then permit you to give a limited list of differential diagnoses that can be restricted further by clinical information. Pulmonary processes are common, and their recognition and differentiation constitute a major portion of chest radiology.

SUMMARY

Diseases that thicken the interstitial support structures of the lung can show four patterns: bronchial, linear, nodular, and honeycombing. While there is a great deal of overlapping, the different patterns can help limit the potential differential diagnoses. The bronchial pattern is most often caused by asthma and cystic fibrosis; the linear pattern is most often seen in granulomatous diseases (sarcoid, tuberculosis), interstitial edema from heart failure, viral and mycoplasmal pneumonia, and lymphangitic distension due to metastatic tumor; the nodular pattern is most often seen in sarcoidosis and metastatic disease; honeycombing is not commonly seen.

Mixed interstitial and alveolar processes are seen when the two appearances are different manifestations of the same disease; when two different diseases are superimposed; and during resolution of an acute alveolar process.

REVIEW QUESTIONS

1. Ring and parallel line shadows represent which of the interstitial lung patterns? What do these shapes represent? What common diseases result in ring and parallel line shadows?

2. What are Kerley's A, B, and C lines? What do they represent anatomically? What are the common diseases resulting in Kerley's lines?

3. The nodular pattern occurs in what common disease?

4. Explain Starling's law of fluid transport.

5. What might happen if you fail to treat a patient with interstitial pulmonary edema?

6. What is the method of choice for diagnosing miliary tuberculosis?

7. Why is the chest radiograph a poor method of diagnosing miliary tuberculosis?

VOCABULARY

bronchiectasis	miliary tuberculosis
connective tissue diseases	pneumoconiosis
cystic fibrosis	primary tuberculosis
honeycombing	sarcoid
Kerley's lines	secondary tuberculosis

SUGGESTIONS FOR FURTHER READING

David S. Feigin. New perspectives on interstitial lung disease. *Radiologic Clinics of North America,* **21**(4): 682–697, 1983.

Michael S. Niederman, Richard A. Matthay. New techniques for the assessment of interstitial lung disease. *Radiologic Clinics of North America,* **21**(4): 667–681, 1983.

I.H. Kerr. Interstitial lung disease: The role of the radiologist. *Clinical Radiology,* **35**:1–7, 1984.

Colleen J. Bergin, Nestor L. Muller. CT in the diagnosis of interstitial lung disease. *American Journal of Roentgenology,* **145**:505–510, 1985.

For additional suggested reading see Chapter 7.

12

ATELECTASIS: DECREASED LUNG VOLUME

KEY CONCEPTS

Radiological

A decrease in lung volume (atelectasis) is a common pattern of lung disease. The decrease in volume can be focal or generalized. Often the radiodensity of the atelectic lung is increased, and it is the shape of the increased lung radiodensity that indicates that the radiodensity is due to atelectasis. When the radiodensity of the atelectic lung is not increased, the identification of a shift in the fissures or of the hili is used to indicate that atelectasis is present. Other signs of atelectasis are listed in the chapter text.

As a lung becomes atelectic, the fissures shift, rotating around the hilar structures; thus a fissure normally seen on the lateral view may be best seen on an oblique or frontal view when the lung is atelectic.

As the fissures shift, they usually remain relatively straight. An outward bulge of a fissure near the hilum, when associated with atelectasis, may indicate the presence of a hilar mass.

Clinical

A decrease in lung volume can be caused by airway obstruction, direct compression of the lung, a lack of surfactant, lung fibrosis, a failure of lung expansion at birth, or a failure of normal lung growth. Bronchial obstruction does not always result in atelectasis because air can pass through the pores of Kohn into the alveoli of an obstructed portion of lung.

OBJECTIVES

When you complete this chapter you will be able to

1. List the radiological signs of atelectasis.
2. Describe the pattern of the shift of the fissures with lobar atelectasis.

3. Identify atelectasis on selected chest radiographs.
4. Identify Golden's reverse S sign and discuss its significance.
5. List the six causes of atelectasis.
6. Differentiate the radiological patterns and clinical causes of a paralyzed hemidiaphragm and a fixed hemidiaphragm.

Focal loss of lung volume is one of the basic patterns of lung pathology. It indicates disease and often points to the type of disease present. Although the term *atelectasis* applies strictly to a lung that has never been completely aerated, it is commonly used to describe focal loss of lung volume acquired during life.

What types of processes can you think of that could cause a focal region of lung to be of decreased volume? There are six general classes:

1. Airway obstruction
2. Lung compression
3. Surfactant absence or loss
4. Lung fibrosis
5. Failure of lung expansion
6. Failure of normal growth

CLASSES OF ATELECTASIS

Airway Obstruction

Bronchial obstruction is the etiology most often mentioned for atelectasis. A tumor filling a bronchus or an aspirated piece of food is a common cause of bronchial obstruction.

Most of the time, however, bronchial obstruction does not cause the lung to lose volume. Why should this be?

There are several reasons. First, consider a mass growing within a bronchus, the bronchus expanding and contracting as the lung inflates and deflates. Initially this mass will have little effect on air exchange; as it gets larger, it will begin to fill the bronchus on expiration, but on inspiration, the bronchus will enlarge and air will rush past the partial obstruction. The first effect of an endobronchial mass is air trapping.

Even when the mass has grown sufficiently to fill the bronchus on both inspiration and expiration, atelectasis frequently still will not occur because of collateral air drift. When a mass obstructs a segmental bronchus, the air can reach the lung ventilated by this bronchus via the *pores of Kohn*. These interalveolar pores permit collateral air to drift into the poorly ventilated lung and prevent atelectasis from occurring. Since collateral air drift is more effective in inspiration than expiration, air trapping will result.

If the mass is in a lobar bronchus, collateral air drift should be blocked by the fissures; however, atelectasis still does not always occur. The reason is that the fissures are often incomplete near the hilum, and these regions of fissure-lack permit collateral drift through the pores of Kohn into the lobe whose bronchus is blocked.

Obstruction of the main right or main left bronchus will result in atelectasis because no collateral air drift occurs between the right and left lungs. Patients with incomplete fissures will occasionally develop atelectasis from bronchial obstruction because fibrosis has blocked the pores of Kohn. Pneumonia with atelectasis may be the first indication of bronchial obstruction because the pneumonic infiltrate has prevented collateral air drift. Less commonly, segmental bronchial obstruction will result in atelectasis for the same reasons.

Since air trapping is the first manifestation of bronchial obstruction, detection of focal air trapping could theoretically be of use in the detection of early lung cancer. In general, this has not become clinically useful because air trapping from chronic bronchitis is quite common in patients who smoke. It has not been possible to differentiate easily those patients with air trapping caused by chronic bronchitis from those with lung cancer.

Case 12-1

This 42-year-old man went to his physician because he had started to cough up blood in his daily phlegm. Figure 12-1 shows his radiographs. What do you see?

There is an area of radiopacity in the upper right lung. This infiltrate extends to a linear margin inferiorly and posteriorly. These margins represent the minor (or horizontal) fissure and the upper portion of the major (or oblique) fissure. As you can see, the horizontal fissure belies its names and is curved in an **S** shape, generally upward. What do you think is going on?

The horizontal fissure is no longer horizontal because the lung above it has lost volume and pulled the fissure

up; the lung in the right upper lobe is atelectic. When fissures are shifted because of atelectasis, they generally retain a near-straight course. In this patient, the fissure is **S** shaped. What might be doing this?

There are several possible explanations: There could be adhesions adjacent to this fissure, preventing it from moving (but none can be seen). There could be infiltrate in the medial portion of the right upper lobe that could not be compressed, but, in general, most infiltrates are peripheral rather than central. Or there could be a mass in the upper portion of the hilum, preventing the fissure from moving in its normal plane. In this case (as in most cases) *Golden's reverse S sign* is the sign of right-upper-lobe atelectasis because of a hilar mass.

Now that you've found the hilar mass and the right-upper-lobe atelectasis, your probable diagnosis is ... cancer. What should you do now?

Return to the film and search for findings that might support or conflict with your diagnosis. In this case, an additional abnormal finding is ...?

The relative elevation of the right hemidiaphragm. What could this be from? Pleural effusion, failure of expansion of the remainder of the lung to fill the space, phrenic nerve paralysis, liver metastases? Each is a possible explanation for this finding.

Pleural effusion would indicate a probable and common site of metastases. The patterns of pleural effusion are discussed in Chapter 15.

Normal lung tissue can usually hyperexpand sufficiently to compensate for the loss of volume from one lobe. With upper-lobe atelectasis, the diaphragm usually remains at or near its normal position. If there is lung disease preventing hyperexpansion (e.g., interstitial lung fibrosis), the hemidiaphragm may be elevated.

The phrenic nerve could be paralyzed. The tumor could have spread to the mediastinum, damaging the phrenic nerve. What would you do to confirm this?

History may suggest more respiratory impairment than the loss of a single lobe would induce. What might you find on physical examination?

Each hemidiaphragm would move appropriately. The paralyzed hemidiaphragm would move in response to the relaxation and contraction of the abdominal-wall musculature.

If that's the case, why did you learn to percuss out the level of the hemidiaphragm in your physical examination course?

To detect a fixed hemidiaphragm. A fixed hemidiaphragm and a paralyzed hemidiaphragm are two different conditions. Paralysis comes about from nerve damage. Fixation results from ...?

Hyperexpansion (emphysema), fibrothorax, splinting caused by irritation from a subphrenic abscess or pleural inflammation.

The only accurate way to detect phrenic nerve paralysis is to study each hemidiaphragm's motion with the fluoroscope. With nerve paralysis, the hemidiaphragms will move synchronously with quiet respiration; but with sniffing or hiccupping (which are specific phrenic

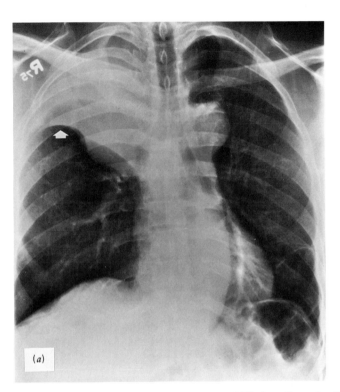
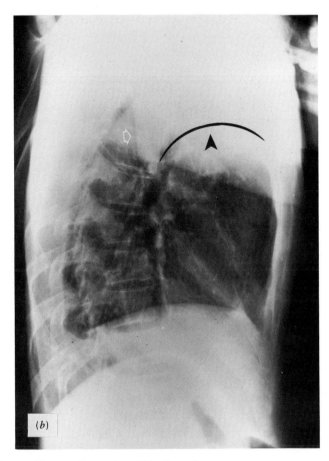

Figure 12-1 PA (*a*) and lateral (*b*) chest films of a 42-year-old man with cough and bloody sputum. Minor fissure at solid arrowhead; major fissure at open arrowhead. On the lateral view, note that the spine is to the left. The lateral view of the chest may be viewed with the spine placed to the right or the left at the preference of the radiologist.

nerve functions), the paralyzed hemidiaphragm will, paradoxically, move upward while the normal hemidiaphragm moves down. Inspiratory and expiratory films will show normal bilateral motion and are not sufficient to exclude this diagnosis.

Could liver metastases cause the hemidiaphragm elevation? Yes, massive liver metastases can cause hemidiaphragm elevation; small metastases will not. If this is the cause, the liver should be palpably large and possibly irregular in margin.

Lung Compression

Lung can lose volume because it is compressed. Focal hyperexpansion of one portion of lung will compress adjacent lung. A pneumothorax or pleural effusion will compress the adjacent lung. A hemidiaphragm elevated by phrenic nerve or abdominal disease will compress the lung. In general, the compressing structure is easily seen and identified.

Surfactant Lack

Surfactant normally functions by changing the surface tension of the alveoli to keep them expanded. Diseases that interfere with the production or function of surfactant permit the alveoli to collapse and permit the lung to become atelectatic. Surfactant lack is a prime cause of the generalized decreased lung volume seen in hyaline membrane disease of the newborn. It is part of the cause of the atelectasis seen in oxygen toxicity, fat emboli syndrome, pulmonary artery embolus, and pneumonia.

Case 12-2

This 23-year-old woman had had an intermittent hacking cough and a cold for a week when she came to our clinic (Fig. 12-2). Five years previously she had been stabbed in the anterior chest. What do you see?

There are metal sutures in the sternum from her transsternum thoracotomy. The right heart border is indistinct. On lateral view, there is a radiodense band crossing the lower heart anteriorly. What do you think is going on?

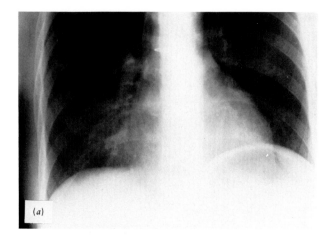

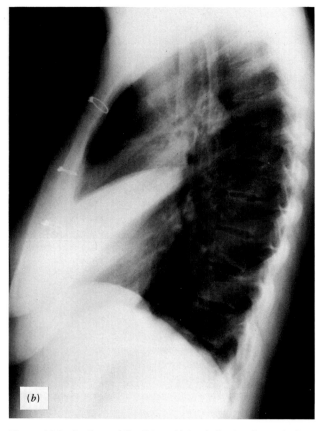

Figure 12-2. Portions of the PA and lateral chest radiographs in a 23-year-old woman with 1 week of cough. There are sutures in the sternum from previous chest surgery required for a stab wound.

The patient has right-middle-lobe atelectasis. What is the etiology?

Probably mycoplasmal or viral pneumonia based on the cough and minimal systemic symptoms. It is also possible that the right-middle-lobe infiltrate resulted from either the stab wound or subsequent surgery. What would you do?

A blood count showed a leukocyte count of 11,500. A

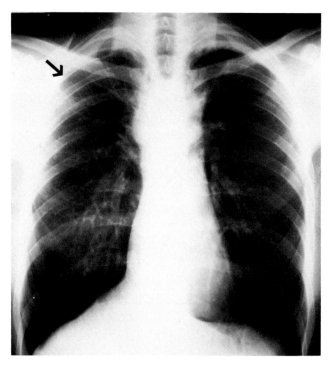

Figure 12-3. Bilateral upper-lobe fibrosis and atelectasis caused by radiation therapy for Hodgkin's disease. The hili are elevated. Mediastinal widening and apical pleural thickening are due to fibrosis caused by the radiation. The minor fissure (arrow) is elevated.

test for cold agglutinins was done (though not necessary) and was positive with a titer of 1:128.

The patient was treated for probable mycoplasmal pneumonia, with erythromycin, and showed clinical improvement in 2 days. The right-middle-lobe atelectasis cleared in 10 days.

Right-middle-lobe infiltrates frequently cause the loss of the silhouette of the right heart border. Mycoplasmal pneumonia is a common cause of a persistent cough associated with other symptoms of a mild upper respiratory infection. Pneumonia can cause atelectasis by interfering with surfactant and by causing airway obstruction.

Lung Fibrosis

Fibrosis causing localized atelectasis is usually due to tuberculosis or irradiation of the lung (Fig. 12-3).

Failure of Lung Expansion: Primary Atelectasis

Primary atelectasis is uncommon and can be seen in infants, where it is caused by bronchial atresia or marked compression of the lung by an adjacent hyperexpanded lobe or an enlarged heart.

Failure of Normal Growth

Severe inflammatory disease of the lung occurring in childhood may prevent normal lung growth. Bronchiolitis obli-

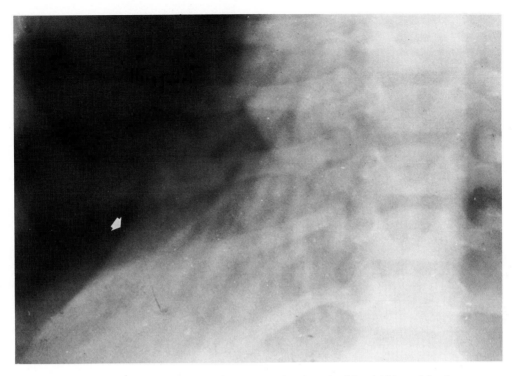

Figure 12-4. This 2-year-old child with bronchiectasis and atelectasis of the right lower lobe demonstrates crowding of the air bronchograms. The visualized bronchi are closer together than normal, indicating the presence of atelectasis. The major fissue (arrow) has been displaced by the atelectasis and can be seen on this frontal view of the chest, another indication of atelectasis.

terans occurring in childhood results in a slightly small hypovascular lung in the adult. The end result is called the Swyer-James or MacLeod syndrome.

Keynotes

- *The pores of Kohn permit air to pass from one alveolus to another.*
- *Because the fissures are incomplete, obstruction of a lobar bronchus may not prevent collateral air drift.*
- *Golden's reverse S sign is usually a sign of a mass causing atelectasis.*
- *A fixed hemidiaphragm results from hyperexpansion, fibrothorax, or splinting from irritation.*
- *Phrenic nerve paralysis can be detected only by fluoroscopy.*

SIGNS OF ATELECTASIS

There are direct and indirect signs of atelectasis. The direct signs demonstrate both the loss of volume and the portion of lung involved by the atelectasis. The indirect signs are signs of volume loss but point less directly to the portion of the lung involved.

Direct Signs	Indirect Signs
Shift of the lung fissures (Figs. 12-1, 12-2, and 12-3)	Smallness of the hermithorax
Shift of hilum (Figs. 12-1 and 12-3)	Crowding of the ribs (this is simulated by chest rotation)
Crowding of lung vessels	Shift of the mediastinum
Crowding of air bronchograms (Fig. 12-4)	Compensatory hyperinflation of adjacent lung
Increased radiodensity in the shrunken lobe (Figs. 12-1, 12-2, and 12-4)	

In looking at the radiograph it is important to look for both direct and indirect signs. Sometimes at first only a single sign is seen, but it leads to further search and more findings that confirm the diagnosis.

Shift of the Fissures

The locations of the normal fissures are drawn on the radiographs in Figure 12-5. The fissures are anchored at the hilum by their bronchial and vascular attachments and are freely movable along their peripheral margins. As volume loss occurs, the fissures both shift and rotate. In upper- or lower-lobe atelectasis, the major fissure, which is usually best seen on the lateral view, will rotate. With moderate volume loss, the major fissure will be best seen on the oblique view; with marked loss of volume, it may become visible on the PA view. With middle-lobe atelectasis the major and minor fissures each move toward the

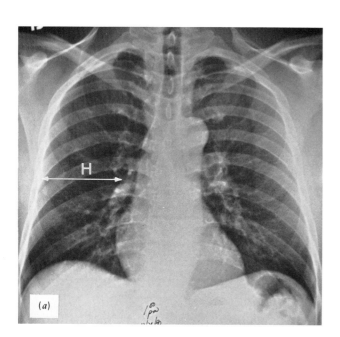

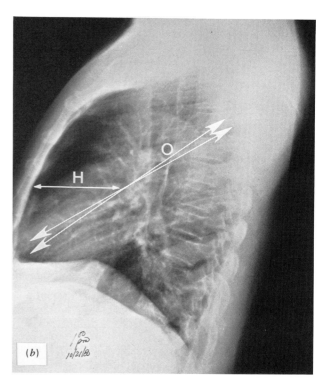

Figure 12-5. Radiograph of a normal chest with the normal locations of the fissures marked. The horizontal, or minor, fissure is labeled "H." The oblique, or major, fissure is labeled "O." The right and left oblique fissures are almost superimposed On the lateral view. (a) PA view. (b) Lateral view.

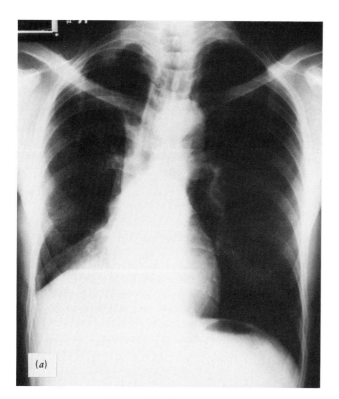

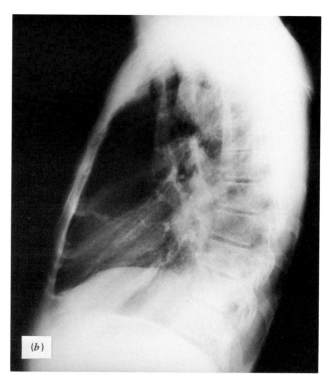

Figure 12-6. These PA and lateral views were obtained on a 53-year-old man with hemoptysis.

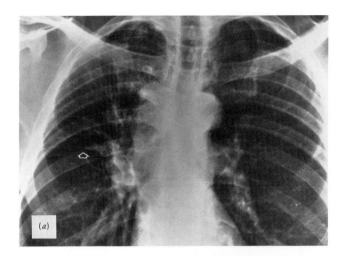
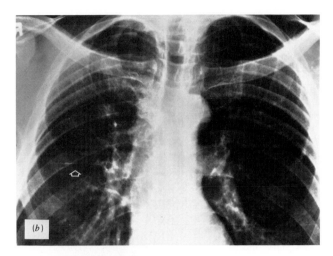
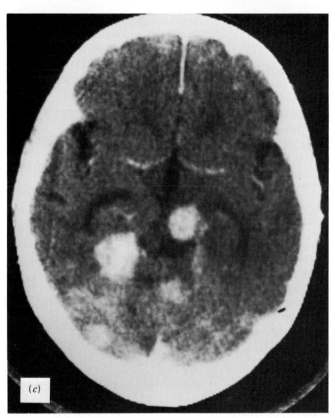

Figure 12-7. (a) PA film obtained when a 62-year-old man was admitted for dizzyness. An arrow indicates the location of the horizontal fissure. (b) Follow-up film obtained after 1 month of therapy. (c) CT scan of the brain, obtained several days after admission, demonstrates several round, white areas, each of which represents a metastasis to the brain.

other, creating a wedge of density. The normal minor fissure can be seen on the PA view, but once shifted, it may be only visible on the lateral view (Fig. 12-2a and b).

When atelectasis is suspected, people often look for the shifted fissure on the same view they would use to find the normal fissure and, not seeing a shifted fissure, assume that no atelectasis is present. If you suspect atelectasis,

always look for the shifted fissue on the PA and lateral views. If you cannot find the fissure, it may be necessary to obtain oblique views to find it.

Case 12-3

Figure 12-6a and b are the PA and lateral views of a 53-year-old man with hemoptysis. What do you see?

There is a small right hemithorax. Adjoining the right heart border is an interface between the opacified right lower lobe and the air-containing right middle lobe. The major fissure has rotated 90°.

With lesser degrees of atelectasis, oblique views may be the best views to demonstrate the fissural shift. This patient had squamous cell cancer obstructing the bronchus.

Increased Radiodensity in the Shape of the Collapsed Lung

Increased radiodensity in the shape of the collapsed lung is usually easily identified on a radiograph. Because of this it is frequently the first radiographic sign of atelectasis. Because it is commonly present, atelectasis unassociated with increased radiodensity is often overlooked. Even in the absence of increased radiodensity, the signs of atelectasis should be looked for.

Case 12-4

Figure 12-7*a* and *b* illustrate the right upper lung of a 62-year-old man who complained of dizzyness. Figure 12-7*a* is a film made at the time of admission; Figure 12-7*b* is a film made after 1 month of therapy. What do you see?

In the first film, the minor fissure is elevated and the right tracheal wall is slightly thickened. Results of a biopsy disclosed oat cell carcinoma. A cerebral CAT scan showed cerebral brain metastases (Fig. 12-7*c*). Chemotherapy resulted in a decrease in the right-upper-lobe atelectasis but with only minimal improvement of the brain symptoms.

It is easy to miss the subtle signs of atelectasis when it is unassociated with increased radiodensity. Fortunately most acute atelectasis results in increased radiodensity, so that almost all patients with bronchial obstruction, pneumonia, or compressive atelectasis will have increased radiodensity. Fibrotic lung may show no increased radiodensity, but usually no specific therapy is required in those cases.

Keynote

• *The fissures both shift and rotate as atelectasis occurs.*

SUMMARY

The focal loss of lung volume indicates the presence of lung or bronchial disease. Atelectasis can be due to airway obstruction, lung compression, lung fibrosis, surfactant disturbances, primary failure of lung expansion, and failure of normal growth. Most acute processes causing atelectasis result in increased radiodensity in the affected lung. Other signs of atelectasis include shifts of the fissures, hili, and mediastinum, the crowding of lung vessels or air bronchograms, and evidence of decreased size of the hemithorax.

REVIEW QUESTIONS

1. Name the processes that can result in focal loss of lung volume.
2. Why does bronchial obstruction not always result in atelectasis?
3. When there is an outward bulge in the margin of the atelectatic lobe, what does it mean?
4. What diseases cause phrenic nerve paralysis? How would you diagnose it?
5. What are the causes of a fixed hemidiaphragm?
6. What does surfactant do?
7. List the direct and then the indirect signs of atelectasis.

VOCABULARY

Golden's reverse S sign   pores of Kohn
surfactant

SUGGESTIONS FOR FURTHER READING

David Nadich et al. CT of lobar collapse. *Seminars in Roentgenology,* **19**(3): 222–235, 1984.

Benjamin Felson, Ed. Lobar collapse. *Seminars in Roentgenology,* **15**(2), 1980.

For additional suggested reading see Chapter 7.

13

RESPIRATORY DISEASE IN THE CHILD

PHILLIP J. HANEY

KEY CONCEPTS

Radiological

Full inspiratory, nonrotated chest radiographs are essential for the proper interpretation of the infant's and the young child's radiographs. The effects of rotation and lung hypoinflation can both be easily confused with the effects of disease and can mask the presence of disease.

Radiographs of the neck, obtained in full inspiration, are used to evaluate for epiglottitis and croup.

Clinical

The diseases seen in infants and young children differ from those seen in older children and adults. Some are seen only in the newborn, others are much more common in the child, and some that can occur in both the child and adult have different radiographic patterns in the child.

The *transient respiratory distress syndrome* of the newborn results from a delay in the clearance of fetal lung fluid. Small pleural effusions can be seen, the fissures are thickened, and increased vascular markings are present. In the usual case, the condition rapidly improves, and the radiograph becomes normal within 24–48 hours.

Hyaline membrane disease (also called "respiratory distress syndrome of the newborn") results from a deficiency of surfactant. The radiographs in this condition demonstrate alveolar collapse with decreased lung volume and a fine granular appearance to the lungs. Air bronchograms are commonly seen.

Pneumothoraces and pneumomediastinum are occasional causes of respiratory distress in the newborn.

In the young child, lower respiratory tract infection demonstrates a pattern of air trapping with increased lung volume associated with focal areas of linear lung atelectasis. The adult pat-

terns of alveolar infiltrates are relatively uncommon in infants and young children.

The child may exhibit respiratory distress after the aspiration of a foreign body. Radiographs and fluoroscopy are useful in identifying secondary findings that imply the presence of a foreign body; the foreign body itself is usually not identified.

Radiographs in the asthmatic patient usually demonstrate lung hyperinflation, sometimes with focal areas of atelectasis. Rapid deterioration in an asthmatic's clinical condition may be due to the development of a pneumothorax or pneumomediastinum.

Epiglottitis is an acute, severe, potentially fatal illness, often producing severe upper airway obstruction. The lateral neck radiograph is the preferred initial method for diagnosing acute epiglottitis. Very early in the course of the disease, the radiograph may be normal, but most of the time it is abnormal.

Symptoms and signs of airway obstruction can also be caused by croup. Radiographs of the neck will demonstrate subglottic narrowing of the upper trachea.

OBJECTIVES

When you complete this chapter you will be able to

1. Select which infant radiographs are taken in full inspiration and are not rotated and thus are suitable for interpretation.
2. Correctly identify radiographs demonstrating transient tachypnea of the newborn, hyaline membrane disease, lower respiratory infection in the young child, asthma, epigottitis, and croup.
3. Describe the common clinical symptoms and signs of each disease listed in Objective 2.

Interpretation of pediatric chest films differs in several important ways from the ideas and techniques involved in reading adult chest films. First, the spectrum of diseases is quite different from that expected in the adult population. The younger the child is, the greater will be the probability of encountering an abnormality exclusive to the pediatric population. Thus it is important to know the patient's age, even down to the number of days in the neonate. Second, the anatomic and physiological changes occurring with growth and development must also be taken into consideration when reading a child's film. The roentgen manifestations of a particular pathological process may not be the same in a child as in the adult. Finally, the techniques used in imaging infants result in unusual findings and may create confusion. It is important, for example, to remember that the films are generally exposed with the patient supine. These concepts are illustrated here by examples of the more common diseases seen on the pediatric chest film, beginning with the patient in the first few hours of life and examining the changing patterns of the next weeks, months, and years.

THE NORMAL NEWBORN'S CHEST RADIOGRAPHY

Figure 13-1 is a normal chest film for a newborn at 1 hour of age.

The Lungs

The alveoli fill with air very rapidly during the first few breaths immediately after birth. The infant generates high negative pleural pressures during this short period of transition to extrauterine life and thereby establishes a functional residual volume. Thus the lungs will appear completely aerated on radiographs several minutes after birth. Notice that the shape of the thorax is different from that of an adult: it tends to be more spherical with a relatively larger AP diameter. This results in a more radiolucent appearance of the lungs. The central hilar bronchovascular structures are much less conspicuous than those of the older child, and the peripheral pulmonary vessels are not at all prominent.

The Mediastinum

The tracheal air column is well seen and overlies the pedicles on the right side of the vertebral bodies. This is the normal position of the trachea, and it should not be mistaken for a mediastinal shift. It occupies this position because the aortic arch lies just to the left of the carina. The arch itself cannot be identified because it is camouflaged by other mediastinal structures; the same is true of the main pulmonary artery. The tracheal air column can be followed downward to the bifurcation into the main-stem bronchi; the right and left main-stem bronchi are easily identified, and air bronchograms are often seen in the first one or two generations of bronchi, especially in the area overlying the left heart shadow.

The upper portion of the mediastinum appears relatively wide in this patient for several reasons. It will al-

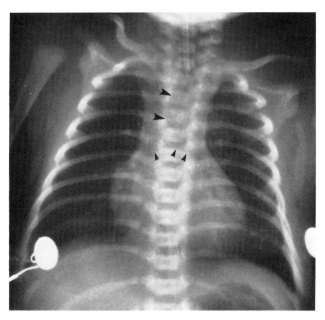

Figure 13-1. A normal neonatal chest. Note the inconspicuous appearance of the pulmonary vascular structures, and the relatively hyperradiolucent appearance of the lung fields. The large arrowheads indicate the right border of the tracheal air column, and the small arrowheads show the inferior surfaces of the right and left main-stem bronchi. An endotracheal tube is positioned in the trachea. The round, dense structures over the lower chest are cardiac monitor leads.

ways look wider when the patient is supine and the x-ray beams travels from anterior to posterior. (This magnification effect also makes the heart look large.) The main cause of the prominent mediastinum, though, is the thymus. This structure lies in the anterior mediastinum and is proportionately larger in the infant's chest than in the older child's. It has thin right and left lobes, which are usually asymmetric in size and shape. Figure 13-2 shows a few of the remarkably diverse appearances of the normal thymus. Whenever there is a question of an unusual mediastinal density or mass in an infant, the thymic shadow is likely to be responsible.

Keynotes

- *The younger the child, the more likely that child's disease will be one seen only in children.*
- *In newborns, an accurate knowledge of the patient's age in days is necessary for correct diagnosis.*
- *The wide mediastinum in the newborn is due to magnification and the presence of the thymus.*

BABY GIRL LAMES

Figure 13-3 shows the chest film of a full-term infant who had a long, difficult delivery and low Apgar scores and was noted to be tachypneic and slightly cyanotic 2 hours after birth. What is the diagnosis?

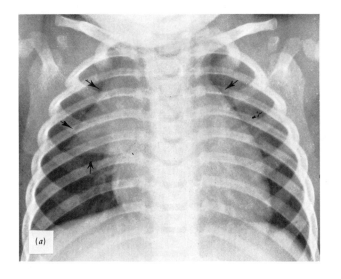

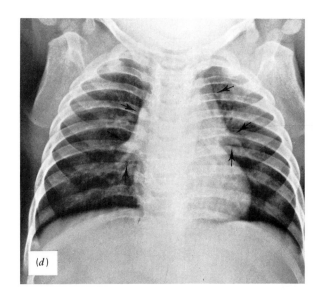

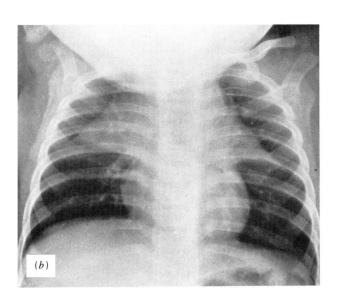

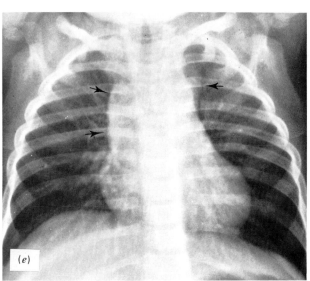

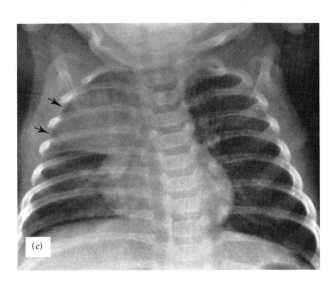

Figure 13-2. A normal thymus. (a) The right lobe of the thymus is indicated by the arrows. Note that it has a triangular configuration, with a fairly flat inferior margin. This appearance has been termed the *sail sign*. It is a typical apparance of the right lobe of the thymus. Note that the left lobe of the thymus, also indicated by arrows, forms a smooth, convex line that makes up the left border of the cardiopericardial silhouette. (b) In this patient there are bilateral sail signs. (c) This patient also has a right thymic sail sign, but in this case the right lobe of the thymus is so large that it extends almost to the right lateral thoracic wall. There is only a thin stripe of air outlining the extreme right lateral border of the thymus (indicated by the arrows). It is important to realize that this is not a pneumonia but a normal appearance of the thymus. (d) This film shows fairly typical appearance of the right and left lobes of the thymus, indicated by arrows. (e) In this film, the right and left lobes of the thymus, indicated by the arrows, also form the interface of the lung with the superior mediastinum. As is often the case in x-rays of infants, the thymus is causing the mediastinum to have a widened appearance.

101

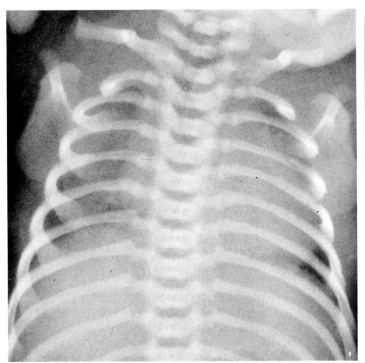

Figure 13-3. Baby Girl Lames's chest radiograph.

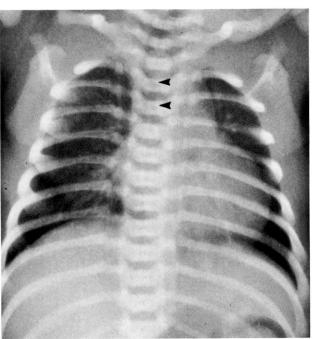

Figure 13-4. Another radiograph of Baby Girl Lames. Note that the lungs are now much better inflated, although this is still not an optimal degree of pulmonary expansion, as you can tell by the fact that the dome of the right hemidiaphragm is only at the level of the right seventh rib posteriorly. The rotation has also been only partially corrected, and it is apparent that the left ribs appear longer than the right ribs. All in all, though, this study represents a marked improvement in technique in comparison to Figure 13-3. The arrowheads show the left border of the tracheal air column.

The heart in this case appears too large, and the lungs look very dense, suggesting heart failure or pneumonia. But, Figure 13-4 shows another film of the same infant taken less than 30 minutes after the first, and this second study is entirely normal. The worrisome findings on the initial film were the result of poor radiographic technique. Rotation and poor inspiration are the chief culprits; every analysis of a pediatric chest film should begin with an assessment of the amount of rotation and adequacy of inspiration.

Note that the ribs on the left (Fig. 13-3) appear elongated compared with those on the right. This is because the baby has rolled over partially onto her left side. The rotation has also caused the heart to overlie the left lung; this appearance simulates cardiomegaly. On a perfectly straight film, the ribs should be symmetrical, appearing just as long on one side as on the other.

The major problem with the film in Figure 13-3, however, is the poor inspiration. Comparison with Figure 13-4 shows that there is simply much less air in the lungs on the first film. This makes the heart look enlarged and causes the lungs to appear very dense. As a rough guide, you can judge the degree of inspiration by looking at the level of the diaphragm. Pulmonary inflation will usually be adequate when the diaphragm is at or below the level of the posterior eighth rib.

Keynote

• *Always check the degree of lung inflation and for rotation before interpreting the radiograph.*

BABY BOY GAYLOR

Baby boy Gaylor is a full-term infant delivered by cesarean section because of cephalopelvic disproportion. He became tachypneic and mildly cyanotic shortly after birth. A frontal chest film obtained at 3 hours of age is shown in Figure 13-5. What radiographic abnormalities are present? What do they represent?

Comparison of this film with Figure 13-4 shows that the lungs are overinflated: both hemithoraces are larger, more expanded, and better aerated than normal. Also, the vascular markings are very prominent and extend farther toward the periphery than do the relatively inconspicuous vascular shadows of the normal chest film. The horizontal line in the right midlung field is the minor fissure, a structure not usually seen on a normal neonatal chest. The presence of fluid in the fissure in this patient accounts for its visualization. There is also fluid in the pleural space; this fluid produces the densities noted at the lateral costophrenic sulci.

It is important to remember that pleural effusion in the supine infant will not produce the same radiographic changes as effusion in the erect adult. In the supine position the fluid layers out posteriorly, between the lung and the back thoracic wall. Some of the fluid may extend ante-

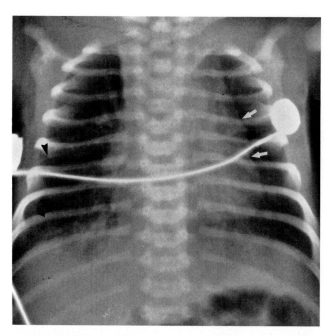

Figure 13-5. Baby boy Gaylor (see text). The large arrowhead indicates the lateral portion of the minor fissure. The small arrowheads show a stripe of increased radiodensity paralleling the right lateral thoracic wall. The white arrows indicate a scalloped appearance of the left cardiopericardiac border. This is produced by the thymus. The scallops are created by indentations of the thymic tissue caused by the anterior costal cartilage.

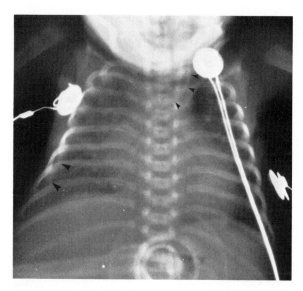

Figure 13-6. This is the film of an infant who had undergone surgery several days previously. The radiograph was obtained because the infant developed tachypnea. Comparisons of the right lung to the left lung indicates that there is an overall increased radiodensity on the right side. As in the previous case, there is also seen a stripe of pleural fluid along the right lateral thoracic wall (large arrowheads). The small arrowheads outline the position of a catheter extending from the left jugular vein to the left brachio cephalic vein. The round concentric structures over the upper abdomen are a gastrostomy tube inserted during surgery. The patient was treated with diuretics, and the radiograph returned to normal the next day. This was a case of pulmonary edema and right pleural effusion caused by fluid overload.

riorly, curving up around the lateral margin of the lung, and produce a dense stripe between the lung and the ribs, as seen in this patient. If there is only a small amount of fluid, however, the thin posterior layer will result only in an overall increased density of the hemithorax. An example of this phenomenon is shown in Figure 13-6.

All of these findings in Baby Gaylor's film are typical of the transient respiratory distress syndrome of the neonate (also known as *transient tachypnea* or the *wet lung syndrome*). The fetal lungs in utero are filled with fluid, which must be eliminated so that the alveoli can fill with air immediately after birth. The fluid escapes through the airways and via the pulmonary veins and lymphatics. Much of the fluid is expressed from the lungs during passage through the birth canal.

Baby Gaylor was not delivered vaginally and so is experiencing delayed resorption of fetal lung fluid. At the time the chest film was exposed, the fluid had entered and dilated the veins and lymphatics, producing the prominent lung markings. Some fluid had collected in the fissure and pleural spaces as well. Fluid in the interstitial spaces tends to narrow the very thin walls of the distal airways, causing air trapping and diffuse overexpansion. Usually, such a condition will rapidly improve and the radiograph will return to normal within 24–48 hours as the last of the pulmonary fluid is resorbed.

While the findings described are fairly typical for retained fetal lung fluid, other problems may also result in a similar accumulation of excess fluid in the lungs. Pulmonary edema can have a similar appearance and may be due to transfusion from a twin or to perinatal asphyxia and myocardial damage or to a patent ductus arteriosus. Polycythemia and hypervolemia caused by transfusion from a twin or the placenta during delivery may also be responsible. Finally, neonatal pneumonia should also be considered; pulmonary infection often masquerades as a more benign process and does not produce the typical pneumonic infiltrates expected in older children and adults. This is an insidious and, if unrecognized, a potentially devastating disease.

Keynote

• *Transient respiratory distress syndrome of the neonate is due to delayed clearing of the fetal lung fluid. Radiographs show increased lung markings, fissural thickening, pleural fluid, and lung hyperinflation.*

BABY GIRL TOWERS

Figure 13-7 is the film of Baby Girl Towers, a premature infant born at 32 weeks' gestational age. She developed grunting breath sounds 2 hours after birth and soon after-

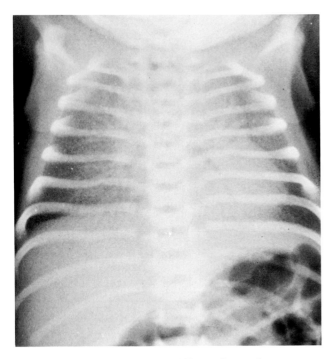

Figure 13-7. Baby girl Towers (see text).

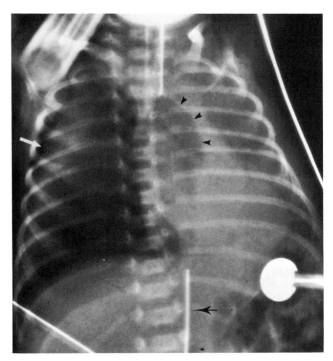

Figure 13-8. Baby boy Glenn (see text). A catheter, indicated by the black arrow, lies in the aorta.

ward became tachypneic and cyanotic. What do you see? What is the diagnosis?

Baby Towers's film shows typical changes of hyaline membrane disease (HMD, or respiratory distress syndrome). This problem results from a deficiency of surfactant, a phospholipid manufactured by the lungs late in gestation. As previously mentioned, the neonate first expands her or his alveoli by strenuously generating high negative pleural pressures. The dilated air-filled alveoli are stabilized by surfactant (a surface-tension–reducing agent). Once expanded, the alveoli remain open in inspiration and expiration, allowing continuous gas exchange. Baby Towers cannot yet produce normal quantities of surfactant; her alveoli therefore collapse on expiration, and as she becomes fatigued, she in unable to expand them even on inspiration.

The chest film reflects these physiological events. Because the process is one of diffuse alveolar collapse, the lungs are poorly inflated. There is also a fine, granular appearance to the lungs. This results from dilated, air-filled distal airways (terminal bronchioles and alveolar ducts), which are interspersed in a sea of atelectatic alveoli. These dilated terminal airway structures are the only sites at which gas exchange can occur. Also note the numerous air bronchograms. The air-filled bronchi are visible because they are embedded in a mass of dense, collapsed alveoli.

Keynote

- *Hyaline membrane disease results from a deficiency of surfactant. Radiographs show lung hypoinflation, a fine, granular lung appearance, and numerous air bronchograms.*

BABY BOY GLENN

Figure 13-8 shows the chest film of Baby Boy Glenn, an infant who developed severe dyspnea and cyanosis several hours after birth. What abnormality is present? How significant are the findings?

This is a typical example of a *tension pneumothorax*. In contrast to the other neonatal problems discussed thus far, this entity constitutes a life-threatening emergency and requires immediate treatment. One of the most important contributions of radiology to the management of neonatal respiratory distress is the detection of abnormalities that will respond to rapid surgical manipulation. The placement of a chest tube in this infant produced a dramatic resolution of his symptoms.

The film itself demonstrates two basic findings: overexpansion of the right hemithorax and hyperradiolucency of the area overlying the right lung. Both changes result from the accumulation of a large amount of air in the right pleural space. The overexpansion can be appreciated from the observation that the right hemithorax is much larger than the left. There is also displacement of the trachea and heart (or mediastinal shift) toward the left side, caused by the tense mass of air ballooning out the right hemithorax to the left side (small arrowheads).

Because the patient is supine when the film is exposed, most of the air rises anterior to the lung and lies between the anterior chest wall and the anterior surface of the lung. The lung on the affected side may be partially or completely collapsed by the pressure. The deflated pulmonary parenchyma tends to retract medially and fall posteri-

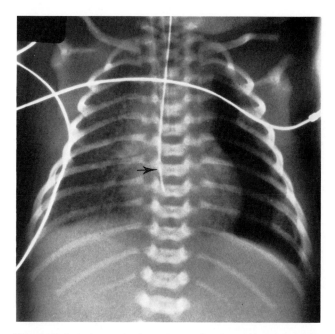

Figure 13-9. Left pneumothorax in an infant being treated for HMD. The right lung shows the typical granular appearance. The left lung is very radiolucent, and there is sharp definition of the left border of the mediastinum, the left side of the heart, and the left hemidiaphragm. Because of the underlying lung disease, the lung has not retracted toward the hilus, as would be expected in the adult. An endotracheal tube is present in the trachea, and the arrow points to a feeding tube positioned in the distal esophagus.

orly, behind the air collection. The distribution of air in the pleural space therefore results in an overall radiolucency to the hemithorax, as opposed to the localized apical collections of air expected in the erect adult.

Figure 13-8 also demonstrates the interface between the partially collapsed lung and the air in the pleural space (white arrow). This appears as a line in the midlung field; the space lateral to the line is very radiolucent (pleural air), and the area medial to the line is more radiodense (pulmonary parenchyma). This line marks the location of the visceral pleura. A pneumothorax can be easily diagnosed when the pulmonary markings end abruptly at the pleural surface and a radiolucent collection of air extends from this surface to the chest wall.

The pneumothorax on Baby Glenn's films was spontaneous, and no underlying chest disease was present. Pneumothorax is also common as a complication of HMD, probably resulting from the high pressures required to ventilate these infants. Figure 13-9 is an example of HMD and associated pneumothorax. This pneumothorax is not under tension, so there is no mediastinal shift, but there is an overall radiolucency on the right compared with the left. Also note that the pleural air tends to outline the mediastinal structures and the hemidiaphragm. Because of the severe HMD, the lungs do not collapse as expected; they are very stiff and may retain their volume despite the presence of large amounts of air in the pleural space.

Figure 13-10 shows another type of abnormal air collection in the infant chest: a *pneumomediastinum.* The diagnosis is best made on the lateral view. Note the very radiolucent area immediately behind the sternum. This is a focal collection of air within the tissue planes of the anterior mediastinum. The frontal view shows the air collection overlying the upper mediastinum. It has pushed the lobes of the thymus out laterally and outlined the medial borders of the thymus. (The medial thymic borders usually blend into the soft tissues of the mediastinum and cannot be seen.) This configuration of the thymus has been termed the *spinnaker sign,* named for a type of sail with a similar shape.

Pneumomediastinum is a generally benign condition often resulting from vigorous resuscitation of the neonate. High ventilatory pressures can rupture alveoli and cause dissection of air centrally along the peribronchial and perivascular sheaths to the mediastinum. Further extension with rupture into the pleural space can produce a pneumothorax; this complication should be anticipated in an infant with pneumomediastinum who requires continued positive pressure ventilation.

Keynote

- *A tension pneumothorax is diagnosed when there is air in the pleural space, when the mediastinum is shifted to the opposite side, and when the opposite lung is not atelectatic. It is a life-threatening emergency.*

BABY BOY SMITH

Figure 13-11 is the chest and upper abdominal examination of Baby Boy Smith. This infant was noted to be dyspneic and cyanotic from birth. Physical examination revealed decreased breath sounds over the left hemithorax and a thin, shallow abdomen. What congenital abnormality is causing this infant's problems?

The figure once again shows a mediastinal shift with displacement of the trachea and heart toward the right, indicating a mass effect on the left. At the base of the left hemithorax there are numerous circular radiolucencies which look like loops of bowel. Very little bowel gas is seen in the abdomen. Baby Smith has a congenital diaphragmatic hernia, a defect in the diaphragm which has allowed abdominal viscera to herniate into the thorax. The herniated bowel acts as a mass much like a tension pneumothorax, compressing normal lung on both the right and left sides and resulting in respiratory distress.

Congenital diaphragmatic hernia is another cause of neonatal respiratory distress amenable to surgical correction. The hernia results from persistence of the pleuroperitoneal sinus, a primitive communication between the thorax and abdomen that normally seals off early in gestation. The defect is usually on the left side and occurs in the posterolateral part of the diaphragm. If the herniation occurs early in gestation, pulmonary growth will slow, the

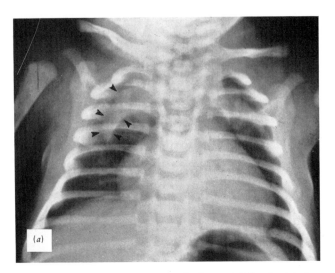

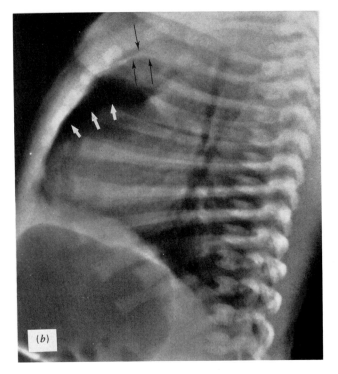

Figure 13-10. Neonatal pneumomediastinum. (*a*) The frontal view of the chest shows the characteristic spinnaker sign. Note that both the lateral and medial borders of the thymus can be seen and are outlined by the arrowheads. A similar finding is present on the left side but is partially obscured by the overlying ribs. (*b*) The lateral view shows that the anterior and superior portions of the mediastinum contain air (the pneumomediastinum), causing this region to appear hyperradiolucent. The anterior border of the heart is indicated by the white arrows; the region extending anteriorly from this point to the sternum is more radiolucent than normal. This can be seen if the area outlined is compared with the posterior costophrenic sulcus. The air anterior to the heart should never be more radiolucent than the region of lung in the posterior sulcus. Also note that the thymus can also be seen outlined with air on the lateral view. This is indicated by the black arrows, which outline a thin tongue of tissue in the anterior mediastinum.

lungs will be hypoplastic at birth, and survival may not be possible even if the hernia is reduced.

MONICA ALLEN

Monica Allen is a 3-month-old who had an uneventful delivery and neonatal course. Her mother brought her to the hospital because of high fever, cough, runny nose, and poor feeding. After examining the child, her pediatrician requested the chest film shown in Figure 13-12. What is your diagnosis?

The most striking finding in the figure is bilateral pulmonary overinflation. Note that the diaphragms are well below the level of the eighth ribs. There is an increase in the AP diameter of the chest on the lateral film as well as wide, deep posterior costophrenic sulci (arrows). There are also short linear radiodensities scattered throughout the lungs (large arrowhead). These radiodensities do not correspond to normal vascular markings; they are areas of subsegmental atelectasis. These findings—overinflation and linear atelectasis—are typical features of lower respiratory tract infections in children. The small arrowheads outline the left lobe of the thymus.

The usual lobar and segmental consolidations seen with adult pneumonias are relatively uncommon in infants. Most lower respiratory tract infections in this age group will produce radiographic changes similar to those of Baby Allen. This is due to anatomic differences between the lungs of infants and those of adults. The distal airways of infants are relatively narrower and more collapsible than those of adults. They also contain more mucus and offer more resistance to the passage of air and fluid. Inflammatory changes in these small airways produce air trapping. Relatively minor degress of infectious narrowing of the bronchioles prevent air from escaping during expiration, although some air can usually flow distally because of the slight dilatation that occurs with inspiration. This results in multiple areas of peripheral air trapping and accounts for the generalized overinflation seen in Figure 13-12. If the airway is completely occluded by inflammation in the wall or by mucus and exudate in the lumen, atelectasis results. This may be linear and subsegmental or in more severe cases may involve entire pulmonary segments and lobes.

Air trapping and atelectasis constitute an age-specific response to pulmonary infection in the infant. Inflammatory changes in the infant's distal airways usually overshadow any alveolar changes. Of course, other signs of pulmonary infection can also be seen. Thickening of the

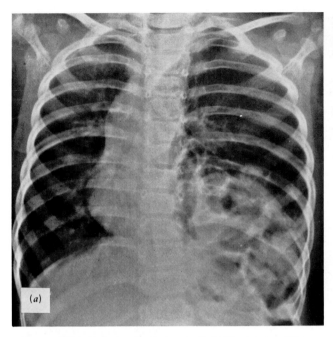

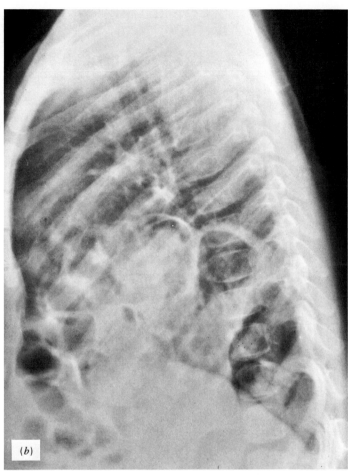

Figure 13-11. Baby boy Smith (see text). (*a*) Frontal view of the chest. (*b*) The lateral view.

bronchial walls produces peribronchial cuffing. Signs of interstitial lung disease, the same as those discussed in Chapter 11, are often present, especially with viral infections. Infants can also develop infectious alveolar consolidations in lobar and segmental distributions, although again such patterns are the exception rather than the rule.

Keynote

- *Pneumonia in young children often shows a radiographic pattern combining overinflation and streaky subsegmental atelectasis.*

DAVID SCOTT

Figure 13-13 is the chest film of David Scott, an 18-month-old boy who was rushed to the hospital by his parents because he suddenly began to wheeze and had difficulty breathing. There had been a party in the house the night before, and David's mother said that there may have been some peanuts lying on the floor. What abnormalities are present on the film? What is the diagnosis?

There is overexpansion of the left lung and shift of the heart and trachea to the right side. The air trapping in this case is not due to infectious narrowing of the bronchus but is the result of a foreign body producing expiratory obstruction and distal overexpansion. David was bronchoscoped, and the remnants of a peanut were removed from the left main-stem bronchus.

Radiography can be very helpful in deciding whether or not a foreign body is present in the airways. Most foreign bodies are not radiopaque, and so we must rely on indirect changes of airway obstruction. The two most important changes are air trapping and atelectasis. These may involve a segment, a lobe, or an entire lung.

The x-ray changes in aspiration may not be as striking as those seen in Figure 13-13. If the foreign body occludes a smaller bronchus, only segmental or lobar emphysema may be noted. It may be necessary to obtain films in inspiration and expiration to enhance and bring out the region of air trapping. Normal, uninvolved lung will lose volume on an expiratory film, but the obstructed region will remain overinflated. Make sure that the radiologist knows what you are looking for so the proper films will be obtained.

Keynote

- *The radiographic signs of bronchial obstruction may be atelectasis, lung hyperinflation, or air trapping. Air trapping may be demonstrated on a film taken in expiration.*

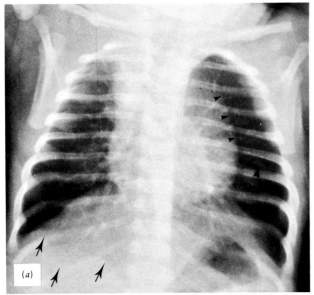

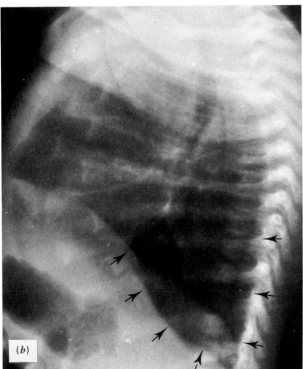

Figure 13-12. Monica Allen (see text).

ASTHMA

Wheezing is a common complaint in the pediatric emergency room, and most cases are not a result of aspirated foreign bodies. Asthma is often responsible. Figure 13-14 is the film of a 5-year-old with asthma. Note that there is once again generalized overinflation; this is the most common finding in acute asthmatic attacks.

The figure also shows a linear area of increased radio-

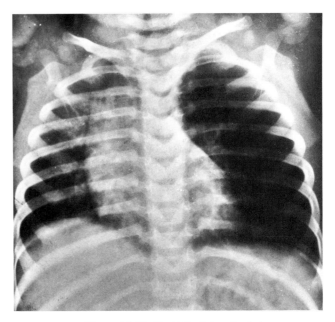

Figure 13-13. David Scott (see text).

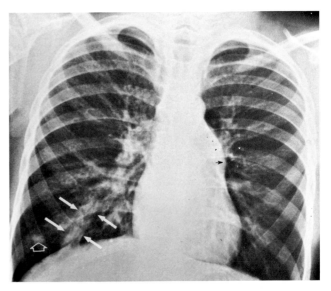

Figure 13-14. Acute asthma. There is bilateral pulmonary overinflation. The white arrows indicate a linear area of increased radiodensity extending from the right hilar region to the right hemidiaphragm. This appearance is the result of a mucous block. The open white arrow shows a small linear area of increased radiodensity that does not appear to be vascular. As discussed in the comments on lower respiratory tract infections, this most likely results from distal areas of subsegmental atelectasis and is a common finding in cases of asthma. The black arrows on the left show the convex appearance of a dilated main pulmonary artery. This is also commonly seen during acute asthmatic attacks.

density at the right lung base. This represents a mucous plug, a large bronchus filled with thick secretions that the asthmatic child cannot spontaneously clear. There may also be regions of pneumonia or atelectasis distal to the impacted airway. It is important in the asthmatic child to

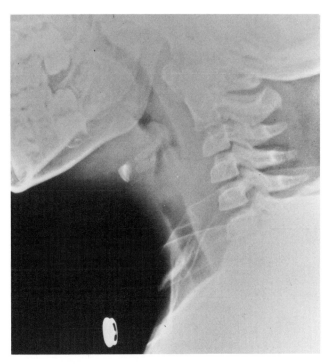

Figure 13-15. Patient Jack London, lateral view of neck.

look for evidence of pneumomediastinum and pneumothorax. These are common complications of asthma and may explain a sudden change in the clinical status.

Keynote

- *In asthma, diffuse lung hyperinflation is the most common finding. Mucous plugs in bronchi and focal regions of atelectasis or pneumonia may be present.*

JACK LONDON

Jack London is a 4-year-old who developed a cold several days ago. His mother explained that Jack seemed to be improving until a few hours earlier, when he suddenly got much worse: He had great difficulty breathing, began drooling, and developed a short, sharp cough. The emergency room house officer took the child to the radiology department and requested the film shown in Figure 13-15. A normal film for comparison is shown in Figure 13-16a. What is your diagnosis?

Figure 13-15 is a lateral view of the soft tissue structures of the neck. It shows a swollen epiglottis typical of acute epiglottitis. This disease is a severe, potentially fatal infection of the tissues immediately above the vocal cords. It is usually caused by a bacterium, *Haemophilus influenzae,* and often produces a rapidly developing severe upper airway obstruction.

The radiographic changes can best be appreciated by comparing our patient's film to the normal neck in Figure 13-16a. The normal epiglottis is a slender structure that

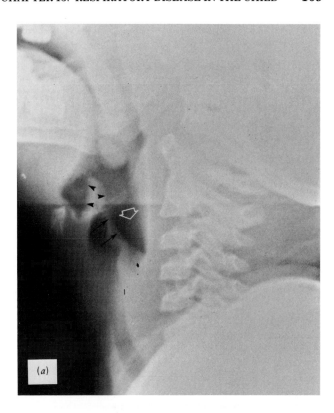

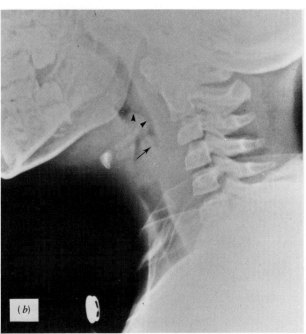

Figure 13-16. (a) A lateral view of a neck. A normal epiglottis is outlined by the small arrowheads. The normal, thin aryepiglottic folds are indicated by the arrows. The open white arrow points into the piriform sinuses immediately behind the folds. Contrast this with (b) acute epiglottis, in which the epiglottis is also outlined by small arrowheads. Note the rounded appearance to the epiglottis and the concomitant thickening of the aryepiglottic folds, indicated by the arrow. The normal airway spaces are partially effaced by the swollen, inflamed supraglottic structures.

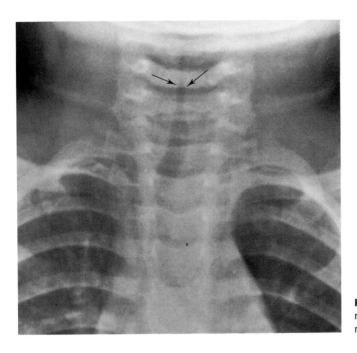

Figure 13-17. Croup. The arrows indicate the immediate subglottic region. Note the tapered narrowing of the airway below the area marked.

becomes thickened, blunted, and deformed in epiglottitis Also note that the fold of tissue extending posteriorly from the epiglottis to the arytenoid cartilage is markedly swollen and thickened and that this is also contributing to the narrowing of the airway. Figure 13-16*b* is this patient's neck with arrows indicating the abnormalities present in Figure 13-15.

The radiograph is the preferred initial method for diagnosing acute epiglottitis. The inflamed epiglottis, if touched by a tongue blade, can throw the hypopharynx into spasm. Occasionally, very early in the disease, the radiograph is normal.

Keynote

• *Acute epiglottitis is best diagnosed by a lateral view of the soft tissues of the neck. Physical examination may result in hypopharyngeal spasm, which can cause death by suffocation.*

CROUP

Symptoms and signs of upper airway obstruction can also be produced by laryngotracheobronchitis (*croup*). This is generally a less severe viral infection of the upper airways that may be difficult to distinguish from epiglottitis clinically. Figure 13-17 is a frontal view of the neck of a patient with croup. Comparison to a normal neck in Figure 13-18 shows that the most prominent radiographic change is in the region immediately below the vocal cords. This part of the airway demonstrates a tapered narrowing compared with the normal configuration in Figure 13-18. The subglottic narrowing is caused by inflammation and edema of the tracheal wall.

In evaluation of upper airway problems, it is important to have both frontal and lateral views. Epiglottitis can involve the subglottic area and produce the changes described with croup on the frontal film. Only by carefully examining the lateral view can the diagnosis be made. It is also important to be sure that you can confidently identify all the pertinent anatomic structures. Poor definition of these structures is often because of an inadequate amount of air in the pharynx and can be remedied by obtaining a film in inspiration.

Keynotes

• *Croup narrows the subglottic portion of the upper trachea.*

• *Epiglottitis can result in subglottic edema, simulating the findings of croup. Croup is best diagnosed on the AP view of the neck; a lateral view is necessary, however, to show that the subglottic narrowing is not due to epiglottitis.*

SUMMARY

The respiratory diseases of young children are varied and often have specific radiographic findings. In the newborn with respiratory distress, the differential possibilities include the transient respiratory distress that results from the delayed clearing of fetal lung fluid, the respiratory distress that results from insufficient surfactant to keep the alveoli expanded, the distress that comes from the compression of lung by a pneumothorax or by herniated gut, and neonatal pneumonias.

In the toddler, aspiration of peanuts or other objects can result in either hyperexpansion or atelectasis. Diffuse

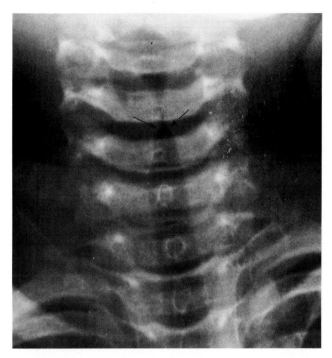

Figure 13-18. A frontal view of a normal neck. The arrows indicate the subglottic region, corresponding to the position marked on Figure 13-17. They also point out the normal "shoulders," which characterize the normal subglottic region. Note the normal caliber of the airway below this region.

chapter emphasized those patterns usually seen only in the young child.

Review Questions

1. What is the cause of the transient respiratory distress syndrome of the newborn? Describe its radiographic findings.
2. What is the cause of hyaline membrane disease? Describe its radiographic findings.
3. What is a tension pneumothorax?
4. How does a pneumomediastinum change the shape of the thymus?
5. What is the usual radiographic pattern of infantile pneumonia?
6. If you thought that a child had bronchial obstruction from an aspirated peanut, what radiographic study would you request?
7. Why is a radiograph used to diagnose acute epiglottitis? Describe its radiographic findings.
8. What is croup? Describe its radiographic findings.

VOCABULARY

croup	transient respiratory distress
epiglottitis	syndrome of the newborn
hyaline membrane disease	transient tachypnea of
pneumomediastinum	the newborn
tension pneumothorax	wet lung syndrome

SUGGESTIONS FOR FURTHER READING

Roderick I. Macpherson, Richard E. Leithiser. Upper airway obstruction in children: An update. *RadioGraphics,* **5**(3): 339–376, 1985.

For additional suggested reading see Chapter 7.

hyperexpansion, sometimes with focal areas of atelectasis, can also result from asthma.

Layngeal obstruction can occur either from the acute epiglottic swelling of epiglottitis or from the subglottic swelling of croup.

In the older child, the alterations on the radiograph resemble those on radiographs of the adult chest. This

14

LUNG DISEASE WITH A NORMAL CHEST RADIOGRAPH

Clinical

The chest radiograph is the screening method of choice for most types of pulmonary disease; there are certain types of lung disease, however, that either cannot be identified on radiographs or can only be identified late in their course. Most patients with pulmonary emboli have normal chest radiographs; for them, the radionuclide lung scan is the diagnostic method of choice. Patients with minimal-to-moderate obstructive pulmonary disease will often have normal chest radiographs; for them, a clinical history followed by selected pulmonary function tests, including measurements of vital capacity and FEV_1, is the diagnostic method of choice. Minimal interstitial lung disease may not be visible. Very early pneumonia may not be seen.

The clinician must judge when a normal radiograph indicates the absense of disease and when a disease is present that does not show on the radiograph.

OBJECTIVES

When you complete this chapter you will be able to

1. List four lung diseases that may demonstrate no radiographic abnormality.
2. List two common and four or more of the uncommon chest radiographic findings in pulmonary emboli.
3. Describe the common clinical findings in a patient with pulmonary emboli and discuss the method of confirming that diagnosis.
4. Describe the findings on chest radiographs of patients with minimal and marked COPD.

The chest radiograph is the common method of screening a patient for lung disease; there are, however, certain types of lung disease that only infrequently result in chest radiograph abnormalities. It is important to be aware of these so that appropriate screening methods can be used for their evaluation. The chest radiograph is a poor screening method for pulmonary emboli, acute and chronic obstructive pulmonary disease, minimal interstitial lung disease, and pulmonary dysfunction from neuromuscular disease of the diaphragmatic or chest wall musculature.

PULMONARY EMBOLI

The main techniques used for screening for pulmonary emboli are clinical history, cardiac exam, electrocardiogram, blood oxygen levels, and perfusion and ventilation lung scans. The patient with a pulmonary embolus often has a history of recent surgery, pregnancy, or recumbancy. He or she may give a history of leg swelling or pain. There is usually an acute onset of chest pain accentuated by deep breathing or of shortness of breath. On examination, a pleural rub may be heard, there may be wide splitting of the Pulmonary second (P_2) heart sound (because of increased pulmonary arterial pressure). In the patient with lung emboli, blood oxygen desaturation will often be present.

The lung scan, described and illustrated in Chapter 7,

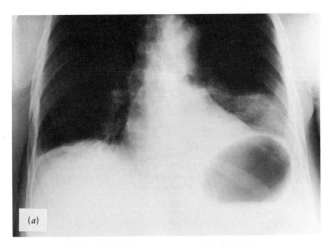

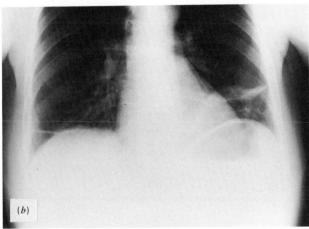

Figure 14-1. (a) Pulmonary emboli. This view of the lower half of a PA chest radiograph demonstrates three findings of pulmonary emboli: infiltrate, a small effusion, and unilateral hemidiaphragmatic elevation. There is alveolar infiltrate in several of the basal segments of the left lower lobe. There is infiltrate partially hidden behind the right hemidiaphragm. There is minimal blunting of the right lateral costophrenic angle caused by a small pleural effusion. There is left hemidiaphragm elevation compatible with hemidiaphragmatic splinting caused by pleuritic pain. (b) Fifteen days later, the bibasilar infiltrates have "melted" into areas of discoid or platelike atelectasis. The sign of pleural effusion has disappeared.

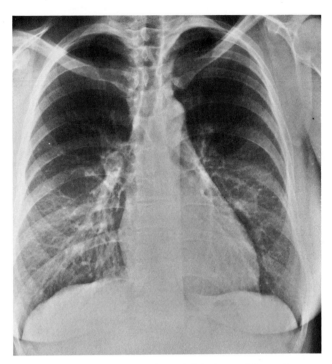

Figure 14-2. Westermark's sign of left lower lobe pulmonary embolus. The left lower lobe is more radiolucent than the right lower lobe. The vessels in the lateral portion of the left lower lobe are substantially smaller than those in the right lower lobe.

is the major confirmatory method for suspected pulmonary emboli. In the patient with pulmonary emboli, the perfusion lung scan will demonstrate one or many focal regions of decreased perfusion, usually in a segmental, subsegmental, or lobar distribution. The ventilation scan done with ^{133}Xe gas will demonstrate normal ventilation in these same regions.

Radiographic Findings in Pulmonary Embolus

Most pulmonary emboli do not result in chest radiograph abnormalities. There is an occasional patient who radiograph is abnormal because of emboli, and it is possible to suggest that this is the diagnosis in some of these patients. The most common chest radiograph finding in the patient with pulmonary emboli is, however, a normal chest radiograph. The second most common (and nonspecific) finding is a small pleural effusion.

Some patients with pulmonary emboli show a segmental or lobar alveolar infiltrate indistinguishable from pneumonia (Fig. 14-1a).

Uncommonly, pulmonary emboli can be suspected because they result in

1. A focal region of decreased lung vascularity (*Westermark's sign* I) (Fig. 14-2).
2. A rapid tapering of the larger pulmonary vessels in a localized segment of the lung (Westermark's sign II).
3. Focal enlargement of the right descending or left main pulmonary artery to greater than 15 mm in women or 17 mm in men.
4. A *Hampton's hump:* a trapezoidal solid-shaped infiltrate, pleural based, with a curved apex pointed toward the hilum (Fig. 10-14).
5. A *melting sign:* As pneumonic alveolar infiltrates resolve, they usually become inhomogeneous, developing focal regions of clearing within the infiltrate. When the alveolar infiltrates from pulmonary emboli clear, they frequently melt—that is, they shrink in size, losing their peripheral density first (Fig. 14-1a and b). This resembles the manner in which an ice cube melts and is called the melting sign.

6. Discoid or subsegmental atelectasis, which can be seen in the lungs in patients with pulmonary emboli (Fig. 14-1*b*).

Keynotes

- *The lung scan is the major confirmatory test for pulmonary emboli.*
- *Most patients with pulmonary emboli have a normal chest radiograph. Small pleural effusions may be present.*

OBSTRUCTIVE PULMONARY DISEASE

The chest radiograph is relatively insensitive in the identification of both acute and chronic obstructive pulmonary disease, for it is abnormal only in those patients already moderately symptomatic from their disease. It is not of use in looking for early disease.

The best method of screening for obstructive pulmonary disease is clinical history, especially as relates to exercise tolerance. The match test is a sensitive screening method, but with false positives: the patient attempts to blow out a match 6 in away from his or her widely open mouth. The best screening test is simple spirometry mea-

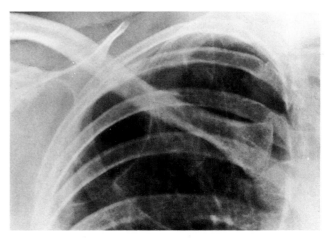

Figure 14-3. This focal view of the right lung apex demonstrates the curved walls of pulmonary blebs.

suring vital capacity and FEV_1 (expiratory volume in the first second of a maximally rapid expiration). Simple machines are available to measure these two parameters of pulmonary function easily and rapidly.

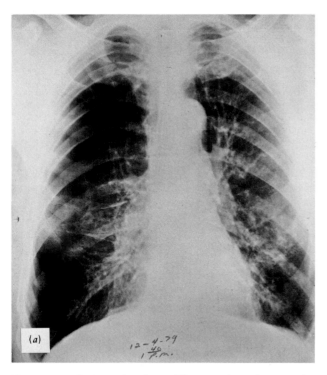

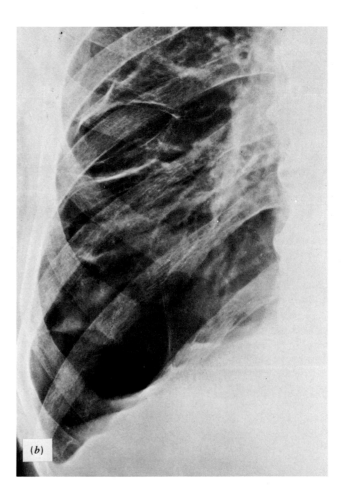

Figure 14-4. Radiographs of two different patients demonstrating several patterns of pulmonary blebs and bullae in far-advanced COPD.

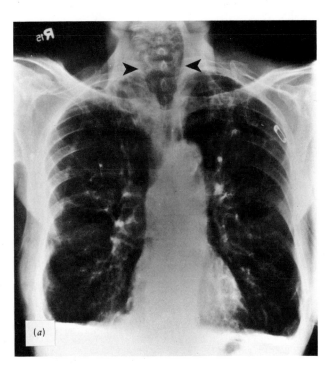 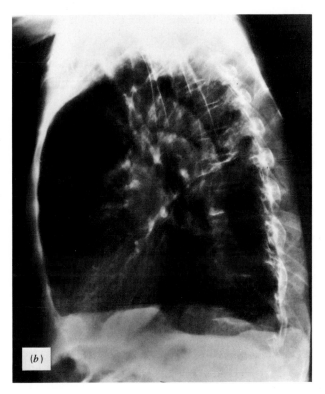

Figure 14-5. Severe COPD demonstrated on PA and lateral views of the chest. The diaphragm is flattened on both the frontal and lateral views. There is increased space between the sternum and the heart because the expansion of the lung has pushed the lung between the sternum and the aorta. The oval radiolucency in the neck overlying the trachea (arrowheads) is a gap left between the hypertrophied sternocleidomastoid muscles: a sign that the patient breathes using his accessory muscles of respiration.

Nuclear Medicine Evaluation Techniques

The ventilation scan can be used both to evaluate regions of the lung without perfusion and to look at regions with air trapping. The patient is instructed to breath an oxygen-xenon 133 mixture for 5 minutes until equilibrium is reached. A static equilibrium image is then obtained, followed by a series of images obtained during the washout of 133Xe that occurs when the patient resumes breathing room air (see Fig. 7-4). Focal regions of air trapping can be thus identified. Regions that do not fill during the equilibration film must be compared with chest radiographs, as regions of alveolar infiltrate will not be normally ventilated.

Chest Radiographic Findings

The chest radiograph is usually of little use in the diagnosis of minimal COPD. Occasionally, the chest radiograph will disclose a few blebs in the lung apex (or less often elsewhere) at a time when the generalized pulmonary function is only minimally decreased (Fig. 14-3). In general, though, the radiograph is abnormal only in the patient with moderate-to-severe disease.

The most common method of detecting COPD is the indentification of blood vessels curved around the margins of intrapulmonary blebs. While this is a specific finding, it is difficult to identify and thus not frequently of help. The identification of blebs and bullae—air-containing sacs within the lung—can be most helpful (Fig. 14-4a and b). These can vary from small to large.

Hyperexpansion is frequently used to evaluate for the presence of emphysema. This hyperexpansion is identified by seeing increased air space between the sternum and the heart on the laterial view and by seeing flattened hemidiaphragms on the lateral view (Fig. 14-5a and b). These findings can be simulated by an occasional normal person who can voluntarily hyperexpand the lungs by taking a really deep breath, so if you see hyperexpansion on a chest radiograph, it is best to confirm this with history or, if that is insufficient, with pulmonary function tests. In general, people who can voluntarily hyperexpand their lungs are under the age of 30 and relatively thin.

Keynote

- *Simple spirometry measuring vital capacity and FEV_1 is the best test for obstructive pulmonary disease.*

DETECTION OF MINIMAL LUNG DISEASE

Imaging techniques are insensitive to the presence of minimal interstitial disease. Minimal sarcoid, tuberculosis, or interstitial fibrosis may be inapparent by imaging techniques until the degree of interstitial disease is moderate. Pulmonary function tests are more sensitive, especially those for blood oxygen levels and diffusion capacity. In some cases, a ^{67}Ga scan shows lung uptake, but it is an unreliable screening test. Early (premetastatic) lung cancer is often too small to be seen on a radiograph.

INAPPROPRIATE TIMING OF IMAGING STUDIES

Lung disease may be inapparent on imaging studies because the amount of disease necessary to cause symptoms may be less than the amount of disease necessary to create an imaging abnormality. This concept was explored in Case 10-2, that of a patient with pneumococcal pneumonia whose chest radiograph was normal at a time when he was severely ill. Similar changes can be seen in patients with active tuberculosis. The disease may not be visible early in the course of the disease because it changes the lung architecture too little to be seen.

SUMMARY

Patients with pulmonary emboli, minimal-to-moderate obstructive pulmonary disease, minimal interstitial disease, early lung cancer, and early pneumonias may show no abnormality on chest radiographs. In diagnosing pulmonary emboli, the radionuclide lung scan is the procedure of choice. Imaging techniques may not help in identifying the other processes listed above.

REVIEW QUESTIONS

1. What does the lung scan done with injected radioactive particles demonstrate?
2. What does the lung scan done with ^{133}Xe gas show?
3. What are the 8 possible radiographic findings of pulmonary emboli?
4. What is the best method for confirming a suspected clinical diagnosis of obstructive pulmonary disease?
5. Other than ordering a biopsy, what is the best method of confirming the diagnosis of minimal interstitial lung disease if the chest radiograph is normal?

Vocabulary

COPD	melting sign
Hampton's hump	Westermark's sign

SUGGESTIONS FOR FURTHER READING

For suggested reading see Chapter 7.

SECTION B

THE PLEURA

The second major category of chest disease discussed is the pleural diseases: pleural effusion, pleural fibrosis, and pneumothoraces. The standard chest radiograph is the main method of analyzing the pleural space. Occasionally sonography is used to localize loculated pleural effusions. Computed tomography is occasionally used to differentiate a pleural fibrotic plaque from a lung mass. Tracer imaging is occasionally used in the evaluation of bloody effusions in looking for pulmonary arterial emboli.

15

PLEURAL EFFUSION

KEY CONCEPTS

Radiological

The pattern that a pleural effusion manifests on radiographs depends on the quantity, viscosity, and site of origin of the fluid; the position of the patient; the presence of pleural adhesions; and the resistance or compliance of the adjacent lung. With the patient upright, the initial collection of fluid, which is between the lung and the hemidiaphragm, is invisible. With greater amounts of fluid, the shape of the base of the lung changes, eventually forming an upward-curved meniscus.

A stiff lung displaces the fluid into the lateral pleural space. An area of atelectatic lung pulls the fluid into the space formerly occupied by the atelectatic lung.

Most pleural effusions shift in position as the patient's position changes. Effusions that are particularly viscous may not shift position. Pleural adhesions may result in loculations that prevent the shifting of the fluid.

Clinical

Pleural effusions are classified into transudates and exudates, based on their protein content, cell count, and lactic dehydrogenase (LDH) levels. In general, *transudates* are caused by increased pulmonary and systemic venous pressure or by a low serum albumen level. *Exudates* are usually caused by infectious, inflammatory, or neoplastic diseases. In some cases, the nature of the fluid can be determined by its appearance on the radiograph; more often, some of the fluid must be removed by thoracentesis for laboratory analysis.

The removal and analysis of pleural fluid in a patient with an undiagnosed illness will often result in the diagnosis being established. When a large pleural effusion interferes with respiration, the removal of the fluid can relieve symptoms.

OBJECTIVES

When you complete this chapter you will be able to

1. List the factors that affect the appearance of pleural effusions.
2. Describe the sequence of radiographic changes seen in an upright patient with increasing amounts of transudate.
3. Describe the appearance of pleural effusions on CT scans.
4. Describe the appearance of pleural effusions in the supine patient.
5. Identify pleural effusions on selected chest radiographic and CT studies.
6. List potential causes of pleural effusions.
7. List the differences between transudates and exudates.

Fluid in the pleural space, once identified, can be removed and analyzed. The characteristics of the fluid can be of great use in diagnosis.

Several patterns can be seen on the chest radiograph of the patient with pleural disease. Because the detection of fluid is important, the recognition of these multiple patterns is also important. Six factors affect the appearance of pleural effusion:

1. Quantity
2. Viscosity
3. Position of the patient
4. Presence of pleural adhesions or loculations
5. Resistance or compliance of the adjacent lung to compression
6. Site of origin of the fluid

Causes

What causes pleural effusion to form? Make a list of the possible causes of effusion and try to group causes according to pathophysiology. There are at least two ways to group the causes of pleural effusion: by general categories of disease or by the pathophysiology as reflected in *Starling's law of fluid transport* (see discussion in Chapter 11).

Categories of Disease

Congenital
  Pulmonary lymphangiectasia
  Transient tachypnea of the newborn
  Erythroblastosis fetalis
Infection
  Pleurisy
    Viral
    Tuberculous
  Empyema
    Spread from pneumonia
    Contaminated wounds
Neoplastic
  Primary
    Mesothelioma
    Sarcoma
  Secondary
    Metastases
      Lung
      Breast
      Ovary, and so on
Traumatic
  Contusion
  Laceration of
    Intercostal vessels
    Lung vessels
    Heart or great vessels
    Thoracic duct
  Secondary to pneumothoraces
Metabolic
  Hypoalbuminemia
    Liver disease
    Nephrotic syndrome
  Uremia
  Hypothyroidism
Toxic
  None known
Collagen-vascular disease
  Rheumatoid lung
  Systemic lupus erythematosis

Starling's Law

Hydrostatic pressure
  Congestive heart failure
  Pulmonary lymphangiectasia
  Pulmonary venous obstruction
  Constrictive pericarditis

Decreased colloid osmotic pressure
  Hypoalbuminemia
    Liver disease
    Kidney disease
Increased capillary permeability
  Infectious
  Traumatic
  Neoplastic
Miscellaneous
  Extravasation from
    Vessels
    Thoracic duct
    Esophagus
    Pancreatic duct
  Decreased resorptive capacity from
    Pneumothorax
    Heart failure
  Secondary to ascites

Keynote

- *Fluids resulting from changes in colloid osmotic pressure and hydrostatic pressure are transudates. Those resulting from changes in capillary permeability are exudates. Protein content, white cell count, and LDH are the main laboratory tests used to differentiate transudate from exudate.*

PATTERNS

Patterns of Accumulation of Transudate in the Upright Patient with Normal Lung and Normal Pleural Space

The normal pleural surface provides a gliding surface between lung and chest wall. With normal respiration, the lung does not completely fill the sulcus surrounding the periphery of the diaphragm, and fluid can collect in this sulcus and be invisible (Fig. 15-1*a* and *b*).

As more fluid accumulates, it usually will collect between the hemidiaphragm and the base of the lung. On the right side, this will initially be undetectable; on the left side, the distance between the stomach bubble and the lung may be increased.

As more fluid accumulates between the hemidiaphragm and the lung, it distorts the shape of the undersurface of the lung, shifting the apex of the curve laterally (Fig. 15-2).

After 200–500 cc of fluid has accumulated between the lung and the hemidiaphragm, it begins to overflow the limits of this subpulmonic space and begins to affect the shape of the lung in the peridiaphragmatic sulcus (Fig. 15-2b).

The initial effect on the pointed margin of the lung is to make it shallower (Fig. 15-1*c*). The fluid then will compress this inferior tongue of the lung, making the point of the lung narrow, and then will make the point of the lung rounded (Fig. 15-1*d*).

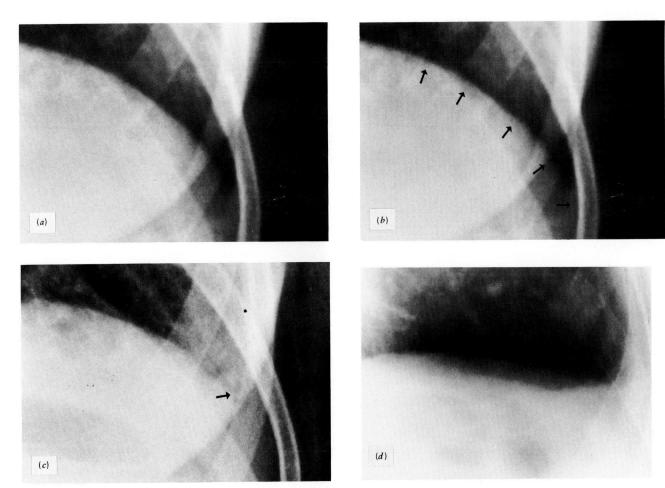

Figure 15-1. (*a*) A normal lateral costophrenic sulcus and left hemidiaphragm shape. (*b*) Arrows indicate the initial locations of pleural effusion; initial pleural effusion collects between the hemidiaphragm and the lung and in the depths of the lateral and posterior costophrenic sulci. The initial collections of pleural fluid are not detectable on upright chest radiographs. (*c*) Larger amounts of pleural fluid result in a filling in of the costophrenic recesses, compressing the lung from its inferior surface and from its sides. (*d*) Still larger amounts of pleural fluid completely fill the costophrenic sulcus and round the tip of the lung.

As more fluid accumulates, the lower margin of the lung assumes an upward curve (Fig. 15-3) and, with large effusions, will encircle the lung.

The pleural effusion assumes this complex pattern of changes because it must press against the lung as it fills the pleural space and because different portions of the lung are more or less compressible. In general, the lung within the sulcus is less compressible than the lung along the broad, flat surfaces. In part, this explains the subpulmonic location and the preservation of the rim of the lung, which sits within the sulcus.

Keynotes

- *The initial collections of pleural fluid, deep in the sulcus and between the hemidiaphragm and lung, are invisible on an upright chest radiograph.*

- *Subpulmonic effusions collecting between the hemidiaphragm and lung shift the apex of the subpulmonic radiodensity laterally.*
- *The shape of the pleural effusion is complex because it must press against a resilient lung.*

Effect of Gravity on the Accumulation of Pleural Effusion

If the pleural fluid is a transudate and the pleural space and lung are normal, the pleural fluid will be freely movable. Thus, if the patient is lying on her or his side, fluid will collect along the lateral pleural margin (Fig. 15-4). The radiographic view used to demonstrate small amounts of pleural effusion, the lateral decubitus view, uses this method for detection of pleural effusion.

When the patient is lying supine, the fluid will accumulate posteriorly and will be projected over the lung, adding diffuse radiodensity to the hemithorax. Since most CT

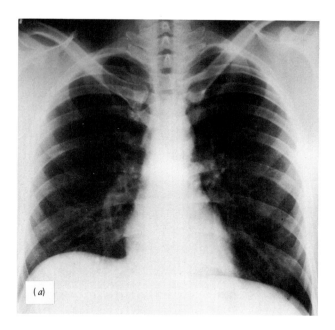

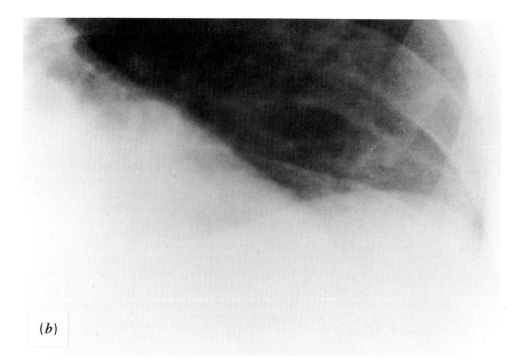

Figure 15-2. The appearance of subpulmonic effusion. (*a*) Normal appearance of the chest in a 23-year-old person. Note the shapes of the right and left lung bases. The appearance of the right (*b*) and left (*c*) lung bases in the same patient when he had moderate pleural fluid collections, mainly in the space between the diaphragm and the lungs.

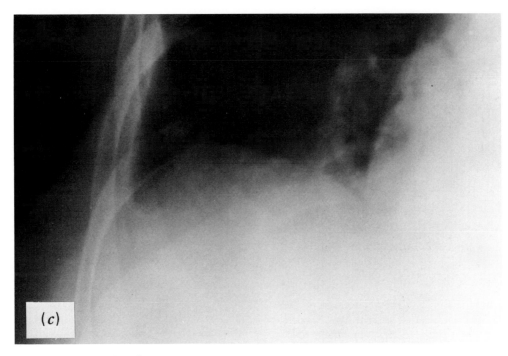

Figure 15-2. (Continued)

scans are done with the patient supine, pleural fluid on CT scans will be layered posteriorly (Fig. 15-5).

When the patient is lying prone, the fluid will collect along the anterior pleural space and can silhouette the heart margin. When the fluid is shifted anteriorly, the lung bases can be evaluated. Change of position is often used to evaluate whether the pleural density is fluid.

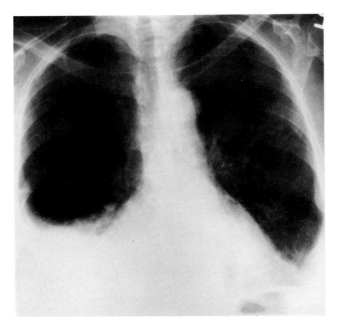

Figure 15-3. Moderate-to-large bilateral pleural effusions, demonstrating the upward curve of the pleural fluid collections.

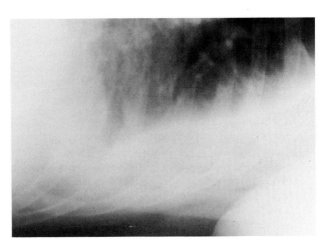

Figure 15-4. A moderate pleural effusion layering along the left side of the chest when the patient lies on his left side. The space between the lung and the ribs is whiter because of the presence of pleural effusion.

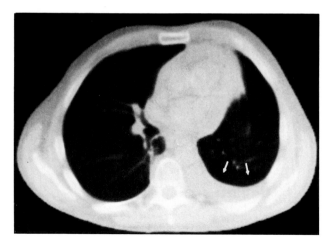

Figure 15-5. Arrows demarcate the left pleural effusion on a CT view of the chest.

Freely moving fluid is easier to remove for testing. Non-moving pleural densities may be pleural fibrosis but can also represent either loculated fluid or thick, viscous exudates.

Case 15-1

The patient is a 22-year-old woman who came to our emergency room with a 5-day history of repeated coughing and chest pain on the left side, a sharp pain occurring with breathing. Her initial film is in Figure 15-6a. What do you see?

There is a small region of alveolar infiltrate in the left lower lobe. How can you tell it's alveolar?

As you follow vessels into the region of density, they disappear. Temperature was 101 °F. Sputum showed many leukocytes with a sparse mixed flora of Gram-negative and Gram-positive organisms. What is your likely diagnosis?

Mycoplasma or viral pneumonia. Positive cold agglutinins titer was 1:64. The treatment was begun with. . .? Erythromycin.

Six weeks later the patient returned for follow-up radiographs, which are in Figure 15-6b. What do you see?

There is now a shallow left costophrenic sulcus, and the space between the base of the lung and the stomach bubble is increased. The infiltrate in the left lower lobe had disappeared. These findings indicate that a small pleural effusion is now present on the left. How could you confirm it?

The lateral decubitus view is shown in figure 15-6c. The left pleural space is thicker with the left side down than with the patient upright.

How much fluid do you think is present? Can you tell?

In general, radiologists can give only a very rough estimate of the amount of fluid present, and errors of 100–400 cc are common.

Case 15-2

RL is an 18-year-old man, a farmer, who was run over by his tractor while planting winter wheat. The tractor ran over his legs, fracturing both his femurs. Figure 15-7a is shortly after admission; Figure 15-7b and c is his chest radiographs taken 5 hours later. What do you see?

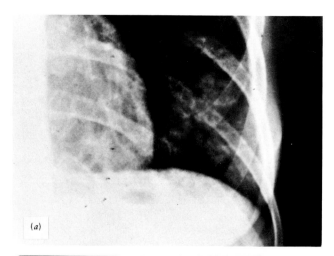

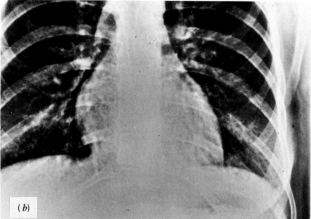

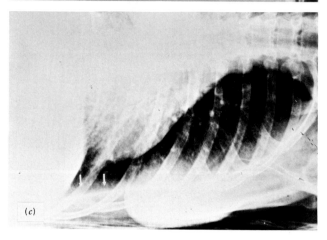

Figure 15-6. Case example. (a) Initial radiograph. (b) Six weeks later. (c) Left lateral decubitus view (taken with the patient's left side down).

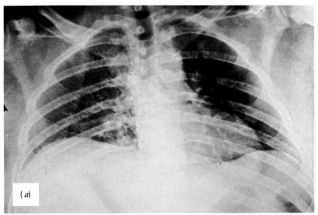

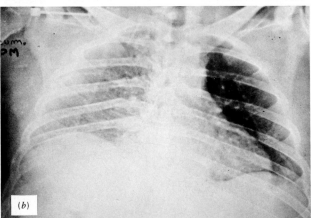

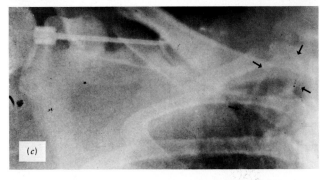

Figure 15-7. (a) A supine view of the chest in this 18-year-old farmer admitted with fractures of both femurs. (b) A follow-up supine radiograph obtained approximately 5 hours later. There is a marked increase in opacification of the right hemithorax. (c) A closeup view of the chest apex on the right side demonstrates the course of the subclavian line (arrows). The course does not follow the normal anatomy of the veins at this site. (Case courtesy of M. Toxopeus, M.D.)

On each film, the right hemithorax is denser than the left, and this density is increasing. What could be doing this?

Each film is taken supine. On the first, the thick pectoral muscle of this right-handed hard-working farmer caused the increased radiodensity. On the second, there is pleural fluid layered posteriorly. Where did it come from?

Look at the closeup in Figure 15-7c. What does it show?

A venous catheter has been placed through the subclavian vein. Its course does not follow the normal venous anatomy of this region—it was placed accidentally into the pleural space. Because the patient was receiving blood through this catheter, any tap of this patient's pleural effusion would have yielded blood, frightened the physicians caring for him, and could have led to an unnecessary thoracotomy.

When you get blood back from a pleural tap, how do you know that you've not punctured a vessel and gotten intravascular blood?

Intravascular blood will clot. Blood in the pleural space will almost always be defibrinated by the motion of the pleura.

Keynotes

- *The lateral decubitus view is a view taken with the patient lying on his or her side with the x-ray beam horizontal.*
- *On a supine view, only large quantities of pleural fluid can be identified. They increase the radiodensity of the hemithorax.*

Effect of Pleural Adhesions or Loculations on the Appearance of Pleural Effusion

Pleural adhesions result in loculated fluid. These demarcated collections of fluid can be single or multiple. Their appearance varies with the location of the adhesion and the amount of fluid. To get some idea of their variable appearance, first consider a patient whose pleural adhesions are primarily in the upper chest (Fig. 15-8a). If the lower pleural space is normal and the cause of the effusion is primarily in the lower lung, the pleural fluid will have the appearance of normal transudate in a normal pleural space. Only when the fluid reaches the region of the adhesion—either because the quantity of fluid is sufficient or because the patient changes position—will the adhesion and loculation become apparent.

Alternatively, if the adhesion is in the upper pleural space but the process causing the effusion is in the upper lung, then the loculation will be visible and the effusion will have the appearance shown in Figure 15-8b. Pleural-based collections showing unusual patterns should be considered to result from loculations of the fluid unless shown to have other causes.

The clinical importance of recognizing loculations is that loculations increase the difficulty of aspirating the fluid. Each small locule may be emptied, but then the needle needs to be adjusted to empty the next locule. CT scans can be quite helpful in localizing the locules of a loculated pleural effusion. Figure 15-9 is the CT scan of a patient with a staphylococcal empyema demonstrating the multiple locules of effusion. The thick rind around the pleural collection is a sign that the effusion is infected. Compare the CT appearance of this empyema with the transudate shown on the CT in Figure 15-5.

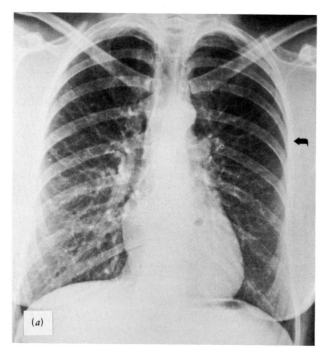

(a)

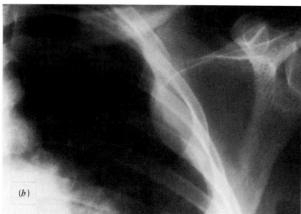

(b)

Figure 15-8. Normal chest radiograph with arrow indicating site of pleural adhesions. (*b*) Loculated effusion, caused by a staphylcoccal empyema, occurring above an adhesion.

Keynote

- *Areas of adhesion between the visceral and parietal pleura limit the spread of fluid, resulting in a variety of unusual locations and patterns for pleural fluid.*

Viscosity of the Fluid

Different types of fluid vary in their viscosity, and this difference can sometimes be recognized by a slow shifting of the shape or location of the fluid as the patient changes position. Very thick fluid may not flow at all, and these viscid effusions may be mistaken for pleural fibrosis. Fig-

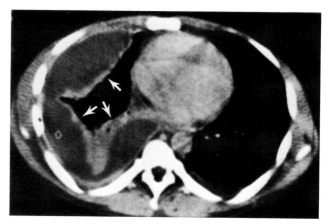

Figure 15-9. A CT scan cross section through the chest. Arrows indicate the location of several of the pleural locules of this staphylococcal empyema. (Courtesy of E. Blum, M.D.)

ure 15-10 is the chest radiograph of a patient with persistent unexplained fever. The pleural density at the left base did not shift with changes in position, and diagnostic taps failed to produce any fluid aspirate. Because of the continued fever and the physician's inability to find another source of fever, a 1-cm drainage opening into the pleural space was cut, and this permitted a pastelike tuberculous pus to be removed. The empyema material was too thick to pass through the 18-gauge needle used in the aspiration attempt.

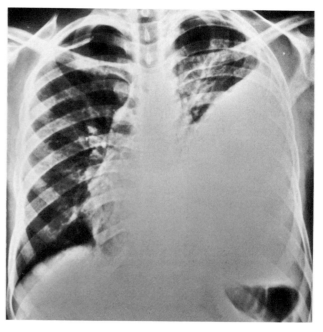

Figure 15-10. This pastelike tuberculous empyema was too viscous to be aspirated through a 16-gauge needle. A 1-cm pleural window was necessary for drainage.

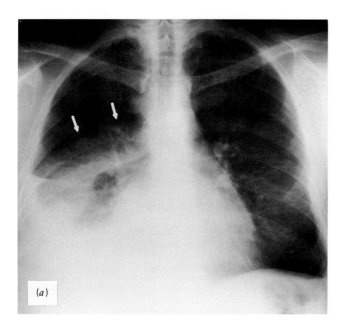

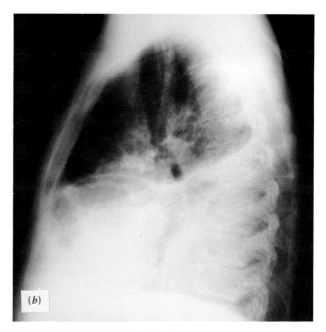

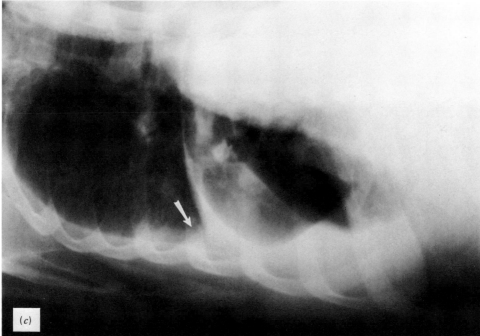

Figure 15-11. Pleural effusion in a 41-year-old man. (*a*) The arrows indicate the superior margin of the major fissure, opacified by fluid within it. The fissure is depressed. Normally the top of the major fissure would project at about the level of the fourth posterior rib. The depressed fissure indicates that the right lower lobe is atelectatic (from cancer). (*b*) The lateral view demonstrates the depressed position of the major fissure. (*c*) The lateral decubitus view demonstrates the preferential collection of the pleural fluid around the atelectatic lower lung. The arrow indicates the "step" in the amount of fluid collected at the lower lobe—upper lobe junction.

Effect of Lung Resistance or Compliance on the Appearance of Pleural Fluid

The radiographs in Figure 15-11*a* and *b* are those of a 41-year-old man with recurrent episodes of dyspnea. What do you see? There are multiple findings on these radiographs. The base of the right lung is elevated, indicating the presence of fluid between the lung and the hemidiaphragm: subpulmonic effusion. There is a curved band of radio-

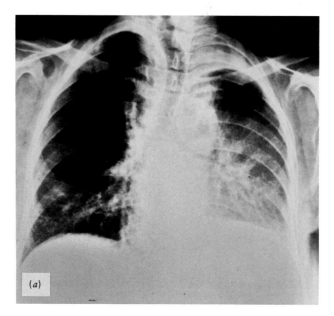

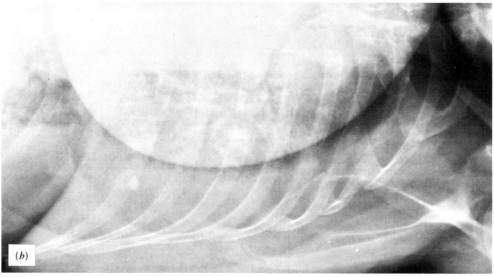

Figure 15-12. Case example 15-3. (a) PA view. (b) Left lateral decubitus view (the patient is lying on her left side).

density crossing the right midlung and representing fluid in the top of the major fissure (arrows). The top of the major fissure is lower than its normal position, which is adjacent to the fourth posterior rib margin, and thus the right lower lung is partially atelectatic.

The lateral view (Fig. 15-11b) demonstrates the effusion and depression of the oblique fissures. Figures 15-11c is the decubitus view. What does the fluid do? The fluid moves freeely into the lateral pleural space, but there is a discontinuity of its margin at the region of the major fissure (arrow). This is due to the loss of volume of the right lower lobe holding additional fluid at this site. The lower lung is less stiff than the upper lung, and the fluid is preferentially held at this level.

Case 15-3

The radiographs in Figure 15-12a and b are those of a 52-year-old woman with hemoptysis. What do you see?

There are several findings. The inferior margin of aerated lung is higher on the left than on the right (the reverse of normal). The left border of the heart cannot be seen (it is silhouetted out), and there is moderate pleural space widening at the apex of the left lung. How do you explain these findings?

There is pleural effusion. The left lateral decubitus chest film shows free movement of fluid within the left hemithorax (Fig. 15-12b). How do you explain the non-visualization of the left of the heart border and the collection of pleural fluid at the left lung apex?

There is left upper lobe atelectasis. The left lung is anchored at the hilum, and thus, as the left lung collapsed, the pleural effusion was displaced superiorly into the apex. What would you do next to evaluate this patient's condition?

There are two ways of investigating. The first is to tap the effusion and study it for tumor cells and bacteria. The second is to use bronchoscopy on the patient. In this case, both were done. An endobronchial carcinoma of the lung was found occluding the left upper lobe bronchus, and metastases from this tumor were found in the pleural space.

Recognition of these unusual patterns of pleural fluid collection aid in the recognition of the underlying lung abnormality.

Effect of Stiff Lung on the Appearance of Pleural Effusion

Stiff lung results in two different patterns of pleural fluid collection. With a stiff lung, the fluid collects in the potential space between the chest volume in inspiration and expiration, thus surrounding the lung in a thin layer (Fig. 15-13a). The more stiff the lung, the more even the layer, the less stiff, the greater the effect of gravity on the location of the fluid (Fig. 15-13b).

In patients with interstitial edema from heart failure, an additional location of effusion is sometimes seen: the *interlobar location*. Fluid visualized mainly in the interlobar location sometimes has a masslike appearance and is called a *fluid pseudotumor* (Fig. 15-14).

Keynote

• *Fluid can collect in an interlobar location when the lung is stiff. This pattern is usually seen in patients with interstitial congestive heart failure.*

Inverted Left Hemidiaphragm Syndrome

While not common, the weight of a large pleural effusion on the left can invert the left hemidiaphragm when the patient is in the upright position. When this occurs, the patient will be severely short of breath because muscular contraction of the diaphragm will shunt air back and forth between the two lungs. When the patient lies down, the weight will be removed from the hemidiaphragm, the hemidiaphragm will revert to its normal position, and respiration will be improved. This phenomenon of platypnea occurs mainly in patients with a pleural effusion resulting from metastatic cancer. When the patient comes to the office, he is usually severely dyspneic. Removal of a few hundred cubic centimeters of effusion relieves his symptoms and permits him to return home.

Keynote

• *In the inverted left hemidiaphragm syndrome, the inversion of the hemidiaphragm results in the patient rebreathing the same air as it passes from right to left to right to left lung.*

SUMMARY

Pleural effusion does show many patterns on the radiograph, some of which indicate the nature of the fluid and some of which reflect abnormalities of the pleura or lung adjacent to the effusion. Their recognition on the radiograph permits a diagnostic tap of the fluid, and its analysis frequently can be helpful in analyzing the cause of a patient's illness.

The small effusion may become visible only when the patient is placed on her or his side. Moderate effusions can blunt the costophrenic angle or can, when larger, result in an upward-curve meniscus.

Pleural adhesions and changes in lung compliance can affect the appearance of the fluid, but these less common appearances of fluid can help in detecting underlying lung disease.

REVIEW QUESTIONS

1. What are the factors that affect the appearance of pleural effusions?
2. Where might the effusion be found in the patient with interstitial congestive heart failure?
3. Describe the sequential changes in the costophrenic angle with increasing quantities of fluid.
4. What is the appearance of pleural effusion in the supine patient?
5. What is a pleural adhesion? How does it affect the appearance of pleural effusion?
6. What is the inverted left hemidiaphragm syndrome? What is its clinical significance?

VOCABULARY

exudate
fluid pseudotumor
interlobar effusion
inverted left hemidiaphragm
  syndrome

platypnea
Starling's law of fluid
  transport
transudate

SUGGESTIONS FOR FURTHER READING

Hamid Sahebjami, Robert G. Landon. Pleural effusion; Pathophysiology and clinical features. *Seminars in Roentgenology*, **12**(4): 269–276, 1977.

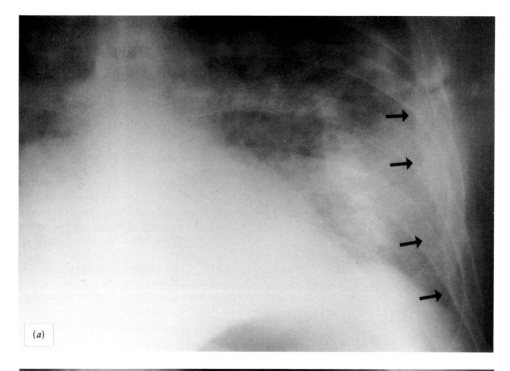

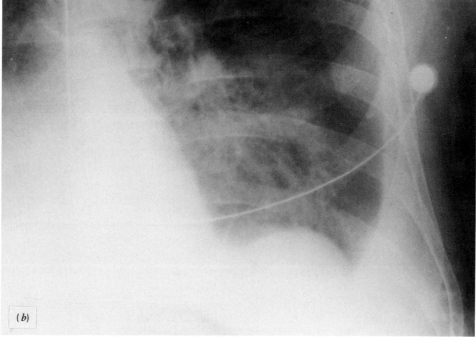

Figure 15-13. The effect of a stiff lung on the appearance of pleural fluid. This patient has severe heart failure. (*a*) When the lung is markedly stiff from interstitial edema, the pleural fluid (arrows) accumulates along the edge of the lung. (*b*) After 24 hours of treatment, the interstitial edema is much decreased, and the fluid shows a more rounded contour. The change in the appearance of the fluid results from the change in the stiffness of the lung.

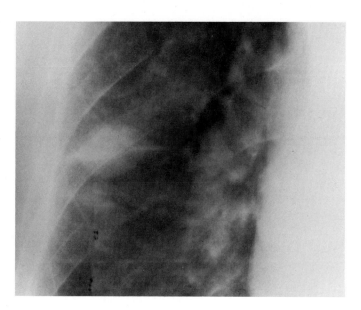

Figure 15-14. An interlobar effusion. In patients with a stiff lung, fluid can accumulate in an interlobar location, simulating a mass. This is sometimes called a fluid pseudotumor. This patient had pulmonary edema from heart failure.

Vernon A. Vix. Roentgenographic manifestations of pleural disease. *Seminars in Roentgenology,* **12**(4): 277–286, 1977.

Michael P. Federle, Alexander S. Mark, Elizabeth S. Guillaumin. CT of subpulmonic pleural effusions and atelectasis: Criteria for differentiation from sub-phrenic fluid. *American Journal of Roentgenology,* **146:**685–689, 1986.

For additional suggested reading see Chapter 7.

16

PLEURAL FIBROSIS

KEY CONCEPTS

Pleural fibrosis is a common cause of blunting of the lateral costophrenic sulcus. Sometimes, the shape of the blunted costophrenic angle will be different from the angle blunting of pleural effusion, permitting the direct diagnosis of pleural fibrosis; when uncertainty is present, a lateral decubitus chest radiograph can be used to demonstrate whether free-moving effusion is present. Pleural calcification usually indicates that the blunting of the angle is caused by fibrosis.

Marked lung hyperinflation can also result in blunting of the costophrenic angles.

OBJECTIVES

When you complete this chapter you will be able to

1. Recognize the classic findings of pleural fibrosis and distinguish them from the pattern of pleural effusion.
2. Correctly classify selected radiographs as demonstrating pleural effusion, pleural fibrosis, or costophrenic angle blunting caused by marked lung hyperinflation.

There is a blunting of the right costophrenic angle in the radiograph in Figure 16-1a. In Figure 16-1b, air under the hemidiaphragm shows the true change of this distorted hemidiaphragm. This pattern differs from those seen in Chapter 15 and represents pleural fibrosis. Most of the time, pleural fibrosis can be distinguished from pleural fluid by differences in the shape of the pleural density. In pleural fibrosis, the shape of the lower margin of lung is often straight, rather than curved. The thickening of the

pleural space laterally often extends higher than one would see with the meniscus of pleural effusion (Figure 16-2). The lateral costophrenic angle is often more severely involved than the posterior angle.

Why does pleural fibrosis attain this different shape? Most processes that cause pleural fibrosis are acute inflammatory processes associated with pleural irritation. Motion of the lung against the pleural is painful and therefore the patient holds the hemidiaphragm in a *splinted* (expiratory) position. In expiration, the lung recedes from the sulcus, placing the inflamed parietal pleura of the hemidiaphragm adjacent to that of the chest wall. Fibrous *adhesions* form between them, filling in the sulcus and maintaining a flattened shape. Sometimes the shape resembles that of a pleural effusion. If the shape is not classical for fibrosis, how could you tell fibrosis from pleural effusion?

Usually pleural fibrosis is confirmed by comparing the current radiograph with old films or by a clinical history incompatible with a pleural effusion. Occasionally a lateral decubitus view of the chest is needed to exclude the presence of free fluid.

Keynote

- *Pleural fibrosis can usually be differentiated from pleural effusion by the shape of the blunting of the costophrenic angle or by comparison of the current film with an old film. Only occasionally is a lateral decubitus film necessary.*

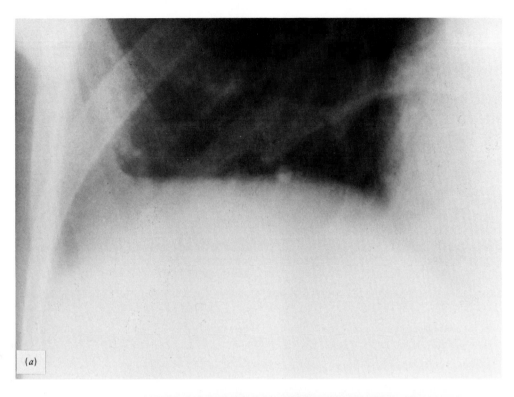

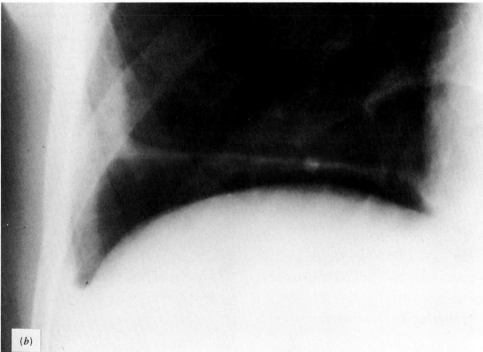

Figure 16-1. (*a*) Blunting of the right lateral costophrenic angle in a pattern indicative of pleural fibrosis. The horizontal shape of the hemidiaphragm does not occur with pleural effusion. (*b*) Air introduced into the abdomen during surgery outlines the undersurface of the hemidiaphragm, confirming the lack of pleural effusion.

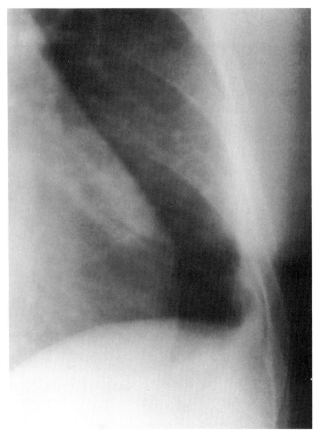

Figure 16-2. Blunting of the left lateral costophrenic sulcus and thickening of the lateral pleural space from pleural fibrosis. This pattern differs from that of pleural effusion because of the distance that the pleural thickening extends above the hemidiaphragm compared with the amount of costophrenic angle blunting present.

PLEURAL CALCIFICATION

The presence of calcification in the pleura is indicative of pleural fibrosis. Figure 16-3 demonstrates the appearance on CT of calcified pleural fibrosis from an old empyema.

BLUNTING OF THE LATERAL COSTOPHRENIC SULCI FROM MARKED LUNG HYPEREXPANSION

Marked lung hyperexpansion and hyperinflation will result in blunting of the lateral costophrenic angles (Fig. 16-4). This occurs in severe chronic obstructive pulmonary disease but can also occasionally be seen in well-trained athletes who take a very deep breath. Blunting of the costophrenic sulcus from lung hyperexpansion can usually be distinguished from pleural effusion and pleural fibrosis because the adjacent hemidiaphragm will show multiple scallops.

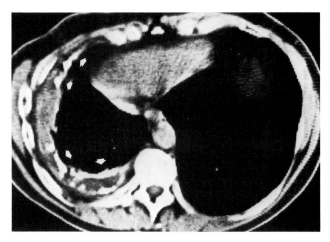

Figure 16-3. Pleural fibrosis with calcification, demonstrated on CT. The thickening of the right pleural space is due to fibrosis. The whiter areas bordering the pleural thickening (arrows) are due to calcification of the fibrosis. (Courtesy of N. Whitley, M.D., University of Maryland Hospital.)

SUMMARY

Pleural fibrosis can often be distinguished from pleural effusion because of its characteristic straighter shape or its extent upward along the lateral chest wall. When the pattern resembles that of pleural effusion, presence of fibrosis can probably be assumed if an old film demonstrates no change in the appearance. Uncommonly, a lateral decubitus view will be necessary to show that free fluid is not present.

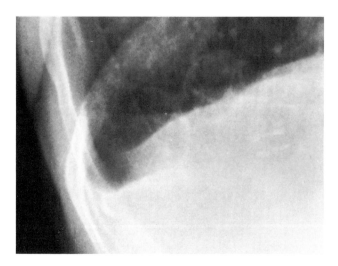

Figure 16-4. Scalloping from hyperinflation. In this patient with severe emphysema, blunting of the right costophrenic angle is present because of marked pressing down on and flattening of the diaphragm. The presence of several scallops in the diaphragm aids in excluding the presence of pleural effusion.

REVIEW QUESTION

1. Describe how the blunting of the lateral costophrenic angle that results from fibrosis is formed.

VOCABULARY

adhesions   splinting

SUGGSTIONS FOR FURTHER READING

For suggested reading see Chapter 7.

17

PNEUMOTHORAX

KEY CONCEPTS

Clinical

Air in the pleural space (a pneumothorax) is a common cause of chest pain and respiratory distress. The clinical effect of a pneumothorax depends on its size and on the underlying lung function. A small pneumothorax in a patient with normal lung function can, without specific treatment, usually be safely followed, watching for increasing size. A small pneumothorax can, however, require urgent treatment if the patient's underlying lung function is compromised. Patients with asthma and COPD can develop pneumothoraces and can show rapid clinical deterioration with even small pneumothoraces.

Large pneumothoraces usually require treatment with a chest tube.

A *tension pneumothorax* is one in which the pressure in the pleural space is increased. This increased pressure can result in mediastinal shift and can interfere with venous return to the heart. When venous return to the heart is decreased, the patient can go into shock and die. A symptomatic tension pneumothorax requires rapid treatment.

Radiological

Small pneumothoraces may be very difficult to recognize because the pleural margin is thin and partially hidden by overlying ribs. A careful search is usually necessary to find it; this search may not be made unless a pneumothorax is suggested by the clinical history.

A tension pneumothorax often results in the mediastinum being shifted away from the side of the pneumothorax. Normal lung will usually collapse in the presence of a tension pneumothorax; lung with air trapping, as in asthma and emphysema, may only partially collapse.

OBJECTIVES

When you complete this chapter you will be able to

1. Identify small, large, and tension pneumothoraces on selected radiographs.
2. List the three signs indicating that a pneumothorax is a tension pneumothorax.
3. Differentiate on selected radiographs among a small pneumothorax, extrapleural fat, and the two types of rib companion shadows.

Case 17-1

Figure 17-1 is the chest radiograph of a 26-year-old woman who experienced the sudden onset of severe shortness of breath and chest pain on the right side. What do you see?

There are almost no lung markings in the right side of the chest, and the heart is shifted into the left side. The patient has a pneumothorax with sufficient pressure in her chest to shift the heart to the opposite side. This type of pneumothorax is called a tension pneumothorax and is a life-threatening emergency. The continued increase of pressure within the pleural space, coupled with the increasing shift of the heart, can decrease venous return to the heart, and the patient can rapidly go into shock and die. The diagnostic features of a tension pneumothorax are

Pneumothorax
Mediastinal shift to the contralateral side
Normal lung (no atelectasis) on the contralateral side

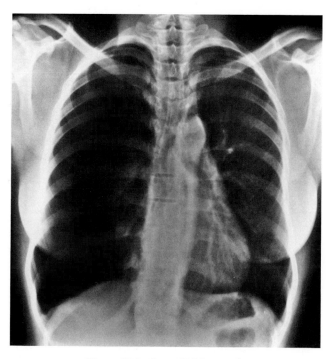

Figure 17-1. Case 17-1 (see text).

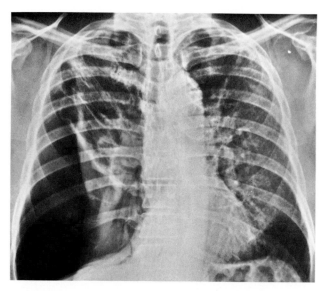

Figure 17-2. Tension pneumothorax with lung and pleural disease. Large blebs are seen in both upper lobes. There is pleural thickening from fibrosis at the right apex, tethering the lung. Despite this tethering, the large pneumothorax at the base of the right chest shifts the heart across the midline into the left side of the chest. This was a spontaneous pneumothorax.

Patients with a pneumothorax on one side and atelectasis on the other will also show a mediastinal shift. When the physical examination is clear-cut and the patient is in severe respiratory distress, treatment should be undertaken without a radiograph. If the patient is stable, a radiograph should be obtained before starting therapy.

Figure 17-2 is the radiograph on a 67-year-old man with pain in the right side of his chest on breathing and with shortness of breath. There is a pneumothorax on the right, but with only limited collapse of the lung. Large blebs are seen in the right and left lungs. The mediastinum is shifted to the left. There is also pleural fibrosis at the right apex that tethers the lung.

This patient also has a tension pneumothorax, but his lung is stiff because of his COPD, and therefore, even the pressure needed to push the mediastinum to the opposite side does not cause complete lung collapse. Patients with COPD already have marginal lung function, and even a small pneumothorax can result in severe distress.

Tension pneumothoraces without complete lung collapse can occur in COPD, asthma, congestive heart failure, interstitial lung fibrosis, and respiratory distress syndrome of the newborn.

THE SMALL PNEUMOTHORAX

The small pneumothorax is detected by recognizing the very thin line of the visceral pleura of the lung bordered by air. Figure 17-3a shows the normal pleural margin, visceral and parietal, with a small amount of extrapleural fat. Figure 17-3b shows the apex of the chest in a patient with a very small pneumothorax. The pleural line is very thin but can be seen with careful study. The major problem in detecting the small pneumothorax is remembering to look for it. Without history, even the best radiologist can miss the pneumothorax. If you think your patient could have a pneumothorax, be certain to mention it on the radiology consultation form.

Some people like to obtain an expiratory film when looking for a pneumothorax. On the expiratory film, the pneumothorax is easier to see for two reasons: the lung is denser in expiration, making it easier to see its margin, and in expiration the air distributes itself closer to the chest apex, making the separation of the lung from the chest wall wider. The expiratory film is almost never necessary. If you look for it, the pneumothorax can be seen or strongly suspected on the inspiratory film. The expiratory film should be obtained only in those cases in which the inspiratory film is equivocal—is the line seen a pleural line or a skin fold? The expiratory radiograph almost always is a waste of film and represents unnecessary x-ray exposure for the patient.

Keynotes

- *A tension pneumothorax is a life-threatening emergency.*
- *A tension pneumothorax can occur without complete collapse of the lung if the lung is stiff.*

Keynote

- *The pleural line bordering a pneumothorax can be seen only with careful study.*

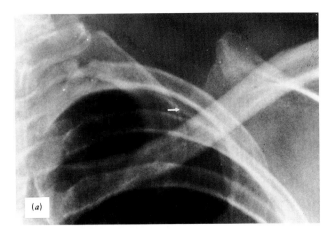

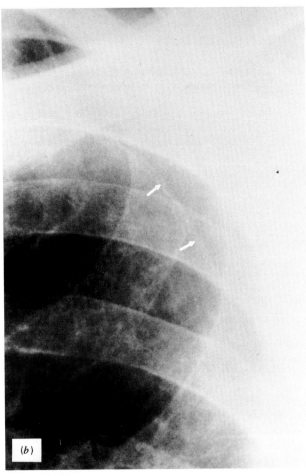

Figure 17-3. (*a*) Normal apical chest appearance. The combined visceral and parietal pleura (arrow) of the lung apex are separated from the chest margin by a radiolucent layer of extrapleural fat. (*b*) Small pneumothorax at the lung apex. The thin line of the visceral pleura of the lung is just visible with air radiolucency above it.

THE PNEUMOTHORAX ON THE SUPINE RADIOGRAPH

Chest radiographs on the sickest patients must be obtained supine because of the patient's inability to sit up. With the patient supine, where do you think the air of a pneumothorax would collect? It collects adjacent to the heart margin and can be recognized as an air radiolucency adjacent to the heart margin (Fig. 17-4). The pneumothorax must be several hundred cubic centimeters in size to be seen by this technique. If small pneumotho-

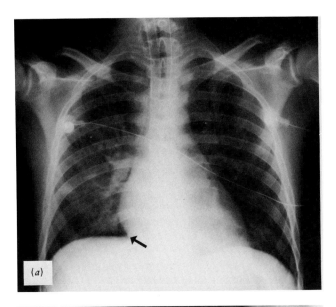

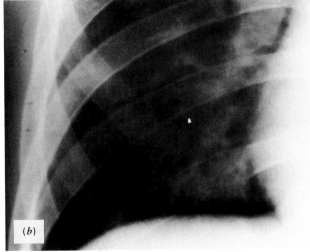

Figure 17-4. Moderate pneumothorax in a supine patient. In the supine position, the free pleural air in the right hemithorax outlines the heart border on the right and the medial portion of the right hemidiaphragm (arrow in *a*). Only moderate-to-large pneumothoraces can be detected on supine radiographs. This pneumothorax resulted from the unsuccessful attempted placement of a subclavian venous line.

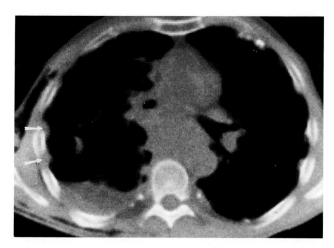

Figure 17-5. CT scan, hydropneumothorax in a patient with pleural metastases of mesothelioma. Air is present in the pleural space on the right, outlining the visceral pleura of the lung. This pneumothorax followed thoracentesis. Pleural nodules are due to the metastases from this malignant mesothelioma (Courtesy N. Whitley, M.D., University of Maryland Hospital.)

races are sought and the patient cannot be examined upright, the best alternate film to obtain is the lateral decubitus chest film positioned to show the edge of the lung that is uppermost.

Keynote

- *The small pneumothorax in the supine patient may be invisible. The large pneumothorax in the supine patient will outline the margin of the heart.*

THE PNEUMOTHORAX ON CT

As on the chest radiograph, the method of identifying a pneumothorax on the chest CT is the identification of the edge of the pleura and the absence of lung markings peripheral to the pleural margin. In Figure 17-5, the pleural edge of the lung is clearly seen in the right hemithorax. No lung markings are seen peripheral to it. Posteriorly, there is a layer of pleural fluid with a sharp interface with the pneumothorax. Compare this finding with the appearance of pleural fluid as shown in Figure 15-5. The horizontal line (called an "air-fluid level") is not seen in a pure hydrothorax and, therefore, is a sign of the coexistence of a pneumothorax and pleural effusion.

The CT scan in Figure 17-5 also demonstrates an additional finding of pleural disease. There are several pleural nodules representing several focal masses of this patient's mesothelioma.

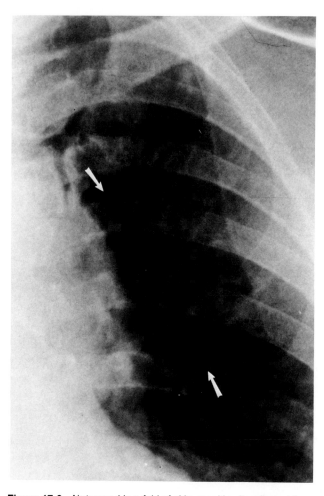

Figure 17-6. Air trapped in a fold of skin, resulting in adjacent lines of radiodensity and radiolucency (arrows). When such lines occur near the edge of the chest, they may simulate pneumothoraces.

RADIODENSITIES SIMULATING PNEUMOTHORAX

Three shadows can be confused with pneumothoraces:

1. One is an extrapleural stripe of fat (shown in Fig. 17-3a), which can be differentiated because the combined band of visceral and parietal pleura is thicker than the single layer of pleura, as shown in Figure 17-3b.
2. Skin folds can also be confused with pneumothoraces, but usually they can be differentiated because of a thick band of radiodensity caused by the thickness of the overfolded skin and subcutaneous tissues adjacent to a line of radiolucency (Fig. 17-6).
3. Companion shadows of ribs can be confused with pneumothoraces. There are two types: a superior-margin skin line that parallels the rib and a more wavy line caused by the lower margin of the flange of the rib (Fig. 17-7). These two shadows can usually be differentiated from a pneumothorax by their simi-

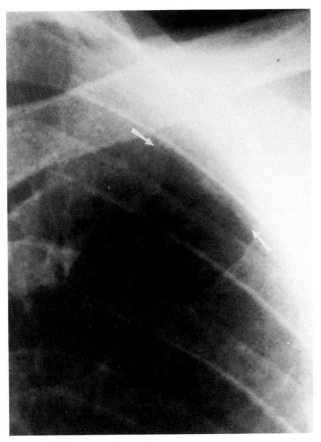

Figure 17-7. A rib companion shadow. The arrows demarcate a rib companion shadow. This shadow is caused by the thin flange at the lower edge of the rib. While it simulates a small pneumothorax, it can usually be differentiated from a pneumothorax because it is parallel to the rib, whereas small pneumothoraces usually run obliquely across the ribs (see Fig. 17-3*b*).

larity of contour to the rib. The contour of the pleural margin in a patient with a pneumothorax does parallel the rib in its medial portion, but laterally the pleural margin usually ceases to be parallel to the rib and parallels the lateral chest wall (Fig. 17-3*b*).

SUMMARY

A small pneumothorax in a patient with healthy lungs is of minimal consequence. The same pneumothorax in a patient with severe lung disease may be life threatening. A large pneumothorax requires immediate treatment. The most important technique for finding the pneumothorax on the radiograph is to look for it. Since they are uncommon and hard to see, it is only by an active search that they can be found. Should you have clinical reasons to suspect a pneumothorax, mention it on the x-ray consultation form to remind both the radiologist and yourself to look for it.

REVIEW QUESTIONS

1. What criteria must be present on a radiograph to diagnose a tension pneumothorax?
2. What is the role of the expiratory chest film in the diagnosis of a pneumothorax?
3. How would you differentiate a skin fold from the pleural line of a pneumothorax?
4. What is the effect of a stiff lung on the appearance of a tension pneumothorax?
5. What is the appearance of a pneumothorax on a supine radiograph?

VOCABULARY

companion shadow   tension pneumothorax
skin folds

SUGGESTIONS FOR FURTHER READING

For suggested reading see Chapter 7.

SECTION C

THE HILUM

The hilum is the most difficult portion of the chest radiograph to evaluate. Composed of vessels, bronchi, and lymph nodes, its variable normal appearance causes many problems for the person attempting to detect its abnormalities. The following chapter attempts to help you differentiate the normal from the abnormal hilum, but remember that even skilled radiologists often have problems evaluating the hili. Be prepared to ask for help when you need it.

18

THE HILUM

KEY CONCEPTS

Clinical

Enlargement of the hilum or hili is abnormal. An increase in the size of the pulmonary veins in the hilum usually indicates the presence of left-sided heart failure or mitral stenosis. Enlargement of one hilum by a mass often indicates the presence of cancer. Enlargement of the hilar lymph nodes often indicates the presence of infection, sarcoidosis, lymphoma, or metastases.

Radiological

The hilum is the portion of the chest in which it is most difficult to differentiate normality from abnormality using imaging techniques. Hilar evaluation is based on criteria of shape, proportionate size, measured size, and radiodensity:

1. Shape. The shape of the normal hilum is that of branching blood vessels. Rounded contours that are not part of vessels may be masses. On CT, contiguous sections may need to be viewed to demonstrate the vascular branching pattern.
2. Proportionate size. On the chest radiograph taken upright, the proportionate size of the hilum is such that the upper portion represents about one-third of the hilar size, the lower portion two-thirds.
3. Absolute size. While there are no absolute measurements, very large hili are usually abnormal. Size measurements are usually not useful in differentiating a normal hilum from a slightly enlarged one.
4. Radiodensity. The radiodensity of the normal hilum reflects the quantity of blood flow through the hilum, and therefore it falls off rapidly as the hilum branches into the upper lobes, more slowly as the hilum branches into the lower lobes. Right and left hilar radiodensity should be similar.

On CT examinations, the radiodensity of the hilum after radiographic contrast administration is an important added criterion. On magnetic resonance imaging, the lack of signal resulting from flowing blood helps in differentiating hilar masses from normal vessels. Abnormalities of the vessels, however, are probably not detectable.

OBJECTIVES

When you complete this chapter you will be able to

1. List the component structures of the hilum and indicate which can be seen by radiographic and CT examinations.
2. Describe the shape, proportionate size, and proportionate radiodensity of the normal hilum.
3. List two main causes of enlargement of the pulmonary veins in the hilum.
4. List one cause of hilar mass and five causes of hilar adenopathy.
5. Differentiate normal from abnormal hili on selected chest radiographs.
6. Differentiate normal from abnormal hili on selected CT sections by comparing the sections with normal sections.

THE NORMAL HILUM ON THE STANDARD CHEST RADIOGRAPH

The normal hilum is composed of pulmonary arteries, pulmonary veins, bronchi, bronchial arteries, lymph nodes, and lymphatic vessels. Of all these structures, only the pulmonary arteries and veins can be identified on the standard radiograph in the normal patient. Showing that only

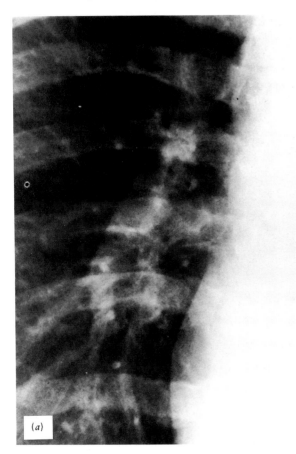 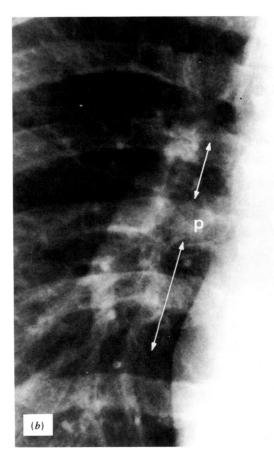

Figure 18-1. (a) Normal right hilum. The vessels can be seen to branch from the central structures into the lung. Note the relationship of the size and radiodensity of the different portions of the hilum. (b) Normal hilum. P-right main pulmonary artery. The one-third/two-thirds, top-to-bottom, proportion of the hilum is indicated with arrows. The differing rates of change in radiodensity above and below the right main pulmonary artery can be observed and compared with subsequent cases.

blood vessels can be identified is the first step in showing that a hilum is normal.

How do you identify the blood vessels that form the hilum? Blood vessels have a characteristic shape; they can be traced toward the periphery, and they show a repetitive branching pattern. The first sign that the hilum is normal is that the margins of the hilum are continuous with structures that branch (Fig. 18-1a).

Anatomically, the lung is larger in the lower chest. With the patient upright, most of the blood flows to the lower lobes. For these reasons, the hilum appears to have most of its substance in the lower portion of the chest: approximately two-thirds of the hilum is below the entry point of the right or left pulmonary artery. This proportionate size is an important criterion of normal (Fig. 18-1b). The right lung receives slightly more blood than the left and is slightly larger. The right hilum is also slightly larger than the left.

Because blood flow is a major component of hilar radiodensity, the normal hilar radiodensity reflects the direction of blood flow (Fig. 18-1). Radiodensity is maximal near the entry of the main pulmonary artery. It falls off

rapidly as the hilum branches into the upper lobe. The branching of the descending pulmonary artery is delayed because of anatomic differences, and there is a segment of the descending pulmonary artery 2–4 cm in length in which the radiodensity is constant until the branching starts. This pattern of radiodensity change is an important determinant of normal.

These three criteria—branching shape, proportional size with two-thirds of hilar substance in the lower lung, and the pattern of radiodensity change—are the main criteria for determining whether a hilum is normal or abnormal. Absolute size is a secondary criterion and is useful only if the hilum is quite large or small. Most subtle masses will not be picked up by detection of size abnormalities.

Keynotes

- *Radiographically, the normal hilum is composed of pulmonary arteries and veins. These are identified by their branching structure.*

- *The top-to-bottom proportion of the hilar substance (one-third/two-thirds) is an important criterion of normal.*

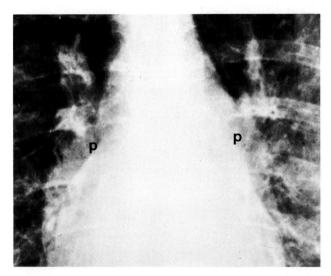

Figure 18-2. Abnormal hili (see text). P-approximate location of the right and left main pulmonary arteries.

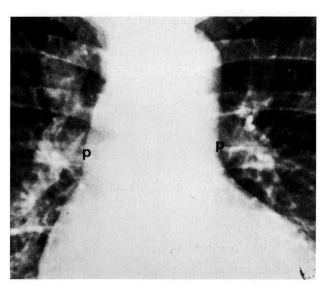

Figure 18-3. Abnormal hilum (see text). P- right and left main pulmonary arteries.

- *The radiodensity of the normal hilum is proportionate to the local blood flow. This radiodensity decreases rapidly toward the top of the hilum and more slowly in the lower portion.*

PATTERNS OF ABNORMALITY

What is wrong with the hili in Figure 18-2? The upper portions are larger, and the upper radiodensity does not fall of as rapidly, but the shape is still the branching shape of blood vessels. This pattern is indicative of increased blood in the upper lungs. This can occur with the patient supine, but if the patient is upright, as in this case, it indicates increased venous pressure.

Anatomically, the upper lung veins contribute their structure to the upper portion of the hilum. The lower lung veins, however, cross inferior to the hilum to reach the left atrium. For this reason, increased venous distention increases the size and radiodensity of the upper portion of the hilum but (at least initially) has little effect on the lower portion. As the venous pressure increases sufficiently, however, the vessels to the lower lung vasoconstrict, accentuating this upward shift of the hilar proportion.

Which processes increase pulmonary venous pressure?

Left-sided congestive heart failure
Mitral stenosis or insufficiency
Left atrial myxoma
Cor triatriatum
Pulmonary venous occlusive disease
Fibrosing mediastinitis

The first two are the most common.

What is wrong with the hila in Figure 18-3? The upper portion of the right hilum is larger; the left is normal. The pattern on the right is not definitely a branching shape. The top to bottom and right to left proportionate sizes are abnormal. The shape is abnormal.

This pattern is indicative of a mass lesion adjacent to the hilum. A mass above the hilum will extend its shadow upward, changing the hilum's proportion and decreasing the rapid falloff in radiodensity normally seen in the upper portion of the hilum. In this case, the pattern was due to a bronchial lesion, bronchogenic carcinoma.

A mass lower in the hilum will increase the radiodensity of that portion of the hilum and, if large enough, will change the hilum's contour as well (as in Figs. 18-4 and 18-5).

What is wrong with the hili in Figure 18-6? The hili are large and lumpy. There are many rounded shadows, none of which seem to extend into branching shadows. Indeed, the branching shadows can be seen faintly superimposed on the rounded shadows. This is the appearance of marked adenopathy. Figures 18-7 and 18-8 demonstrate the appearance of lesser degrees of adenopathy. See the differentials for bilateral and unilateral adenopathy:

Bilateral Hilar Adenopathy

Sarcoid
Lymphoma
Viral infections
    Adenovirus
    Infectious mononucleosis
Metastases from
    Oat cell carcinoma
    Renal cell cancer
    Melanoma
    Breast cancer

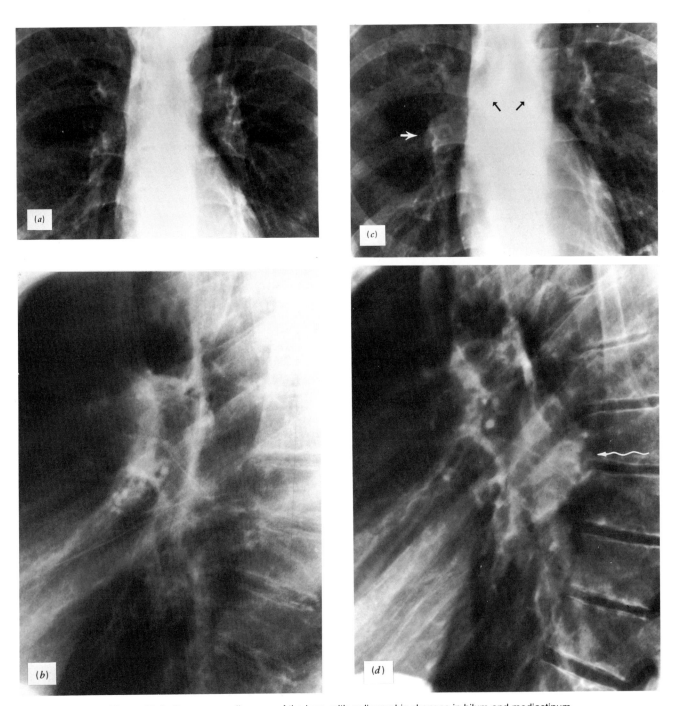

Figure 18-4. Squamous cell cancer of the lung, with radiographic changes in hilum and mediastinum developing over an 11-month period. (*a, b*) PA and lateral views of essentially normal hili and mediastinum. (*c, d*) PA and lateral views 11 months later. There is a focal area of increased radiodensity and a more rounded contour to the midportion of the right hilum (*c*, white arrow). There is increased radiodensity and slight widening of the angle between the right and left bronchi (*c*, two black arrows). On the lateral view, a new mass can be seen lying between the hilar shadow and the spine (*d*, white wavy arrow).

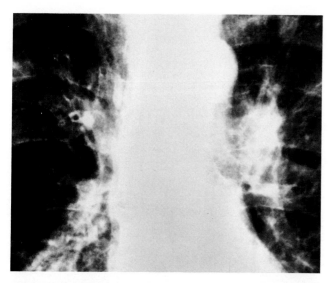

Figure 18-5. Left hilar lymph node mass from oat cell cancer of the lung. The increased radiodensity of the left hilum and its somewhat rounded shape are indicative of the enlarged hilar lymph node. Comparisons of the two sides is most helpful in detecting hilar abnormalities.

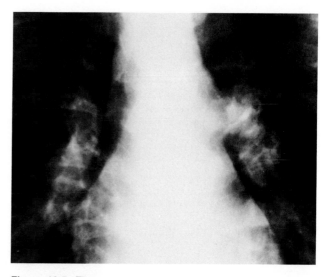

Figure 18-7. There are smaller rounded lymph nodes in this 18-year-old patient with sarcoid. The nodes can be detected because the contour of the hili is not that of branching vessels alone but contains the rounded contours of lymph nodes.

Unilateral Hilar Adenopathy

Primary tuberculosis

Atypical mycobacterial infection

Tularemia

Lymphoma

Sarcoid

Metastases (see above)

Hili in Congenital Heart Disease and Pulmonary Hypertension

In certain types of congenital heart disease, the blood flow through the lungs may be decreased or increased. When this change in flow is great enough, the hilar size will reflect the abnormal level of flow, being small when the flow is markedly decreased and large if the flow is markedly increased. When pulmonary arterial hypertension is present, the hilar vessels will be enlarged, but the peripheral vessels remain small. In each of these cases, although the hili will appear abnormal in size, their shape will still

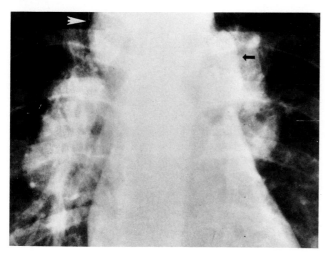

Figure 18-6. Sarcoid with adenopathy in both hili and the mediastinum. The hili are rounded and lumpy. There is a bulge in the left side of the mediastinum near the pulmonary artery (black arrow) caused by adenopathy, and there is widening of the right paratracheal region (white arrow), also from adenopathy.

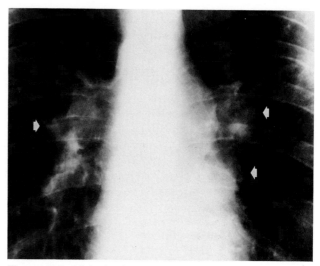

Figure 18-8. Minimal adenopathy in the hili. There are several rounded areas (arrows) in the hili that represent minimal adenopathy in this 32-year-old man with sarcoid.

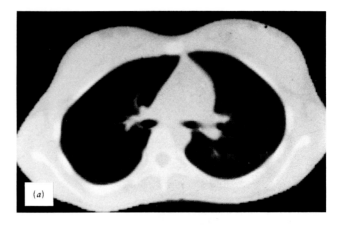

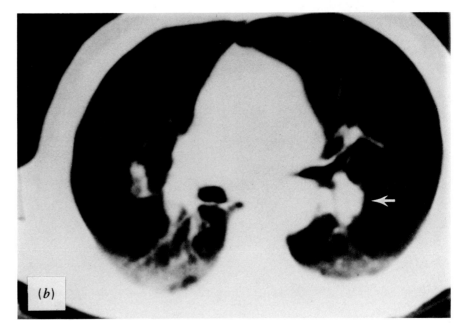

Figure 18-9. (a) A CT scan through normal hili, demonstrating the normal size and appearance of the hilar vessels and lung vessels at this level. (b) A CT scan through approximately the same level in a 56-year-old man. In comparison, the pulmonary arteries are substantially larger (because of pulmonary arterial hypertension), the lung vessels are more widely spaced (as they course around lung bullae), and there is an extra radiodensity (arrow) in the posterior left hilum (representing a primary squamous cell lung cancer arising in a hilar bronchus).

be that of branching vessels with no additional contour changes. These patterns of vascular change are more completely discussed in Chapter 22.

Keynotes

- *The pulmonary veins contribute to the shape of the upper portion of the hilum but bypass the lower portion.*
- *A hilar mass may change the proportionate size of the hilum.*
- *A hilar mass may increase the hilar radiodensity focally or diffusely.*
- *Chronic changes in blood flow and chronic increases in pulmonary arterial pressure can change the size of the pulmonary vessels in the hilum. Increased flow and increased pressure increase the hilar vessel size; decreased flow decreases the hilar vessel size.*

THE CT SCAN IN THE DIAGNOSIS OF HILAR ABNORMALITIES

Both traditional and computed tomography can be of use in confirming or excluding the presence of hilar masses. The principle used is the same as that used on the conventional chest radiograph: a questioned area must be shown to be neither a pumonary artery nor a pulmonary vein. On CT this is done by knowing the precise anatomy of the vessels of the hili and their relationship to the hilar bronchi.

This CT anatomy is complex and beyond the scope of this book; the student can, however, evaluate CT studies of the hili by comparing a suspected abnormal section with a section from a normal patient taken at the same level. As an example of the technique, compare the normal section in Figure 18-9a with the patient's section shown in Figure 18-9b. What abnormalities and differences do you see?

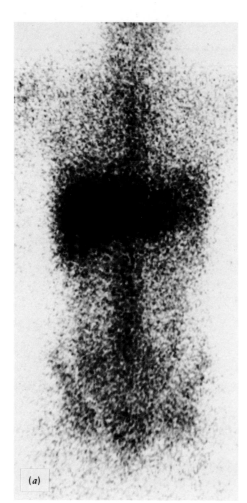 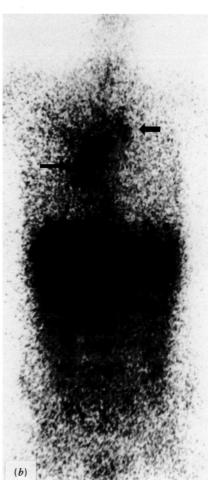

Figure 18-10. (a) A ^{67}Ga scan of a normal torso. The band of increased radiodensity in the center of the image is the liver activity. (b) A ^{67}Ga scan of the torso in a patient with lymphoma being evaluated for the extent of disease. Increased activity is seen in the hili and mediastinum (arrows) as well as in the area just below the liver. These areas of increased activity represent areas of lymphoma in lymph nodes.

Comparing the two figures, the pulmonary arteries are larger in Figure 18-9b, the lung vessels are distorted as they pass around pulmonary bullae, and there is a mass lying just posterior to the left hilum. This patient has severe emphysema that distorts the lung vessels, large pulmonary arteries from pulmonary arterial hypertension, and a bronchogenic cancer lying just posterior to the left pulmonary artery.

When it is not possible to decide whether a possible hilar mass seen on CT is a mass or a vessel, sometimes the problem can be solved by the rapid injection of intravenous contrast medium, a medicine that will make the blood vessels more opaque.

Keynotes

- *Comparison of a known normal with a suspected abnormal CT scan can assist the novice in interpreting CT scans of the hili.*
- *The rapid injection of radiographic contrast medium can opacify hilar vessels sufficiently so that they can be differentiated from hilar masses.*

MAGNETIC RESONANCE IMAGING AND THE HILUM

As MRI techniques become defined and as more machines become available, it seems likely that MRI will play an important role in the evaluation of the possible hilar mass. Currently, the likely application seems to be in the evaluation of the hilum still not adequately evaluated by CT. Magnetic resonance imaging has a major advantage over CT in differentiating vessels from masses because, with properly selected imaging parameters, a flow-void phenomenon is seen. This flow-void phenomenon is an absence of signal coming from flowing blood because the protons in the blood that have been aligned and then perturbed by the machine will have flowed away from the imaged slice during the time needed for imaging. This will leave a void of image signal where blood is flowing. Because no flow occurs in solid masses, masses can be easily differentiated from vessels. One of the likely applications of MRI will therefore be the evaluation of the equivocal hilar mass, with its use probably being limited to those patients with an equivocal CT scan.

Keynote

• *The flow-void phenomenon on MRI is the result of blood flowing out of and into the imaging field between the tissue activation and tissue-emitting phases of imaging. Because the blood in the image field is not activated (because new, nonactivated blood has replaced the activated blood that had been in the field), no imaging signal is received from flowing blood, and the image is therefore black or void of signal.*

NUCLEAR MEDICINE TECHNIQUES IN THE EVALUATION OF HILAR AND MEDIASTINAL MASSES

Nuclear medicine techniques play only a limited role in the evaluation of the hili and mediastinum. Gallium 67 imaging can demonstrate increased hilar and mediastinal uptake in most patients with hilar and mediastinal lymphoma and in some patients with metastatic lung cancer. Though not commonly used to evaluate a known or suspected mass, ^{67}Ga imaging is used for the staging of lymphoma. Figure 18-10*a* is a ^{67}Ga scan of a normal torso. The area of increased activity in the midtorso is from activity in the liver and spleen. In Figure 18-10*b,* the area of increased activity in the midchest is from hilar and mediastinal adenopathy in a patient with lymphoma.

SUMMARY

The evaluation of the hili for masses depends on differentiating a mass from a normal hilar blood vessel. On the standard chest radiograph, look for the normal branching pattern of vessels, the radiodensity changes reflecting the predominant lower lobe direction of blood flow, the proportionate top-to-bottom size of one-third to two-thirds, and the right-to-left hilar proportions (right slightly larger than left). Overall size alone is not an adequate criterion. On CT, the same criteria apply, but it is easier for the novice to compare normal CT sections to the equivalent sections of the patient being studied.

As sufficient machines become available, it is likely that MRI will have a limited, but important, role in the evaluation of the hilum still equivocal after CT scanning. The flow-void phenomenon will prove most useful in the evaluation of suspected hilar masses.

REVIEW QUESTIONS

1. What is the shape of the normal hilum?
2. What are the potential effects of a small mass on the radiodensity of the hilum?
3. What is the effect of mitral valve stenosis on the appearance of the hilum?
4. What are the common causes of bilateral hilar adenopathy? Of unilateral hilar adenopathy?
5. What types of processes can change the size of the pulmonary arteries?
6. How might you determine whether a hilum seen on a CT image is normal or abnormal?
7. What is the flow-void phenomenon?

VOCABULARY

cor triatriatum	mitral stenosis
infectious mononucleosis	oat cell carcinoma
left atrial myxoma	sarcoidosis
lymphoma	tularemia
melanoma	

SUGGESTIONS FOR FURTHER READING

Robert G. Levitt, et al. Magnetic resonance imaging of mediastinal and hilar masses: Comparison with CT. *American Journal of Roentgenology,* **145:**9–14, 1985.

Gary M. Glazer et al. Imaging the pulmonary hilum: A prospective comparative study in patients with lung cancer. *American Journal of Roentgenology,* **145:**245–248, 1985.

For additional suggested reading see Chapter 7.

SECTION D

The Heart

The next six chapters discuss the imaging methods used in evaluating the patient with heart disease. Chapter 19 is a guide to the proper selection of imaging techniques. In it are described the advantages and disadvantages of each technique. Chapter 20 discusses the application of nuclear medicine imaging to heart disease. Chapter 21 discusses in depth echocardiography, including techniques of ultrasonography beyond those described in Chapter 6.

Chapters 22, 23, and 24 discuss the evaluation of heart disease on the chest radiograph. Chapter 22 describes the changes in pulmonary vascularity seen in the patient with heart disease. Chapter 23 discusses the findings in the patient with diseased cardiac valves. Chapter 24 describes the findings in patients with cardiac chamber or generalized cardiac enlargement.

19

THE HEART: METHODS OF STUDY

KEY CONCEPTS

Clinical

Each of the methods for evaluating the heart has specific advantages and disadvantages. Selecting among the techniques is based on a careful history and physical examination.

The physical examination is best for the detection of heart murmurs and is useful in the evaluation of heart size, right-sided heart failure, and alveolar pulmonary edema.

The electrocardiogram is best for the evaluation of conduction disturbances and muscular hypertrophy and can be useful or misleading in the evaluation of myocardial ischemia.

The standard radiograph is best for the evaluation of left-sided heart failure and can be used to estimate pulmonary venous pressure. It can be used to screen cardiac size and chamber enlargement and may be abnormal with valvular disease.

Conventional radiographic angiography is best for coronary artery anatomy and in the evaluation of cardiac shunts and malformations. This last application may be replaced by MRI.

Echocardiography is best for the evaluation of pericardial effusions, cardiac valve disease, and idiopathic hypertrophic subaortic stenosis. It partially evaluates cardiac chamber enlargement.

Nuclear medicine imaging is best for evaluating the location of cardiac ischemia, for localizing myocardial infarcts, and for estimating the ejection fraction.

OBJECTIVES

When you complete this chapter and Chapters 20–24 you will be able to

1. List the major indications for use of each of the methods of imaging the heart.
2. Describe the method for the evaluation of patients with

a. Intermittent cardiac chest pain.
b. A suspected acute myocardial infarct.
c. Suspected mitral or aortic valve stenosis.
d. Palpitations.
e. Suspected heart failure.
f. Suspected pericarditis.
g. Suspected idiopathic subaortic stenosis.

There are many methods available for evaluating cardiac function and disease. Selection of the appropriate one for your patient depends on a careful assessment of the patient's clinical history and a knowledge of the capabilities of each method of study.

As in much of medicine, a careful clinical history is the foundation of all subsequent studies. Physical examination, the standard radiograph, radiographic angiography, heart catheterization, cardiac ultrasound imaging, nuclear medicine imaging, angiography, and electrocardiography each has its proper place in accurate diagnosis. The information sought may be anatomic detail or evidence of physiological disturbance. Each modality of study is detailed below.

Keynote

- *The choice of imaging study should be based on the clinical history and physical examination.*

PHYSICAL EXAMINATION

    Best for
        Detection of murmurs
            (Indicators of valvular disease and shunts)
    Useful for evaluation of
        Heart size
        Right-sided heart failure
        Alveolar pulmonary edema (severe left-sided heart
            failure)
    Sometimes useful for
        Pericardial effusion
        Conduction disturbances

Keynote

• *The physical examination is of major use in detection of murmurs and in the estimation of heart size.*

ELECTROCARDIOGRAM

    Best for
        Conduction disturbances
        Muscular hypertrophy
        Ischemia
        Acute pericarditis
    Useful in evaluation of
        Heart size

Keynote

• *The electrocardiogram is of major use in the detection of conduction disturbances and often demonstrates muscle hypertrophy and myocardial ischemia.*

STANDARD RADIOGRAPH

    Best for
        Left-sided heart failure
        Estimate of pulmonary venous pressure
        Chamber enlargement (especially of the left atrium)
        Cardiac size
        Valvular disease
            Especially valvular calcification
        Large shunts
    Useful for
        Size of right and left venticles
    Not useful for evaluation of
        Myocardial ischemia
        Muscular hypertrophy

Keynote

• *The main use of the chest radiograph is in the detection of left-sided heart failure.*

CONVENTIONAL RADIOGRAPHIC ANGIOGRAPHY

    Best for
        Coronary artery anatomy
        Shunt anatomy
        Chamber anatomy
        Complex congenital malformations
    Useful for
        Valvular anatomy
            Size of opening
        Degree of muscular contraction
        Ejection fraction
        Constrictive pericarditis

Keynote

• *The main use of cardiac angiography is in the evaluation of the coronary arteries.*

HEART CATHETERIZATION WITH PRESSURE MEASUREMENTS AND/OR DYE DILUTION CURVES

    Best for
        Degree of valvular stenosis
        Size of shunt flow
        Estimate of cardiac output and ejection fraction

CARDIAC ULTRASOUND (ECHOCARDIOGRAPHY)

    Gives information on
        Pericardial effusion
        Constrictive pericarditis
        Wall motion
        Valve motion
        Idiopathic hypertrophic subaortic stenosis

Keynote

• *Cardiac ultrasound is used most often in the evaluation for pericardial effusions and valvular abnormalities.*

NUCLEAR MEDICINE IMAGING

    Gives information on
        Vascular supply to heart (regions perfused)

Regions of ischemia
Myocardial wall contractility
Estimate of ejection fraction

Keynote

• *Nuclear medicine imaging is used mainly in evaluating areas of myocardial ischemia and for calculation of the ejection fraction.*

NUCLEAR MEDICINE IMAGING FLOW STUDY

Gives information on
Moderate-to-large intracardiac and extracardiac shunts

CLINICAL CHEMISTRY

Gives information on
Infarction (enzymes serum glutamic-oxaloacetic trans aminase (SGOT), creatine phosphokinase (CPK), LDH)
Interstitial edema (decreased arterial Po_2)

MAGNETIC RESONANCE IMAGING

The future clinical role for MRI of the heart is uncertain. Because of the excellent demonstration of the walls of the heart and of the great vessels that results from the flow-void effect of flowing blood in the heart chambers and great vessels, MRI seems likely to prove of great benefit in the evaluation of congenital abnormalities of cardiac structure. (see Chapter 5) While additional applications are likely to be developed, the further clinical role of MRI of the heart is uncertain.

SUMMARY

The advantages and disadvantages of the common methods used for evaluating cardiac function and anatomy have been briefly reviewed. The imaging techniques—nuclear medicine imaging, echocardiography, and radiography are discussed in more detail in the next five chapters.

REVIEW QUESTIONS

1. List the major uses of the following methods of imaging the heart:
   a. The chest radiograph
   b. Radiographic angiography
   c. Cardiac ultrasound
   d. Nuclear medicine imaging
   e. Magnetic resonance imaging

2. Describe the method of evaluation of a patient with
   a. Intermittent cardiac chest pain
   b. Suspected mitral or aortic valve stenosis
   c. Palpitations
   d. Left-sided heart failure

VOCABULARY

cardiac ejection fraction	LDH
constrictive pericarditis	myocardial ischemia
CPK	pericarditis
electrocardiogram	SGOT
idiopathic hypertrophic subaortic stenosis	

SUGGESTIONS FOR FURTHER READING FOR CHAPTERS 19 TO 24

A Textbook of Radiological Diagnosis, 5th Ed. Vol. 2, *The Cardiovascular System*, John B. Partridge (Ed.). W.B. Saunders: Philadelphia. 1985.

Marvin L. Daves. *Cardiac Roentgenology*. Year Book Medical Publishers: Chicago. 1981.

Charles B. Higgins. Overview of M.R. of the heart. *American Journal of Roentgenology,* **146:**907–918, 1986.

20

NUCLEAR MEDICINE IMAGING OF THE HEART

KEY CONCEPTS

Clinical

Radiotracers image the heart using three different methods: blood pool imaging, in which blood cells or plasma are labeled; myocardial perfusion studies, in which an agent extracted from the blood by heart muscle is used to demonstrate the portions of heart muscle being perfused; and myocardial infarct imaging, in which agents that bind to necrotic heart muscle are used.

Blood pool imaging is used to measure the ejection fraction of the heart by measuring the radioactivity of the left ventricle in systole and diastole and calculating

$$\text{Estimated ejection fraction} = \frac{\text{Diastole activity} - \text{Systole activity}}{\text{diastole activity}}$$

Usually, the measured activity is averaged over many cardiac cycles, a method called a *MUGA scan*. MUGA stands for *MU*lti-*G*ated *A*cquisition.

In some cases a single pass is recorded looking for intracardiac shunts.

Myocardial perfusion studies are usually performed with thalium 201, an agent extracted from blood by heart muscle activity. The method is usually used to look for myocardial ischemia during an exercise stress test.

Myocardial infarct studies use agents that attach to regions of injured tissue. They permit confirmation that a recent infarction has taken place and permit localization of the infarct.

OBJECTIVES

When you complete this chapter you will be able to

1. Calculate the ejection fraction, given the measurements obtained during a MUGA scan.
2. Define *MUGA* and explain what the letters in it mean.
3. List the clinical uses of blood pool cardiac scans, myocardial perfusion scans, and infarct scans.
4. List the agents used for blood pool scans, myocardial perfusion scans, and infarct scans.

Three different methods are used in nuclear medicine imaging of the heart:

Blood pool imaging of the left ventricular cavity
Myocardial perfusion imaging
Myocardial infarction imaging

BLOOD POOL IMAGING OF THE LEFT VENTRICULAR CAVITY

The blood pool within the body can be imaged either by labeling the plasma, by injecting technetium Te 99m albumen aggregates, or by labeling red blood cells. Because the chambers of the heart contain more blood per unit volume than their surrounding organs, it is possible to image the chambers. The left ventricle is usually the chamber chosen for careful evaluation.

156

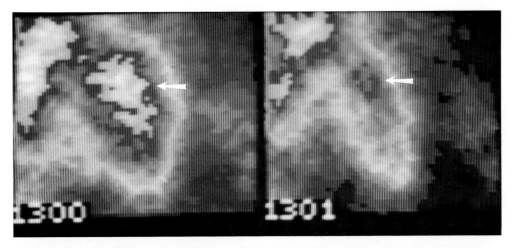

Figure 20-1. Two frames from a MUGA scan: left, diastole; right, systole. The intense white area on the central portion of the end-diastolic image (left arrow) represents intense radioactivity in the left ventricular chamber. On the end-systolic view (right) the intense activity is gone. The darker area (arrow) represents residual activity in the left ventricular cavity. The ejection fraction can be estimated by comparing the two images. (Courtesy of M. Vaccaro, M.D.)

MUGA Study: Measuring the Ejection Fraction

The more commonly performed studies using blood pool imaging are called MUGA studies. The *MUltiGated Acquisition* studies are obtained by using a simultaneous electrocardiogram to select the times during the cardiac cycle when data will be recorded (the electrocardiogram opens and closes the gate for the recording of data). In general, images from multiple cardiac cycles are accumulated, with separate recordings being made for end systole and end diastole.

These images of left ventricular chamber volume and shape obtained when the ventricular volume is at its largest and smallest size are then used to measure the ejection fraction of blood from the ventricle and to look for regions of the ventricular wall with abnormally decreased or paradoxical motion. Figure 20-1 demonstrates images of the heart obtained at end systole and end diastole. The radioactivity in the region of the left ventricle in each cardiac phase can be measured. The ejection fraction is equal to the activity of

$$\text{estimated EF} = \frac{\text{Diastole} - \text{Systole}}{\text{diastole}}$$

The Single-Pass Image

Blood pool imaging is also used in single-pass studies. The passage of a radiotracer through the cardiac chambers can be imaged and is useful in looking for intracardiac shunts. A normal single-pass image is shown in Figure 20-2.

Keynote

• MUGA stands for multigated acquisition. In the MUGA study, multiple cardiac cycles are recorded. These are matched up by cuing the image recorder to record only during selected portions of the cardiac cycle. This cuing is controlled by the electrocardiogram.

MYOCARDIAL PERFUSION IMAGING

Thalium 201 injected intravenously will accumulate in regions of the myocardium with normal blood perfusion. The test for regions of myocardial ischemia is usually performed by injecting the ^{201}Tl at a time of maximal exercise stress, then making an image. Regions of decreased perfusion show as defects in the ringlike structure of the left ventricle (Fig. 20-3a). If a defect is found, the image is repeated 4 hours later, when redistribution of the isotope will have occurred. If the site of decreased ^{201}Tl has become active, there was transient ischemia of that portion of the heart segment (Fig. 20-3b); if the site of decreased ^{201}Tl activity remains decreased, the ischemia is fixed— and represents a region of old or new infarction.

Keynotes

• Thalium^{201} will accumulate in regions of the myocardium with normal blood flow.

• The injection of ^{201}Tl during periods of maximal exercise stress will demonstrate regions of transient myocardial ischemia.

MYOCARDIAL INFARCT IMAGING

Technetium 99m phosphate complexes accumulate in regions of bone turnover and in regions of tissue necrosis. Usually used as a bone-scanning agent, technetium can

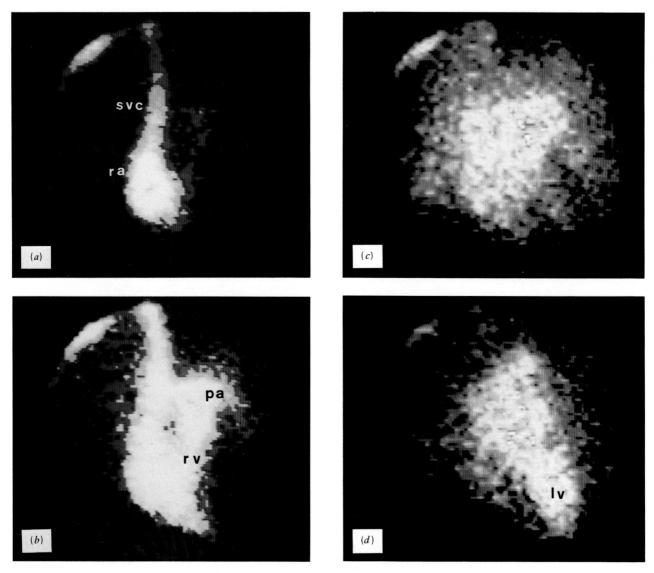

Figure 20-2. Image of a single pass of radioactivity through the heart. Sequential images: (a) superior vena cava (svc) and right atrium (ra), (b) right ventricle (rv) and pulmonary artery (pa) added to image in a of superior vena cava and right atrium, (c) activity in the lungs, (d) activity in the left ventricle (lv). (Courtesy of M. Vaccaro, M.D.)

also be used to imaged regions of tissue necrosis such as sites of myocardial infarction (Fig. 20-4). Its usual use is to further evaluate regions of persistently decreased ^{201}Tl activity seen during myocardial perfusion imaging. Foci of persistent decreased ^{201}Tl activity that accumulate activity with ^{99m}Tc phosphate complexes are regions of acute infarction. Regions without ^{99m}Tc phosphate complex uptake are regions of old infarction.

Keynote

• *Technetium Tc 99m pyrophosphate will accumulate in regions of tissue necrosis such as regions of acute myocardial infarction.*

NUCLEAR MEDICINE IMAGING STUDIES' CLINICAL ROLE IN THE EVALUATION OF CARDIAC DISEASE

These techniques are recent developments in the science of imaging, and their precise clinical role is still being defined. They can be of great use in the following situations.

1. Suspected cardiac angina with a normal stress electrocardiogram
2. Atypical chest pain, possibly cardiac in origin; normal stress electrocardiogram
3. Suspected cardiac angina, patient unable to achieve maximal exercise during stress electrocardiogram

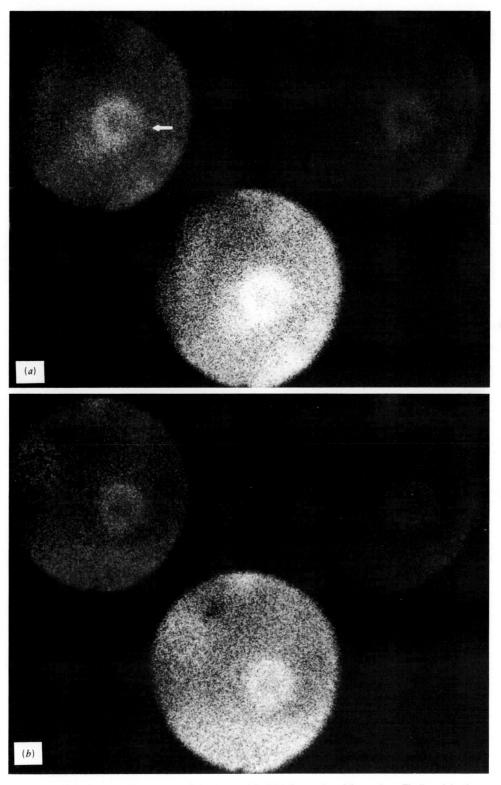

Figure 20-3. Thalium 201 images of the heart. (*a*) 40° left anterior oblique view. Thalium injection during maximal exercise stress. The three images are obtained with different intensity settings, but all are simultaneous. A defect is seen in the ring near the cardiac apex (arrow), indicating a region of decreased perfusion. (*b*) Repeat image obtained 2 hours later shows filling in of the ring with normal activity, indicating that the process affecting the heart resulted in ischemia that was transitory. (Courtesy of M. Vaccaro, M.D.)

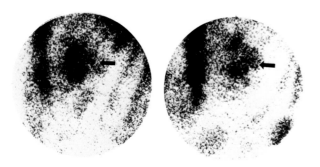

Figure 20-4. Technetium Tc99m MDP (phosphate complex) image of the myocardium with increased activity indicating a large infarct (arrow). The vertical dark band to the left of the images is the sternum. The oblique dark bands are the ribs. (Courtesy of M. Vaccaro, M.D.)

because of fatigue or for other reasons; normal stress electrocardiogram

4. Suspected cardiac angina or infarction in a patient in whom a cardiac conduction defect decreases the ability of the electrocardiogram to detect ischemia or infarction.

Summary

Three different methods are used for nuclear medicine imaging of the heart: blood pool imaging, myocardial perfusion imaging, and myocardial infarction imaging. There are two types of blood pool imaging: the single-pass technique, useful in the evaluation of intracardiac shunts, and the MUGA scan, useful in the evaluation of ventricular wall motion and in the estimation of the ejection fraction. Myocardial perfusion imaging is done with ^{201}Tl, an isotope that is actively concentrated in myocardial cells. Images obtained during exercise can demonstrate regions of ischemia.

Myocardial infarction imaging is done with technetium Tc99m pyrophosphate, an agent that accumulates in regions of tissue necrosis. It can be used to image acute myocardial infarcts.

REVIEW QUESTIONS

1. What are the main techniques for nuclear medicine imaging of the heart?
2. What does MUGA mean?
3. What is a MUGA scan?
4. Describe the single-pass technique of cardiac imaging.
5. How can nuclear medicine images be used to show regions of myocardial ischemia?
6. How can nuclear medicine images be used to show regions of myocardial infarction?
7. How would you differentiate an infarct from a region of myocardial ischemia using only ^{201}Tl as your tracer?

VOCABULARY

blood pool scan
ejection fraction
infarct scan

MUGA scan
single-pass technique

SUGGESTIONS FOR FURTHER READING

For suggested reading see Chapter 19.

21

ECHOCARDIOGRAPHY

YU-CHEN LEE

KEY CONCEPTS

Clinical

Echocardiography is the evaluation of the heart using high-frequency sound waves. It is an important noninvasive method for looking at the heart valves, muscle wall thickness, and motion, chamber size, and at thrombi and tumors. It is the procedure of choice in evaluating patients for pericardial effusion, and various congenital heart diseases.

Imaging

Two different methods of imaging the heart are in common use. The traditional method of echocardiography uses a continuous-strip recording of cardiac motion, called an *M-mode display*. This method provides much information about the heart, but its image does not resemble the anatomic shape of the heart and is thus more difficult to learn and interpret. The newer method is a two-dimensional image of the heart that more closely resembles cardiac anatomy.

In addition to the two imaging methods, Doppler evaluation of flow velocity can be added to the image, aiding in interpretation.

The intravenous injection of saline or indocyanine increases the echoes in the heart chambers and can be used to evaluate for abnormal pathways of blood flow. The usefulness of these methods is greatly enhanced by Doppler color flow mapping.

OBJECTIVES

When you complete this chapter you will be able to

1. Describe the differences between an M-mode and a two-dimensional echocardiogram.

2. Differentiate a normal mitral valve echogram from one revealing mitral stenosis or mitral valve prolapse.

3. Identify the cardiac structure on an M-mode echogram and two-dimensional echograms.

4. Diagnose aortic stenosis on selected two-dimensional echograms.

5. Diagnose valvular vegetations on selected M-mode and two-dimensional echograms.

6. Identify an atrial myxoma on M-mode and two-dimensional echograms.

7. Identify pericardial effusions on selected M-mode and two-dimensional echograms.

8. Measure cardiac chamber size and wall thickness and identify wall motion abnormalities.

Echocardiography has become an important diagnostic tool in cardiovascular diseases. It is based on the use of sonar, which was developed between the first and second world wars for detection of underwater objects.

Using sound waves to locate cardiac structures and to study their motions was first attempted by Inge Edler and his colleagues in Sweden during the early 1950s. It was not until the 1970s, however, when a major technological breakthrough took place, that echocardiography became a routine diagnostic procedure. This chapter describes some of the basic principles of ultrasound and presents some typical examples that show the usefulness of echocardiography.

BASIC PRINCIPLES

Ultrasound has a frequency greater than 20,000 c/s and is inaudible to the human ear. Echocardiography uses ultra-

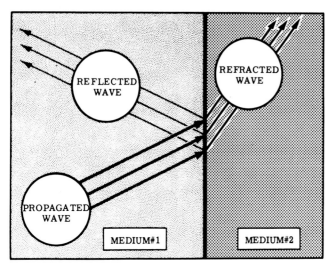

Figure 21-1. Ultrasound is reflected and refracted by an interface between two media of different acoustic impedance. The amount of ultrasound reflected or refracted depends upon the angle at which the ultrasound beam hits the interface. (From Feigenbaum H.: *Echocardiography,* 2nd Ed. Reproduced by permission of Lea & Febiger, Philadelphia, 1976.)

sound of 2–5 *mega hertz* (1 mH = 1,000,000 cs). Generation and detection of ultrasound is carried out by a *transducer,* which contains a *piezoelectric crystal*. This crystal possesses a property of being able to convert electrical energy into sound waves and vice versa. The echocardiographic transducer transmits very brief ultrasound pulses, each 1 microsecond in duration, at a rate of approximately 1,000/ s, which enables a discrete echo to return. The ultrasound beam is directed toward the area to be studied. Part of an ultrasonic wave is reflected whenever it crosses a boundary between tissues having different *acoustic impedances* (Fig. 21-1). The time delay between transmission of the wave and the return of the echo depends on the propagation velocity and the path length. The velocity of sound is fairly constant for human soft tissues. The distance from the transmission point to the reflecting boundary can be determined automatically by measuring the echo delay.

An oscilloscope is used to display the ultrasound echoes. Initially, permanent records that duplicate the oscilloscopic image were obtained by taking a Polaroid photographs. To overcome the disadvantage of being able to record only a few cardiac cycles at a time, it is now universal practice to use a continuous-strip chart recorder, which is commonly known as M-mode display. This display plots distance against time and records signals from moving cardiac structures as wavy lines. Although extremely useful clinically, the recording obtained by the M-mode display provides what has been referred to as "an icepick view of the heart," for it does not resemble the actual configuration of the heart. More recently, real-time two-dimensional echocardiography, which provides spatial anatomic information about cardiac structures, has been developed, and recordings from these newer systems resemble heart structures.

The two commonly used imaging systems are mechanical sector scanners and electronically steered or phased-array sector scanners. A mechanical sector scanner uses a rotating scan head that contains a single or multiple transducers spinning around inside a small dome filled with liquid. As each transducer passes over the scan head, it transmits pulses and receives echoes. The echo signals are displayed on the oscilloscope (Fig. 21-2). The phased-array sector scanner is the most advanced type; it steers the ultrasound beam electronically without moving the transducer.

Keynotes

- *1 Hz = 1 c/s. 1 mh = 1,000,000 c/s.*
- *Piezoelectric crystal: a crystal that converts electrical energy into sound waves and vice versa.*
- *M-mode display: a display that plots distance against time as a continuous recorded strip.*

CLINICAL APPLICATIONS

M-mode echocardiography alone or combined with two-dimensional echocardiography has been shown to have diagnostic value with many cardiac lesions, some examples of which are mitral stenosis, pericardial effusion, prolapse of the valves, valvular aortic stenosis or insufficiency, hypertrophic subaortic stenosis, vegetation of the valves, and intracardiac mass. The size of all cardiac chambers, thickness of the ventricular wall and interventricular septum, and ventricular function can be estimated with reasonable accuracy. Two-dimensional echocardiography is especially useful in detecting segmental ventricular wall motion abnormalities or ventricular aneurysm. Echocardiography is highly useful in the diagnosis of congenital heart lesions, such as atrial septal defect, atrioventricular canal, Fallot's tetralogy, transposition of the great vessels, and Ebstein's anomaly. The use of the contrast method expanded the ability to detect intracardiac shunt. This method consists of injection of indocyanine or normal saline into peripheral veins, which will produce excellent echo targets, enabling detection of abnormal blood flow. Recent introduction of ultrasonic Doppler techniques in combination with two-dimensional echocardiography further enhances cardiovascular diagnostic ability. *Doppler ultrasound techniques* furnish data about the velocity of blood flow in the heart and great vessels. Measurement of the velocity of blood flow is based on the Doppler shift principle, which states that if a sound beam strikes a moving target, the reflected wave has a different frequency from the incident wave such that the change in frequency is proportional to the velocity of the moving target. When partial obstruction to blood flow is present, the velocity of flow increases. The increase in velocity requires a pressure drop across the obstruction. The pressure drop can be calculated from Bernoulli's equation:

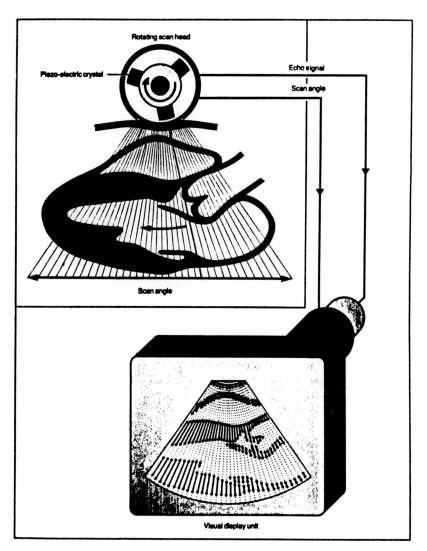

Figure 21-2. The principle of a mechanical sector scanner. (From Leech G., Kisslo J.: *Geigy: An Introduction to Echocardiography,* 2nd Ser. Unit 1, *Two-Dimensional Echocardiography in the Normal Heart.* Reproduced by permission of Medi-Cine Ltd., London 1981.)

$$\text{Pressure drop} = 4 \times V^2,$$

where V is maximal velocity across the obstruction. Because echocardiography is noninvasive and does not cause damage to the tissues, serial studies can be performed in following the progression of a disease process or evaluating the results of therapy. It is important to know, however, the indications for use as well as the limitations of this technique. Misinterpretation or overinterpretation of echocardiograms constitutes a real and serious hazards.

Keynotes

- *Contrast methods in echocardiography: indocyanine or normal saline injected intravenously will result in a cloud of echoes when it reaches the heart, thus serving to enhance the echogenicity of the blood.*
- *The Doppler technique measures the velocity of blood flow and the pressure gradient across the valves and detects the direction of blood flow throughout the cardiac cycle.*

ECHOCARDIOGRAPHIC EXAMINATION

The usefulness of echocardiography largely depends on the quality of the records. Therefore, echocardiographic recordings must be made by highly skilled personnel, usually a well-trained technician. The patient is studied in the supine or left lateral position with the transducer placed against the anterior chest wall between the second and fifth intercostal spaces and within 3–4 cm to the left of the sternal border. The exact location and direction of the ultrasound beam varies according to the individual patient. Sometimes it is advantageous to place the transducer in the suprasternal notch or subcostal area. A conducting gel is applied over the skin to eliminate air from the space between the transducer and chest wall. In adult echocardiography, a 2.25-MH transducer is commonly used. In infants and young children, a transducer with a frequency of 3.5 or 5.0 MH is preferred. Figures 21-3 and 21-4 demonstrate the M-mode echocardiographic recording as the transducer is directed from the apex to the base of the heart.

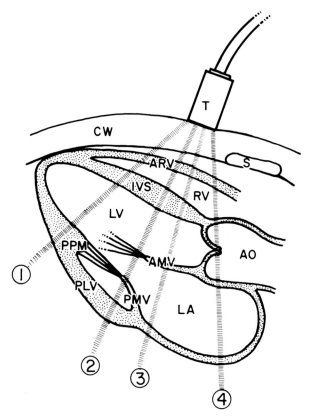

Figure 21-3. A cross section of the heart showing the structures through which the ultrasonic beam passes as it is directed from the apex toward the base of the heart. CW = chest wall, T = transducer, S = sternum, ARV = anterior right ventricular wall, RV = right ventricular cavity, IVS = interventricular septum, LV = left ventricle, PPM = posterior papillary muscle, PLV = posterior left ventricular wall, AMV = anterior mitral valve, PMV = posterior mitral valve, AO = aorta, LA = left atrium. (From Feigenbaum H: Clinical applications of echocardiography. Pro*gress in Cardiovascular Diseases,* 14:531, 1972. Reproduced by permission of Grune & Stratton, New York.)

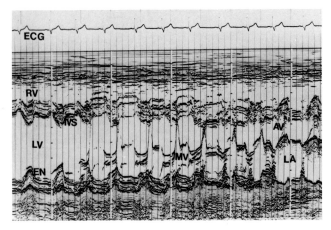

Figure 21-4. M-mode scan from the apex to the base of the heart. EN = endocardium, AV = aortic valve. For other abbreviations, see Figure 21-3. The horizontal lines, distance markers, are 1 cm apart. The vertical lines, time markers, are 0.2 second apart.

Two-dimensional echocardiographic examination is performed in a number of cross-sectional planes through the heart. These include the *parasternal long axis* of the heart (Fig. 21-5); the serial *parasternal short axis* of the left ventricle from the apex (Fig. 21-6) to the base (Fig. 21-7); the *apical four-chamber view* (Fig. 21-8); and the *apical two-chamber view,* which demonstrates the left ventricle and left atrium. Other structures, such as the pulmonary artery, aorta, and inferior vena cava, may be visualized by placing the transducer at appropriate positions.

HEART VALVES AND THEIR DISEASES

Mitral Valve

Normal Mitral Valve. The echoes from the mitral valve are among the easiest to recognize and record because of their distinctive pattern of motion. In fact, the earliest clinical application of echocardiography was detection of mitral stenosis. The mitral valve echoes are also very useful in the evaluation of certain other pathological conditions. The normal mitral valve undergoes a series of movements during diastole, as shown in Figure 21-9. Shortly after the end of the left ventricular systole, the mitral valve leaflets swing open in opposite directions as left atrial pressure exceeds that of the left ventricle (Fig. 21-9, point D). Maximum excursion of the anterior leaflet occurs at point E. As the blood empties rapidly into the left ventricle, partial closure of the valve occurs (E–F segment in the figure). With atrial systole, the valve leaflets again swing apart (point A indicates the peak of atrial systole), and finally, the valve closes at the beginning of ventricular systole (point C).

Mitral Stenosis. Echocardiography is an important adjunct in diagnosing *mitral stenosis* and in determining its severity. In mitral stenosis (Fig. 21-10), because of a narrowed mitral orifice, rapid filling of the left ventricle will be hindered and the early diastolic closing velocity of the mitral valve (E–F slope) is reduced. The amplitude of the a-wave is reduced in the presence of sinus rhythm, and the a-wave will be absent if *atrial fibrillation* is present. The posterior mitral leaflet usually moves anteriorly during diastole as a result of fusion of the commissure from scarring and adhesion. The M-mode echocardiogram shown in Figure 21-10 is a typical example of moderate mitral stenosis. The mitral leaflets are not calcified, and the anterior leaflet may show marked doming, giving the appearance of normal excursion of the anterior leaflet. This type of mitral valve may benefit from *mitral commissurotomy.* On the other hand, the M-mode echocardiogram shown in Figure 21-11 shows heavily calcified mitral valve leaflets and is an example of severe mitral stenosis. This type of mitral valve will not benefit from a mitral commissurotomy and requires a prosthetic valve.

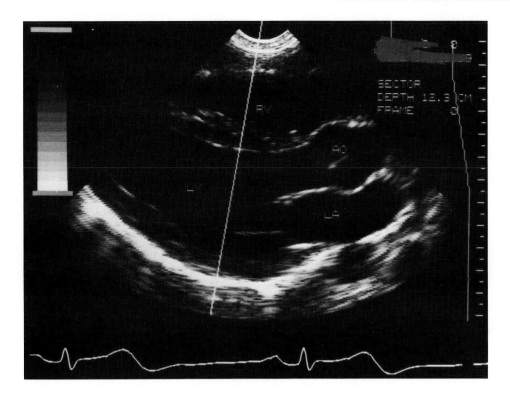

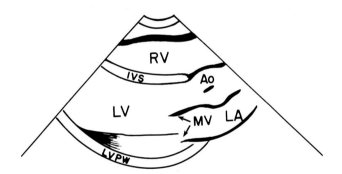

Figure 21-5. Two-dimensional echocardiogram (2-D), parasternal long-axis image, diastole. Aortic valve is closed; mitral valve is open. LVPW = left ventricular posterior wall.

Two-dimensional echocardiography, especially in combination with Doppler ultrasonic techniques, is very useful in estimating the size of the mitral valve opening (Figs. 21-12 and 21-13).

Mitral Insufficiency. Echocardiography has not proven to be a sensitive tool for the diagnosis of *mitral insufficiency* except for the presence of specific causes such as *mitral valve prolapse* (Fig. 21-14) or flail mitral valve. Initially, it was thought that in patients with mitral insufficiency, the E–F slope of the anterior mitral leaflet and total amplitude of the mitral valve opening were greater than normal. Subsequently, these findings were found not to be specific to mitral insufficiency. If, however, the patient has a mitral systolic murmur and the echocardiogram shows the above findings together with enlargment of the left atrium and left ventricle, the diagnosis of hemodynamically significant mitral insufficiency is highly probable. Doppler ultrasound techniques are highly useful, allowing recording of the regurgitation flow in the left atrium.

Mitral Annular Calcification. Calcification of the mitral annulus is frequently associated with aortic valve sclerosis and aortic root thickening among patients of advanced age. This condition may produce mitral insufficiency and, rarely, mitral stenosis or atrioventricular conduction disturbance. *Mitral annular calcification* can be seen on M-mode echocardiogram as a dense band of echoes between the posterior mitral leaflet and the posterior left ventricular wall (Fig. 21-15). A two-dimensional echocardiogram

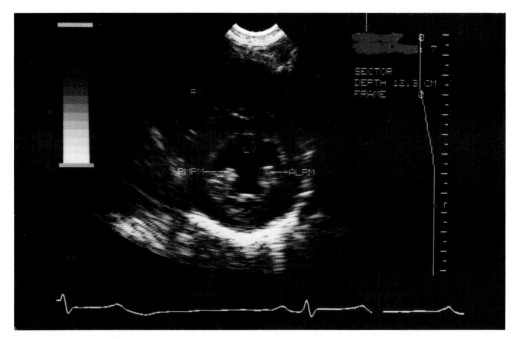

Figure 21-6. 2-D, parasternal short-axis image at papillary muscle level. PMPM-posteromedial papillary muscle, ALPM-anterolateral papillary muscle.

shows more exactly the location and extent of annular calcification.

Mitral Valve Prolapse. *Midsystolic clicks* and late systolic murmurs are well known clinical findings of mitral valve prolapse. The incidence of this syndrome is reported to be about 6% in women, and contrary to the earlier reports, the incidence in men is probably close to that in women. Most of these patients are asymptomatic. Up to 10%, however, may have complications, such as atrial or ventricular arrhythmia, endocarditis, embolic phenomena, atypical chest pain, severe mitral insufficiency, congestive heart failure, and, rarely, sudden death. With prolapse of the mitral valve, the normal gradual anterior movement of the mitral valve on the M-mode is disrupted by posterior movement during mid or late systole (Fig. 21-14). This is best demonstrated at the junction between the left ventricle and left atrium. In some cases, the mitral leaflets may appear redundant. Two-dimensional parasternal long-axis and apical four-chamber views (Fig. 21-16) are commonly used for recording mitral valve prolapse.

Aortic Valve and Root

Echocardiography, when combined with clinical findings, is useful in the diagnosis of diseases of the aortic valve and aortic root. Conditions in which echocardiography may supply diagnostic clues are valvular aortic stenosis, aortic insufficiency, *bicuspid aortic valve, vegetation,* dissecting aneurysm of the aortic root, and aneurysm of the sinus of Valsalva.

Normal Aortic Valve. Figure 21-17 shows the M-mode echogram of a normal aortic valve and aortic root. During ventricular systole, the aortic valve opens and appears as a boxlike configuration. The anterior aortic valve echo originates from the right coronary cusp, whereas the posterior aortic valve echo originates from the noncoronary cusp. The left coronary cusp is not visualized by the M-mode echogram. During diastole, the aortic valve closes, and the cusps form a linear echo approximately halfway between the anterior and posterior aortic walls. The aortic walls and the aortic valve cusps move upward and parallel to each other during systole. The parasternal short-axis view of the two-dimensional echocardiogram often demonstrates all three aortic cusps (Fig 21-7).

Valvular Aortic Stenosis. The diagnosis of valvular *aortic stenosis* is suggested by the presence of multiple echoes from the thickened, deformed aortic cusps. When the aortic valve is severely calcified, the aortic valve opening may be markedly reduced (Fig. 21-18). Hypertrophy of the left ventricle provides additional important evidence of aortic stenosis if other causes of left ventricular hypertrophy are absent (Fig. 21-18). It should be noted that even if the aortic valve is significantly calcified, there may be no pressure gradient across the aortic valve. On the other hand, in children or young adults, calcification is usually absent, and the severely stenotic aortic valve may appear to have a normal valve opening by M-mode echocardiogram because echoes are more readily recorded from the wide part of the domed valve than from the stenotic orifice at the tip. In such cases, two-dimensional echocardio-

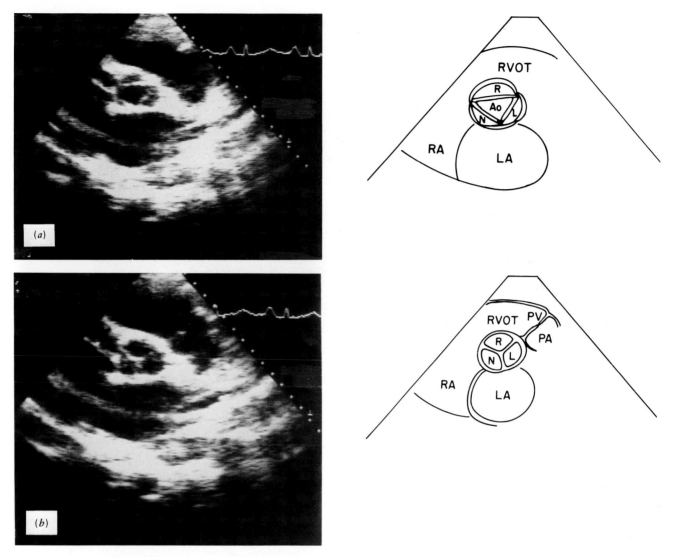

Figure 21-7. 2-D echogram, parasternal short-axis image at the level of the aortic valve. Aortic valve is open in systole (*a*), closed in diastole (*b*). R = right coronary cusp, L = left coronary cusp, N = noncoronary cusp, LA = left atrium, RVOT = right ventricular outflow tract.

graphy is helpful in demonstrating the *domed aortic valve,* enabling correct diagnosis (Fig. 21-19). Recently, Doppler ultrasound techniques have been shown to be useful in the quantitation of the transvalvular pressure gradient in patients with aortic stenosis.

Aortic Insufficiency. Echocardiographic evidence of *aortic insufficiency* is often indirect inasmuch as the echogram of the aortic valve may appear normal. In aortic insufficiency, columns of regurgitant blood reenter the left ventricle, which may cause high-frequency vibrations of the anterior mitral valve during diastole (Fig. 21-20). If such vibrations are seen on the anterior mitral valve as well as on the left side of the interventricular septum in diastole, the diagnosis of aortic insufficiency is virtually certain. The vibrations must be differentiated from a recording artifact caused by sensitive recorders; this artifact is usu-

ally seen throughout the entire cardiac cycle. Doppler ultrasound techniques are very helpful in demonstrating aortic regurgitation. Patients with hemodynamically significant aortic insufficiency usually demonstrate dilatation of the left ventricle, and it has been suggested that echocardiography may be a valuable adjunct in following the progression of the disease.

Bicuspid Aortic Valve. *Bicuspid aortic valve* is a congenital abnormality that may predispose a person to bacterial endocarditis or calcific aortic stenosis in the later years of life. The finding of eccentricity of the diastolic aortic valve echo (Fig. 21-21) is one of the echocardiographic criteria for this anomaly. Another sign of this anomaly is the multiple diastolic echoes coming from the wavy edge of the redundant cusp (Fig. 21-21). These criteria may, however, cause false normal as well as abnormal results. Two-

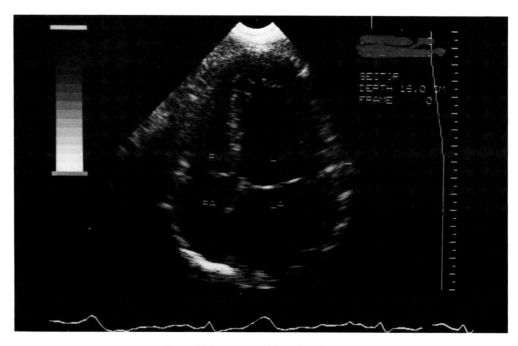

Figure 21-8. 2-D, apical four-chamber view.

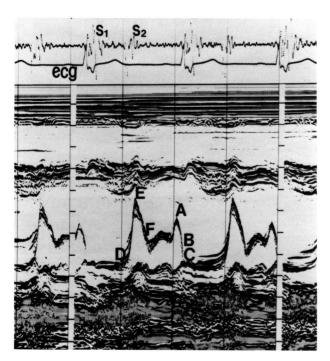

Figure 21-9. M-mode echogram of a mitral valve; ecg = electrocardiogram, S₁ = first heart sound, S₂ = second heart sound.

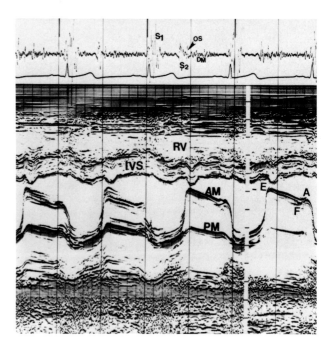

Figure 21-10. M-mode echocardiogram of a patient with moderate mitral stenosis. E–F slope is reduced; a-wave of the anterior mitral valve (AM) is small; posterior mitral valve (PM) moves anteriorly and parallel with anterior mitral valve. Both leaflets are slightly thickened; excursion of the anterior mitral valve remains normal. Phonocardiogram showed an opening snap (OS) followed by a diastolic murmur (DM).

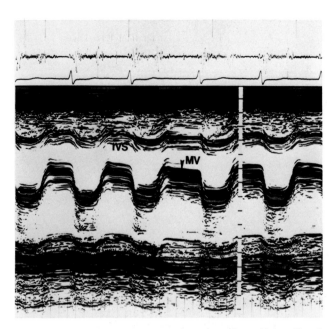

Figure 21-11. M-mode echocardiogram of a patient with heavily calcified severe mitral stenosis. Electrocardiogram shows atrial fibrillation.

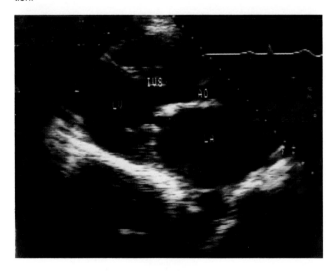

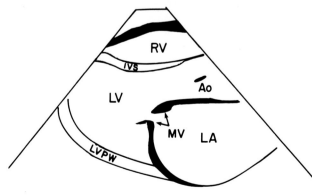

Figure 21-12. Parasternal long-axis view of a patient with mitral stenosis in diastole. The anterior mitral valve is domed, and the mitral valve opening is stenotic.

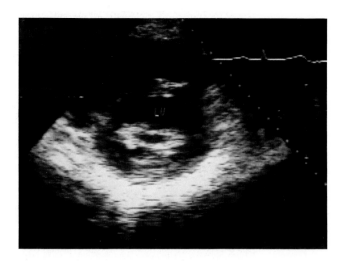

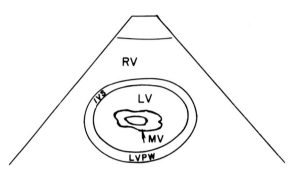

Figure 21-13. Parasternal short-axis view of the same patient in diastole. The mitral valve area was estimated as 1.3cm².

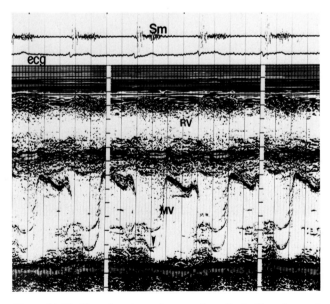

Figure 21-14. M-mode echocardiogram of a patient with prolapse of the mitral valve. The arrowhead indicates posterior movement of the mitral valve in mid and late systole. The phonocardiogram showed a mid-to-late systolic murmur (SM).

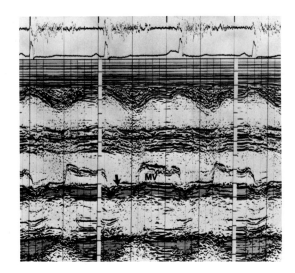

Figure 21-15. M-mode echocardiogram of a patient with mitral annular calcification (arrow).

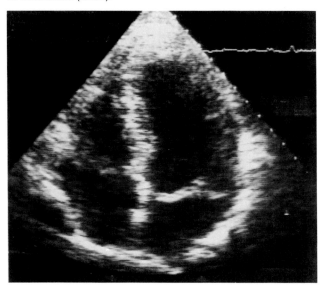

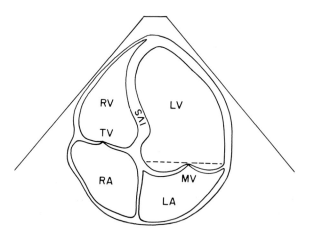

Figure 21-16. Apical four-chamber image of a patient with mitral valve prolapse, demonstrating both mitral leaflets extending beyond the plane of the mitral annulus (dotted line). TV=tricuspid valve. (Compare with Fig. 21-8.)

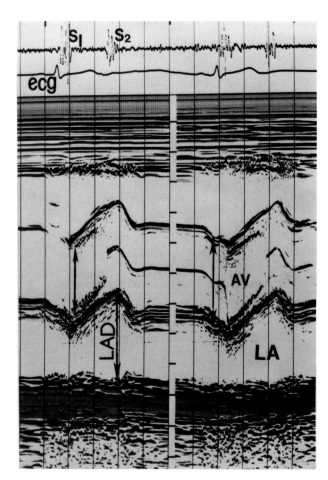

Figure 21-17. M-mode echogram of a normal aortic valve. The aortic valve opens as a boxlike appearance in systole and becomes a linear echo in the center of the aortic root in diastole. Arrows on the left indicate separation of the aortic cusps; arrows on the right indicate the aortic root. LAD = left atrial dimension.

dimensional echocardiography is often more reliable in detecting bicuspid aortic valves (Fig. 21-22).

Tricuspid and Pulmonic Valves

The tricuspid and pulmonic valves are more difficult to record than the mitral and aortic valves in normal adults by M-mode echocardiography. Two-dimensional echocardiography overcomes many of the difficulties.

Tricuspid Valve. The tricuspid valve is located anteriorly and medially with respect to the mitral echoes. Although the anatomic structure of the tricuspid valve differs from that of the mitral valve, its echocardiographic appearance is similar (Fig. 21-23).

Pulmonic Valve. Figure 21-24 shows a normal M-mode echogram of the pulmonic valve. Atrial systole causes a posterior dip marked "a" in late diastole. In valvular pulmonic stenosis, because of the increased force of right atrial contraction and elevated right ventricular end-diastolic pressure, the amplitude of the a-wave is increased.

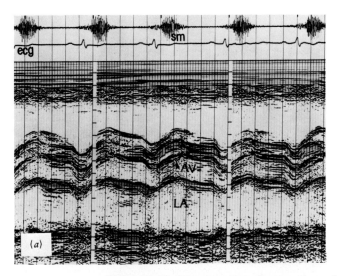
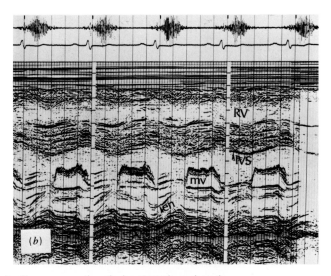

Figure 21-18. M-mode echocardiogram of a patient with severe aortic valvular stenosis and aortic insufficiency. (*a*) The aortic valve is heavily calcified. (*b*) The interventricular septum and the left ventricular posterior wall are markedly hypertrophied. High-frequency vibrations seen over the anterior mitral valve in diastole are suggestive of aortic insufficiency.

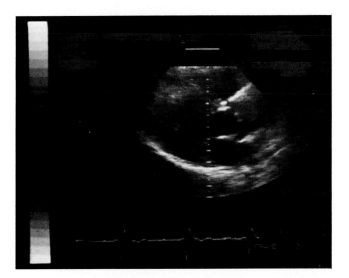
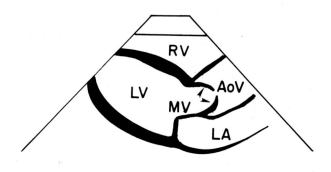

Figure 21-19. 2-D echogram of congenital aortic valvular stenosis. Note the doming of the valve (arrows) with a small opening in systole. AoV = aortic valve.

On the other hand, with *pulmonary hypertension,* because of the elevated pulmonary artery diastolic pressure, the effect of the atrial contraction on the movement of the pulmonic valve is attenuated, which results in decreased amplitude of the a-wave. Other findings of pulmonary hypertension include a flattened slope of the diastolic closure echo and a midsystolic notching of the pulmonic valve. Unfortunately, there are some false normal as well as abnormal results with these findings. Recently, Doppler ultrasound techniques have been reported to be highly useful in detecting pulmonary hypertension.

Vegetative Endocarditis

Echocardiography has provided a valuable contribution in the diagnosis and management of patients with *endocarditis.* Valvular *vegetations* of sufficient size (2 mm or greater) may be detected by either M-mode or two-dimensional echocardiography. The sensitivity of echocardiography in detecting bacterial vegetations has been reported to range from 34% to 70%. Characteristically, M-mode echocardiography shows shaggy, nonuniform echoes on the involved valve in systole, diastole, or both (Fig. 21-25, 21-26, and 21-27). Two-dimensional echocardiography

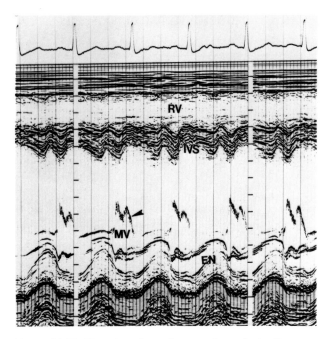

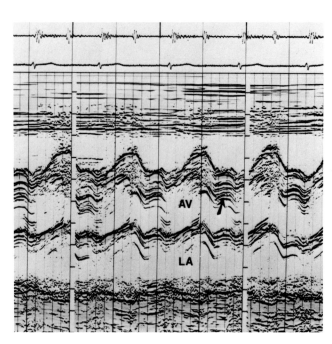

Figure 21-20. M-mode echocardiogram of a patient with severe aortic insufficiency. There are high-frequency vibrations on the mitral valve in diastole (arrowhead). The left ventricle is markedly dilated.

Figure 21-21. M-mode echocardiogram of a bicuspid aortic valve. The diastolic echoes (arrow) are multiple and eccentric.

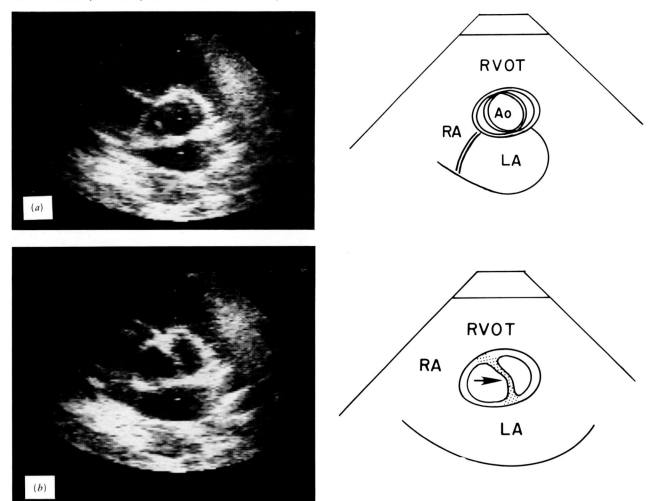

Figure 21-22. Parasternal short-axis view of the aortic valve from a patient with bicuspid aortic valve, in systole (a) and diastole (b). Only two aortic cusps are seen.

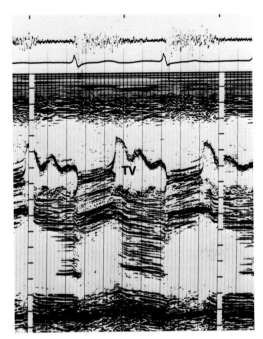

Figure 21-23. M-mode echocardiogram of the tricuspid valve, which resembles the mitral valve.

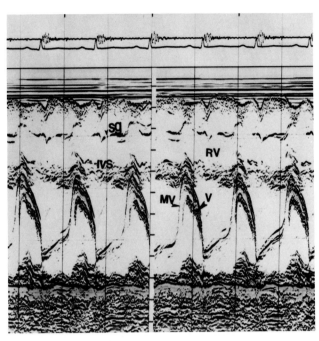

Figure 21-25. M-mode echocardiogram from a patient with bacterial endocarditis. A vegetation (V) is seen on the anterior mitral valve in diastole. A Swan-Ganz (sg) catheter is present in the right ventricle.

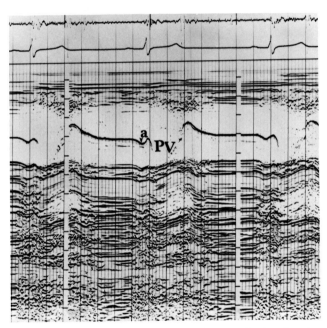

Figure 21-24. M-mode echocardiogram of a normal pulmonic valve (PV).

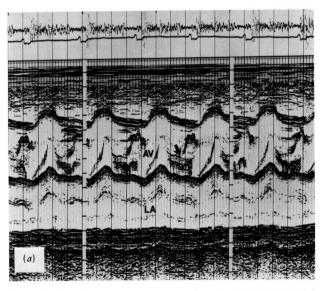

Figure 21-26. M-mode echocardiogram from a patient with bacterial endocarditis of the aortic valve. (a) Arrow indicates a vegetation. (b) This patient had aortic insufficiency, as evidenced by the presence of the high-frequency vibrations on the anterior mitral valve and on the left side of the interventricular septum in diastole. The mitral valve closes (arrowhead) considerably ahead of the QRS complex of the simultaneously taken ECG. This finding suggests very high diastolic pressure in the left ventricle.

has been shown to be very useful in assessing the location and size of the vegetation (Fig. 21-28). Premature closure of the mitral valve seen in association with acute aortic valve insufficiency because of aortic valve endocarditis is an ominous sign, indicating marked elevation of the left ventricular end-diastolic pressure (Fig. 21-26). It should

be stressed that failure to detect vegetations by echocardiography cannot exclude the diagnosis of endocarditis.

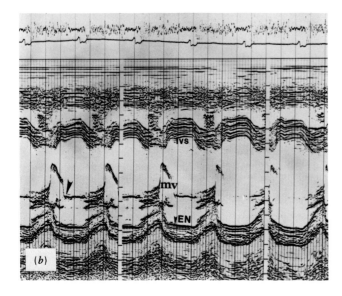

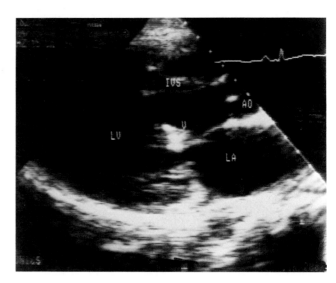

Figure 21-28. Parasternal long-axis view in diastole. A vegetation (V) is seen on the anterior mitral leaflet.

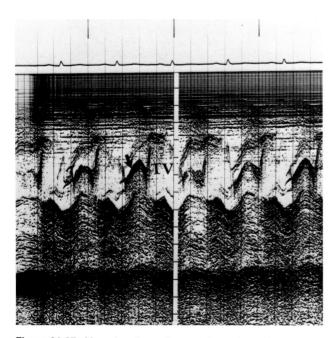

Figure 21-27. M-mode echocardiogram of a patient with a vegetation on the tricuspid valve (arrow).

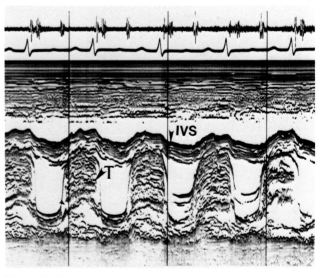

Figure 21-29. M-mode echocardiogram from a patient with a left atrial myxoma (T). A small echo-free space is seen before the tumor echoes (smaller arrowhead), which indicates the time gap between the mitral valve opening and prolapse of the tumor through the mitral valve.

Keynotes

- M-mode echocardiographic findings of mitral stenosis include: reduced early diastolic closing velocity of the anterior mitral valve (E–F slope), reduced or absent a-waves, anterior motion of the posterior leaflet of the mitral valve, and a thickened or calcified valve.
- Mitral commissurotomy: Cutting or tearing open of the fused commissures of the stenotic mitral valve. This procedure is best done when the mitral valve is not heavily calcified.

- Calcification of the mitral annulus is usually seen in patients of advanced age.
- Mitral valve prolapse is a common condition, usually asymptomatic, but it is occasionally associated with severe complications.
- Echocardiographic findings suggestive of aortic stenosis include multiple echoes from thickened, deformed cusps; reduced opening of the aortic valve; hypertrophy of the left ventricle; and demonstration of a pressure gradient across the aortic valve by Doppler method.

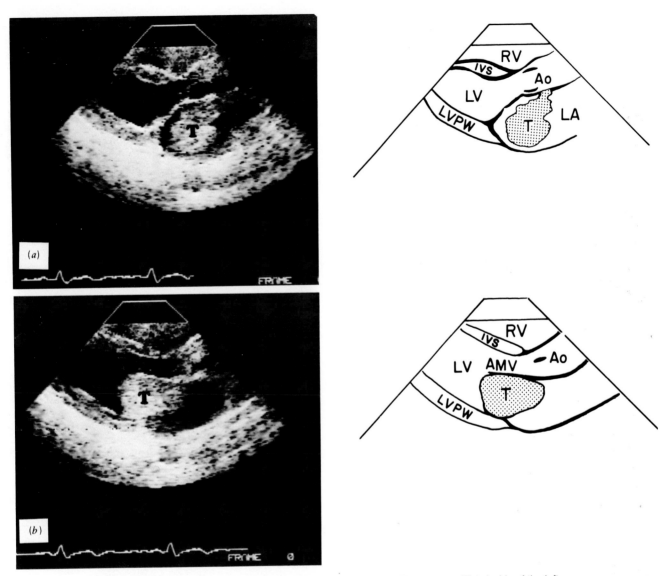

Figure 21-30. Parasternal long-axis view of a left atrial myxoma. The myxoma (T) is inside of the left atrium in systole (a) and protrudes into the left ventricle through the mitral valve in diastole (b).

- *Echocardiographic findings suggestive of aortic insufficiency include high-frequency vibrations of the anterior mitral leaflet and occasionally of the left side of the interventricular septum, dilatation of the left ventricle, and Doppler demonstration of regurgitant blood flow.*
- *The valvular vegetations of endocarditis can be detected by M-mode or two-dimensional echocardiography when they are 2 mm or greater in size.*

ATRIAL MYXOMAS

Atrial myxoma is the most common cardiac tumor and more often occurs in the left atrium than in the right. It is usually pedunculated and attached to the atrial septum via a stalk. The clinical symptoms and signs may mimic those of mitral stenosis or bacterial endocarditis. Systemic

emboli are the most serious complications. Typically, M-mode echocardiography reveals multiple tumor echoes posterior to the anterior mitral valve leaflet during diastole. Noted at the beginning of diastole is a small echo-free space, which represents the time interval between the opening of the mitral valve and tumor prolapsing across the mitral valve (Fig. 21-29). Two-dimensional echocardiography not only is more sensitive in the detection of the tumor but can provide better information about its size and location (Fig. 21-30).

Keynotes

- *Atrial myxoma is the most common cardiac tumor.*
- *The typical echocardiographic appearance of an atrial myxoma is the presence of multiple echoes behind the anterior mitral valve in*

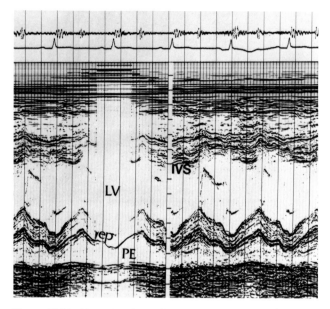

Figure 21-31. M-mode echocardiogram of a patient with a moderate amount of posterior pericardial effusion (PE); ep = epicardium.

diastole and is more easily seen on two-dimensional than on M-mode echocardiography.

PERICARDIAL EFFUSION

Echocardiography is the procedure of choice for the detection of *pericardial effusion.* It is accurate, reliable, and rapid; can be done at the patient's bedside; and may be repeated as often as necessary. Normally the posterior left ventricular epicardium and pericardium appear as a single moving echo. In the presence of an effusion, the fluid is seen as an echo-free space between these two structures (Fig. 21-31). Similar echo free spaces may be found between the anterior right ventricular epicardium and pericardium if a larger effusion is present. It is necessary to record the echocardiogram at various gain settings in order to identify the endocardial, epicardial, and pericardial echoes. The accuracy of this technique depends on the proficiency of the technician performing the examination. Two-dimensional echocardiography provides complimentary information in the diagnosis, localization, and quantitation of pericardial effusion (Fig. 21-32).

Keynotes

- *Echocardiography is the procedure of choice for the detection of pericardial effusion.*
- *Pericardial effusion appears as echo-free space between the epicardium and the pericardium.*

HYPERTROPHIC SUBAORTIC STENOSIS

Hypertrophic subaortic stenosis is a form of *hypertrophic cardiomyopathy* in which there is hypertrophy of the interventricular septum and obstruction of the left ventricular outflow. Echocardiography is the procedure of choice for the diagnosis of this entity. The characteristic findings include asymmetric hypertrophy of the interventricular septum and *systolic anterior motion (SAM)* of the mitral valve (Fig. 21-33). The aortic valve echogram may show midsystolic closure and subsequent reopening (Fig. 21-34). In patients with hypertrophic subaortic stenosis, the out-

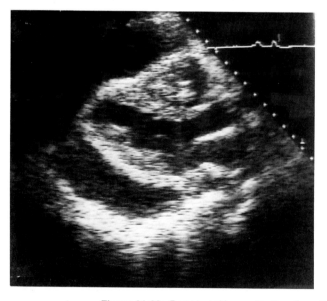

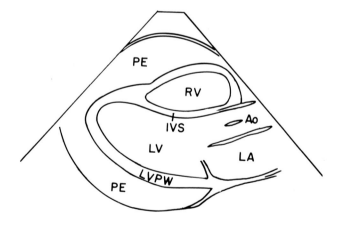

Figure 21-32. Parasternal long-axis view of a patient with large pericardial effusion (PE).

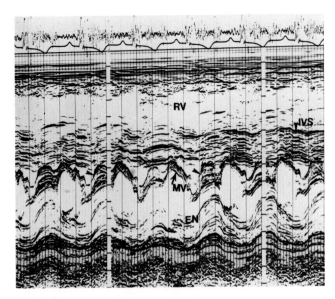

Figure 21-33. M-mode echocardiogram of a patient with hypertrophic subaortic stenosis. The IVS is markedly thickened. The left ventricular posterior wall is also hypertrophied but not as much as the IVS. SAM of the mitral valve (arrow) is clearly seen.

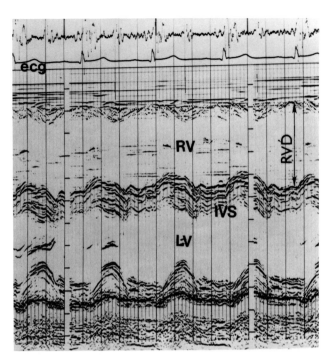

Figure 21-35. M-mode echocardiogram from a patient with secundum type of atrial septal defect. The RV is dilated (3.7 cm); the IVS moves paradoxically.

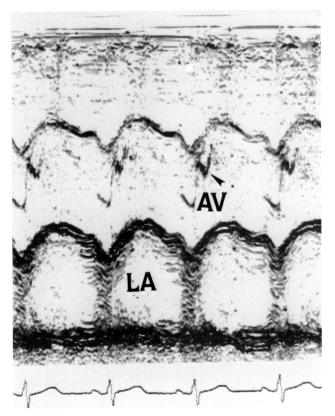

Figure 21-34. Aortic valve echogram of a patient with hypertrophic subaortic stenosis. During midsystole, the aortic valve closes partially (arrowhead) because of the subvalvular obstruction; it then reopens.

flow obstruction may not be present at rest, and SAM of the mitral valve may only occur after a compensatory pause following a ventricular premature beat or with Valsalva manuever or administration of *amyl nitrate* or *isoproterenol*. Occasionally, SAM of the the mitral valve is seen in patients with exaggerated posterior left ventricular wall motion who otherwise have no evidence of hypertrophic subaortic stenosis. There are other forms of nonobstructive hypertrophic cardiomyopathy, and the distribution of hypertrophy may exhibit marked variation. Echocardiography is highly useful in providing a definite diagnosis.

Keynote

- *Characteristic echocardiographic findings in hypertrophic subaortic stenosis include asymmetric hypertrophy of the interventricular septum and SAM of the mitral valve. Midsystolic closure and subsequent reopening of the aortic valve leaflets may also be seen.*

RIGHT VENTRICULAR VOLUME OVERLOAD

Right ventricular volume overload (RVVO) is caused by many cardiac lesions such as *atrial septal defect, tricuspid insufficiency, pulmonic insufficiency,* and *anomalous pulmonary venous return.* Characteristic echocardiographic findings include increased right ventricular dimensions

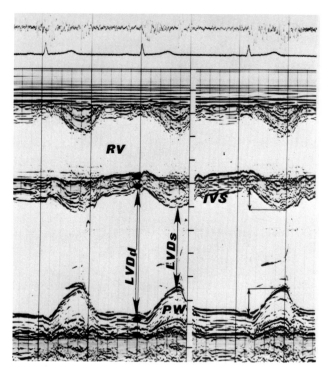

Figure 21-36. M-mode echocardiogram of the normal left ventricle. The left ventricular internal dimension in end diastole (LVDd) is measured from the left side of the IVS to the endocardium of the left ventricular posterior wall (PW) at the peak of the QRS complex of the simultaneously taken electrocardiogram. The left ventricular internal dimension in systole (LVDs) is measured at the point corresponding to the peak posterior motion of the IVS. Short arrows indicate the thickness of the IVS and PW. The excursion of the IVS (normal 5–9 mm) and PW (normal 9–14 mm) is indicated by the small arrows on the right side of the figure.

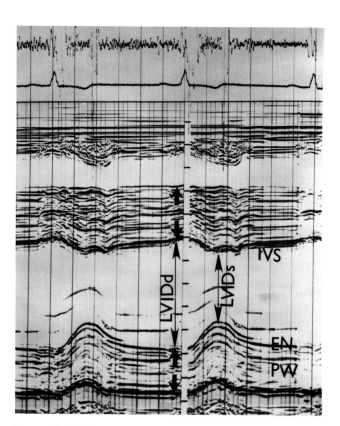

Figure 21-37. M-mode echocardiogram of a patient with marked left ventricular hypertrophy. The thickness of the IVS is 22 mm and PW is 20 mm (whereas normal for both is 7–11 mm).

and abnormal interventricular septal (IVS) motion (Fig. 21-35). In normal hearts, the movement of the IVS is opposite in direction to that of the left ventricular posterior wall in systole. In RVVO, systolic motion of the IVS is in synchrony with the left ventricular posterior wall. The mechanism of the abnormal pattern of the septal motion in RVVO has been the subject of many investigations. Several investigators have concluded that the combination of right ventricular dilatation and an exaggerated anterior motion of the entire heart are responsible for the paradoxical motion. More recent studies using two-dimensional echocardiography indicate that the increased diastolic filling of the right ventricle causes a shift of the septum toward the left ventricle. With ventricular systole, this shift is rapidly corrected, and the septum moves anteriorly toward the right ventricle. In atrial septal defect, 75–90% of the patients exhibit abnormal IVS motion. It should be noted that abnormalities of the IVS motion may be seen in patients with left bundle-branch block, after open heart surgery or constrictive pericarditis. Therefore, you should not make the diagnosis of RVVO in those patients who have abnormalities of the IVS motion in the

absence of right ventricular dilatation. Two-dimensional echocardiography, especially combined with contrast echocardiography, plays an important role in the diagnosis of atrial septal defect. Doppler ultrasound techniques are very useful in detecting tricuspid insufficiency that may not be apparent clinically.

Keynote

- *Right ventricular volume overload results in increased size of the right ventricle and an abnormal motion of the IVS, which moves in the same direction as the posterior wall of the left ventricle.*

LEFT VENTRICLE

M-mode echocardiography has been used extensively in the evaluation of left ventricular anatomy and function. Although there is a considerable disagreement concerning the reliability of M-mode echocardiography in assessing the left ventricle, this technique is often very useful clinically. The introduction of two-dimensional echocardiography has further enhanced the usefulness of this application.

Measurements of the left ventricular internal dimension at end systole (LVIDs), left ventricular internal di-

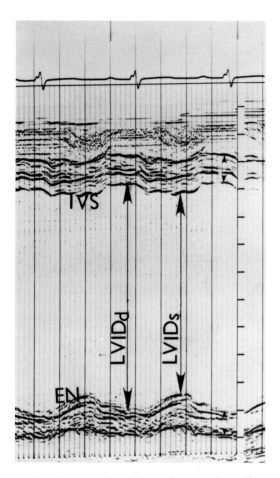

Figure 21-38. M-mode echocardiogram from a patient with congestive cardiomyopathy and left ventricular dilation. LVIDd is 8.2 cm. The excursion of the IVS and PW is decreased; their thickness (small arrowheads) is normal.

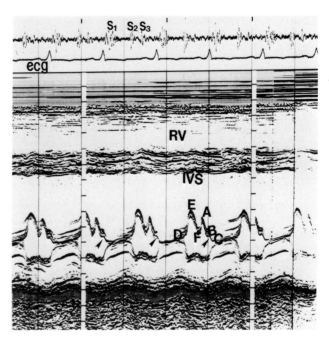

Figure 21-39. M-mode echocardiogram from a patient with left ventricular failure. The left ventricle is dilated (6.7 cm); IVS and PW are hypokinetic. The mitral valve opening is diminished, and the distance between the E point of the anterior mitral valve and the left side of the IVS is 2.4 cm (upper limit of normal is 0.6–1.0 cm). In addition, the A–C slope is interrupted (B bump), and the PR–AC interval is short (less than 60 ms).

mension at end diastole (LVIDd), and thickness and motion of the interventricular septum and left ventricular wall can be made by left ventricular echogram (Fig. 21-36). Left ventricular echocardiography is useful in detecting left ventricular hypertrophy (Fig. 21-37), left ventricular dilatation or *congestive cardiomyopathy* (Figs. 21-38 and 21-39), segmental wall abnormality seen in coronary artery disease (Figs. 21-40 and 21-41), and mural thrombus (Fig. 21-42).

It has been shown empirically that the cubed left ventricular internal dimensions, LVIDd^3 and LVIDs^3, correlate reasonably well with angiographic left ventricular end-diastolic and end-systolic volume. *Stroke volume* is LVIDd^3 minus LVIDs^3, and the *ejection fraction* is stroke volume divided by LVIDd^3. These formulas are based on the assumptions that the left ventricle is ellipsoid in shape, the long axis is twice the short axis, the echocardiographic LVID approximates the minor axis, and the ventricle contracts uniformly. But M-mode echocardiograms reveal only a small part of the left ventricle, and many drawbacks exist. In the presence of segmental wall motion abnormalities, the data obtained by these formulas may

be grossly inaccurate. For example, in a patient with infarction of the apical segment of the left ventricle, the M-mode beam may traverse the normal myocardium at the base of the heart, resulting in overestimation of the left ventricular function.

The mitral valve echogram is also valuable in the evaluation of left ventricular function. In the presence of left ventricular failure, the mitral valve opening is decreased, resulting in increased distance between the E point of the anterior mitral valve and the interventricular septum (Fig. 21-39). It should be noted that decreased mitral valve excursion may be seen in patients with aortic insufficiency who do not have heart failure. Other helpful findings of left ventricular failure are interruption of the A–C slope of the anterior mitral valve (B bump) and shortened PR–AC measurement (less than 60 ms). The PR interval is obtained from the simultaneously taken electrocardiogram; the A–C slope is the interval between the A and C points of the anterior mitral valve (Fig. 21-39). This measurement is not reliable when the PR interval is less than 150 ms.

The recent development of two-dimensional echocardiography permits real-time tomographic evaluation of a large portion of the left ventricle throughout the cardiac cycle and has greatly enhanced the capability of echocardiographic evaluation of left ventricular anatomy and function. There is a significant agreement among evaluations of regional wall motion by two-dimensional echocardiogra-

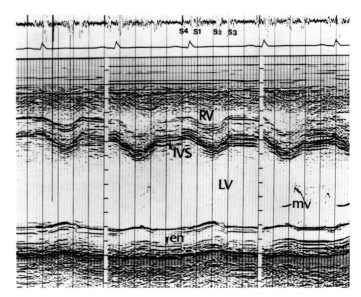

Figure 21-40. M-mode echocardiogram from a patient with infarction of the posterobasal segment of the left ventricle. The systolic motion of the left ventricular posterior wall at the level of the mitral valve is markedly diminished, whereas the systolic motion of the IVS is hyperdynamic.

phy, by radionuclide angiography, and by contrast ventriculography.

Keynotes

- *Echocardiographic measurement of left ventricular size in systole and diastole can be used to measure stroke volume and the ejection fraction. Because of the assumptions made in deriving these measurements, inaccuracies can result when there are segmental ventricular wall motion abnormalities.*

- *The echocardiogram, especially the two-dimensional echocardiogram, is very useful in the evaluation of ventricular anatomy, function, and wall motion abnormalities.*

SUMMARY

The echocardiogram demonstrates the anatomy and function of the heart. Information can be recorded in M-mode or two-dimensional images, and these images can be enhanced by the use of contrast agents and Doppler echocardiography. The technique is most useful in the evaluation of various congenital as well as acquired heart diseases such as mitral stenosis, mitral valve prolapse, aortic stenosis and insufficiency, hypertrophic subaortic stenosis, pericardial effusion, atrial myxoma, vegetation of the valves, hypertrophy or dilatation of the ventricles, ventricular failure or aneurysm, and RVVO. The specific echocardiographic findings of each of these are discussed in this chapter.

REVIEW QUESTIONS

1. What is the basic principle of echocardiography?
2. Describe the M-mode scans from the apex to the base of the heart.
3. Describe various 2-D echocardiographic views of the heart.
4. Describe normal echograms of the mitral valve; of the aortic valve; of the tricuspid valve; of the pulmonic valve.
5. What are the findings of mitral stenosis?
6. What are the findings of aortic stenosis?
7. Does the calcified aortic valve always indicate the presence of aortic stenosis?
8. What are the findings of mitral insufficiency?

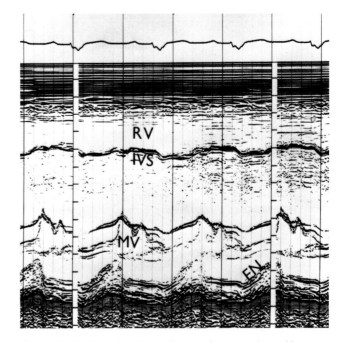

Figure 21-41. M-mode echocardiogram from a patient with extensive infarction of the IVS. The IVS is markedly scarred, thin, and hypodynamic. There is increased distance between the E point of the anterior mitral valve to the left side of the IVS and the presence of a B bump. These findings indicate left ventricular failure.

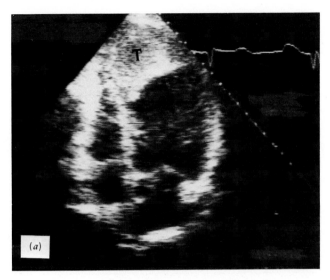
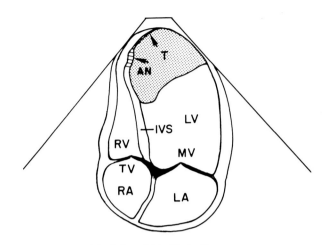

Figure 21-42. Apical four-chamber view of a patient with an aneurysm of the left ventricle filled with a large thrombus (T). Arrows indicate the aneurysm (AN).

9. What are the findings of aortic insufficiency?
10. What is the mitral valve prolapse syndrome? Describe its echocardiographic findings.
11. What is mitral annulus calcification? Describe its echocardiographic findings.
12. What are the findings of endocarditis?
13. What is the significance of early closure of the mitral valve in patients with endocarditis of the aortic valve?
14. Do negative echocardiographic findings rule out the diagnosis of endocarditis?
15. What is an atrial myxoma? Describe its echocardiographic findings.
16. How can a pericardial effusion be identified?
17. What are the findings and causes of RVVO?
18. What are the findings of hypertrophic subaortic stenosis?
19. How can one calculate stroke volume and ejection fraction of the left ventricle?
20. Describe the findings of left ventricular failure.

VOCABULARY

acoustic impedance
amyl nitrate
aneurysm
anomalous venous return
aortic insufficiency
aortic stenosis
apical four-chamber
apical two-chamber
asymmetric hypertrophy

left ventricular end-systolic dimension
megahertz
midsystolic click
mitral annular calcification
mitral commissurotomy
mitral insufficiency
mitral stenosis
mitral valve prolapse

atrial fibrillation
atrial myxoma
atrial septal defect
bicuspid aortic valve
congestive cardiomyopathy
domed aortic valve
Doppler ultrasound techniques
ejection fraction
end-diastolic pressure
endocarditis
hypertrophic cardiomyopathy
hypertrophic subaortic stenosis
isoproterenol
left ventricular end-diastolic dimension

M-mode display
mural thrombus
paradoxical interventricular septal motion
parasternal long-axis
parasternal short-axis
pericardial effusion
piezoelectric crystal
pulmonary hypertension
pulmonic insufficiency
right ventricular volume overload (RVVO)
stroke volume
systolic anterior motion
tricuspid insufficiency
Valsalva's maneuver

SUGGESTIONS FOR FURTHER READING

H. Feigenbaum. *Echocardiography*, 4th Ed. Lea & Febiger: Philadelphia. 1986.

A. Labovitz, G. Williams. *Doppler Echocardiography*. Lea & Febiger: Philadelphia. 1985.

B. Berger. *Doppler Echocardiography in Heart Disease*. Dekker: New York. 1987.

For additional suggested reading see Chapter 19.

22

EVALUATING THE HEART ON THE CHEST RADIOGRAPH: PULMONARY VASCULARITY

KEY CONCEPTS

Clinical

The early changes of congestive heart failure often produce no detectable change on physical examination. The earliest changes of vascular redistribution and interstitial edema are silent. Alveolar edema and cardiac enlargement can be detected on physical examination but are later findings.

Mitral valve stenosis can be associated with palpitations, sometimes caused by atrial fibrillation. The chest radiograph can diagnosis only some patients with mitral stenosis; in others, the chest radiograph is normal.

Increased pulmonary blood flow can be a normal finding in pregnancy but can also be due to fever, anemia, and several types of congenital heart disease.

Radiological

An evaluation of the pulmonary vascularity is the first step in evaluating the chest radiograph of a patient with heart disease. With the patient upright, the maximal flow and predominant vessel size is seen in the lower lobes.

With *increased pulmonary venous pressure,* the upper lobe vessels become larger, and after a certain level of pressure increases, the lower-lobe vessels decrease in size. This shift in vessel size is reflected both in the peripheral vessels and in the central hilar vessels.

As the pulmonary venous pressure increases, the flow through the lymphatic channels also increases, and eventually there is sufficient lymphatic flow to be seen. The lymphatic flow can be seen as thickening of the fissures and as thickening of the interlobular septa.

Radiographs can detect major changes in the amount of pulmo-

nary blood flow, either increased or decreased. These changes of flow are reflected in the increased or decreased size of the hili and the increased or decreased size of the more peripheral pulmonary vessels.

OBJECTIVES

When you complete this chapter you will be able to

1. Identify on selected radiographs the patterns of vessel and lymphatic change that indicate increased pulmonary venous pressure.
2. Describe the sequential patterns resulting from increasing pulmonary venous pressure.
3. List the two common causes of increased pulmonary venous pressure.
4. Identify on selected chest radiographs the pattern of increase pulmonary blood flow.
5. List one normal cause of increased blood flow.
6. List four diseases that cause increased pulmonary blood flow.
7. Describe the pattern of decreased pulmonary blood flow.

An evaluation of the pulmonary vascularity is the first step in evaluating the chest radiograph in the patient suspected of having cardiac disease. Two general types of changes in pulmonary vascularity occur. There can be changes in pressure or blood flow.

Increases in pressure in the pulmonary arterial or venous system.

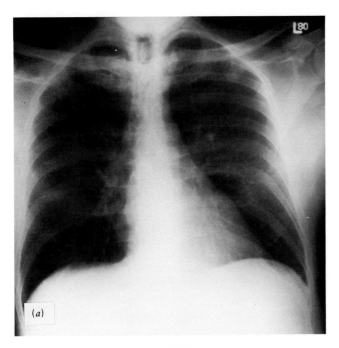

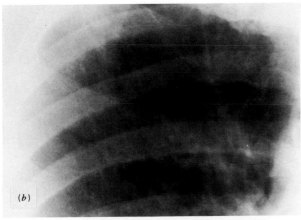

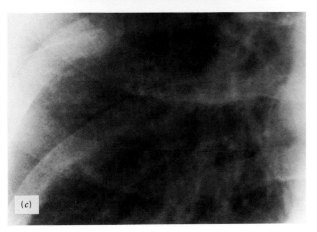

Figure 22-1. Normal pulmonary vascularity with the patient upright. The size of the upper and lower lobe vessels should be compared. With the patient upright, the lower lung vessels should be larger than the upper lung vessels. (*a*) PA view of the chest. (*b*) Focal view of the upper lung vessels. (*c*) Focal view of the lower lung vessels.

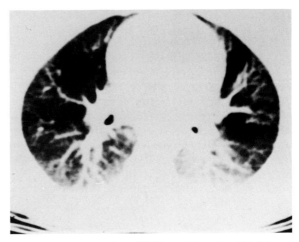

Figure 22-2. Lung vessels on CT. The relative size of blood vessels can also be detected on CT examinations of the chest. The vessel size is affected by gravity. Because most chest CTs are done with the patient supine, the more dependant vessels are posterior, and therefore, the posterior vessels are larger than the anterior ones. On a supine standard chest film, the smaller anterior and larger posterior vessels are superimposed; therefore, on a supine chest radiograph, the vessels size seen by comparing the lung apex and base will be about the same.

Changes in total flow through the lungs (increases and decreases)

NORMAL PULMONARY VASCULARITY

With the patient upright, most of the blood flowing through the lungs courses through the lower lobes. In part this is the effect of gravity and is reflected in the relative size of the upper and lower lung pulmonary vessels: The upper lung vessels are smaller; the lower lung vessels are larger (Figs. 22-1 and 22-2).

Blood passing through the lung moves through both arteries and veins. In much of the lung, it is not possible or necessary to distinguish artery from vein. Only at the hilum is the structure of the arteries and veins sufficiently different to permit differentiation. Pulmonary veins contribute to the upper portion of the hilar vascular shadow as they course toward the left atrium. The lower-lung veins generally run inferior to the hilum, horizontally toward the left atrium. This horizontal course permits their identification. Distention of the pulmonary veins will increase the size of the vascular structures at the superior portion of the hilum, and as discussed in Chapter 18, this change in the top-to-bottom proportional size aids in the recognition of pulmonary venous pressure increases.

As the pulmonary blood vessels branch, each branch becomes smaller. The general effect of this branching is a slow, repetitive decrease in vessel size toward the periphery of the lung. Rapid tapering implies either pulmonary arterial hypertension or vascular occlusion.

This normal, gentle tapering of the pulmonary vessels results in vessels that are just visible in the outer 2 cm of lung. These small vessels in the lung periphery will be visible only when the film technique has stopped respiratory motion. With motion or long exposure times, blurring of these peripheral vessels will occur, making them invisible. Care must be taken in using older texbooks of radiology because older technical methods used longer exposure times and some older books contain statements that vessels cannot be seen in normal people in the outer one-third of the lung or in the outer 2 cm of lung. With modern technique, vessels can occasionally be seen within a few millimeters of the pleural margin, and this does not imply increased vascularity.

Keynote

• *On the normal upright chest radiograph, the lower lung vessels are larger than the upper lung vessels.*

CHANGES OF INCREASED PULMONARY VENOUS PRESSURE

Pulmonary venous hypertension occurs in

Left-sided congestive heart failure
Mitral valve stenosis, insufficiency, or both

and more rarely in

Left atrial myxoma
Pulmonary venous occlusive disease
Cor triatriatum

It can be recognized by the detection of changes in the normal lower lung predominance in pulmonary blood flow (Fig. 22-1).

Minimal increases in pulmonary venous pressure result in an increase in the size of the upper lung pulmonary vessels so that they equal in size the lower lung vessels (Fig. 22-3). It is often difficult to judge these minor changes in vessel size between the upper and lower lung. The size estimate is best made in the lateral portion of the lower and upper lung because of anatomic differences in branching; the vessels of the lower hilum branch more peripherally than those of the upper portion of the hilum. The region inferior to the hilum is thus often deceptive. It can be difficult to look from the top to the bottom of the chest, ignoring vessels in the middle, and accurately compare vessel size. While learning to look carefully, it can be helpful to use a cut-out piece of paper with two holes, top and bottom, superimposed on the chest radiograph to compare the vessel size.

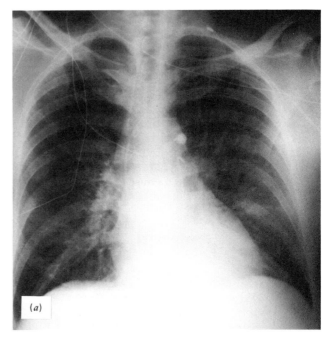

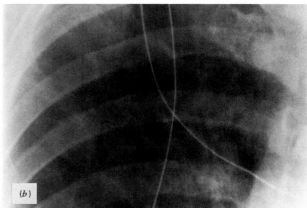

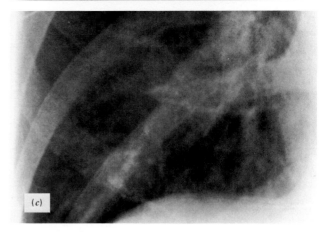

Figure 22-3. A mild increase in pulmonary venous pressure results in greater equality between the upper and lower lung vessels. This radiograph is of the same patient as in Figure 22-1. (*a*) PA view of the chest. (*b*) Focal view of the upper lung vessels. (*c*) Focal view of the lower lung vessels.

With moderate pulmonary venous pressure increases, the upper lung vessels can exceed the size of the lower lung vessels (Fig. 22-4). The lower lung vessels actively decrease in size as the pressure in the veins increases. The reason for this vascular contraction is uncertain, but it is a common occurrence with moderate elevation of the venous pressure.

When the pressure in the pulmonary veins becomes markedly elevated, the fluid in the lymphatic channels becomes visible. With each rise in venous pressure, the lymphatic channels have had to carry increasing amounts of interstitial fluid. This is because the normal resorption of interstitial fluid on the venule side of the capillary depends on the lower hydrostatic pressure in the venous circulation. When less fluid is resorbed, more remains to be removed by the lymphatic vessels (a more detailed explanation of Starling's law of the fluid transport is given in Chapter 11).

The increased lymphatic flow is first visible along the fissures as it passes through the subpleural lymphatic system toward the hilar nodes (see Fig. 11-9 a and b). With increasing lymphatic flow, the interlobular septa become visible. First described by Peter Kerley and called "*Kerley's lines*," Kerley's A lines are near the apex of the lung and near the upper portion of the hilum (Fig. 22-5 a and b); Kerley's B lines are more common and are seen near the lung bases (Figs. 22-5c and 22-6). The superimposition of multiple, visible lymphatic channels toward the center of the lungs result in recticular lines called Kerley's C lines.

With increasing pulmonary venous pressure, the pressure in the interstitium of the lung eventually exceeds the resistance to permeability of the alveolar lining cells and surfactant, and the fluid flows into the alveoli, creating alveolar infiltrates of edema (Fig. 22-5). In some patients these are in a *batwing* or *butterfly* pattern (Fig. 22-7).

Keynotes

- *The common causes of increased pulmonary venous pressure are left-sided heart failure and mitral valve stenosis or insufficiency.*
- *The pulmonary venous pressure is increased when, on a film taken upright, the lower lobe vessels are no longer larger than the upper lobe vessels.*
- *With sufficient increases in pulmonary venous pressure, increased lymphatic flow becomes visible.*
- *Increased lymphatic flow can be seen as thickened fissures and thickened interlobular septa. Sometimes Kerley's lines are called septal lines.*

Case 22-1

JS came to our emergency room, ashen pale and sweaty, with the complaint that there was "someone" sitting on his chest who would not get off. "I'm going to die." On physical examination, his pulse was 96, pressure 150/100 mm Hg, and an S$_3$ gallop was present. The lungs

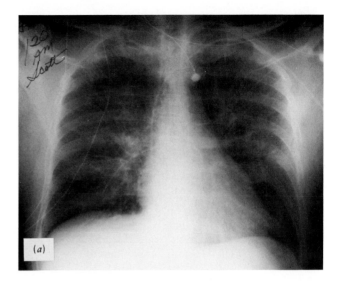

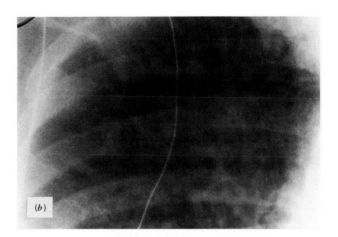

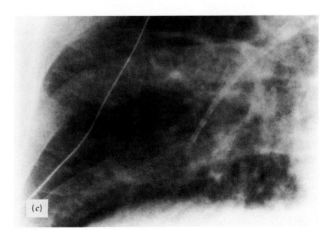

Figure 22-4. Moderate increase in pulmonary venous pressure. The upper lobe vessels are now larger than the lower lobe vessels. The lower lung vessels are now probably smaller than in Figures 22-1 and 22-3. (*a*) PA view of the chest. (*b*) Focal view of the upper lung vessels. (*c*) Focal view of the lower lung vessels.

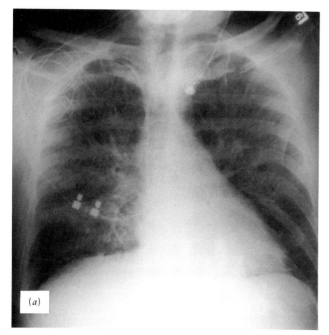

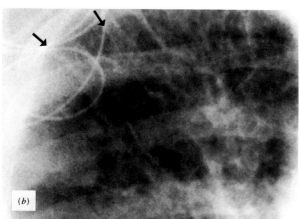

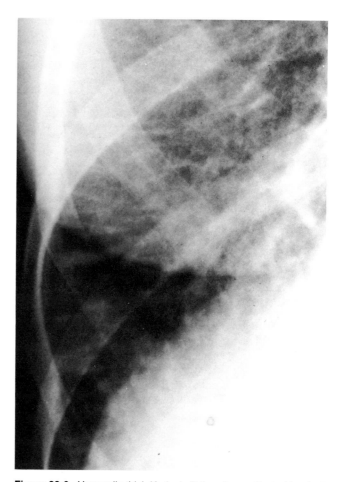

Figure 22-6. Unusually thick Kerley's B lines in a patient with mitral valve stenosis. In this patient, these lines are due to chronic edema and probably interstitial fibrosis.

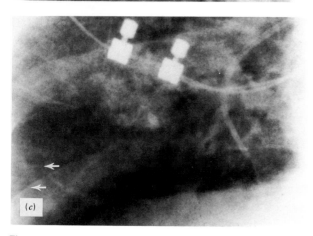

Figure 22-5. Marked increase in pulmonary venous pressure. Kerley's A, B, and C lines are now present. The lower lobe vessels are barely visible because of spasm. (*a*) PA view of the chest. (*b*) Focal view of the upper lungs. Arrows mark some of the Kerley's A lines. (*c*) Focal view of the lower lung. Alveolar infiltrate silhouettes some of the vessels in the middle of this field. Kerley's A lines are at the edge of the picture (arrows). The extra lines in the right side of the picture are the so-called Kerley's C lines.

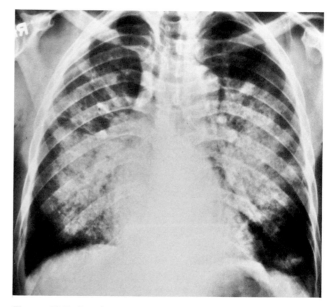

Figure 22-7. Batwing pattern of alveolar pulmonary edema. The patient was uremic from chronic renal failure and also had acute congestive heart failure.

186

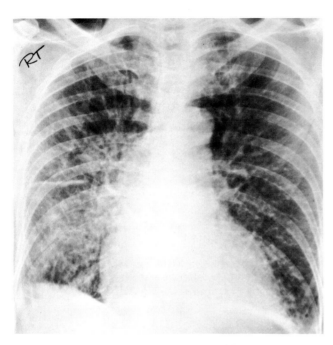

Figure 22-8. Case example 22-1.

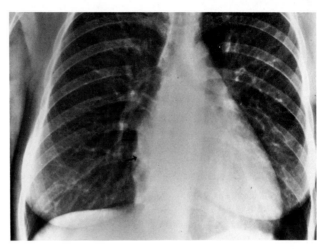

Figure 22-9. Case example 22-2.

were clear. A chest radiograph obtained on his way to the intensive care unit is shown in Figure 22-8. What does it show?

The heart is slightly enlarged. The upper lung vessels are larger than those in the lower lung. Extra lines can be seen in the periphery of the lung base: Kerley's B lines. What do you think is happening?

His heart is failing and he has developed interstitial edema. His history suggests he probably has had an acute myocardial infarction.

How should he be treated?

For pulmonary edema. One method of treatment is to start cardiac monitoring, administer a potent diuretic such as furosemide, and start nasal oxygen.

Interstitial edema cannot be heard on physical examination. Any patient clinically suspected of having possible cardiac decompensation should have either a chest radiograph or blood oxygen level measurements to exclude interstitial edema. If interstitial edema is not recognized and treated, alveolar edema will often develop, and this will result in an increased likelihood of death.

Keynote

- *This patient's sense of impending doom was probably related to hypoxia.*

Case 22-2

This 33-year-old woman has had recurrent *palpitations* during which her heart was "racing." At these times

she has become short of breath and has had to stop and rest until she felt better. On examination her pulse was 110 and irregular. Her chest radiograph is shown in Figure 22-9. What does it show? The upper lobe vessels are larger than those at the lung base. The proportion of the hili is shifted superiorly. Kerley's B lines are present at the lung bases. The heart border on the left is straight. Arrows mark an extra heart contour. What do you think is going on?

These are clear signs of increased pulmonary venous pressure, but in this case, the history points to a chronic intermittent condition rather than acute heart failure. The straightening of the heart border on the left and the extra contour are signs of left atrial enlargement. The patient has mitral stenosis and the heart rhythm is due to atrial fibrillation.

This patient demonstrates the increased size of the upper lung vessels that can occur in patients with mitral stenosis. In addition, minimal left atrial enlargement is present. Not all patients with mitral stenosis demonstrate these findings. Some patients with mitral stenosis severe enough to require surgical treatment will either have normal chest radiographs or demonstrate only minimal upper lung vessel enlargement with no signs of left atrial enlargement. Processes resulting in heart muscle hypertrophy may be invisible on standard radiographs (see Chapter 24).

CHANGES IN PULMONARY ARTERIAL HYPERTENSION

Pulmonary arterial hypertension can be caused by chronic lung disease, chronic or recurrent pulmonary venous hypertension, chronic increases in pulmonary blood flow, and large or recurrent pulmonary emboli. Idiopathic pulmonary hypertension can be seen in young women. The radiographic pattern consists of large central pulmonary arteries that taper rapidly as they extend toward the periphery.

CHANGES IN PULMONARY BLOOD FLOW

Blood flow through the lungs can be increased or decreased in many diseases. Minor changes in flow usually cannot be recognized, but changes in the range of a 2-fold or 2.5-fold magnitude can often be detected. Changes in flow are reflected in changes both in the size of the hili and in the size of the peripheral pulmonary vessels. In general the small hili of marked decreased flow permit its diagnosis. Increased flow is more difficult to recognize.

Changes of Increased Pulmonary Blood Flow

The normal pulmonary vessels are just barely visible in the outer 2 cm of the lungs. Vessels easily seen in the lung periphery are abnormal (Fig. 22-10). If they branch (and thus are not lymphatic channels or septa), their easy recognition indicates increased pulmonary flow. Conditions resulting in increased flow recognizable on a chest radiograph include

Pregnancy

Fever

Anemia

Arteriovenous shunts

Left-to-right cardiac or extracardiac shunts
    Atrial and ventricular septal defects
    Persistent ductus arteriosis

Lesions permitting the mixture of right and left heart blood (*admixture lesions*)
    Truncus arteriosus
    Tricuspid atresia
    Transposition of the great vessels

Case 22-3

BT is a 27-year-old man found to have a positive tuberculin skin test during a screening program at his place of employment. Because the test was positive, the chest radiograph shown in Figure 22-11 was obtained. What do you see?

The lung vessels in the periphery of the lung are enlarged. They can be easily seen in the outer few centimeters of the lung. The hili are of normal size. The heart is enlarged, its apex displaced above the hemidia-

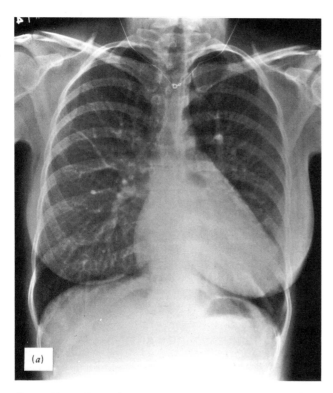

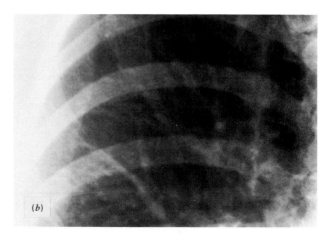

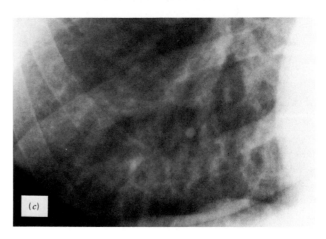

Figure 22-10. The pattern of increased pulmonary blood flow. In this 28-year-old woman with an atrial septal defect, the pulmonary blood vessels are larger than normal, with the lower lung vessels larger than the upper lung vessels. (*a*) PA chest radiograph. (*b*) Focal view of the upper lung vessels. (*c*) Focal view of the lower lung vessels.

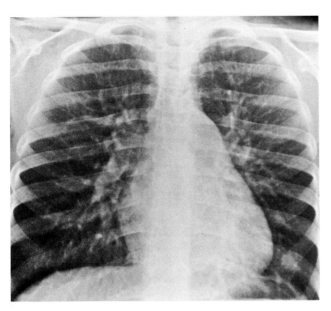

Figure 22-11. Case example 22-3.

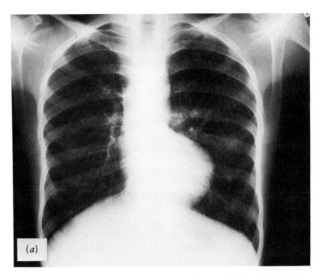

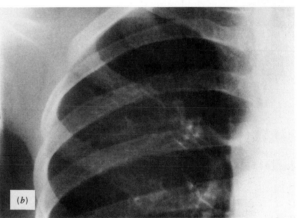

Figure 22-12. The pattern of decreased pulmonary blood flow. This 18-year-old man has Fallot's tetralogy with shunting of blood from the right to the left side of the heart. The blood vessels in the hili and lungs are smaller than usual. (*a*) PA chest radiograph. (*b*) Focal view of the upper lung vessels.

phragm. The left border of the heart is straightened with a separate bulge for the pulmonary artery. The cardiac findings are compatible with right ventricular enlargement associated with clockwise rotation of the heart. What disease do you think is causing the increased pulmonary blood flow and the right ventricular enlargement?

This 27-year-old asymptomatic man has a left-to-right shunt, probably an atrial septal defect. What should you do now?

Take a history and do a physical examination and an electrocardiogram. There are no cardiac symptoms. Physical examination is normal except for a retrosternal heave and a midsystolic heart murmur just to the left of the sternum. The electrocardiogram reveals right ventricular hypertrophy. All these findings are compatible with an atrial septal defect. What should you do now for your patient?

Cardiac catheterization should be done to calculate the degree of shunt and the level of pulmonary arterial pressure. If the shunt is 2:1 or greater and there is no pulmonary hypertension, open heart surgery with repair of the atrial septal defect is usually indicated. This surgery carries the best prognosis if done before cardiac symptoms and pulmonary arterial hypertension occur.

Decreased Blood Flow through the Lungs

Figure 22-12 is the radiograph of an 18-year-old man. The hili are very small, the pulmonary vessels thin and widely separated. The pattern is that of a marked decreased in pulmonary vascularity. This patient has cyanotic congenital heart disease. The vessels seen in the right lung proved to be bronchial arteries rather than pulmonary arteries.

SUMMARY

An evaluation of the distribution of pulmonary blood vessels can tell you how the heart is functioning or failing; an evaluation of how much blood is flowing through the lungs may indicate the presence of cardiac or systemic disease. The evaluation of pulmonary vascularity is often the key to understanding your patients' cardiac disease.

In the normal lung (with the patient upright), the vessels in the lower lung are larger than those in the upper lung. With increased flow, the vessels at the periphery of the lungs are larger; with decreased flow, the hili and the peripheral vessels are smaller. When there is left-sided heart failure, the vessels in the upper lungs get larger, and those in the lower lungs get smaller. With marked elevation of the pulmonary venous pressure, interstitial edema occurs, with the appearance of Kerley's lines. Alveolar edema occurs with severe heart failure.

REVIEW QUESTION

1. Describe the relative size of the pulmonary blood vessels in the normal upright patient and in the patient with left-sided heart failure.
2. What are the more common diseases that result in increased pulmonary venous pressure?
3. What pattern is seen when the blood flow through the lungs is increased?
4. What common conditions result in increased pulmonary blood flow?
5. What is the radiographic appearance of decreased blood flow?
6. In what condition or conditions is bronchial artery circulation increased?

VOCABULARY

admixture lesions
arteriovenous shunt
atrial septal defect
palpitations
pulmonary venous occlusive disease
batwing edema
butterfly edema
cor triatriatum
increased pulmonary venous pressure
Kerley's lines
left atrial myxoma
mitral valve stenosis
septal lines
transposition of the great vessels
tricuspid atresia
truncus arteriosus
ventricular septal defect

SUGGESTIONS FOR FURTHER READING

Ronald G. Grainger. The pulmonary circulation. *Clinical Radiology*, **36**:103–116, 1985.

For additional suggested reading see Chapter 19.

23

EVALUATING THE HEART ON THE CHEST RADIOGRAPH: CARDIAC VALVULAR DISEASE

KEY CONCEPTS

Clinical

The patient suspected of having cardiac valvular disease based on clinical history or cardiac auscultation is usually best evaluated by cardiac ultrasound and may need cardiac catheterization.

The patient with aortic valve stenosis may have symptoms of angina and dyspnea on exertion, syncope, and arrhythmias. If the pressure gradient across the aortic valve is sufficiently high, valve replacement may be indicated.

Radiological

The radiological signs of cardiac valvular disease include changes in pulmonary vascularity, the presence of valvular calcification, dilation of the aorta or pulmonary artery, and dilation or hypertrophy of the adjacent cardiac chambers. Apart from valvular calcification, the valve itself is not seen; thus the diagnosis of valvular disease is usually inferred from the other findings.

Mitral valve disease often produces the changes of pulmonary venous hypertension; the valve may be calcified; and enlargement of the left atrium (and left ventricle in mitral insufficiency) may be seen.

With aortic stenosis, dilation of the ascending aorta and valve calcification may be seen. With aortic insufficiency, dilation of the left ventricle and of the aorta may be present.

OBJECTIVES

When you complete this chapter you will be able to

1. List the four main types of radiological findings of the patient with cardiac valvular disease.
2. List the major clinical and radiological findings seen in a patient with mitral stenosis.

3. List the major clinical and radiological findings seen in a patient with aortic valve stenosis.

Cardiac valvular disease can be evaluated both by the chest radiograph and by cardiac ultrasound (echocardiography). Of the two, cardiac ultrasound gives more precise information, but is obtained only in the patient in whom valvular disease is already suspected. The chest radiograph is used for screening for a large number of diseases, and since it can demonstrate cardiac valvular disease, an understanding of what it can tell you about valvular disease is important.

Valvular disease can be detected on the chest radiograph because of

1. Its effect on the pulmonary vascularity
2. The presence of valvular calcification
3. Its effect on the pulmonary artery or aorta
4. Its effect on the cardiac chambers on either side of the valve

---

Keynote

- *When cardiac valvular disease is suspected, physical examination and echocardiography are the examinations of choice.*

PULMONARY VASCULARITY AND VALVULAR DISEASE

Mitral valve stenosis and insufficiency commonly result in pulmonary venous hypertension which can be detected because pulmonary venous hypertension increases the relative size of the upper lung pulmonary vessels and of the upper portion of the hili. For a full discussion see Chapters 18 and 22.

RECOGNITION OF VALVULAR CALCIFICATION

Calcification of the aortic valve is best seen on the lateral view (Fig. 23-1). Mitral valve calcification can be seen on either the frontal or lateral view (Fig. 23-2). Calcification can occur in either the leaflets or the annulus of the valve. Aortic valve calcification implies the probable presence of aortic stenosis. Mitral leaflet calcification usually indicates mitral stenosis. Calcification of the mitral valve annulus (Fig. 22-3) is a degeneration phenomenon occurring in elderly patients and is often associated with defects in the electrical conduction of the heart.

Valvular calcification is most easily identified on fluoroscopy, where the rapid motion of the calcium helps to separate its shadow from overlying lung markings. On standard radiographs it is harder to identify. When calcification is identified on the lateral view, it is sometimes useful to draw a line from the hilar bronchi to the apex of the heart (Figs. 23-1 and 23-2b). Calcifications anterior to that line usually are in the aortic valve; those posterior to it, usually in the mitral valve.

Keynotes

- *Calcification of the aortic valve is best seen on the lateral view. Calcification of the mitral valve can be seen on either the frontal or lateral view.*
- *The rapid motion of valvular calcifications can be seen on fluoroscopy, aiding in their detection.*
- *Calcifications anterior to the hilar bronchus–cardiac apex line usually are in the aortic valve; those behind it, usually in the mitral valve.*

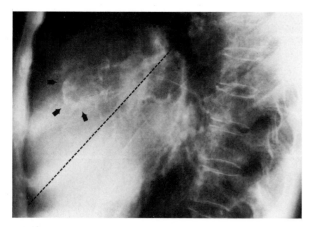

Figure 23-1. Portion of a lateral chest radiograph showing aortic valve calcification (arrows). A dotted line runs from the hilar bronchi to the cardiac apex.

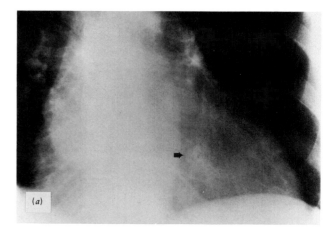

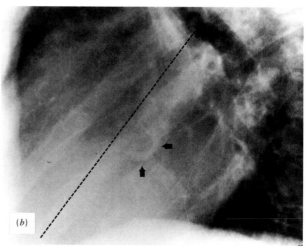

Figure 23-2. Mitral valve calcification (arrows). (*a*) Frontal view. (*b*) Lateral view; a dotted line runs from the hilar bronchi to the cardiac apex.

POSTSTENOTIC DILATION OF GREAT VESSELS

The jet of blood flowing through a stenotic valve and the turbulence it produces often result in the dilation of the vessel distal to the stenotic valve. This distention can be identified in the postvalvular portion of the aorta in a patient with aortic stenosis and in the main pulmonary artery in a patient with stenosis of the pulmonic valve.

Case 23-1

FJ is a 28-year-old man who decided to start jogging and passed out during his first block. A loud systolic murmur was present at the base of the heart. His radiograph is in Figure 23-4. What do you see?

The pulmonary vascularity is normal, the heart is of normal size; the ascending aorta, however, protrudes from the mediastinum whereas the descending aorta is not dilated. The lateral view shows slight filling in of the retrosternal clear space. What do you think the patient's problem is?

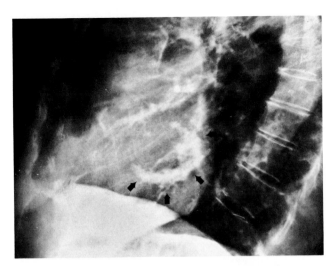

Figure 23-3. Mitral annulus calcification (arrows).

He has aortic stenosis. What symptoms are associated with this disease?

Slowly progressive decrease in exercise ability, angina and dyspnea on exertion, syncope, arrhythmias, sudden death. What should you do for him? Evaluate the degree of stenosis and degree of myocardial hypertrophy with an echocardiogram, electrocardiogram, and with heart catheterization to evaluate the pressure gradient. If the disease is severe enough, aortic valve replacement is indicated. In this patient a 50 mm Hg gradient was present, and the valve was replaced with a prosthesis.

In some patients, the poststenotic dilation of the aorta is best seen on the frontal view; in others it is best seen on the lateral view. Both views should be studied.

Keynote

• *The ascending aorta may show poststenotic dilation in aortic stenosis.*

SUMMARY

There are both direct and indirect radiographic signs of cardiac valve disease. Valvular calcification is the direct sign. Both aortic and mitral calcifications can be seen on the lateral view. Mitral valve calcification can sometimes be seen on the frontal view. Fluoroscopy aids in the recognition of valvular calcification, permitting it to be distinguished from superimposed lung markings.

Indirect signs are not specific for valve disease but are the only signs present in a majority of patients. Mitral valve disease results in increased pulmonary venous pressure and in an increase in the size of the left atrium. Aortic stenosis can result in dilation of the ascending aorta and hypertrophy of the left ventricle. Pulmonic stenosis can result in dilation of the main pulmonary artery.

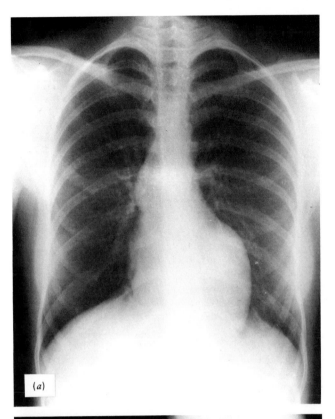

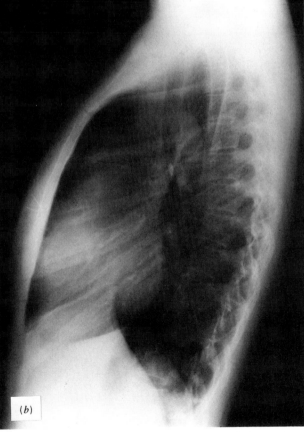

Figure 23-4. Case 23-1. (a) Frontal view. (b) Lateral view.

When suspected clinically, valvular disease is best confirmed and delineated by echocardiography.

REVIEW QUESTIONS

1. What is the effect of mitral valve disease on the pulmonary vascularity?
2. There are four cardiac valves. Calcification in some of these valves can be seen on the lateral view. For some it can be seen on the frontal view. Which view would you use to demonstrate aortic calcification? Which view would you use to look for mitral calcification?
3. Why does fluoroscopy help in the visualization of valvular calcification?
4. What is the usual clinical significance of
   Mitral valve calcification?
   Mitral annulus calcification?
   Aortic valve calcification?
5. A line drawn on the lateral chest film from the hilar bronchi to the cardiac apex is useful in determining which valve is calcified. Which valve lies in front of and which behind this line?
6. In which diseases is post stenotic dilation of a great vessel seen?
7. What symptoms occur in the patient with aortic valve stenosis?

VOCABULARY

angina

arrhythmia

dyspnea

mitral annulus calcification

syncope

SUGGESTIONS FOR FURTHER READING

Acquired valvular disease of the heart. *Seminars in Roentgenology,* **14**(2), 1979.

For additional suggested reading see Chapter 19.

24

EVALUATING THE HEART ON THE CHEST RADIOGRAPH: CARDIAC AND HEART CHAMBER ENLARGEMENT

KEY CONCEPTS

Clinical

The heart can respond to disease in two ways: muscle can hypertrophy and chambers can dilate. Muscle hypertrophy is best detected by an electrocardiogram but in some cases is better identified by an echocardiogram.

Myocardial hypertrophy usually results from a gradual increase in the pressure within the heart, such as that seen with developing arterial hypertension or from an increasingly stenotic valve. An idiopathic form of myocardial hypertrophy, idiopathic hypertrophic subaortic stenosis, is usually best detected by echocardiography.

Cardiac chamber dilation usually results from weakening of the myocardium, often caused by ischemia or myocarditis and less commonly by increasing volume overload as in valvular insufficiency.

Radiological

Generalized cardiomegaly is usually determined by measurement of the *cardiothoracic ratio:* the ratio of the transverse diameter of the heart to the transverse diameter of the lungs at the level of the right hemidiaphragm. On a PA, good-inspiratory radiograph taken upright, the normal ratio is less than 50%. A ratio greater than 50% can result from cardiomegaly and pericardial effusion. The measurement becomes an inaccurate predictor of cardiomegaly and pericardial effusion when the lungs are hypoinflated. Sometimes large amounts of pericardial and epicardial fat will increase the cardiothoracic ratio.

Left atrial enlargement results in straightening of the heart border on the left and results in a double density of the enlarged left atrium superimposed on the heart shadow.

Right ventricular enlargement can elevate the cardiac apex, straighten the heart border on the left, and partially fill in the retrosternal space.

Left ventricular enlargement tends to push the cardiac apex inferiorly and results in a rounded bulging of the lateral and posterior borders of the left side of the heart.

OBJECTIVES

When you complete this chapter you will be able to

1. Identify the location of the cardiac chambers on normal PA and lateral chest radiographs.
2. List four findings indicating probable left atrial enlargement.
3. Correctly identify patients with a large left atrium on selected chest radiographs.
4. Calculate the cardiothoracic ratio and interpret its meaning on selected chest radiographs.
5. Correctly identify right ventricular enlargement on selected chest radiographs.
6. Describe the radiographic changes of left ventricular enlargement.
7. List three causes of myocardial hypertrophy.
8. List five causes of cardiac chamber dilation.

The myocardium responds to disease in two distinct, but overlapping, ways: it can dilate or it can hypertrophy. Myocardial hypertrophy occurs mainly as the response to slow increases in pressure as a result of either hypertension (pulmonary or systemic) or a slowly developing stenosis of a valve. Most of the time, chamber hypertrophy is invisible on the standard radiograph. It will result, however, in increased voltage on the electrocardiogram, and when it is sufficiently increased, it can be recognized as increased wall thickness on an echocardiogram.

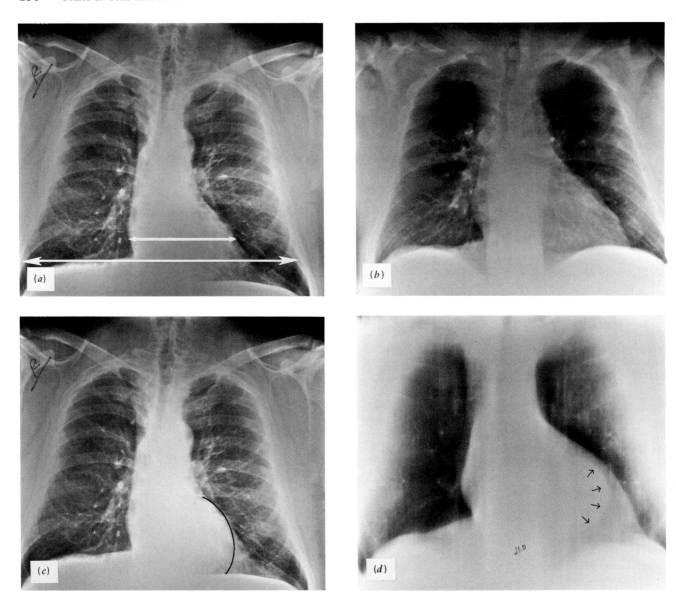

Figure 24-1. Normal heart in different views. (*a*) PA view in good inspiration. The arrows demonstrate a "short-cut" method for the measurement of the cardiothoracic ratio. (*b*) The same patient with poor expansion of the lungs. The heart shadow extends further from side to side, simulating cardiomegaly. (*c*) The same view as in *a*. The curved line demonstrates the method of approximating the true edge of the heart, excluding the fat pad. (*d*) A conventional tomogram through the heart demonstrates the junction (arrows) between the water-radiodensity heart and the combined epicardial and extrapericardial fat. Although this is not a valid clinical use for tomography, it is used here to demonstrate the proportion of the "cardiac" silhouette that is from fat rather than heart.

Cardiac dilation can affect either the entire heart or specific chambers. It results either from myocardial disease (myocardiopathy, myocarditis, infarction) resulting in decreased contractility or from a chronic increase in the volume of blood handled by the heart (shunts, insufficient valves).

Keynotes

- *The myocardium can hypertrophy or dilate in response to disease.*

- *Hypertrophy is a response to a slow increase in the pressure load on the heart.*
- *Dilation results from an increased volume load or decreased contractility of the cardiac muscle.*

GENERALIZED CARDIAC ENLARGEMENT

The cardiac silhouette seen on the radiograph is composed of five structures, each of which contributes to its transverse diameter: the heart, the epicardial fat, the pericardial space, the pericardium, and the extrapericardial fat pad. The usual method of judging the overall cardiac size is to compare the transverse diameter of the heart shadow to the transverse diameter of the inner margin of the rib cage (Fig. 24-1a). When this ratio is less than 50%, generalized cardiomegaly is considered to be absent. When it is greater than 50%, a more careful evaluation of the shape and character of the cardiac shadow must be made.

Lung Hypoinflation

Hypoinflated lungs will push the heart into a more transverse position, simulating cardiac enlargement (Fig. 24-1b). The hypoinflation can be recognized by noting the upward curve of each hemidiaphragm. The lack of cardiac enlargement can be judged by observing the relatively narrow height of the heart. With generalized cardiomegaly, the heart enlarges in all three planes: side to side, top to bottom, and front to back. Hypoinflation does not increase the top-to-bottom size.

Extra Pericardial and Epicardial Fat

Extrapericardial fat and *epicardial fat* are always present and can simulate cardiac enlargement. More fat tends to be present in obese patients and in those with chronic corticosteroid excess. In general, the likely heart margin can be extrapolated by using the upper lateral margin of the left side of the heart as the start of the arc of the heart; by completing the arc, you can judge where the heart margin probably lies (Fig. 24-1c). In Figure 24-1d, a tomogram of the chest reveals the actual water-density heart sitting within the more radiolucent extrapericardial and epicardial fat layer and illustrates the type of curve the apex of the heart usually has. If any question persists as to the presence or absence of cardiac enlargement after interpretation of the standard radiograph, a careful physical examination with observation and palpation of the point of maximum cardiac impulse should resolve the question. It is also useful to remember that fat people tend to have more extrapericardial fat and tend to take shallower breaths; therefore it is useful to be somewhat skeptical of the cardiac size visible on the radiograph in fat people and to seek clinical confirmation of this finding.

Pericardial Effusion

Pericardial effusion simulates diffuse cardiomegaly. Any large cardiac shadow that shows no signs of specific cardiac chamber enlargement should be given a dual interpretation of cardiomegaly and/or pericardial effusion. When suspected, the best method of confirming or excluding the presence of pericardial fluid is the echocardiogram (Chapter 21).

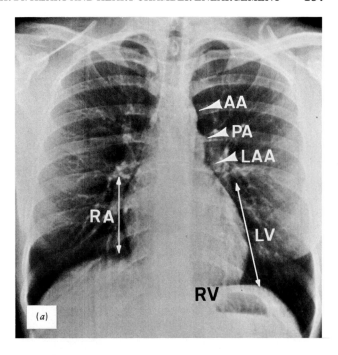

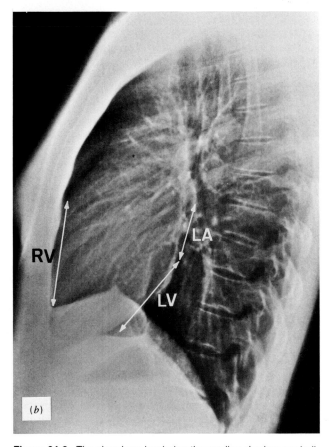

Figure 24-2. The chambers bordering the cardiac shadow are indicated on these normal PA (*a*) and lateral (*b*) chest radiographs. RA = right atrium, RV = right ventricle, LA = left atrium, LAA = left atrial appendage, LV = left ventricle, PA = main pulmonary artery, AA = aorta and aortic arch.

SPECIFIC CHAMBER ENLARGEMENT

Figure 24-2 illustrates the location of each of the normal heart chambers. There are specific radiographic signs of enlargement of the left atrium and of the right and left ventricles. Of these, the signs for enlargement of the left atrium are the most specific.

Left Atrial Enlargement

Left Heart Border Straightening. The signs of left atrial enlargement are quite good but occasionally confusing. If you refer to Figure 24-2 a of the normal heart contours, you will see that the region of the left atrial appendage is normally concave. As the left atrial appendage enlarges, it tends to progressively fill in that portion of the cardiac contour, straightening it and then bulging it outward, making it convex (Fig. 24-3a and b)

Two other processes can also make the left side of the heart border straight or minimally convex, and these both do it by rotating the heart in a clockwise direction, bringing the pulmonary outflow tract to a border-forming position. These are right ventricular enlargement and a common skeletal abnormality—pectus excavatum—in which the sternum is depressed, pushing on the heart and often rotating it.

Double Density. The second finding in left atrial enlargement is the *double density*, or double contour, of the right side of the heart margin (Figs. 24-3 and 22-9). The left atrium normally sits behind and medial to the right atrial margin. Normally, the contour of the posterior heart is relatively smooth. As the left atrium enlarges, it bulges posteriorly, and its right margin becomes visible behind the right atrial margin. This is a very good sign of left atrial enlargement, but it is sometimes confused with tortuosity of the ascending aorta (Fig. 24-4a), which can appear to be a second curved contour superimposed on the right atrium. The aortic shadow, however, starts at the midpoint of the right atrial shadow, rather than lower.

Carinal Angle. The enlarging left atrium also has an identifiable effect on the tracheal bifurcation. Sitting just inferior to the tracheal bifurcation, the large left atrium will widen the carinal angle between the right and left bronchi and elevate the left main bronchus. This elevation is also stimulated by a lordotic projection of the chest, so care must be used in applying it.

Displacement of the Esophagus. The enlarged left atrium will also push back on the esophagus, indenting and often

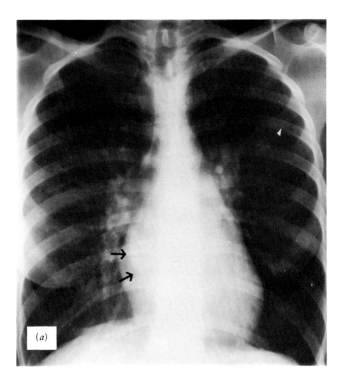

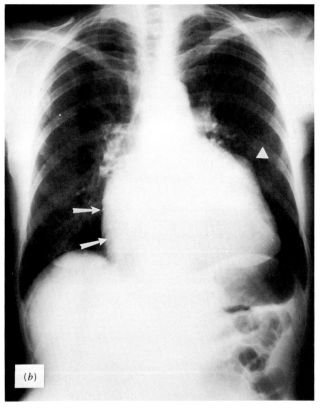

Figure 24-3. Examples of left atrial enlargement. (*a*) Straightening of the left side of the heart border, from enlargement of the left atrial appendage; double density of the left atrium (arrows). (*b*) The left atrial appendage protrudes from the left side of the heart border (arrowhead). The double density is almost superimposed on the right side of the heart border (arrows).

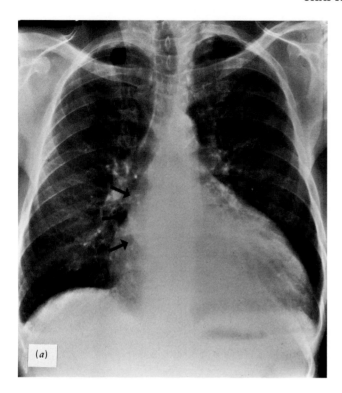

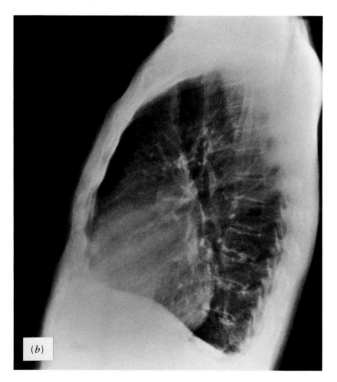

Figure 24-4. Aortic insufficiency with left ventricular enlargement and tortuosity of the ascending aorta. Arrows (a) demarcate the ascending aorta.

displacing it. Views are sometimes taken with barium in the esophagus to better detect this left atrial bulge.

Right Ventricular Enlargement

The right ventricle lies anteriorly and inferiorly in the heart (Fig. 24-2). It rests against the sternum, the left anterior chest wall, and the diaphragm. As it enlarges, it presses against these structures, elevating the cardiac apex and pushing the apex of the heart posteriorly (Fig. 24-5). It also rotates the heart in a clockwise fashion, sometimes straightening the left side of the heart border. The retrosternal space is often filled in by the enlarged pulmonary artery.

Left Ventricular Enlargement

The left ventricle is located in the posterior and superior portion of the heart (Fig. 24-2). As it enlarges, it tends to push the apex of the heart inferiorly and to bulge out along the superior and posterior cardiac margin (Figs. 24-4 and 24-6).

Keynotes

- *Left atrial enlargement straightens the left side of the heart border, creates a double density of the right side of the heart, splays the carina, elevates the left main bronchus, and indents and displaces the esophagus.*
- *Enlargement of the right ventricle elevates the apex of the heart and pushes it back.*
- *Enlargement of the left ventricle rounds the left side of the heart border laterally and posteriorly and pushes the cardiac apex down.*

SUMMARY

The myocardium can respond to disease by hypertrophy or dilation. Hypertrophy usually cannot be detected on radiographs but can be evaluated by electrocardiography and echocardiography. Dilation can be evaluated by radiography and echocardiography. Cardiac chamber dilation can result from decreased contractility or from a chronic increase in the volume of blood the heart has to handle.

Generalized cardiomegaly is detected by measuring the cardiothoracic ratio. A ratio less than 50% indicates that generalized cardiac enlargement is not present. A ratio greater than 50% can be due to cardiac enlargement, pericardial effusion, a film taken in incomplete inspiration, or an increased amount of extrapericardial fat.

When the left atrium enlarges, it fills in the normally concave portion of the upper left border of the heart, straightening it and then causing it to bulge outward. Often a second radiodensity is seen superimposed on the right atrial portion of the heart. The carina can be splayed and the left main bronchus elevated. The esophagus can be indented.

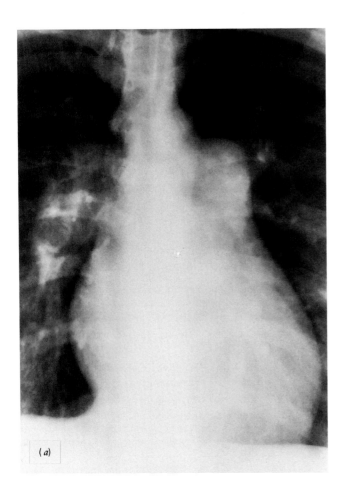
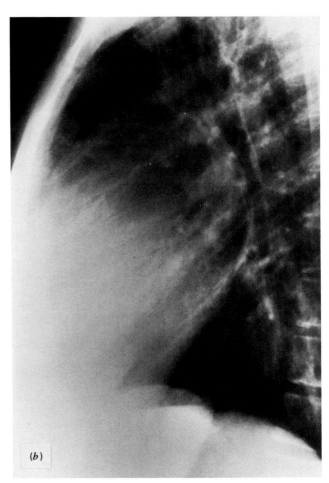

Figure 24-5. Right ventricular enlargement in a patient with pulmonary hypertension. The rounded apex of the heart with the apex projected above the diaphragm (a) and the filling in of the retrosternal space (b) are signs of right ventricular enlargement. Note the markedly enlarged main pulmonary artery on the PA view. This patient had an untreated atrial septal defect for many years, eventually developing pulmonary arterial hypertension.

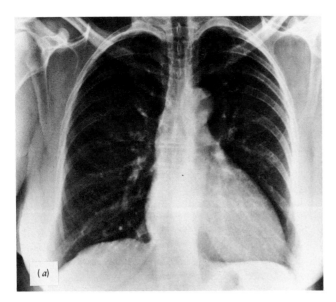
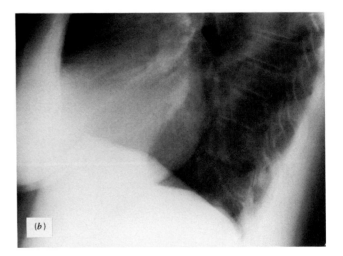

Figure 24-6. Left ventricular enlargement caused by ischemic cardiomyopathy. The rounding of the left side of the heart border combined with the relatively inferior placement of the apex of the heart on the PA view (a) and the low posterior bulge of the heart on the lateral view (b) are signs of left ventricular enlargement.

Right ventricular enlargement pushes the apex of the heart up and back. Left ventricular enlargement pushes the apex of the heart down and rounds the left lateral border of the heart.

The detection of localized cardiac chamber enlargement can aid in the detection of valvular disease, myocardial disease, and peripheral vascular disease.

The proper evaluation of the patient with heart disease requires a careful history and physical. Based on the type of cardiac disease suspected, an electrocardiogram, a chest radiograph, an echocardiogram, or a nuclear medicine imaging study may be needed. The evaluation of the conditions of the patient with complex cardiac malformations and the one who might benefit from surgical correction of a defect may require heart catheterization with or without angiography for precise anatomic information.

REVIEW QUESTIONS

1. What are the two basic ways in which the myocardium can respond to disease?
2. How is myocardial hypertrophy best detected?
3. What is the cardiothoracic ratio? What is its normal limit? What is the meaning of an enlarged cardiothoracic ratio?
4. How can you distinguish pericardial effusion from cardiomegaly?
5. What are the specific signs of left atrial enlargement?
6. What symptoms can be seen in the patient with mitral stenosis?
7. What is an insufficient valve? What effect does it have on the heart?
8. What is a stenotic valve? What effect does it have on the heart?
9. What are the radiographic findings in right ventricular enlargement?
10. What are the radiographic findings in left ventricular enlargement?

VOCABULARY

cardiothoracic ratio

double density sign

epicardial fat

idiopathic hypertrophic subaortic stenosis

extrapericardial fat

myocarditis

myocardiopathy

pectus excavatum

SUGGESTIONS FOR FURTHER READING

For suggested reading see Chapter 19.

SECTION E

THE BREAST

Chapter 25 discusses mammography, the radiology of the breast. Breast cancer is the most common cancer in women, accounting for one-quarter of all cancer in women and one-fifth of all cancer deaths in women. There are over 100,000 new cases of breast cancer each year. Mammography is important both as a major screening method for early cancer and as a technique for evaluating a palpable lump or known breast cancer.

In addition to breast cancer, there are other diseases of the breast that can be evaluated with mammography. Chapter 25 discusses these along with the methods recommended for breast cancer screening.

25

MAMMOGRAPHY

ERLINDA McCREA

KEY CONCEPTS

Clinical

Mammography is used mainly in the evaluation of women with suspected or known breast cancer, in screening women with known risk factors for the development of breast cancer, and increasingly in the screening of asymptomatic women over the age of 40. As a screening test, it should be combined with monthly breast self-examination and annual breast physical examination by a trained medical worker (nurse, physician, or physician's assistant).

Screening of asymptomatic women without known risk factors for developing breast cancer should consist of a baseline mammogram at age 40, with follow-up examinations at 1- to 2-year intervals. Annual mammography is recommended for women over the age of 50.

Risk factors for breast cancer indicate the need for an earlier start of screening. Women with these risk factors should be trained in breast self-examination, be examined by a trained medical worker annually starting at age 25, and have annual mammograms starting at age 35. Those at increased risk for the development of breast cancer are women who have one or more of the following risk factors. They are nulliparous or first became pregnant at age 28 or later, have a mother or sister with breast cancer, or have had a previous biopsy revealing ductal hyperplasia.

Radiological

There are two methods of mammography: one uses a film-screen combination; the other uses the Xerox method. Both methods use low doses of radiation. Mammograms can detect both benign and malignant disease. Sometimes the diagnosis of a benign mass is definite and a biopsy is not necessary; more often a biopsy is necessary to exclude cancer. There are specific mammographic signs of cancer, but many small cancers overlap the patterns seen in benign disease. Radiographic signs suggesting probable cancer include masses with irregular or spiculated margins, masses with ill-defined margins, microcalcifications, and secondary signs such as skin thickening, skin retraction, and increased vascularity.

Small, nonpalpable masses can be localized for a guided biopsy by the placement of a localizing needle under radiographic guidance.

OBJECTIVES

When you complete this chapter you will be able to

1. List the four risk factors for the development of breast cancer.
2. List the three types of examination that constitute appropriate screening for breast cancer.
3. List the frequency of screening mammography in women with and without specific risk factors for breast cancer.
4. List the four mammographic findings that indicate that a breast mass probably represents cancer.
5. Describe what you would tell a patient who is concerned about the risk from the radiation used for mammography.
6. Identify solitary masses on selected mammograms and indicate which have specific findings indicating the probable presence of cancer.

Mammography is the radiology of the breast. It is used for the diagnosis of breast disease and the identification and localization of breast cancer. This chapter discusses the indications for mammography, the current techniques, the mammographic patterns of breast disease, and the controversy concerning the hazard of breast tissue exposure to radiation.

INDICATIONS FOR MAMMOGRAPHY

Who should and should not have mammography? Although mammography can help in the identification of many breast disorders, its main use is in the evaluation of suspected or known breast cancer. It is also recommended as a screening test for asymptomatic women. Mammography is used in:

1. Screening patients in certain high-risk groups for breast cancer
2. Screening women without risk factors for breast cancer
3. Evaluating a clinically palpable mass
4. Evaluating the opposite breast in a patient with known cancer in one breast, looking for a nonpalpable second primary
5. Following remaining breast tissue after the removal of a tumor

Screening of Patients with Increased Breast Cancer Risk

Those at increased risk have one or more of the following risk factors. They

Are nulliparous

First became pregnant at age 28 or later

Have a mother or sister with breast cancer

Have had a previous biopsy revealing ductal hyperplasia

These women should be instructed in breast self-examination; should be examined by a physician annually, probably starting at age 25; and should have mammographic examinations annually starting at age 35.

In the woman with a previous breast cancer, the opposite breast should be examined by x-ray 6 months after surgery and yearly thereafter. Up to 16% of these patients will develop cancer in the remaining breast, half of which occurs within 6 years after mastectomy.

Is Screening for Breast Cancer Worthwhile? The BCDDP (Breast Cancer Detection Demonstration Projects) (Baker 1982) is a screening program established in the United States in 1973 using 29 different centers throughout the country, to determine the usefulness and efficacy of mammography. Recent results indicate the superiority of mammography over physical examination in detecting nonpalpable or occult cancers:

Mammography, 95%

Physical examination, 33%

A baseline mammogram is now recommended at age 40 (an earlier age is preferable in high-risk patients), with follow-up examination at 1- to 2-year intervals determined by analysis of physical and mammographic findings and other risk factors. For women over 50 years of age, annual mammography is currently recommended (Mammography Guidelines, 1983).

Other Uses

Mammography can also be of value in certain situations such as:

1. In the patient with pendulous breasts that are difficult to examine
2. In the presence of signs like skin ulceration, retraction or dimpling, and nipple discharge or retraction without an associated palpable mass
3. When metastases are present in a patient with an unknown primary cancer and the possibility that an occult breast cancer exists or when an equivocal mammogram was previously done

---

Keynotes

- *Mammography has a key role in the diagnosis of early breast cancer and in the evaluation of the opposite breast in a patient with breast cancer.*
- *Mammography should be used in the patient with any of the high-risk factors for breast cancer. These are patients who are (1) nulliparous, (2) first became pregnant at age 28 or later, (3) have a mother or sister with breast cancer, (4) have had a previous biopsy revealing ductal hyperplasia.*
- *All women should have a baseline mammogram between ages 35 and 40, with follow-up mammograms every 1–2 years to age 50, and then annually.*

HOW MAMMOGRAPHY IS PERFORMED

There are two mammography methods, both requiring radiation exposure. One method uses film-screen combinations (Fig. 25-1); the other uses the Xerox method (Fig. 25-2). Both techniques use low diagnostic doses of radiation. Xeromammography uses a photoconductive surface and electrostatic charges, resulting in a blue-toned permanent image on plastic-coated paper for viewing and storage. The advantage of the Xerox method is its property of edge enhancement, wherein the contrast of differences in tissue radiodensities is greatly enhanced, resulting in an optimal technique for breast examination. Either method is acceptable; low levels of radiation are used with resultant good image quality.

Keynote

- *There are two main methods of mammography: xerography and radiography.*

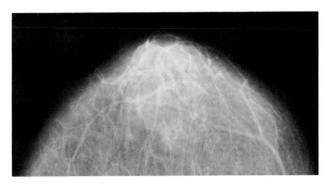

Figure 25-1. Plain-film mammogram of a normal fatty postmenopausal breast.

THE ISSUE OF HAZARD FROM THE RADIATION IN MAMMOGRAPHY

Much has been written about the carcinogenic effects of radiation exposure of breast tissue. When mammography first came into general use in the early 1960s, doses were quite high, sometimes as much as 4–8 R at skin surface. A study published in the early 1970s, indicated possible carcinogenic effects. The data used were, however, derived from high-radiation sources such as Hiroshima victims (the atom bomb), multiple fluoroscopic examinations of the chest in women with tuberculosis and undergoing treatment, radiotherapy for patients with acne, and so forth. Current techniques use much lower doses, 1 rad or less per breast (two views) per study, and therefore, the earlier studies of carcinogenesis are no longer applicable (*Mammography,* 1982). Linear extrapolation to low doses is too simple an explanation when there are many factors, several still unknown, involved in the development of breast cancer. "Mammography has been used clinically for 20 years, yet there is not one proven case of breast cancer association with mammography," according to Sickles (1977).

Let us look at this issue in another way. The age-adjusted incidence for breast cancer in American women is 70/1,000/year, or 7%. Using linear extrapolation, a single mammographic examination, delivery of 1 rad per breast, increases the lifetime risk of developing breast cancer from 70/1,000/year to 70.7/1,000/year, or from 7% to 7.07%. As Moskowitz (1978) reported in JAMA, "The probability that a 35 year old woman will die an accidental death is 13 to 25 times as great as the possibility that she will die of mammography induced breast cancer. If a woman is a 1 to 1½ pack per day smoker for 30 years, her chance of dying of lung cancer is 60 to 113 times greater than her chance of dying of induced breast cancer." Therefore, when mammography is indicated, the risk of this theoretically possible complication of the radiation should not prevent one from using the examination.

Keynote

- *The hazard of the radiation used in mammography, if it exists at all, is much less than the risk of missing an early breast cancer.*

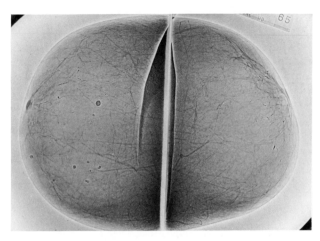

Figure 25-2. Xerographic mammogram of postmenopausal fatty breasts with benign calcifications within the ducts bilaterally.

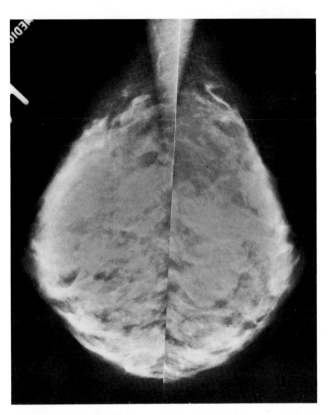

Figure 25-3. A palpable mass, left, in a 31-year-old woman, difficult to evaluate because of the increased radiodensity of the normal glandular tissue. The mass is not seen.

MAMMOGRAPHIC FEATURES OF BREAST DISEASE

Breast tissue varies in appearance according to age, number of pregnancies, and underlying disease within the breast (parenchymal disease). Women below the age of 35 generally have more glandular tissue and hence are "denser" and more difficult to interpret (Fig. 25-3).

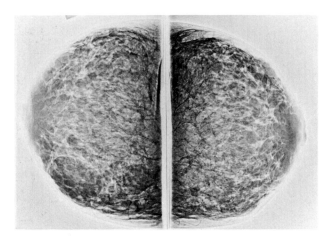

Figure 25-4. Severe mammary dysplasia (with fibrocystic disease, adenosis, and papillomatosis), difficult to interpret. Malignancy cannot be excluded.

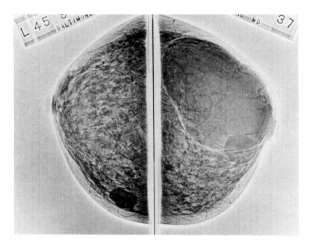

Figure 25-5. Mammogram of a 37-year-old woman with bilateral lumps. A huge fibroadenoma was removed on the right.

Women 40 years and older develop fatty replacement of normal glandular tissue and become less radiodense, revealing abnormalities more readily (Fig. 25-2).

Mammary dysplasia is a common term you will encounter in mammographic reports. It is a general condition wherein breast tissue appears radiodense, that is, more blue in the Xerox technique or more white in the film-screen technique when compared with normal breast. This is because of a mixed histologic picture of fibrocystic disease, adenosis, fibrosis, and papillomatosis. The first three are present at the beginning of breast development, often coexist, tend to regress with age and pregnancies, and are symmetrical bilaterally (Fig. 25-4). Depending on the degree of involvement, the increase in radiodensity of breast tissue may obscure an underlying cancer, especially the minimal or occult cancers (defined as less than 1 cm in diameter and difficult to palpate on physical examination). The breast with dysplasia often presents difficulty in interpretation for the mammographer. A clinically palpable lesion in the presence of a normal mammogram, particularly with radiodense breasts, should not prevent a clinician from performing a biopsy to exclude cancer.

Benign Breast Conditions and How They Appear on Mammography

Fibroadenoma. The most common benign tumor, fibroadenoma is seen in young women from teens to 40 years of age. It usually presents as a smooth, firm, and freely movable mass. There are multiple masses in 35% of cases. It can occur unilaterally or bilaterally (Fig. 25-5). Giant fibroadenomas are often seen in the younger patient, and lactating adenomas can occur after pregnancy.

On a mammogram, a fibroadenoma is easily recognized as a smooth-mass radiodensity with most of its margins visible (Fig. 25-5). When it is solitary and some of its borders are not well defined, it may be difficult to differentiate from malignancy and a biopsy may be necessary. In time, coarse and thick calcifications appear in the mass radiodensity and are diagnostic (Fig. 25-6).

Cysts. Cysts tend to involve an older age group than fibroadenoma. History is helpful in that rapid fluctuation in size, appearance, and number is characteristic and makes serial examinations, both physical and radiographic, quite important and helpful. Cysts are often tender, freely movable, and multiple.

On a mammogram, the margins are sharp around an oval or round mass (Fig. 25-7). Overlapping structures may obscure portions of the margins (as in fibroadenoma), but the absence of signs of malignancy should go against

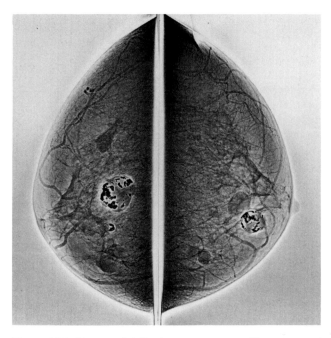

Figure 25-6. Many well-defined masses, some with coarse and thick calcifications, indicating fibroadenomas.

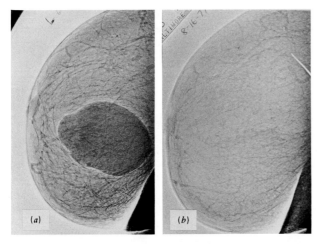

Figure 25-7. Well-defined oval mass suggests a cyst; confirmed by aspiration on follow-up. (*a*) Before aspiration of cyst. (*b*) After aspiration.

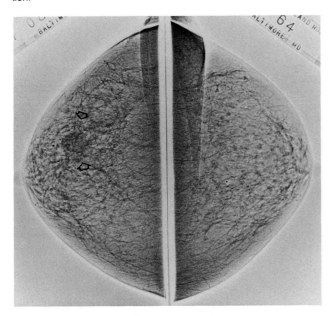

Figure 25-8. A poorly marginated mass lateral to the nipple (arrows) in a patient with mammary dysplasia. Suggests cancer; proven to be an abscess.

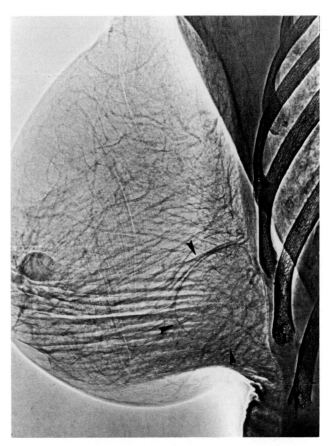

Figure 25-9. Ringlike radiodensity indicates the outer margin of a lipoma, with decreased radiodensity from fat (arrowheads).

the diagnosis of cancer. Occasionally, it may be difficult to differentiate a cyst from a well-marginated cancer. Ultrasonography and aspiration can be both diagnostic and therapeutic.

Abscess. Abscesses may be acute or chronic, with the chronic type usually subareolar or close to the nipple. The acute variety can occur anywhere, with the clinical and radiographic findings quite similar to those of a cancer and requiring a biopsy for confirmation (Fig. 25-8).

Lipomas and Galactoceles. Readily recognizable on mammograms because their fat content gives them a radiodensity less than that of normal breast tissue are both lipomas

and galactoceles. (Galactoceles are milk-containing retention cysts.) (Fig. 25-9).

Fat Necrosis. Fat necrosis results from trauma, either accidental or surgical. There are several mammographic appearances, most of which are benign and easy to recognize. On occasion, however, the appearance may mimic a cancer, requiring a biopsy to confirm a benign process, especially in the absence of a history of trauma (Fig. 25-10).

Sclerosing Adenosis. Usually a symmetrical and bilateral condition, in sclerosing adenosis there is hyperplasia or overgrowth of terminal ductules and connective tissue. Minute calcifications (microcalcifications) are often present in a scattered fashion. This condition causes an increase in the normal breast radiodensity, and where there is asymmetry, which is not uncommon, malignancy might be suspected, necessitating a biopsy to exclude cancer.

Biopsy Scars. many women will have biopsies to rule out cancer at some time in their lives. As the area heals, it may leave an actual masslike scar so that physically and mammographically a tumor cannot be excluded (Fig. 25-11).

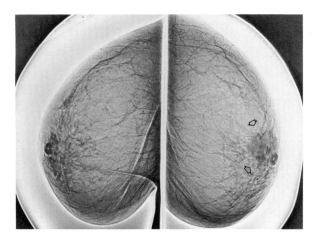

Figure 25-10. A subareolar mass (arrows) with poorly defined margins, which suggests cancer but is proved, on biopsy, to be fat necrosis.

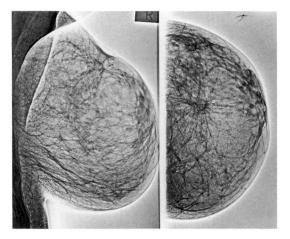

Figure 25-11. An upper-outer-quadrant mass with spiculated margins and skin dimpling, which suggests cancer; proven to be a biopsy scar.

Keynotes

- *Mammary dysplasia is a common condition that interferes with the diagnosis of early breast cancer. Although mammograms are more sensitive than physical examination of the breast for the detection of cancer, a mammogram that does not show cancer should not prevent the clinician from performing a biopsy of a clinically suspect breast nodule.*

- *Fibroadenomas are common benign tumors of the breast seen in young women.*

- *Cysts occur in middle-aged and older women. A sonogram of the nodule found on mammography can usually diagnose the cyst; when mammographic diagnosis is probable, needle aspiration of the cyst can be both diagnostic and therapeutic.*

- *Biopsy scars can be confused with cancer, and rebiopsy may be necessary.*

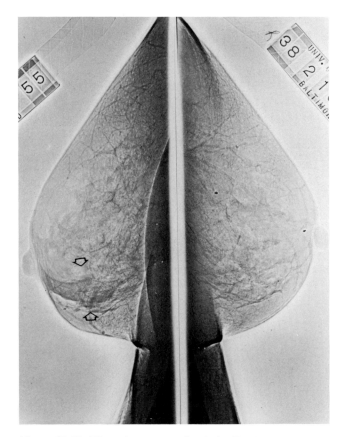

Figure 25-12. Bilateral mammary dysplasia. Focal asymmetric increased radiodensity in lower quadrant of left breast (arrows) proved to be intraductal cancer.

Breast Cancer

As you can see, there are many conditions that mimic cancer and may require an excisional biopsy and histologic examination to exclude breast cancer. This leads us to the next question: How does breast cancer appear on mammograms? Of all malignancies, 80–90% are evident by their mass radiodensity. The appearance is variable, ranging from a subtle asymmetric increase in radiodensity in a focal area in one part of a breast (Fig. 25-12) to an obvious mass (Fig. 25-13).

Scirrhous cancers are the malignancies most easily recognizable on mammograms. They have irregular margins because of an associated desmoplastic reaction surrounding the tumor, are highly aggressive and locally invasive, and therefore tend to feel larger clinically than their radiographic images appear (Fig. 25-13). Well-defined and nodular cancers, such as *colloid carcinomas* (Fig. 25-14), tend to feel the same size as their mammographic dimensions indicate and have a more favorable clinical prognosis. Obvious cancers may also show skin dimpling, nipple retraction, and spiculation, which are easily identified clinically and mammographically (Fig. 25-15).

Most cancers tend to be infiltrative and appear poorly marginated, whereas benign tumors appear mammographically and pathologically well-defined, with sharper

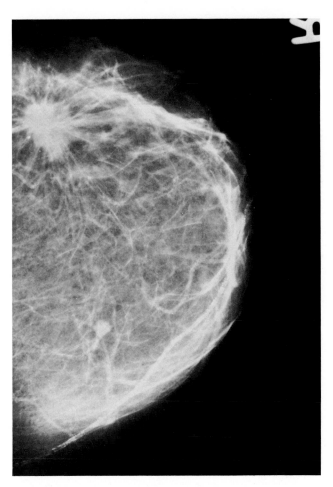

Figure 25-13. Scirrhous (infiltrating ductal) cancer with irregular margins and surrounding distortion.

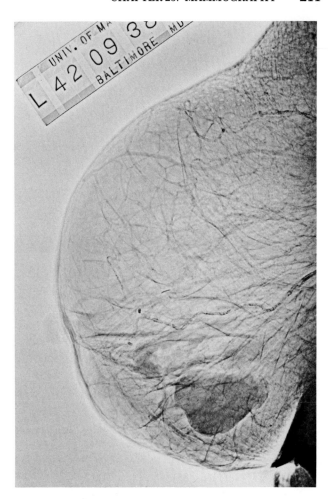

Figure 25-14. A smoother, lobulated mass suggesting a benign lesion but which proved to be a colloid cancer.

margins. Occasionally, however, well-circumscribed cancers like medullary and colloid carcinomas can resemble benign tumors. It is wise, therefore, to perform excisional biopsy of solitary masses, particularly in women who are at risk for cancer, regardless of the clinical and mammographic features.

Microcalcifications are present in as many as 40% of cancers and may be the only finding (i.e., there is no associated mass) in 16% of cases (Fig. 25-16). These appear dark blue on xerography or white on radiographs, are small (0.1–2.0 mm), and are usually clustered in groups of 5–20, although they can also be widely scattered, as in comedocarcinoma (Fig. 25-17).

The Small Nonpalpable Cancer. Mammograms can detect small cancers but do not always localize them precisely. Biopsy of these nonpalpable lesions can be difficult. Preoperative mammograms do detect but do not always localize small cancers for these reasons: the mammogram is performed with the breast compressed away from the chest wall and the patient in an upright position most of the time, whereas surgery is done with the breast flattened on the chest wall while the patient is supine. You can understand,

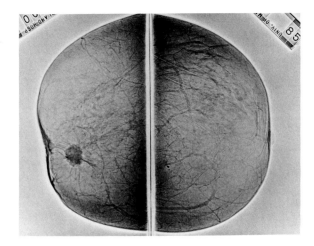

Figure 25-15. Scirrhous (infiltrating ductal) cancer showing nipple retraction from an obvious mass with irregular margins and distortion of surrounding breast tissue, left.

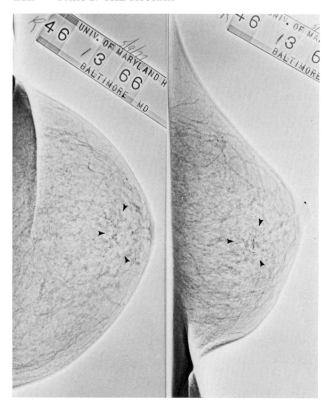

Figure 25-16. This cluster of microcalcifications inferior and posterior to the nipple without mass radiodensity was proven to be an intraductal carcinoma (arrowheads).

then, the discrepancy between the physical examination and subsequent surgery. "Blind" biopsy can thus miss the lesion, resulting in extension of the biopsy incision, prolonging anesthesia time, and increasing postsurgical scarring.

Needle Localization.   Needle localization is now the method of choice for precise localization for biopsy of nonpalpable breast lesions. There are various techniques described. The goal is to resect the smallest amount of breast tissue that includes the suspicious area. No complications have been reported. The basic principle is the percutaneous insertion of a metallic marker, either a needle or a wire, into the breast in as close proximity to the suspicious area as is possible. The position of the marker is verified mammographically during the procedure (Fig. 25-18). The marker may be left in place (after being snugly taped in place to prevent removal), or a dye can be injected through the needle and the needle removed. Either the needle or dye can then be used as a visual guide by the surgeon. Using dye, the biopsy must be done within 1 hour of the procedure to prevent the diffusion of dye into the surrounding tissues, obscuring the precise area of suspicion.

Specimen Radiography.   Resection of the suspected abnormal area can be confirmed by specimen radiography. The surgical specimen is radiographed to confirm the removal of the suspicious lesion (Fig. 25-19). This is particularly useful when calcifications are present. Specimen radiography, like needle localization, obviously requires close cooperation between the mammographer, the surgeon, and the pathologist for optimal results.

Keynotes

- *Of cancers of the breast, 80–90% show increased radiodensity from the mass, varying from subtle increases in radiodensity to definite focal masses.*
- *Breast cancers can appear spiculated and poorly defined or well defined on the mammogram.*
- *Microcalcifications are present in many breast cancers and may be the only sign of breast cancer in up to 16% of cancers.*
- *Needle localization of nonpalpable breast masses should be performed in the radiology department before a biopsy.*
- *Radiographs of the resected specimen (specimen radiography) can be used to confirm that the mammographically suspect lesion has been resected at surgery.*

SUMMARY

Breast cancer remains the leading cause of morbidity and death in women. Combined physical examination and mammography have proven useful in the detection of early breast cancer. An improved salvage rate does occur with mammography alone. The usefulness of mammography is directly proportional to the quality of the procedure.

Screening programs such as those conducted by BCDDP have proven the value of detection of minimal cancers, which comprise one-third of the cancers discovered. Mammography is the primary method for detecting these cancers, especially in women over 50 years old and in women whose physical examination is less reliable. In these early cancers, which are clinically nonpalpable, 70–80% of the axillary nodes were without metastases, indicating local disease without distant spread.

The routine use of mammography has also been beneficial in women over the age of 50 and in patients with a high risk of developing breast cancer.

REVIEW QUESTIONS

1. What are the risk factors for breast cancer occurrence?
2. Can you describe the method of breast self-examination to a patient?
3. What is the recommended frequency for screening mammography in patients not having specific risk factors other than being female?
4. What is the detection rate of mammography for minimal breast cancer?
5. What are the two main methods of mammography?
6. What is the magnitude of the risk of the radiation used in mammography?
7. What is mammary dysplasia?

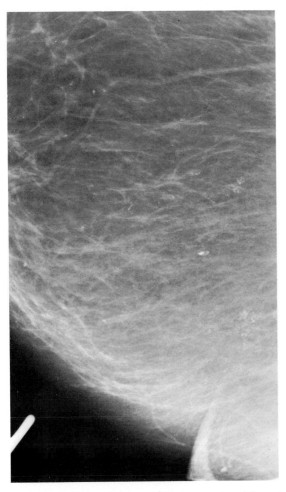

Figure 25-17. These clusters of calcifications scattered throughout breast proved to be intraductal in situ carcinoma.

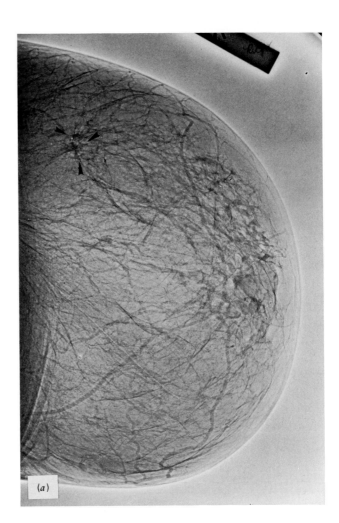

(a)

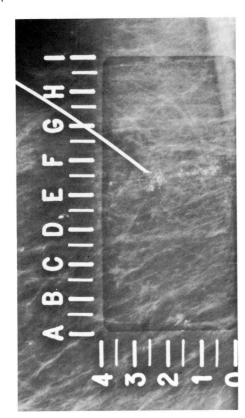

Figure 25-18. A cluster of calcifications without palpable mass is localized by needle and verified with a mammogram; proven to be ductal cancer.

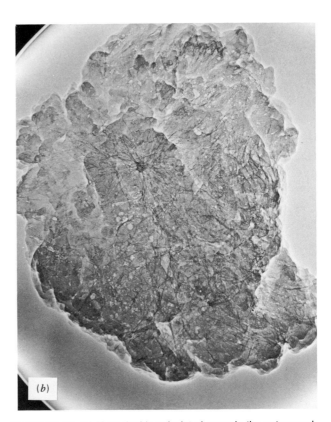

(b)

Figure 25-19. (a) Nonpalpable spiculated mass in the outer quadrant (arrowheads). (b) Specimen radiograph confirms removal after a "blind" biopsy. Infiltrating ductal carcinoma proven.

8. What is a fibroadenoma, and how would you establish the diagnosis?

9. What is a breast cyst, and how would you establish the diagnosis?

10. What is the role of microcalcifications in the diagnosis of breast cancer?

11. What is the usual appearance of breast cancer on mammograms?

12. How is needle localization used in the treatment of breast cancer?

13. What is specimen radiography, and what is its role in the treatment of breast cancer?

VOCABULARY

adenosis	mammary dysplasia
colloid carcinoma	medullary carcinoma
fat necrosis	papillomatosis
fibroadenoma	scirrhous cancer
fibrocystic disease	sclerosing adenosis
galactocele	xeromammography

SUGGESTIONS FOR FURTHER READING

L.H. Baker et al. Breast Cancer Detection Demonstration Project: 5-year summary report. *CA*, **32**:194–225, 1982.

Mammography guidelines 1983: Background statement and update of cancer-related checkup guidelines for breast cancer detection in asymptomatic women age 40 to 49. *CA*, **33**:255, 1983.

Mammography 1982: A statement of the American Cancer Society. *CA*, **32**:226–230, 1982.

E.A. Sickles. Benefits and risks of screening mammography. *Western Journal of Medicine*, 70–71, Jan. 1977.

M. Moskowitz. Mammography in medical practice. *JAMA*, **240**:1898–1899, 1978.

PART 2

THE ABDOMEN

The next 20 chapters survey the role of imaging techniques in the evaluation of the abdominal organs. Because of the complexity of abdominal disease and the difficulty of establishing an accurate diagosis by physical examination, the imaging techniques are often critical in the evaluation of the patient with abdominal complaints.

Multiple techniques are available for imaging the abdomen and its organs. Because the choice of imaging procedures is wide and the cost of a procedure done by mistake is high, an understanding of the differences among these procedures and their individual roles is important. Chapter 26 discusses the types of exams that can be performed.

In addition, because of the complexity and hazards of abdominal surgery, the role of the radiologist as an interventionist in abdominal and retroperitoneal disease has been growing. Imaging guidance can permit the percutaneous biopsy of organs, the drainage of abscesses, the dilation of strictures, and even the percutaneous removal of gallstones. As appropriate, some of these techniques are discussed in various chapters in Part 2.

Part 2 is divided into two sections. The traditional division would have been into the evaluation of the plain (non-contrast-enhanced) abdominal radiograph and the barium studies, but in the late 1980s this division no longer makes sense. These chapters are divided, therefore, into those about methods that evaluate the abdomen based on shape and appearance of the lumen of the gastrointestinal tract when it is opacified with contrast media (Chapters 34 through 45) and those about techniques that use other methods of evaluating the abdomen and its contents (Chapters 27 through 33).

SECTION A

INTRODUCTION TO THE ABDOMINAL EXAM

Chapter 26 discusses the types of studies that are available for evaluating the abdomen and its contents and the clinical role of each. Chapters 27 through 33 discuss the application of the various studies to diseases seen in the abdomen based on the fundamental patterns of normality and disease that can be evaluated on these studies: fat, calcium, air in the bowel, air free in the peritoneum, masses, vessels, and abdominal fluid collections. The basic types of abnormality are demonstrated, as appropriate, using radiography, CT, nuclear medicine studies, and ultrasonography.

26

ABDOMINAL IMAGING: THE CHOICE OF EXAM

KEY CONCEPTS

The abdominal radiograph is useful in the detection of intra-abdominal calcifications, the evaluation of the size of the major abdominal and retroperitoneal organs, and evaluation of the bowel for distension and decreased peristaltic emptying. In patients with acute abdominal pain, a chest film taken in the upright position is helpful because abdominal diseases can result in reactive changes in the chest and because lower lobe pneumonia can produce symptoms of abdominal pain.

The abdominal sonogram is useful in the evaluation of the liver, gallbladder, common bile duct, kidneys, aorta, and female pelvic organs. Masses can be detected and often characterized; abscesses can be located; gallstones and common bile duct dilation can be identified.

The abdominal CT is used in the evaluation of the liver, kidneys, pancreas, and spleen for enlargement, masses, and inflammatory diseases such as pancreatitis and for severe forms of renal infection.

Nuclear medicine techniques are used mainly in the evaluation of gallbladder disease, liver dysfunction, and liver masses and less often in the evaluation of gastrointestinal bleeding and in evaluation for intra-abdominal abscesses.

Magnetic resonance imaging has currently a limited role in studying the abdomen and is mainly of research interest at this time.

OBJECTIVES

When you complete this chapter you will be able to

1. List the major techniques used to image the abdomen and give two types of diseases for which each technique is useful.
2. List the advantages of the supine abdominal film, the upright abdominal film, the lateral decubitus abdominal film, and the upright chest film obtained in the evaluation of acute abdominal pain.
3. List five organs that can be evaluated by the abdominal sonogram.
4. List five organs that can be evaluated by the abdominal CT.
5. List three of the nuclear medicine techniques that are useful in the evaluation of abdominal disease.

ABDOMINAL RADIOGRAPH

Abdominal radiographs can be taken with the patient lying supine, (Fig. 26-1a), with the patient upright (Fig. 26-1b), or with the patient lying on his or her side. On the radiograph, the major abdominal organs can usually be identified because they are outlined by fat or filled with air. The liver, spleen, kidneys, bladder, stomach, and bowel can be studied (Fig. 26-1c).

The supine abdominal view is best for evaluating organ size, organ calcification, and ascites. The upright view helps in evaluating bowel abnormalities; the detection of air-fluid levels (Figure 26-1b and d) may help in determining that a loop of bowel is distended. The abdominal view with the patient on her or his side (the lateral decubitus view) can substitute for the upright view and can also be used to look for free intra-abdominal air.

It is often helpful to obtain an upright chest radiograph in the patient with acute abdominal pain because:

The radiograph aids in the identification of free intra-abdominal air.

Some abdominal disease results in pleural effusions.

Sometimes a lower lobe pneumonia may cause abdominal pain.

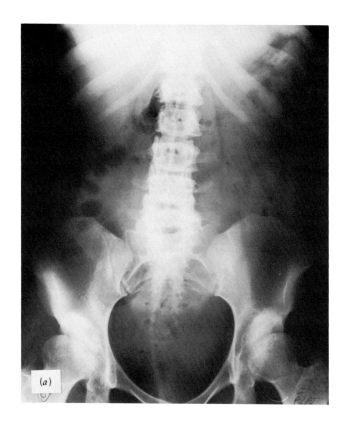

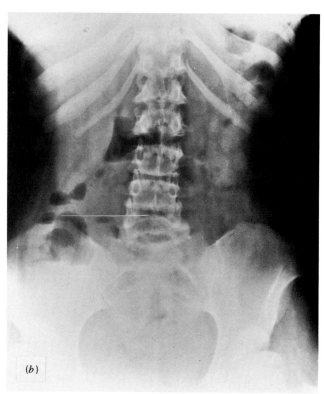

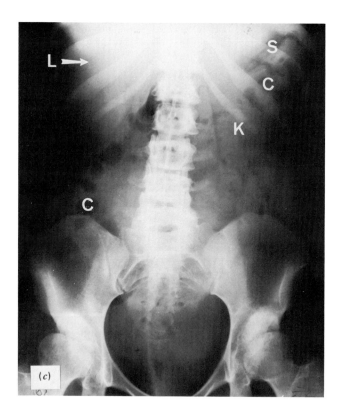

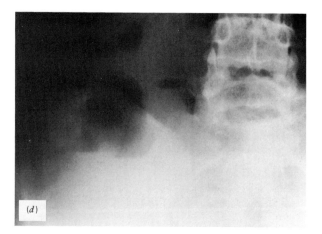

Figure 26-1. Abdominal radiographs taken in supine and upright positions. (*a*) Supine abdominal view. Fat and air permit the identification of some of the intra-abdominal organs, some of which are labeled in *c*. (*b*) Upright abdominal view. The delineation of the fat margins is less clear, but the bowel air is somewhat easier to see, and air fluid levels can be seen. (*c*) Same view as in *a*, but with some of the abdominal organs identified. L = liver, K = spleen, C = colon, S = stomach. Minimal deformity of the hip joints in this patient is secondary to mild congenital displacement of the hips. (*d*) This focal view of the right lower quadrant of the abdomen demonstrates multiple air-fluid levels. This is abnormal and in this patient is due to an adjacent inflammatory process: a tuboovarian abscess. These sentinel loops caused by the adjacent inflammatory process are discussed further in Chapter 33.

ABDOMINAL SONOGRAM

The abdominal sonogram consists of a series of longitudinal and transverse images of the abdomen. Images can be made of structures composed of soft tissue, fluid, and fat (Fig. 26-2). More than a minimal amount of air or calcium stops the sound waves, resulting in a region of intense sound reverberation with an echo-free region distal to the site of marked echogenicity. This property of *acoustic "shadowing"* can be most useful in identifying calcifications, biliary calculi (Fig. 26-3), and air within abscesses.

Tissue interfaces between water, fat, fibrous tissue, and fluid-filled spaces permit images of abdominal organs to be made. The liver, gallbladder, kidneys, aorta, inferior vena cava, and female reproductive organs can be well demonstrated by this technique (Fig. 26-2 and 26-4). Masses in or adjacent to these organs and fluid collections (e.g., abscesses and hematomas) can usually be seen. The technique can be useful in the evaluation of the pancreas and spleen, but the ability to visualize these organs is slightly less than

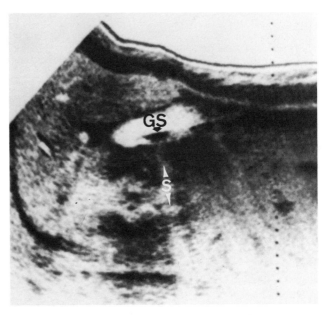

Figure 26-3. Sonogram demonstrating gallstones (GS) with acoustic shadow (S).

that afforded by CT (for the spleen and pancreas) and nuclear medicine imaging (for the spleen).

Sonography can be quite useful in the search for a hidden intra-abdominal abscess. It is not generally of use in imaging the bowel.

ABDOMINAL COMPUTED TOMOGRAM

The computed tomogram consists of a series of images made at the level of the suspected abnormality. Differences between air, fat, water, and soft tissue permit images to be made (Fig. 26-5a). Often a contrast medium is given by mouth to outline the upper gastrointestinal system (Fig. 26-5b) and by rectum to outline the colon and rectum. Intravenous contrast medium can be used to increase the radiodensity of structures with blood perfusion and to demonstrate the kidney and urinary systems (Fig. 26-5a).

Computed tomography can be used to image the liver, spleen, peritoneal space, kidneys, aorta, retroperitoneal nodes, pancreas, and bladder. It is not usually used to visualize the gallbladder or the bowel. It is of greatest use in looking for masses and fluid collections in the abdomen and retroperitoneum.

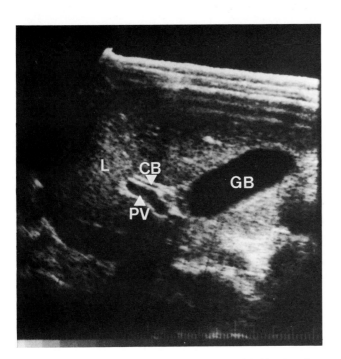

Figure 26-2. Sonogram of a normal liver and gallbladder. L = liver, GB = gall bladder, CB = common bile duct, PV = portal vein. The gallbladder is echo free. (Courtesy Morgan Dunne, M.D.)

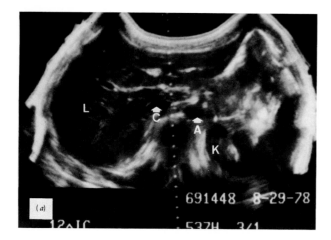

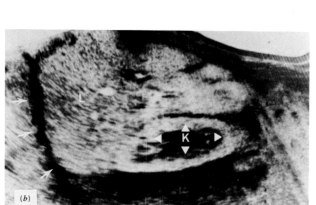

Figure 26-4. Sonographic views of a normal abdomen. (*a*) Transverse view through the upper abdomen. The liver (L), aorta (A), inferior vena cava (C), and left kidney (K) are labeled. The liver fills much of the right side of the abdomen and contains portal and hepatic venous channels that are sonolucent. The aorta and vena cava are ovoid and sonolucent. The kidney is a sonolucent horseshoe-shaped rim of renal parenchyma with an echogenic central sinus. (Courtesy M. Dunne, M.D.) (*b*) Longitudinal view through the right upper abdomen. The liver (L) and right kidney (K) are labeled. The liver fills much of the central portion of the image and is limited superiorly by the curved echogenic right hemidiaphragm (arrows). The kidney is ovoid with a sonolucent parenchyma, indicated by arrowheads, and an echogenic sinus (K) in its center. (Courtesy R. Sanders, M.D.)

Keynote

- *Computed tomography is of greatest use in looking for masses and fluid collections in the abdomen and retroperitoneum.*

NUCLEAR MEDICINE IMAGING TECHNIQUES IN THE ABDOMEN

Nuclear medicine imaging studies yield both anatomic and physiological information. Images can be made of the liver and spleen, using technetium Tc 99m sulfur colloid

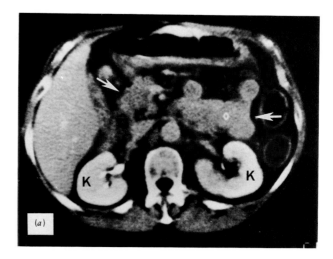

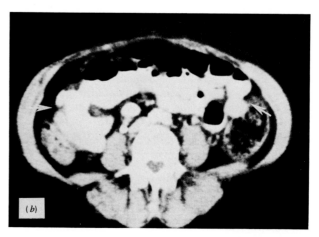

Figure 26-5. CT of a normal abdomen. (*a*) Nonopacified bowel (arrows) could be confused with a soft tissue mass. The kidneys (K) are whiter than the liver because they have been opacified by the injection of an iodine-containing medicine that is excreted by the kidneys—an intravenous radiographic contrast medium. (*b*) The bowel has now been opacified by a swallowed contrast medium. The bowel (arrows) appears whiter because of the contrast medium.

particles to label the phagocytic cells of the reticuloendothelial system. This results in anatomic information about the liver and spleen (Fig. 26-6). Masses can be identified within the liver (Fig. 26-7).

Technetium Tc 99m iminodiacetic acid derivatives (IDA) compounds can be used to image the liver, showing the pathway of bile synthesis and excretion. Hepatocytes and the biliary tree are visualized (Fig. 26-8). Timed studies can be used to evaluate for biliary obstruction. Failure of filling of the gallbladder can be used to indicate the probability of cystic duct obstruction with acute cholecystitis.

Sodium pertechnetate Tc 99m can be used to image gastric mucosa and is of occasional use in patients with suspected ectopic gastric mucosa in a Meckel's diverticulum.

Nuclear medicine imaging studies are greatly useful in evaluating the condition of the patient with suspected ma-

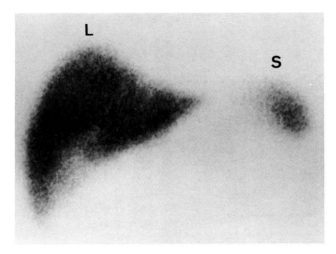

Figure 26-6. Technetium Tc 99m sulfur colloid nuclear medicine scan of a normal liver and spleen, frontal view. L = liver, S = spleen. Multiple views are normally taken.

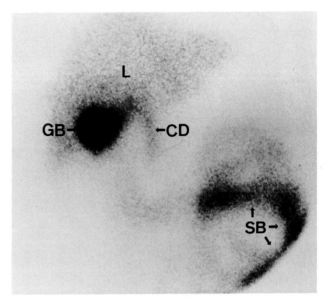

Figure 26-8. Technetium Tc 99m disida scan of the biliary tract, normal study, 45-min image. L = liver, GB = gallbladder, CD = common bile duct, SB = small bowel.

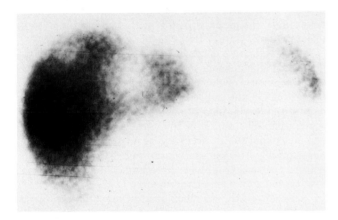

Figure 26-7. Technetium Tc 99m sulfur colloid nuclear medicine scan of the liver in a patient with metastatic colon cancer. The white, rounded areas within the liver are the metastases.

jor lower gastrointestinal tract bleeding (Fig. 26-9). Because many patients with lower gastrointestinal tract bleeding stop bleeding spontaneously, the nuclear medicine study demonstrates which patients are still bleeding and therefore require arteriography.

Renal imaging can either use agents that attach to the renal tubular cells (^{99m}Tc-labeled 2,3-dimercaptosuccinic acid (DMSA)) or agents that are glomerular filtrates (^{99m}Tc-labeled Diethylenetriaminepentaacetic acid (DTPA)) or agents that rely on both glomerular filtration and tubular excretion (iodohippurate sodium I 131). These techniques are discussed in Chapter 49.

Gallium citrate Ga 67 can be used both for the localization of lymphomatous or inflamed lymph nodes and for the localization of intra-abdominal abscesses (Fig. 26-10).

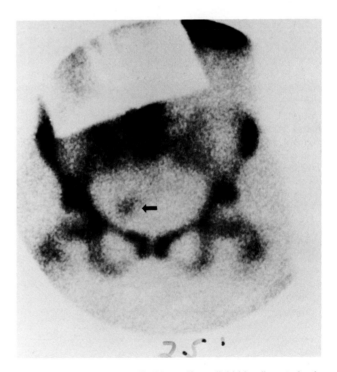

Figure 26-9. Technetium Tc 99m sulfur colloid bleeding study. An arrow marks a collection of radioactivity that shouldn't be seen. This was a bleeding site in a sigmoid colon diverticulum.

Keynote

• *Nuclear medicine imaging studies can image the liver and spleen, biliary tract, kidneys, and some abnormal lymph nodes.*

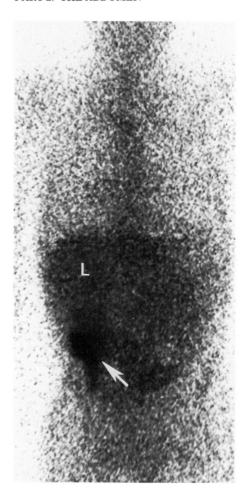

Figure 26-10. Gallium citrate Ga 67 scan of the torso (see Fig. 18-10*a* for normal comparison). The area of increased ^{67}Ga uptake (arrow) just inferior to the liver (L) is due to a subhepatic abscess secondary to a ruptured appendix treated 6 weeks before.

ANGIOGRAPHY IN THE ABDOMEN

With improvements in the imaging techniques using sonography, CT, and nuclear medicine imaging, the need for abdominal angiography has decreased. Its current role is in the evaluation of vascular disease (occlusive disease, aneurysms, periarteritis nodosa), preresection evaluation of renal cancer, and the evaluation and treatment of major upper and lower gastrointestinal tract bleeding.

Keynote

• *The patient with gastrointestinal tract bleeding can sometimes be treated via an angiographic catheter, either by embolic occlusion of the bleeding vessel or by the perfusion of vasoconstrictors.*

MAGNETIC RESONANCE IMAGING OF THE ABDOMEN

Magnetic resonance imaging of the abdominal organs can be done with visualization of the liver, spleen, kidneys,

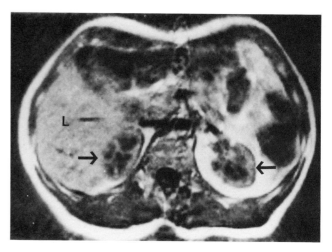

Figure 26-11. MRI transverse view through the upper abdomen. The liver (L) and kidneys (arrows) are well seen The renal cortex can be differentiated from the medulla.

pancreas, and major vessels (Fig. 26-11). The bowel itself is poorly seen because of its motion during the imaging process. Currently, it does not appear that MRI will offer advantages compared with CT in the evaluation of most abdominal complaints, with the following exceptions:

1. Visualization of major blood vessels. Because of the flow-void phenomenon, it is probable that MRI will be a useful method of evaluating aneurysms and atherosclerotic narrowings of the major abdominal vessels. It is not yet determinable whether or to what extent it will replace the sonographic evaluation of the aorta and whether it is of sufficient diagnostic accuracy to replaced major-vessel angiography. Preliminary results suggest that it might be able to replace the preoperative angiogram in a patient with an abdominal aortic aneurysm.

2. Because MRI can image in different planes in the body (Fig. 26-12), it may prove useful in evaluating pelvic masses and fluid collections and abscesses occurring just below or just above the diaphragm. Current imaging techniques often leave the surgeon or interventionist radiologist uncertain if a fluid collection is pleural or abdominal or both. Because the approaches to subdiaphragmatic and supradiaphragmatic abscesses are different, more accurate diagnosis should improve the care of the patient. MRI may provide this important information.

Keynote

• *Currently, MRI has only limited applications in the abdomen. Its main applications are likely to be based on its ability to visualize the major vessels and to image in multiple planes. The ability to image in multiple planes is likely to have its greatest utility in the pelvis and peridiaphragmatic areas.*

SELECTING THE PROPER IMAGING STUDY

Because there are so many methods in use for studying the abdomen, it is easy to choose the wrong one. Because the

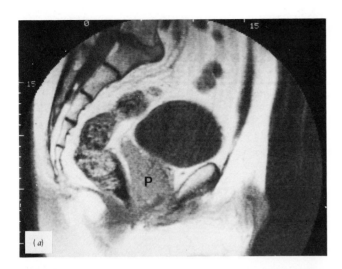

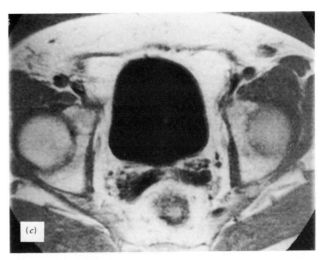

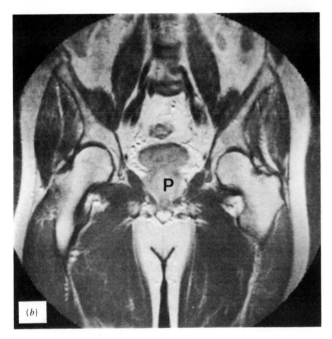

Figure 26-12. MR images of benign prostatic hypertrophy imaged in three planes. The prostate is labeled P. (*a*) Sagittal plane. (*b*) Coronal plane. (*c*) Transverse or axial view of the bladder, above the level of the prostate. (All courtesy C. Citrin, M.D.)

cost of using the wrong study can be high (both in missed diagnosis and dollars), selection of the proper study or studies is most important. (Chapters 27 through 45 discuss the abdominal organs and their diseases and the applications of the different imaging techniques to each organ's investigation.)

In some parts of the body, the imaging techniques for each suspected disease are well established; in others, disagreement remains as to the best choice of modalities. These chapters present one choice for interpreting radiographs and caring for patients. It represents a personal method of clinical care, rather than the only acceptable method. The choice reflects the balanced skills in these modalities in one particular institution. Should your institution have more skilled imaging specialists in one modality than in another, this should affect your choice of imaging technique.

SUMMARY

The abdominal radiograph obtained with the patient supine can be used to evaluate organ size, calcifications, and ascites. The upright view helps in evaluating bowel abnormalities by allowing the detection of air-fluid levels and helping to determine bowel distension. In the patient with acute abdominal pain, an upright chest radiograph can aid in detecting free intra-abdominal air.

The abdominal sonogram is used to evaluate the major abdominal organs, including the biliary system, liver, kidneys, aorta, and female reproductive organs. It is also useful in evaluating intra-abdominal fluid collections and abscesses.

The computed tomogram of the abdomen is used to image the liver, spleen, peritoneal spaces, pancreas, aorta, retroperitoneal lymph node regions, and bladder. It is helpful in evaluating masses and fluid collections in the abdomen.

Nuclear medicine procedures are used to image the liver, spleen, biliary tract, gallbladder, and kidneys. These techniques can be used in the evaluation of masses, acute cholecystitis, and traumatic injuries. Nuclear medicine techniques are also used in the evaluation of suspected major gastrointestinal tract bleeding, to confirm the active bleeding and as a guide to angiography.

Angiography is used in evaluating vascular diseases including the evaluation of ischemic disease and aneurysms, and in the evaluation and treatment of major hemorrhage.

Chapters 27 through 45 discuss the types of studies in greater detail and describe their applications in the evaluation of diseases.

REVIEW QUESTIONS

1. What is the supine abdominal view best for demonstrating?
2. The supine and upright views are used for evaluating which abdominal organs?
3. Describe how a lateral decubitus view is obtained.
4. Which abdominal organs can be studied by the sonogram? By the computed tomogram?
5. Which abdominal organs can nuclear medicine imaging study?

VOCABULARY

acoustic shadow	phagocytic cells
periarteritis nodosa	reticuloendothelial system

SUGGESTIONS FOR FURTHER READING FOR CHAPTERS 26 TO 33

J. Frimann-Dahl. *Roentgen Examinations in Acute Abdominal Diseases*. Charles C. Thomas: Springfield. 1974. (Classic text)

Charles D. Johnson, Reed P. Rice. The acute abdomen: Plain radiographic evaluation. *RadioGraphics,* **5**(2): 259–272, 1985.

George R. Leopold. The acute abdomen: Ultrasonography. *RadioGraphics,* **5**(2): 273–283, 1985.

Leonard M. Freeman, Letty G. Lutzker, Heidi S. Weissman. The acute abdomen: Radionuclide imaging. *RadioGraphics,* **5**(2): 285–306, 1985.

Michael P. Federle. The acute abdomen: Computed tomography. *RadioGraphics,* **5**(2): 307–322, 1985.

27

ABDOMINAL FAT

KEY CONCEPTS

Radiological

Fat surrounds the retroperitoneal organs and parts of some of the intra-abdominal organs. The difference in the radiodensity and echogenicity of fat compared with that of the contained organ defines the boundary of these organs, permitting the evaluation of their size and shape.

Fat can infiltrate organs when they are diseased, decreasing their radiodensity and increasing their sonographic echogenicity. This pattern of change is seen most often in fatty infiltration of the liver.

Fat can fill in the space left as organs are removed or as they atrophy. This increased fat can be used as a confirmatory sign of organ absence or atrophy.

Fat can be infiltrated by edema, tumor, or infection, increasing its radiodensity. The sonographic appearance of infiltration can be that of increased or decreased echogenicity. Air can infiltrate fat, usually via dissection from an open wound and less often from air in the mediastinum or from gas produced by infection.

Fat can be decreased or absent in the patient who is malnourished or who has catabolized fat during a severe chronic illness. Evaluation by CT and plain radiography in patients with little abdominal and retroperitoneal fat may be limited by the lack of visualization of the borders of abdominal organs. Usually, a sufficient boundary exists for sonographic evaluation.

Clinical

Fat infiltration into the liver can occur with alcoholic liver disease and less often with acute malnutrition (as after surgery).

Fat can become edematous, appearing the same as water on imaging studies, with decreased serum albumen, when injured, and when inflamed.

OBJECTIVES

When you complete this chapter you will be able to

1. Identify regions of fat on radiographic, CT, sonographic, and MRI images of the abdomen.
2. Detect fatty infiltration of the liver on selected CT images.
3. Detect air infiltration of fat on radiographs and CT images.

In the abdomen, fat both outlines many of the organs and is affected by their diseases. In techniques using x-ray photons, fat serves as a region of differing radiodensity, different from the structures it surrounds (Figs. 27-1 and 27-2). Fat is one of the basic radiodensities (of air, fat, water, bone, and metal) and is intermediate in radiodensity between air and water. When fat outlines water-radiodensity abdominal organs, it permits their identification because of the difference in radiodensity.

When high-frequency sound waves are used to make the image, the fat surrounding the organ contributes to the marginal echos that outline the edge of organs. Fat ranges from being minimally to moderately echogenic (Fig. 27-3).

When radiofrequency waves are used to perturb protons in a strong magnetic field, the protons in fat respond differently from the protons in the abdominal organs, permitting visualization of the outline of the organs (Fig. 27-4) and the estimation of the amount of fat contained within them.

Keynote

• *The fat surrounding the abdominal organs serves as an area of different radiodensity, permitting their margins to be seen.*

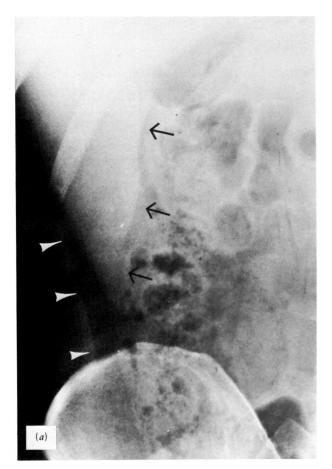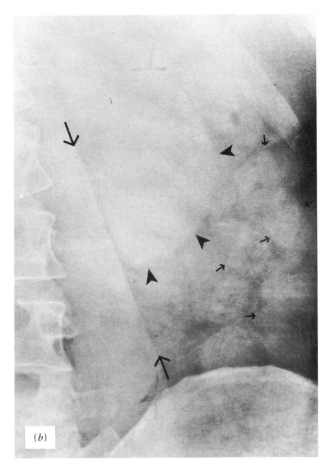

Figure 27-1. (a) Normal right upper abdomen on conventional radiograph. The liver edge (black arrows) is outlined by fat. This edge is the posterior margin of the liver. The anterior portion that you can palpate when you examine a patient is usually lower but cannot be seen on radiographs. The white arrowheads mark the flank stripe (or properitoneal fat). This band of fat can become edematous from adjacent intra-abdominal or retroperitoneal inflammatory processes or secondary to retroperitoneal hemorrhage in the posterior pararenal space. (b) Normal left side of the mid-abdomen on conventional radiograph. The bowel loops can be seen outlined by fat (small arrows). The psoas muscle margin is outlined by fat (large arrows). As with the flank stripe, inflammatory processes adjacent to the psoas margin can smudge or eliminate it; the psoas margin is often not visible, however, in normal people. The lower margin of the left kidney is also seen outlined by fat (arrowheads).

LOCATION OF ABDOMINAL FAT

Intraperitoneal Fat

Within the peritoneal cavity, there is usually a large amount of fat attached to the mesentery of the bowel and to the omentum. This fat surrounds the bowel and may permit its identification (Fig. 27-1b). It lies against the dome of the bladder, and its displacement permits the identification of intra-abdominal fluid (explained in Chapter 32). It also forms part of the liver margin and can be displaced by intra-abdominal fluid.

Extraperitoneal Fat

Surrounding the peritoneum is a layer of fat. Posteriorly, the fat layer is moderately thick; laterally and anteriorly it is moderately thin. Many of the intra-abdominal organs lie with their posterior margins embedded in this retroperitoneal fat. The posterior portion of the liver can be identified in this way (Fig. 27-1a, 27-2, 27-3 and 27-4). The kidneys are enveloped by this fat (Figs. 27-1b, 27-2, 27-3, and 27-4), delineating their margins. The kidneys also contain fat within the centrally located renal sinus, resulting in some central radiolucency within the kidney

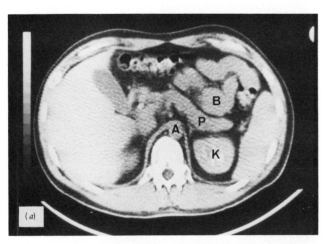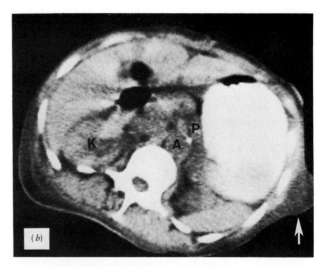

Figure 27-2. (a) CT of the normal midabdomen. The abdominal and retroperitoneal organs are outlined by fat. K = left kidney, P = body and tail of the pancreas, B = small bowel loops, A = aorta. (Courtesy Morgan Dunne, M.D.) (b) This emaciated uremic patient lacks sufficient retroperitoneal fat to outline the abdominal organs. The right kidney (K) is only faintly delimited by fat. The pancreas (P) is only partially demarcated from the aorta (A). Because the patient is uremic, the body fat (arrow) is reticulated from fat edema. Compare the appearance of the body fat with that in a. (Courtesy Nancy Whitley, M.D., University of Maryland Hospital.)

on techniques using x-rays and increased echogenicity on sonograms.

The thin layer of fat laterally forms the margin of the peritoneum and is called the flank stripe, or properitoneal fat (Fig. 27-1a). Its radiolucency can be affected by several types of disease.

Keynotes

- *The displacement of omental and mesenteric fat permits the identification of intra-abdominal fluid.*
- *Only the posterior portions of the liver and spleen lie in fat. The liver edge seen on a radiograph is the posterior fat.*

HOW DISEASE AFFECTS FAT

Fat can be affected in five different ways by disease:

1. It can be displaced.
2. It can become edematous.
3. It can become air containing.
4. It can become infiltrated by tumor or infection.
5. It can be catabolized and be absent.

Fat can also infiltrate organs, such as the liver, as a sign of disease and can fill in the spaces left when organs atrophy or are surgically removed.

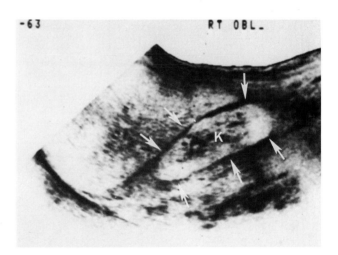

Figure 27-3. Sonogram through the right side of the upper abdomen, longitudinal section. The kidney (K) is surrounded by its echogenic capsule and retroperitoneal fat (arrows). The central echos within the center of the kidney are due to fat and the collecting system within the renal sinus. (Courtesy Roger Sanders, M.D.)

Fat Displacement

The fat within the peritoneum is attached both to the mesentery and to the omentum. When free intraperitoneal fluid (*ascites*) is present, this fat will be displaced from its normal position, both because fat is lighter than waterlike fluid and because the fat attached to the bowel will be pulled to the most superior region of the abdomen by air in the bowel lumen. This displacement of fat is used to identify the presence of ascites and is discussed in Chapter 32.

Edematous Fat

Normal fat is more radiolucent than water and appears to be a darker gray (Fig. 27-2a). When injured, inflamed, or infected, it becomes edematous and has water radiodensity (Fig. 27-5). When the serum protein level falls sufficiently, fat can become edematous.

Minimal edema makes the fat reticulated: multiple lines appear within the radiolucent fat. Moderate edema changes the fat to water radiodensity and makes the margin of water-density organs indistinct.

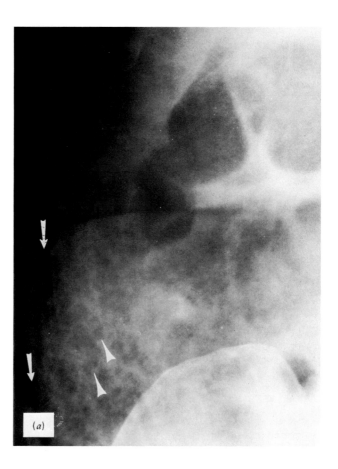

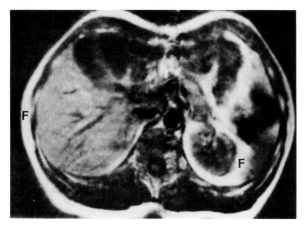

Figure 27-4. MRI section through the liver and left kidney. Fat (F) appearing white on this image outlines the left kidney and portions of the liver. Part of the whiteness of the liver is due to its fat content.

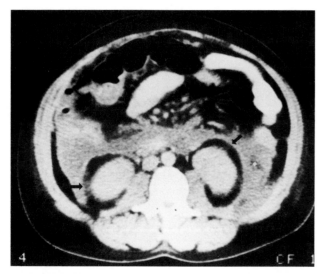

Figure 27-5. This patient with pancreatitis demonstrates edematous fat and fluid collections in the retroperitoneal spaces. The fat around the kidneys is partially spared by the process and remains radiolucent, but with focal areas (arrows) of edema. Compare this with Figure 27-2a.

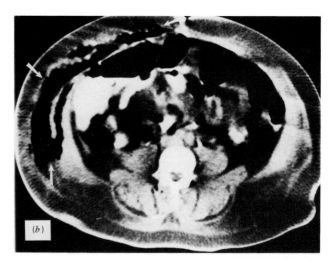

Figure 27-6. Air in fat. (a) This focal view of the right lower part of the abdomen and abdominal wall demonstrates streaks of air (white arrows) within the layers of the abdominal wall. When seen en face, the bubbles of air in the abdominal fat appear as focal radiolucencies (arrowheads). (b) The CT image through the midabdomen demonstrates extraperitoneal air (arrows) separating the layers of fat (compare the right and left sides). This patient had unexplained fever 3 days after a right inguinal hernia repair. Aspiration and Gram stain of material from the abdominal wall demonstrated Gram-negative rods that proved to be *Escherichia coli*.

Air in Fat

Air can dissect into fat from surgery or from chest wall injuries. Uncommonly, air will accumulate in fat because of an infection with a gas-forming organism (Fig. 27-6)

Tumor Infiltration

Tumor infiltration will change fat to water radiodensity. The obliteration of fat around an abdominal organ is a useful sign for demonstrating tumor infiltration on CT.

Increased Fat in Disease

Certain diseases result in fatty replacement of normal tissue. In the abdomen this is most commonly seen in the acute fatty liver of alcoholism. The fat can be recognized on CT as increased radiolucency of the organ (Fig. 27-7). On sonography, patients with an acutely fatty liver will have a generalized increase in echos in the liver.

When organs atrophy or are surgically removed, fat often fills in the space that is left. The presence of increased fat indicates that there has been a loss of tissue but does not identify its cause. This process of fatty replacement is most often seen in the renal sinus, where the size of the renal sinus is increased and of fat radiolucency on

studies using x-rays. Sonograms demonstrate an enlargement of the renal sinus echos within the center of the renal image.

Keynotes

- *Disease can displace fat or infiltrate fat with fluid or air.*
- *Injured or infected fat is often of water radiodensity.*

SUMMARY

Many organs in the abdomen are easier to evaluate because they are surrounded by fat. This fat has a different echogenicity and radiodensity than the organ. Imaging techniques using x-rays (radiography and CT) are less accurate if the patient is emaciated or edematous.

Disease can affect fat in five ways: the fat can be displaced; it can be infiltrated with fluid (edema) or with tumor, permeated with air, or catabolized and absent. An evaluation of the intra- and extraperitoneal fat is part of the evaluation of the patient with abdominal disease.

REVIEW QUESTIONS

1. Compare the radiodensity of fat with that of the other intra-abdominal organs.
2. Which abdominal organs are enveloped by fat? Which have only their posterior margins surrounded by fat?
3. How echogenic is fat?
4. How is fat used to identify ascites?
5. What happens to the radiodensity of fat when it's injured?

VOCABULARY

ascites	flank stripe
edema	properitoneal fat

SUGGESTIONS FOR FURTHER READING

A.K. Dixon, R.C. Nightingale. Abnormal fat: A useful marker of intra-abdominal disease at computed tomography. *Clinical Radiology,* **35:** 469–473, 1984.

For additional suggested reading see Chapter 26.

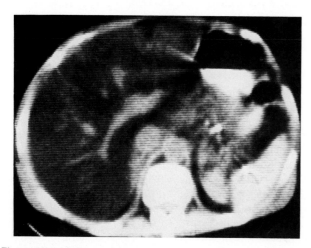

Figure 27-7. CT in a patient with a fatty liver secondary to alcoholism. The liver is more radiolucent (blacker) than normal, and the water-radiodensity venous channels stand out distinctly within the radiolucent fat. Compare this appearance with that in Figure 27-2a. (Courtesy of Nancy Whitley, M.D., University of Maryland Hospital.)

28

CALCIUM DEPOSITS IN THE ABDOMEN

KEY CONCEPTS

Radiological

Focal calcium deposits in the abdominal organs appear whiter on radiographs and CT scans because of their increased radiodensity.

On sonograms, calcium deposits appear as foci of increased echogenicity, with increased blackness or whiteness, depending on whether the black-on-white or the white-on-black image format is used. When they are sufficiently large, calcium deposits produce a sonic shadow: because they reflect all the sound waves directed at them, no sound passes through and therefore no echos distal to the calcification are produced.

When there is a rapid and active deposition of calcium, ^{99m}Tc phosphate complex bone scans can demonstrate increased activity at the site of calcifications.

Clinical

When calcifications are identified on abdominal radiographs, their etiology should be determined. Some calcifications are due to benign degenerative processes; others can be associated with severe symptoms that require treatment.

Calcium can form as concretions (stones) within the lumina of organs and can be associated with symptoms. Renal and biliary calculi and appendicoliths are examples.

Calcium can collect in both benign and malignant tumors and their metastases. Uterine fibroid tumors and ovarian dermoid cysts commonly contain calcium deposits. Some colon cancers and an occasional ovarian cancer contain foci of calcification.

Vascular calcifications can be unimportant when they occur in veins (*phleboliths*) or as minimal arterial calcification in the elderly (a result of atherosclerosis). Sometimes arterial calcification occurs prematurely and requires evaluation. Calcified aneurysms can be detected.

Calcification in the pancreas is often a sign of chronic pancreatitis. Vas deferens calcification is often a sign of diabetes.

OBJECTIVES

When you complete this chapter you will be able to

1. Identify calcium deposits in the abdomen on selected radiographs, CT scans, and sonograms.
2. Detect aortic aneurysms, vas deferens calcification, urinary and biliary calculi, and calcified tumors on selected radiographs and CT scans.
3. List two benign and two malignant tumors that can calcify.
4. Describe the calcifications that can occur in chronic pancreatitis and diabetes.
5. Describe the appearance of and correctly detect phleboliths on abdominal radiographs.
6. Indicate the clinical significance of appendicoliths.

Small quantities of calcium are present in every cell; deposits of calcium large enough to be imaged are normally found however, only within the bone. Calcium elsewhere is usually a sign of disease or degeneration of tissues because of aging. These calcium deposits can be identified on the standard radiograph or on transmission computed tomograms as more radiodense (whiter) regions (Fig. 28-1 and 28-2). On sonography, calcium deposits are markedly echogenic (Fig. 28-3). A small amount of calcium results in multiple echos and a region of *sonic shadowing* beyond the calcium. (Sonic shadowing describes regions of lack of echo beyond regions of marked echogenicity. They occur either with calcium deposits or with foci of air.)

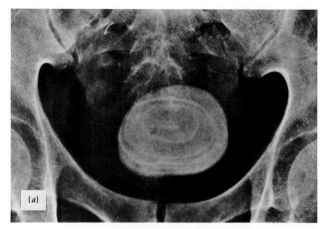
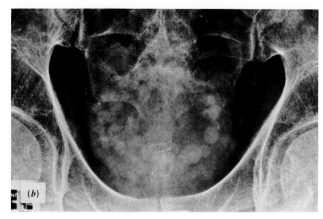

Figure 28-1. Calcified bladder calculi. (*a*) This large, densely calcified, layered bladder calculus is more radiodense than the bones of the pelvis. (*b*) Many faintly calcified bladder calculi are seen in the bladder. The radiodensity of calculi depend on how much calcium they contain and how thick they are. (Both courtesy M. Vaccaro, M.D.)

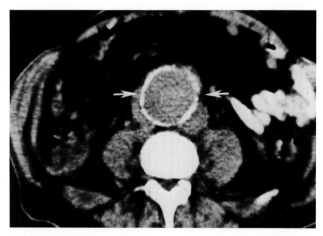

Figure 28-2. The white ring (arrows) in the center of this midabdominal CT is the calcified rim of an abdominal aortic aneurysm. Calcium appears whiter on CT scans because it is more radiodense than the surrounding tissues.

Less commonly calcium deposits in soft tissues will be demonstrated on nuclear medicine imaging studies using bone-seeking agents (99mTc phosphate complexes, 67Ga, and strontium isotopes). This is more likely to occur with acute tissue necrosis than with chronic calcific deposits.

Keynotes

- *Calcium deposits, other than in bone, are usually indicative of disease or degenerative change resulting from aging.*
- *Calcium deposits are*
  "White" on radiography and CT
  Echogenic with sonic shadowing on sonography
  Active in some cases on 99mTc phosphate complex nuclear medicine imaging scans

---

LOCATION OF ABNORMAL DEPOSITS

Calcium deposits in bone are normal; all others are abnormal. When calcium in seen in the abdomen, its etiology is usually established by noting its location within the abdomen and the shape of the calcification. When the calcification could indicate the need for treatment, as it does with urinary and biliary calcifications, then additional tests may be necessary to confirm its location.

Common Sites

Vascular Calcification. Arterial calcification is usually recognized as a line or lines of calcium that may branch (Fig. 28-4). Splenic artery calcification is curved rather than straight. Calcification commonly occurs in aorta and iliac arteries, less commonly in superior mesenteric and renal arteries.

Indications of Aneurysms. An aortic aneurysm is demonstrated by calcium in opposite walls more than 3.5 cm apart. Splenic and renal aneurysms are revealed by curvilinear calcification outlining part of the sphere.

Venous Calcifications. Venous calcifications (phleboliths) are commonly seen in the pelvis in adults and usually are of no clinical significance. Uncommonly they can outline a scrotal varicocele. They are rounded, often with a radiolucent center (arrows in Fig. 28-5).

Gynecologic Calcifications. Uterine fibroids often calcify in a speckled or solid pattern (Fig. 28-6). Ovarian dermoid cysts often contain calcification that may contain toothlike regions (Fig. 28-3).

Andropathic Calcifications. Vas deferens calcification is often a sign of diabetes (Fig. 28-7).

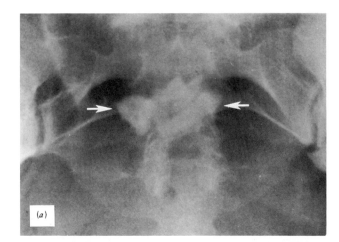

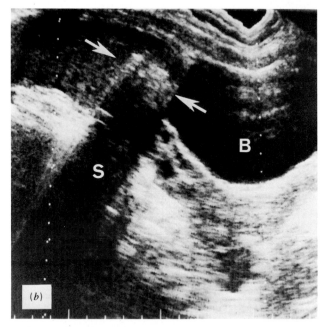

Figure 28-3. Calcifications in a dermoid cyst of the ovary. (*a*) This focal view of the pelvis demonstrates focal calcifications (arrows) overlying the sacrum. The calcifications in dermoid cysts often resemble teeth or portions of a mandible with teeth. There is a faint resemblance here to tooth-shaped projections. (*b*) This longitudinal sonographic view demonstrates the bladder (B) containing reverberation echos. Just above the bladder there is an echogenic structure (arrows) with shadowing (S) inferior to it.

Biliary Calcifications. Approximately 20% of gallstones calcify. They may be laminated, faceted, or fissured (Fig. 28-8).

Urinary Calcifications. Renal, ureteral, and bladder stones can calcify. Although 80% contain calcium, only 50% contain enough calcium to be identified.

Pancreatic Calcifications. Pancreatic calcifications (Fig. 28-9) usually indicate chronic pancreatitis. These calcifica-

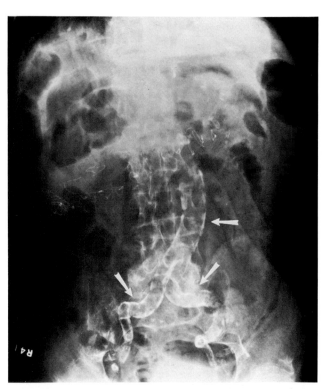

Figure 28-4. This abdominal radiograph demonstrates marked atherosclerotic calcification of the abdominal aorta and iliac arteries (arrows).

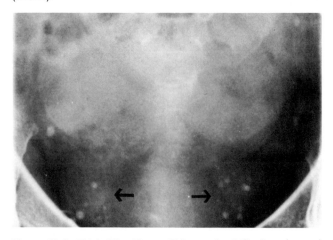

Figure 28-5. Phleboliths. The multiple small calcifications (arrows) are small calcified thrombi in pelvic veins. They are of no clinical significance.

tions are clinically important both to explain recurrent abdominal pain and because the patient with chronic pancreatitis may not have an elevated serum amylase level during an attack of superimposed acute pancreatitis.

Adrenal Calcification. Calcification of the adrenal glands (Fig. 28-10) is often a sign of adrenal insuffciency (Addison's disease).

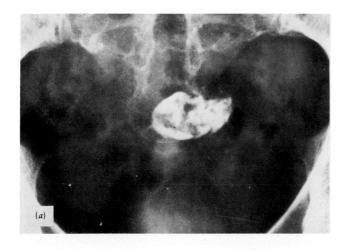

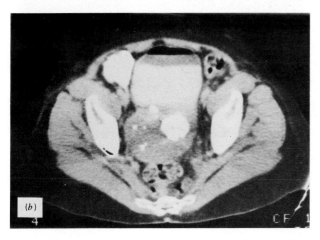

Figure 28-6. Uterine fibroid calcifications. (*a*) Calcified uterine fibroid on a standard radiograph. (*b*) Calcified uterine fibroid on a CT scan of the pelvis.

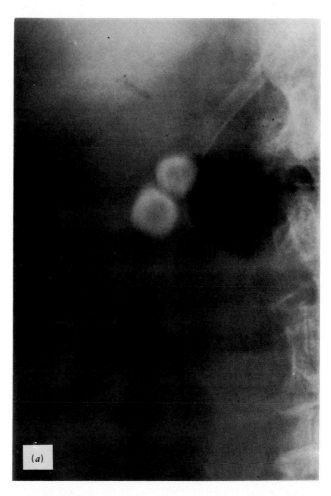

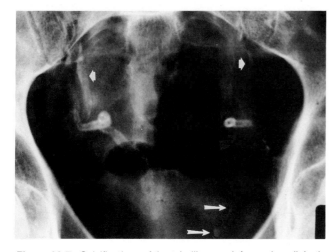

Figure 28-7. Calcifications of the tubelike vas deferens in a diabetic male patient. Long arrows mark phleboliths. Short arrows mark faint calcifications in the iliac arteries.

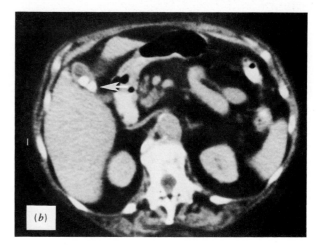

Figure 28-8. Biliary calculi. (*a*) Focal view from the right upper quadrant of the abdomen demonstrates two white, rounded gallstones. (*b*) An upper abdominal CT section in the same patient demonstrates the appearance of these gallstones (arrow) on CT.

235

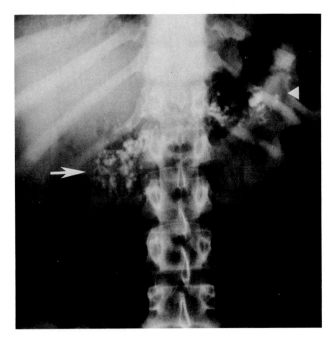

Figure 28-9. Pancreatic calcifications in a 47-year-old man with chronic pancreatitis. An arrow demarcates the head of the pancreas. An arrowhead points to the tail of the pancreas.

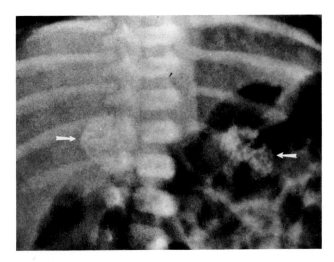

Figure 28-10. Focal calcifications in the adrenal glands (arrows) in this infant are secondary to adrenal hemorrhage occurring at birth.

Appendix. Appendicoliths usually indicate either the presence of appendicitis or that appendicitis will soon develop.

Tumor Calcification. Certain tumors contain calcium. The bone-forming (osteogenic) sarcomas are obvious, but in addition some bowel cancers (Fig. 28-11) and some ovarian cancers can contain calcium, which aids in the identification of both the primary tumor and its metastases.

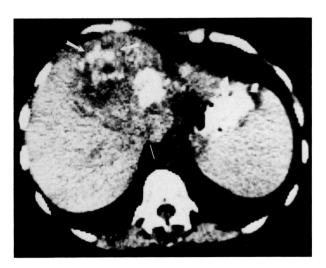

Figure 28-11. A CT scan through the liver demonstrates calcifications (arrows) within metastases within the liver of this 57-year-old man with metastatic colon cancer.

Keynotes

- *If the calcified walls of the aorta are more than 3.5 cm apart, an aneurysm is present.*
- *Phleboliths are common calcifications in pelvic veins. They often have a radiolucent center.*
- *Vas deferens calcification is often a sign of diabetes.*
- *Pancreatic calcifications usually indicate chronic pancreatitis.*
- *An appendicolith is a calcified stone in the appendix. Patients with appendicoliths often have or will soon have appendicitis.*

SUMMARY

The identification of calcifications is an important aid in the diagnosis of abdominal disease. Calcium deposits can be identified on radiography, CT, and sonography. Some acute calcifications can be identified as regions of increased tracer uptake on scans done with ^{99m}Tc phosphate complexes.

Vascular calcifications can aid in the diagnosis of aneurysms. Uterine fibroids and ovarian dermoid cysts often contain calcium. Vas deferens calcification is often a sign of diabetes. Some biliary and urinary calculi are calcified. Pancreatic calcifications usually indicate chronic pancreatitis. Adrenal calcification is associated with adrenal insufficiency. Calcified stones (appendicoliths) usually indicate the presence of appendicitis.

REVIEW QUESTIONS

1. What is the appearance of calcium on
   a. Radiography?
   b. Computed tomography?
   c. Sonography?
   d. Technetium 99m phosphate complex scans?

2. How might you recognize an abdominal aortic aneurysm?
3. What is the significance of phleboliths?
4. Name two common gynecologic calcifications.
5. What is the significance of vas deferens calcification?
6. What percentage of biliary calculi calcify? What percentage of renal calculi calcify?
7. What is the clinical significance of pancreatic calcification?
8. What is the significance of an appendicolith?

VOCABULARY

Addison's disease

aneurysm

phlebolith

sonic shadowing

appendicolith

dermoid cysts

pancreatitis

uterine fibroids

varicocele

vas deferens

SUGGESTIONS FOR FURTHER READING

For suggested reading see Chapter 26.

29

THE IMPORTANCE OF AIR IN THE ABDOMEN

KEY CONCEPTS

Radiological

Focal collections of air in the abdomen appear as blacker areas (areas of increased radiolucency) on radiographic and CT examinations. Often, if the collection is large enough, an air-fluid level will be present because most of the processes that result in abdominal air also result in the presence of collections of abdominal fluid.

On sonograms, air is markedly echogenic. Increased echos will be present at sites of air collection, with sonic shadowing distal to the air collection, unless the air collection is very small. On sonographic examinations, both air and calcium collections are very echogenic and result in sonic shadowing. Sometimes, they can be differentiated because calcium deposits sometimes have a defined sonographically recognizable shape, whereas air collections are poorly defined by sonography. Usually, however, they cannot be accurately differentiated.

Air, unless it is contained in a smaller structure, will rise to the highest portion of the abdomen. When the patient is upright, air will collect just below the diaphragm or under the liver edge. With the patient supine, air will collect anteriorly and can outline the falciform ligament. With a person lying on the left side, air will collect between the liver and the right abdominal wall. Large amounts of air may outline bowel loops.

Abscesses may contain air and debris; a mixture of air, fluid, and debris; or fluid and debris only. The diagnosis of an abscess requires both the demonstration of the fluid component and the evidence of infection.

The fluid component can be demonstrated by CT or ultrasound. The detection on radiographs or CT images of an air-fluid level or of bubbles of air within a structure is most helpful in detection of an abscess. Radiographs, CT, and sonography cannot, however, determine that the fluid collection is infected. For this purpose, these techniques may be combined with galium citrate

Ga 67 or indium 111 leukocyte scanning for confirmation of the presence of inflammation or infection.

Clinical

Abdominal air not contained in the bowel is always abnormal in a man and usually abnormal in a woman.

Air can result from a perforation of the bowel, from iatrogenic causes such as surgery, and from infections with gas-forming organisms such as *Escherichia coli* and Clostridia.

Air within the wall of the bowel is usually a sign of bowel necrosis but can be seen as a relatively benign finding. Air in the portal venous system of the liver is usually a sign of bowel necrosis.

Air in the biliary system can be seen after biliary tract surgery or, uncommonly, with biliary tract infections.

OBJECTIVES

When you complete this chapter you will be able to

1. Identify air collections on selected abdominal radiographs and CT examination.
2. Identify free intra-abdominal air on selected radiographs and CT scans.
3. List the three major categories of causes of free intra-abdominal air.
4. Discuss the method of evaluation of a suspected intra-abdominal abscess.
5. Describe the difference in significance of air in the biliary system and air within the portal venous system of the liver.

Air within a nondilated stomach, small bowel, or colon is normal. Infrequently, small amounts of air are seen in the peritoneal cavity of normal women. All other abdominal air is abnormal and is indicative of disease or recent abdominal surgery.

RECOGNIZING AIR COLLECTIONS

On the standard radiograph and on a transmission computed tomogram, air shows a region of increased radiolucency compared with surrounding fat- or water-radiodensity structures (Fig. 29-1). Though its grayness will vary with the settings used on the machine, air usually will be black or dark gray on the image. Most helpful in identifying air collections is the presence of an *air-fluid level* (Figs. 29-2 and 29-3). This is frequently present because most diseases that result in the presence of abnormal air collections also result in fluid collections. These straight lines of radiodensity change can be identified on radiographs taken with a horizontally directed beam (the kind used for an upright or decubitus film) and on most transmission computed tomographic views.

On the sonogram, air is markedly echogenic. Minimal amounts result in intense echos; moderate amounts result in marked echos with sonic shadowing. Large amounts of air interrupt the sound beam and result in multiple echos without intrinsic shape (Fig. 29-4). Abdominal air collec-

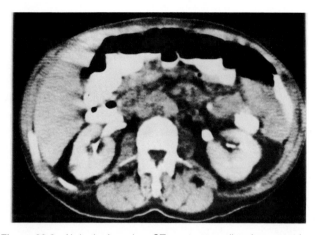

Figure 29-2. Air in the bowel on CT; contrast medium is present in the colon, with long air-fluid levels. Contrast medium is also present in the renal collecting system. The margin of the aorta is indistinct because there is minimal adenopathy in the retroperitoneal nodes.

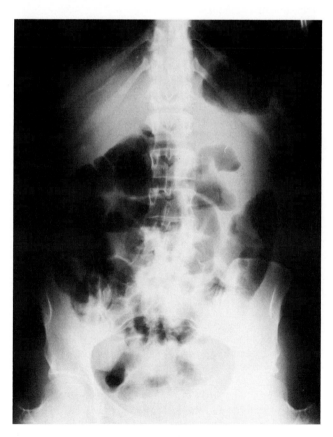

Figure 29-1. Air is seen in the stomach and in the small and large bowel in this 28-year-old woman with an adynamic ileus secondary to peritonitis. The air within the bowel appears dark gray to black.

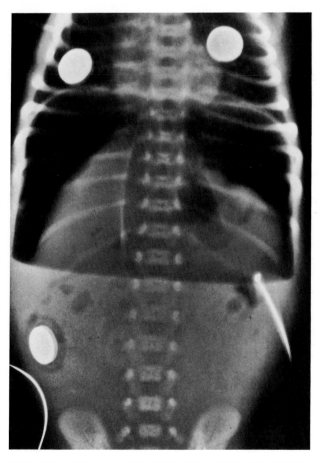

Figure 29-3. Upright view. This infant with a rupture of the stomach demonstrates a straight air-fluid level where the air and fluid in the peritoneal cavity meet.

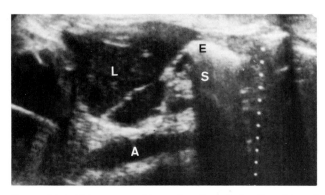

Figure 29-4. This sonographic section through the liver (L) and aorta (A) demonstrates amorphous echos (E) inferior to the liver with shadowing (S). This is the appearance on sonography of large collections of air. (Courtesy of M. Dunne, M.D.)

tions cannot be directly identified by nuclear medicine imaging techniques.

Keynotes

- *An air-fluid level is the sharp demarcation between adjacent collections of air and fluid. Its sharp margin can be seen when the x-ray beam is tangential to the demarcated edge.*
- *Air is markedly echogenic and can result in sonic shadowing.*
- *A sonic shadow occurs when the transmission of sound is stopped. The lack of sound transmission distal to the area of stoppage is the sonic shadow.*

ABNORMAL AIR COLLECTIONS

Free Intraperitoneal Air

Air not contained in the gastrointestinal system and free within the peritoneal cavity can be recognized on the radiograph and transmission computed tomogram because it outlines margins of structures not normally outlined by air.

Free Air on the Radiograph Taken Upright. On an upright radiograph, free air collects under the hemidiaphragm or under the liver edge (Fig. 29-5). The best radiograph for identification of free intraperitoneal air is the upright film taken with chest radiographic technique with the x-ray beam centered at the level of the diaphragm. It can take up to 5 minutes for small amounts of air to collect under the diaphragm, but with proper technique, as little as 1 cc can be identified.

Free Air on a Radiograph Taken with the Left Side Down. Many patients with acute perforations of a viscus are hypotensive and cannot stand for the upright view. A view taken with the left side down (a lateral decubitus view) using a horizontally directed x-ray beam can show small amounts of free intraperitoneal air. The air collects

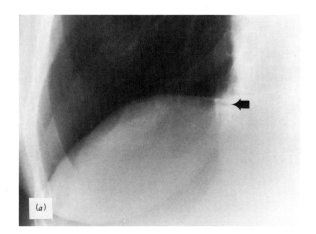

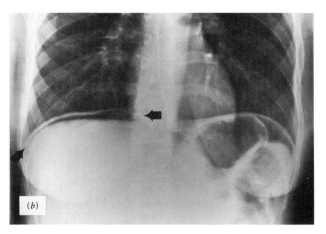

Figure 29-5. Free abdominal air. (*a*) Minimal air (arrow) is seen under the right hemidiaphragm in this patient with an acutely perforated duodenal ulcer. This was the only radiographic sign of this surgical emergency. (*b*) Moderate amounts of free air are seen under the diaphragm (arrows) in this patient shortly after abdominal surgery.

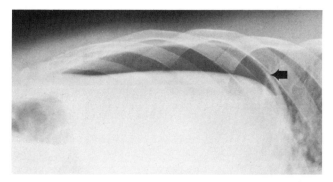

Figure 29-6. Focal view of the right upper quadrant of the abdomen, a left lateral decubitus view, demonstrates free abdominal air (arrow) located between the liver and the abdominal wall.

between the liver and the lateral abdominal wall (Fig. 29-6). The film technique should be adjusted to be slightly darker than the usual chest radiographic technique. Standard abdominal technique is often too dark, and small amounts of air may be invisible.

Air on a Radiograph Taken in the Supine Position. In the supine position, air will lie adjacent to the anterior abdominal wall and will outline remnants of the umbilical vein, arteries, and urachus. Of these the only one commonly identified is the peritoneal fold over the fibrotic remnant of the umbilical vein: the *falciform ligament,* it is imaged as a white streak running from the umbilicus to the porta hepatis (Fig. 29-7).

With large amounts of free air, the outer margin of bowel loops can also be shown outlined by air (Fig. 29-8).

Free Air on the Transmission Computed Tomogram. Air free within the peritoneal cavity will collect along the anterior peritoneal wall, where it can outline the falciform ligament and the outer margins of bowel loops. It is some-

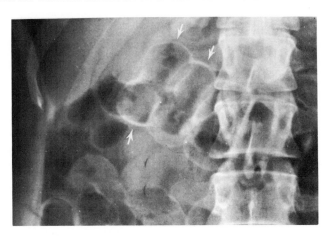

Figure 29-8. Both the inner and outer walls of bowel loops can be seen (arrows), demonstrating the presence of free intraperitoneal air in this postoperative patient.

times difficult to decide if small amounts of air are contained within the bowel. A repeat section obtained with the patient lying on the left side should show the displacement of free intraperitoneal air to the space between the liver and the peritoneal wall.

Free Intraperitoneal Air Causes. Free intraperitoneal air can result from

> Perforation of
> > Stomach
> > Duodenal ulcer
> > Colon
> > Small bowel (rare)
> > Appendix (rare)
> Infections
> > Peritonitis with gas forming organisms
> > > *E. coli*
> > > Clostridia
> Iatrogenic
> > Surgery
> > Paracentesis (needle taps)
> > Following air insufflation to test for fallopian tubal patency (*Rubin test*).

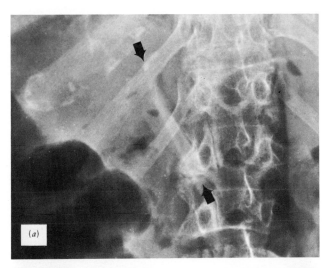

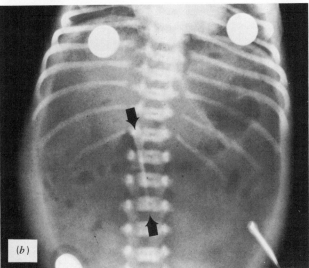

Figure 29-7. Demonstration of the falciform ligament outlined by free peritoneal air on supine radiographs. (*a*) Focal view of the right upper quadrant of the abdomen. Arrows localize the falciform ligament. (*b*) Focal view of the upper abdomen in an infant with rupture of the stomach. Arrows localize the falciform ligament. (The upright view of this infant's abdomen is Fig. 29-3.)

Keynotes

- *Air free within the peritoneal cavity outlines structures normally not seen: the undersurface of the diaphragm, the liver, the outer wall of the bowel, and the margins of the falciform ligament and peritoneum.*

- *It may take up to 5 minutes for small amounts of air to shift to outline the diaphragm or peritoneal margin.*

- *A decubitus view is a view taken with the patient lying down with a horizontally directed x-ray beam.*

- *The falciform ligament is the peritoneal fold over the obliterated umbilical vein.*

- *With the patient supine, free intraperitoneal air outlines the falciform ligament. The falciform ligament can be seen on radiographs or computed tomograms.*

Air in Abscesses

An abscess cavity may be filled with fluid or with a mixture of air and fluid. When air is present in an abscess, it may accumulate in one bubble, resulting in a sharp air-fluid level, or it may form many small bubbles scattered through the abscess fluid (Fig. 29-9).

The major problem encountered in diagnosis is being certain that the air and fluid seen are in an abscess rather than in the bowel. This can be easily done when the bowel contains air. A contrast medium must sometimes be given to outline the stomach, small bowel, and colon to aid in their localization.

Sonography can also help to identify abscesses, for they often have many internal echos. If air is contained within the abscess in small bubbles, these bubbles will cause focal regions of intense echogenicity and sonic shadowing. The sonographer can also have difficulty differentiating abscesses from bowel but, if skilled, can usually differentiate them by making multiple images in different directions and by using a real-time machine to look for changes in bowel shape caused by peristalsis.

Gallium citrate Ga 67 can also be used to image the location of abscesses. Its localization in the abscess depends on its uptake by leukocytes and bacteria. Unfortunately ^{67}Ga also accumulates in the colon, and this colonic accumulation may simulate an abscess. Alternatively, an abscess may not be recognized, because the tracer localization is assumed to be in feces. Indium 111–labeled white blood cells can also be used to localize abscesses.

Interrelationship of the Differing Imaging Modalities in the Identification of an Abscess. When the clinical setting is appropriate, two separate features of an abscess must be confirmed to diagnose an abscess: there must be an inflammatory (infectious) process, and there must be a collection of fluid to be drained. The gallium citrate Ga 67 scan is a sensitive test for the identification of an inflammatory process, but it cannot tell whether an abscess cavity is present and drainable. Both CT and sonography can localize fluid collections in abnormal locations, but often they cannot tell whether the process is infected. Only when air is admixed with the localized collection of fluid is an abscess probable. But many abscesses will not contain air, making it impossible to distinguish a sterile from an infected fluid collection. For this reason a patient may require both a CT or a sonogram and a gallium citrate Ga 67 scan.

Keynote

- *An abscess may contain no air, a few small bubbles of air, or one large bubble of air.*

Air Within the Wall of the Bowel

Air within the wall of the bowel is usually a sign of bowel necrosis. It occurs most frequently in the newborn with necrotizing enterocolitis but can be seen at any age. The

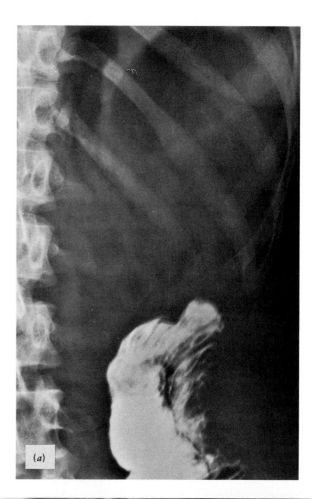

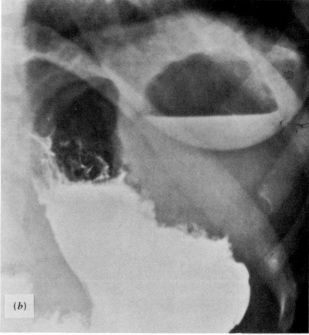

Figure 29-9. Left subphrenic abscess. Air lies between the stomach (opacified with barium) and the left hemidiaphragm. (*a*) Supine view. (*b*) Upright view. An air-fluid level is seen in the abscess.

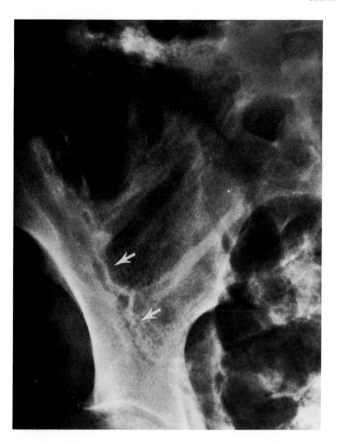

Figure 29-10. Focal view of the right lower quadrant of the abdomen. Air (arrows) is seen in the wall of the cecum in this patient with bowel infarction caused by a decrease in the flow of blood in the superior mesenteric artery (superior mesenteric artery ischemia).

patient shown in Figure 29-10 has superior mesenteric artery–induced bowel ischemia with necrosis of the bowel wall. Occasionally, air can be seen in the wall of the bowel as a benign condition called *pneumatosis coli*. But serious illness should always be considered when bowel wall air is found.

Biliary Air

Air in the biliary tree can be seen after biliary tract surgery or occasionally with biliary tract infection.

Hepatic Venous Air

Air in the hepatic veins can be a sign of bowel necrosis. It is seen in some newborns with necrotizing enterocolitis and is a sign of potential poor prognosis.

SUMMARY

Air in the abdomen can be identified on radiographs, computed tomograms, and sonograms. On the radiograph and computed tomogram, air appears blacker than its surrounding tissues. Air-fluid levels often aid in its identification. On sonograms, air is intensely echogenic and can result in sonic shadowing.

Air in nondilated bowel is normal. Air free within the peritoneal cavity in men is always abnormal and in women often abnormal. Small amounts of air rise to the highest location and depending on the patient's position, can outline the diaphragm, inferior edge of the liver, peritoneal margin, or falciform ligament.

Air in an abscess can have one large bubble or many small bubbles.

REVIEW QUESTIONS

1. What are the five basic radiodensities? Which is the most radiolucent?
2. What is an air-fluid level?
3. What is the appearance of small and large quantities of air on sonograms?
4. If you want to demonstrate small quantities of air free in the peritoneal cavity, how would you do it?
5. What are several causes of free intraperitoneal air?
6. How might you identify an intra-abdominal abscess?

VOCABULARY

air-fluid level	paracentesis
decubitus view	Rubin test
falciform ligament	sonic shadowing

SUGGESTIONS FOR FURTHER READING

For suggested reading see Chapter 26.

30

THE ABDOMINAL VESSELS

KEY CONCEPTS

Radiological

Nuclear medicine tracers can be injected and viewed serially to evaluate flow in vessels. Complete obstruction, and partial obstruction sufficient to slow flow, can be detected. This technique is used mainly in the evaluation of suspected renal artery stenosis and suspected superior vena cava syndrome.

Sonograms can detect both the lumen and the outer wall of a larger vessel. This permits the identification of larger plaques and thrombi that may be within the vessel. This technique is used mainly in the evaluation of the abdominal aorta. It is also used in the evaluation of the carotid arteries and, to a lesser extent, other peripheral arteries. When used to evaluate the carotid arteries, small plaques and some ulcerations in plaques can be detected.

CT exams performed with an intravascular contrast medium can demonstrate both the vessel lumen and its outer wall. Thrombi within the vessel can be detected.

Angiography is useful in evaluating both small and large vessels in the abdomen. It demonstrates the lumen of the vessel but does not demonstrate the vessel's outer wall. It may fail to demonstrate an aneurysm where the lumen is partially filled with a clot. It is the best method of looking at smaller vessels and gives the most detailed information about the anatomy of the lumina of vessels. It is used mainly as a confirmatory study before abdominal aortic aneurysm surgery and in planning for the resection of some abdominal and retroperitoneal tumors.

Magnetic resonance imaging shows promise in its ability to evaluate the abdominal vessels and may partially replace angiography, once the technique is more fully developed.

Clinical

Imaging techniques are used to evaluate abdominal vessels for vascular obstruction and aneurysms and in the evaluation of some abdominal and retroperitoneal masses. When vascular obstruction is found in midsized arteries, treatment by an interventional radiologist using balloon angioplasty can relieve obstruction and restore flow.

OBJECTIVES

When you complete this chapter you will be able to

1. Identify vessels on selected nuclear medicine, ultrasound, angiography, CT, and MRI examinations.
2. Identify luminal narrowing on selected angiograms.
3. Identify abdominal aortic aneurysms on selected angiograms, ultrasound exams, and CT examinations.

APPEARANCE OF NORMAL VESSELS

Each of the imaging modalities can be used to evaluate the intra-abdominal vessels. Nuclear medicine flow studies can be done with any radiopharmaceutical that can pass through the lung capillaries. Multiple images can be made, and major disturbances can be detected (Fig. 30-1).

On sonography the larger vessels have a sonolucent lumen and echogenic wall (Fig. 30-2). Both the lumen and inner and outer portions of the wall can be seen. Sonographic Doppler studies can demonstrate differences in flow rate. The Doppler effect is a shift in the frequency of high-frequency sound waves that results when the sound is reflected from a moving stream of blood. The shift of ultrasonic frequency can be equated to the speed of blood

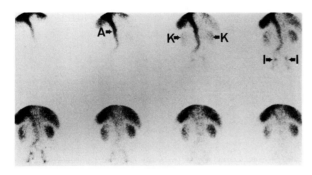

Figure 30-1. A normal nuclear medicine flow study of the abdominal vessels. Serial images are recorded. First seen is the aorta (A), followed by activity in the kidneys (K) and then by the iliac arteries (I). Compare this with figure 30-4.

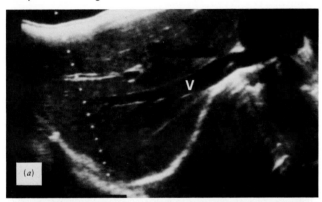

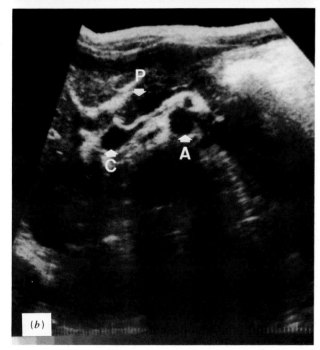

Figure 30-2. (a) This sonographic view of the liver demonstrates the hepatic veins (V) within the liver. The lumina of the vessels have no echo signal. (Courtesy M. Dunne, M.D.) (b) This cross-sectional sonographic view demonstrates the aorta (A), the inferior vena cava (C), and a small portion of the portal vein (P). The lumina of the vessels are echo free. (Courtesy M. Dunne, M.D.)

flow, thereby indicating the site and severity of vessel narrowing.

On the computed tomogram, a large vessel will have a homogeneous lumen and a smooth wall (Fig. 30-3). On the angiogram, a contrast medium is injected into the lumen of a vessel, defining precisely its luminal anatomy (Fig. 30-4). The outer margin of the vessel is not usually identified.

On MRI, large vessels can be evaluated because of the flow-void phenomenon. When the appropriate echo sequences are chosen, flowing blood will not create a signal, leaving the vessel lumen devoid of image while the surrounding tissues are seen (see Chapter 5). Areas of clot and luminal narrowing can be identified. The clinical role of MRI in the evaluation of the abdominal vessels has not yet been established.

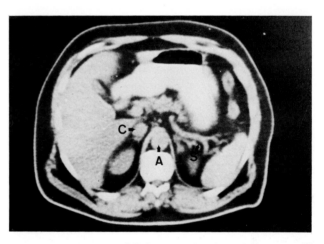

Figure 30-3. Abdominal CT demonstrating the splenic artery (S) with some of its branches. The abdominal aorta (A) and inferior vena cava (C) are seen in cross section. (Courtesy N. Whitley, M.D., University of Maryland Hospital.)

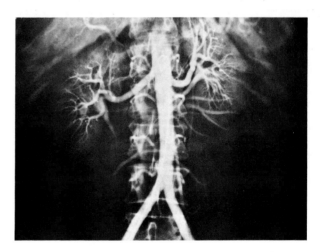

Figure 30-4. Abdominal aortogram, normal appearance. The aorta has been opacified by radiographic contrast medium injected through a catheter. (Courtesy S. Cisternino, M.D.)

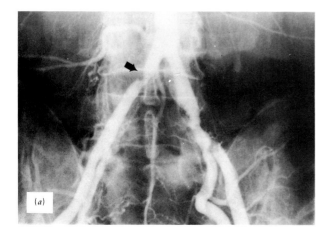

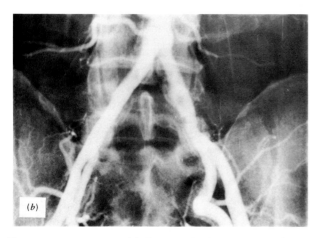

Figure 30-5. Angioplasty. (*a*) The preangioplasty angiogram demonstrates a focal narrowing (arrow) of the right common iliac artery. (*b*) The postangioplasty angiogram demonstrates that the narrowing is no longer present.

Keynotes

- *A nuclear medicine flow study is done by serially recording the passage of the radioactive tracer through a region of the body.*
- *With sonography, both the inner and outer walls of the vessel can be seen.*
- *The angiogram demonstrates the luminal anatomy. The wall itself is not seen.*

DISEASE OF BLOOD VESSELS

Imaging studies can be used to evaluate the presence and severity of vascular disease.

Obstruction

The nuclear medicine flow study can disclose moderate-to-severe vascular obstruction, which is reflected in a delay in the movement of the tracer through the vessels. The angio-gram can demonstrate luminal narrowing and slowed flow (Fig. 30-5*a*). The Doppler sonogram can demonstrate changes in flow rate.

Angioplasty

Focal areas of vessel narrowing can be treated by the interventional radiologist with balloon catheters. These catheters are passed through the arterial system until they are positioned at the site of vessel narrowing. The balloon is then inflated, dilating the focal narrowing of the vessel. Figure 30-5 demonstrates the before-and-after appearance of balloon dilation of the iliac artery.

Focal infusions of streptokinase have also been used experimentally in small arteries to reopen acutely thrombosed and obstructed vessels.

Aneurysms

The angiogram, the sonogram, and the computed tomogram can each show aneurysms (Fig. 30-6). Two main types of aneurysms are seen: *fusiform aneurysms* (diffusely widened vessels) and *sacular aneurysms* (focal rounded regions of vascular widening). The basic criterion is enlargement of the vessels beyond limits of normal variation. For example, widening of the abdominal aorta beyond 3.5 cm is diagnostic of an aneurysm.

In general, sonography is the preferred method of diagnosis for fusiform aneurysm, with CT the second choice. Angiography is better for sacular aneurysms but is less reliable for fusiform aneurysms because these frequently contain a blood clot, which narrows the lumen. Thus the lumen demonstrated does not necessarily represent the true diameter of the vessel being evaluated.

New Vessels and Tumor Vessels

New vessels (neovascularity) can form in response to both benign and malignant processes. Vessels can grow in the tissue formed around abscesses and hematomas. Growing neoplasms, both benign and malignant, develop new vessels as they grow. In some cases the pattern of the new vessels indicates that a process is likely to be malignant. Patterns of tumor vascularity that suggest malignancy are vessels that have areas of widening and narrowing and vessels with a sudden change in diameter suggesting that they are encased with tumor. In a few benign tumors, the pattern of the new vessels strongly suggests the specific diagnosis. In general, however, the specific patterns of neovascularity have become much less important in diagnosis since the development of CT. Angiography of tumors is now mainly used for surgical planning, for presurgical chemotherapy, and for the presurgical occlusion of tumor vessels to reduce surgical blood loss.

Vascular Displacement by a Mass

Masses commonly displace adjacent blood vessels, and this displacement can be used to identify and localize the mass. Sonography, CT, and angiography can each be used for

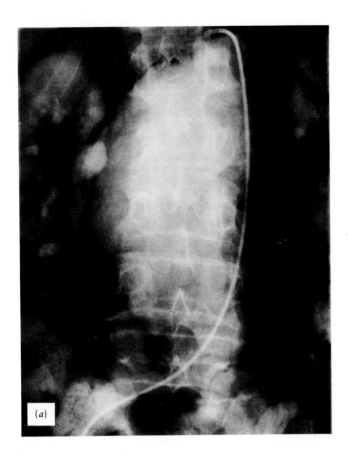

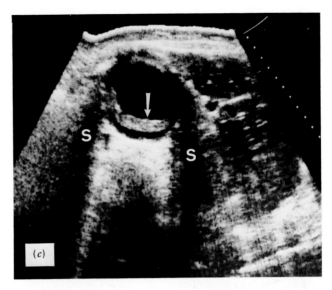

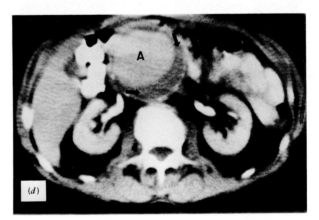

Figure 30-6. Fusiform abdominal aortic aneurysm demonstrated by angiography, sonography, and CT. (*a*) This large aneurysm is demonstrated by catheter angiography. Compare its appearance with that in Figure 30-4. (*b*) Longitudinal sonogram through the aneurysm. The echogenic area (arrow) in the posterior portion of the aneurysm is a clot. Many abdominal aortic aneurysms contain clots. (*c*) Transverse sonogram through the aneurysm. The posteriorly placed clot is easily seen. The sonic shadowing (S) is due to aortic calcification. (*d*) CT through the midabdomen again demonstrates this abdominal aortic aneurysm. Radiographic contrast has been given to opacify the aortic lumen (A). The region of lesser radiodensity surrounding it (arrows) is the blood clot. Because a blood clot will prevent the angiogram from demonstrating the maximal diameter of the aorta, sonography and CT better demonstrate the true diameter of the aorta.

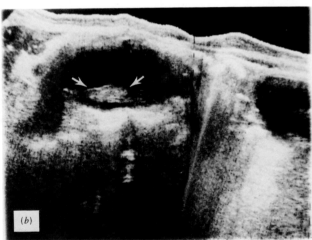

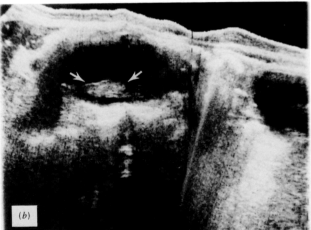

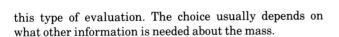

this type of evaluation. The choice usually depends on what other information is needed about the mass.

Arteritis

Arteriography can be used to define and diagnose several forms of arteritis including periarteritis nodosa, fibromuscular dysplasia, and Takayasu's arteritis.

Keynotes

- *Nuclear medicine flow studies and angiograms can demonstrate obstruction as slowed or absent flow.*
- *Fusiform aneurysms show dilation of the entire circumference of the lumen. Sacular aneurysms arise as an outpouching from the wall; the main lumen of the vessels is usually nearly normal.*

• *Periarteritis nodosa:* an inflammatory disease of small arteries resulting in focal areas of microaneurysm formation and focal areas of obstruction.
• *Fibromuscular dysplasia:* a disease of blood vessel walls. In areas where the wall is thickened, the lumen is narrowed; where the wall is thin, focal areas of dilation occur.
• *Takayasu's arteritis:* inflammatory occlusion of the origin of large vessels from the aorta.

SUMMARY

The abdominal vessels can be studied by nuclear medicine flow studies, sonography, CT, and angiography. The paths of movement of blood can be seen on nuclear medicine flow studies and angiography. The structure of the large vessels can be seen best by sonography and slightly less well by CT. Luminal shape and the structure of small vessels is best studied by angiography.

Vascular obstruction is well demonstrated by nuclear medicine, Doppler flow studies, and angiography. Fusiform aneurysms are best demonstrated by sonography. Sacular aneurysms and arteritis are best studied by angiography.

REVIEW QUESTIONS

1. Describe how a nuclear medicine flow study is done.
2. What is the appearance of large vessels on sonography? On CT?
3. What is the best way to demonstrate a fusiform aneurysm of the abdominal aorta?
4. How might you demonstrate obstruction of the left common iliac artery?
5. How might you diagnose arteritis?
6. What problem might be encountered in diagnosing an aortic aneurysm by angiography?

VOCABULARY

aneurysm
fibromuscular dysplasia
flow study
fusiform aneurysm
neovascularity

periarteritis nodosa
sacular aneurysm
Takayasu's arteritis
tumor vascularity

SUGGESTIONS FOR FURTHER READING

For suggested reading see Chapter 26.

31

ABDOMINAL MASSES

KEY CONCEPTS

Radiological

The two stages in the evaluation of an abdominal mass are (1) finding it and (2) determining if it represents focal hypertrophy, focal swelling, a cyst, a hematoma, or a neoplasm.

A mass can be suspected and partially localized based on the history, a physical examination, and clinical analysis. Initial confirmation or detection of a mass is usually best done with CT or ultrasound. When the mass is in the lumen or wall of the bowel, barium studies such as the upper gastrointestinal tract (GI) series and barium enema are usually preferable.

When the mass could represent focal hypertrophy, a physiological imaging method that labels that tissue (such as a nuclear medicine technique) is often the procedure of choice. Labeling techniques exist for hepatic, splenic, renal, and biliary tissues. Nuclear medicine techniques can also be used to label inflammatory tissue.

When the mass most likely represents a cyst or pseudocyst, ultrasound examination is usually preferred with CT available as an alternative.

When an abscess is suspected, two types of methods can be used. The first uses nuclear medicine techniques to localize areas of inflammation; agents can be gallium citrate Ga 67 or indium 111–labeled white blood cells. The second is to look for the mass caused by the abscess, using either ultrasonography or CT.

Clinical

Those aspects of the patient's clinical history that suggest the possible presence of an abdominal mass include

1. A sense of heaviness or fullness in the abdomen
2. Involuntary weight loss
3. Blood seen in urine, feces, or vomitus

4. Malaise or new onset of depression in middle age
5. Unexplained fever

Clinical signs include migratory thrombophlebitis (seen in pancreatic carcinoma), a palpable mass, and certain skin rashes.

The clinical symptoms and signs should be used to suggest the probable organ involved and the type of process suspected. This clinical evaluation should then be used to guide the selection of the most appropriate test. The careful selection of the best test is the key to controlling costs.

OBJECTIVES

When you complete this chapter you will be able to

1. List five symptoms that could indicate the presence of an abdominal mass.
2. List three clinical signs of a possible abdominal mass.
3. Indicate the appropriate imaging method for the following suspected masses: focal hypertrophy of the kidney, intrahepatic abscess, pancreatic carcinoma, renal cyst, and carcinoma of the stomach.

Much of abdominal imaging is concerned with the identification and diagnosis of abdominal masses. Masses can be focal hypertrophy of normal tissue, focal swelling from inflammation or edema, benign tumors, fluid-filled cysts, hematomas, malignant neoplasms, and abscesses. Imaging methods used in a properly chosen sequence can often precisely determine the diagnosis. Masses located in specific organs are discussed later in separate chapters, but it is important to have an overview of the methods. There are two overlapping processes:

Finding the mass
Diagnosing the mass

Keynote

• First, find the mass; second, figure out what it is.

FINDING THE MASS

Clinical suspicion often guides the search for a mass. A history of prolonged weight loss may suggest malignancy; symptoms of gastric irritation may point to the stomach; migratory thrombophlebitis may suggest pancreatic carcinoma. A mass may be palpable. Blood may be found in the urine or feces, pointing to disease in those organs systems. The suspected diagnosis guides the direction of search. For example:

Suspected	First Study
Renal cancer	Intravenous urogram
Bladder cancer	Cystoscopy
Stomach cancer	Upper GI series
Colon cancer	Sigmoidoscopy, then an air-contrast barium enema
Pancreatic cancer	Transmission computed tomography
Liver cancer (hepatoma)	Liver scans (nuclear medicine or CT imaging)
Gynecological mass	Sonogram

These are discussed in more detail in later chapters.

Keynote

• Clinical suspicion should guide the search for the mass.

DIAGNOSING THE MASS

The imaging analysis of each mass must demonstrate whether it is

A focal enlargement of a normal portion of an organ
A benign fluid-filled cyst
An abscess
A neoplasm, benign or malignant

Diagnosing Focal Enlargement of an Otherwise Normal Organ

Focal enlargement can be due to normal variants in growth or to hypertrophy resulting from disease elsewhere in the same organ. Two main methods are used. When the focal enlargement is due to variation in normal growth, the overall structure of the organ may be distorted in a typical configuration. One of the most common focal regions of masslike anomaly is the kidney (Fig. 31-1a). Perhaps 5% of people show a focal thickening of cortical tissue within the central portion of the kidney. These "pseudotumors" can often be specifically diagnosed because they usually occur between the upper and middle pole of the kidney, and they usually have shorter than normal calyces and infundibula draining them. If oblique views confirm that the infundibula are anatomically short (Fig. 31-1b), the diagnosis is established and further evaluation is not necessary. If only a single view is available, care must be taken because a mass can displace a long calyx, making it appear foreshortened on a single view.

The second method of showing that a mass is an enlarged but otherwise normal portion of the involved organ is by using a method of specifically identifying the structure of the organ and showing that the questioned mass has essentially normal structure. This is best done by a nuclear medicine image using a pharmacological marker for the cells localized in that organ.

In the liver, agents that are phagocytosed by Kupffer's cells can be used. The agent usually used is technetium Tc 99m sulfur colloid particles. This results in tracer activity in regions of the liver with normal Kupffer's cell function (Fig. 31-2).

For the kidney, a substance interacting with renal tubular cells can be used. Technetium Tc 99m DMSA attaches to renal tubular cells that show on this tracer imaging study as regions of normal uptake. Technetium Tc 99m stannous glucoheptanate gives similar information (Fig. 31-3).

In some cases, an angiogram must be used to study the vascular architecture of the organ to be certain that only normal tissue is present, but because of the danger of complications from angiography, nuclear medicine imaging studies are preferred when they are suitable.

Diagnosing Benign Fluid-filled Cysts

Cysts in the kidney and liver are so common as to be considered normal. They usually cause no symptoms. Mesenteric cysts and ovarian cysts may cause symptoms. Pancreatic pseudocysts are quite common after pancreatitis and can be associated with the prolongation of symptoms of acute pancreatitis. Some cysts need no treatment. Others may require draining or excision.

Confirming that a mass is a cyst is usually best done with sonography. A mass with no internal echoes; a smooth, well-defined margin; and good transmission of sound through the lesion is cystic (Fig. 31-4). Multiple views are necessary, and it is important to be sure that the wall of the cyst distant from the transducer is well seen.

Transmission computed tomography is almost as good as sonography in establishing the fluid-filled nature of a mass, but it is more expensive and is, therefore, the second choice. On CT, a cyst will appear filled with homogeneous water-density material and will not change its ra-

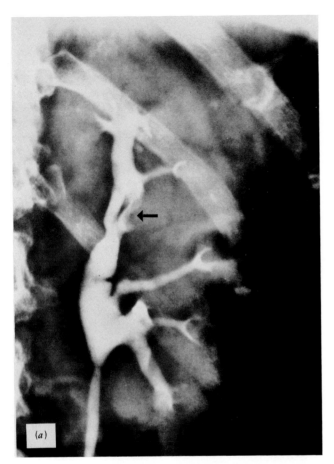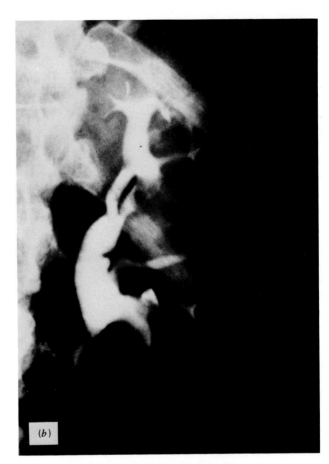

Figure 31-1. Renal pseudotumor. (*a*) AP view demonstrates a separation between the upper and mid collecting system suggestive of a mass. A short or displaced calyx (arrow) is present. (*b*) An oblique view confirms that the calyx developed abnormally short, indicating that a normal renal variant (the renal pseudotumor) is present.

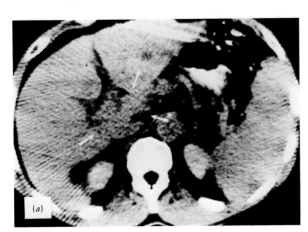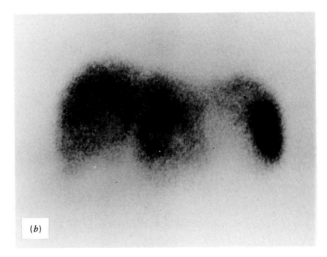

Figure 31-2. Focal hepatic hypertrophy. (*a*) A possible mass in the portahepatis (arrows) is seen on CT. (*b*) A technetium Tc 99m sulfur colloid liver scan demonstrates that this mass functions as normal liver and therefore represents focal hypertrophy of the caudate lobe.

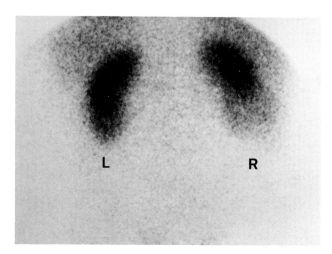

Figure 31-3. A technetium Tc 99m glucoheptanate scan of the kidneys demonstrates asymmetry. The right kidney (R) on this posterior view is shorter than the left (L) and demonstrates decreased activity inferiorly. This patient had a possible renal mass on intravenous urography. This mass proved to be a renal cell cancer.

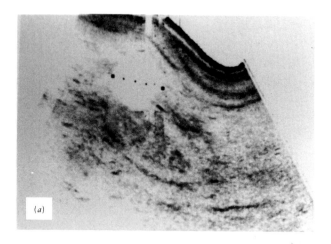

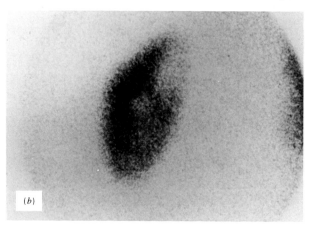

Figure 31-4. A benign renal cyst. (a) Demonstrated by sonography. The lack of internal echos, the well-defined walls, and the increased through transmission of sound all indicate the cystic nature of this renal mass. (b) A technetium Tc 99m DMSA scan demonstrates a focal lack of activity at the site of the renal cyst.

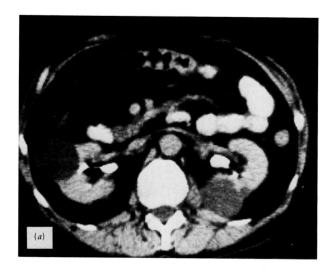

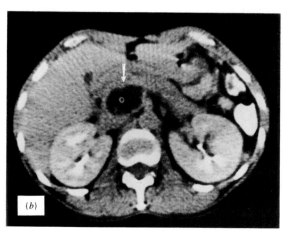

Figure 31-5. (a) Bilateral renal cysts on CT. They demonstrate a homogeneous appearance, well-defined walls, and a sharp demarcation from the adjacent renal substance. (Courtesy N. Whitley, M.D.) (b) A pancreatic pseudocyst (arrow) is demonstrated within the pancreatic head.

diodensity after administration of intravenously injected radiographic contrast medium (Fig. 31-5). In some cases, conventional tomography done immediately after the injection of a high dose of intravenous contrast medium may define specific diagnostic criteria for a cyst, but great care is needed for performance and interpretation of this study.

Needle Puncture of Cyst Lesions. Should any doubt be present after an appropriate imaging study that the mass in question might not be a cyst, a needle puncture with aspiration and analysis of the fluid can be performed, using ultrasound or CT to guide the aspiration or biopsy.

Diagnosing an Abscess

Sometimes the clinical history and findings are so strongly suggestive of an abscess that additional imaging studies are not needed. If additional confirmation is needed, there are two types of imaging studies that can be done. The first uses a pathophysiological approach. When gallium citrate Ga 67 is injected intravenously, it labels leukocytes, transferin, and bacteria, which then localize in the abscess (Fig. 31-6). (A similar study can be performed using ^{111}In-labeled white blood cells.) The major disadvantages of gallium citrate Ga 67 are

1. The need to wait 24–72 hours before diagnostic images can be obtained
2. The accumulation of tracer activity in the colon, possibly simulating an abscess
3. The need for cleaning enemas to clean the colon
4. The accumulation of tracer in surgical scars

The major disadvantage of the ^{111}In study is its currently higher cost.

The second type of study is anatomic localization of an extra intestinal fluid or air-fluid collection. This localization is usually best done with sonography or transmission CT but is occasionally possible on standard abdominal radiographs.

Diagnosing a Neoplasm

Nongastrointestinal   Neoplasms. Nongastrointestinal neoplasms are usually diagnosed by exclusion, by showing that a mass is not a benign cyst or hypertrophied but otherwise normal tissue. The diagnosis of an abscess can usually be excluded because the patient with an abscess has a clinical history suggestive of abscess (fever, chills, recent surgery); if this is lacking, specific tests for abscess need not be performed.

Sometimes an angiogram can be used to show the fine vessels within a neoplastic mass, permitting the diagnosis of benign neoplasm. This can occur with hepatic adenomas and hepatic hemangiomas. Conversely, an angiogram can demonstrate an irregular tangle of vessels indicative of malignancy (Fig. 31-7).

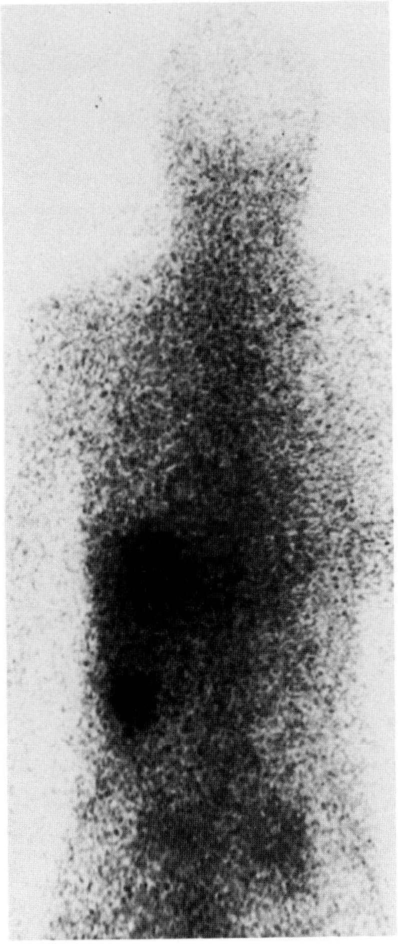

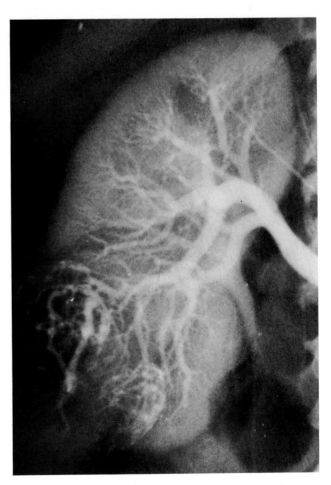

Figure 31-6. A subhepatic abscess is demonstrated on this ^{67}Ga scan as an area of increased activity inferior to the liver. This patient was febrile 4 days after surgery on a ruptured appendix, and this increased activity was from an abscess.

Figure 31-7. Renal cell cancer demonstrated by angiography (same patient as in Figure 31-3). The varying size of the vessels, their tortuosity, and areas of focal dilation are indicative of the malignant nature of this mass. Benign masses usually have more uniform vessel size and distribution.

Gastrointestinal Neoplasms. Differentiating benign from malignant neoplasms in the GI tract is discussed in Chapter 36.

Keynotes

- *Renal pseudotumors can often be directly diagnosed because they occur between the upper and middle collecting system and have short calyces draining them.*
- *Nuclear medicine imaging techniques permit a pharmacological approach to the identification of selected tissues.*
- *Confirming that a mass is a cyst is best done by sonography.*
- *An abscess is an infected fluid collection.*
- *Sonography and CT can both demonstrate that there is a fluid collection present, but ⁶⁷Ga scanning can show that infection is present in the fluid.*

SUMMARY

There are two processes used in evaluating a suspected abdominal mass; first, finding it, and second, deciding what it is. The finding of the abdominal mass is based on the careful selection of appropriate imaging studies based on a carefully derived clinical suspicion. Random searches are expensive and may not be productive. Clinical history, physical findings, and laboratory tests may each point to the organ system likely to be involved. The imaging technique chosen is based on the organ system thought likely to be involved.

Deciding what a mass is depends first on identifying what organ it arises from and second on deciding whether it represents hypertrophied but otherwise normal tissue, focal swelling, a cyst, a hematoma, an abscess, or a neoplastic mass. Hypertrophied but otherwise normal tissue is usually best evaluated by using a nuclear medicine imaging technique. Physiological labels exist for liver, spleen, bone marrow, kidney, and the biliary tree. The diagnosis of a cyst or pseudocyst is usually best done by sonography, but it can also be done by CT. The diagnosis of an abscess depends on demonstrating a fluid collection and showing that it is infected. A combination of ^{67}Ga scanning with sonography or CT may be necessary. Masses that are shown not to be hypertrophied but otherwise normal tissue, cysts, hematomas, or abscesses should be suspected of being neoplastic and should be considered for possible resection.

REVIEW QUESTIONS

1. How can imaging techniques be used to show that a mass is a focal area of hypertrophied but otherwise normal tissue?
2. How can a mass be shown to be a cyst?
3. A 50-year-old man has a high fever 1 week after a cholecystectomy. How would you discover if he had an abscess?
4. What technical problems limit the use of ^{67}Ga scanning in the diagnosis of abscesses?

VOCABULARY

cystoscopy   Kupffer's cells

SUGGESTIONS FOR FURTHER READING

For suggested reading see Chapter 26.

32

THE PERITONEUM

KEY CONCEPTS

Radiological

Peritoneal fluid can be detected on plain abdominal radiographs, ultrasound studies, and CT. On the plain abdominal radiograph, moderate amounts of ascitic fluid can be detected by noting the displacement of mesenteric fat from around the bladder and by medial displacement of bowel loops toward the midabdomen. The ultrasound images can detect small-to-large amounts of fluid as sonolucent areas behind the bladder or uterus and between the liver and kidney. The computed tomogram can demonstrate small-to-large amounts of fluid as a homogeneous collection of water-radiodensity material within the peritoneal cavity. Sometimes tumor nodules can be detected within the ascitic fluid, indicating its cause.

Clinical

Clinical symptoms of ascitic fluid depend on its quantity, etiology, and location. Small amounts of transudate may be undetectable and asymptomatic. Small amounts of inflammatory fluid can cause pain. Large amounts of ascitic fluid can result in a complaint of fullness or swelling and can usually be detected on physical examination.

Inflammatory fluid in the greater peritoneal sac often results in pain, tenderness, rebound tenderness, and guarding. Inflammatory fluid in the pelvis can result in pain and tenderness, with no guarding. Inflammatory fluid in the lesser peritoneal sac can result in pain; tenderness may be limited or absent; guarding and rebound tenderness are usually absent.

The spread of fluid through the peritoneal cavity can result in symptoms and signs far removed from the site of origin. Tumors can spread through the peritoneal space to the pelvis or subhepatic space. Blood will collect in the pelvis and under the diaphragm, sometimes resulting in pain referred to the shoulder. Abscesses caused by a ruptured viscus may be manifest distant to the site of rupture. Understanding these pathways of spread can help in finding a hidden abscess or unsuspected metastasis.

The causes of ascites can be understood as manifestations of changes in the balance in Starling's law of fluid transport.

OBJECTIVES

When you complete this chapter you will be able to

1. Identify ascitic fluid on selected plain abdominal radiographs, sonograms, and CT images.
2. Explain the pathogenesis of the shoulder pain in a ruptured ectopic pregnancy.
3. Explain the process resulting in a Blumer's shelf or a Krukenberg tumor.
4. List the likely locations of abscess formation following appendicitis with rupture.

Many diseases occurring in the abdomen have associated abnormalities of the peritoneum. Guarding, or abdominal rigidity, from a perforated ulcer; ascites from liver failure; blood from a ruptured spleen or ectopic (tubal) pregnancy are but a few of these diseases. Imaging techniques are useful in detecting the presence of peritoneal fluid or metastases that have spread through the peritoneal cavities. Certain peritoneal abnormalities are best found on physical examination, others by aspiration from the peritoneal cavity; the imaging techniques can be most useful, however, in finding peritoneal abnormalities while they are still limited in extent.

Clinically, the peritoneum is best divided into three portions:

Greater sac

Lesser sac

Pelvic cavity

Physical examination is of most help in the greater peritoneal sac; guarding and rigidity of the abdominal musculature are important signs of peritoneal irritation. In the pelvis, physical examination and imaging share the task of evaluation. Because of its pathway of innervation, inflammatory processes in the pelvis result in little or no guarding or rigidity. Palpation is an important method for the finding and evaluation of pelvic masses.

The lesser sac is a relatively silent portion of the abdomen on physical examination; disease can be extensive and severe with only limited findings. When inflammation is isolated in the lesser sac, it does not result in rigidity; tenderness may be limited and may not fully indicate the severity of the patient's disease. Imaging techniques are most helpful in this region of the peritoneal cavity. Fortunately for patients, disease in the lesser sac is usually coexistent with disease in the greater sac, with the clinical signs of greater sac disease predominating.

Keynotes

- *A division of the peritoneal cavity into greater sac, lesser sac, and pelvis is clinically useful.*
- *Signs of inflammatory disease in the greater peritoneal sac include guarding, rebound tenderness, and muscular rigidity.*
- *Pelvic inflammation processes result in little or no guarding or rigidity.*
- *Lesser sac inflammatory disease can result in few objective signs of disease.*

IDENTIFICATION OF INTRAPERITONEAL FLUID

Intraperitoneal fluid, when it is moderate in amount, can be recognized by physical examination: as a fluid wave or a shifting dullness. Smaller amounts of fluid can be recognized on the standard radiograph, the sonogram, and the CT. Intraperitoneal abscesses often cannot be localized by physical examination. Standard radiography is seldom helpful, though an occasional abscess may show mottled air or an air-fluid level. Sonography, CT, and nuclear medicine imaging with gallium citrate Ga 67 each can be used to look for localized peritoneal abscesses. These techniques are often equally effective, but each has its drawbacks. Sonography and CT can demonstrate fluid collections, but in many cases, they cannot determine whether the fluid collection is infected. Gallium citrate Ga 67 can confirm the probable presence of infection but does not indicate whether there is a fluid collection present and drainable. In most cases, the sonography or CT demonstration of a fluid collection in a patient with a suspected abscess is sufficient diagnosis for treatment. Only when there are several fluid collections present does the use of gallium citrate Ga 67 become necessary.

Free fluid within the peritoneal cavity will gravitate to the most dependent portion. With the patient supine, the most dependent portion of the peritoneal cavity is the pelvis adjacent to the rectum (the pouch of Douglas in women, the retrovesical space in men). Fluid produced anywhere in the peritoneal cavity can appear as pelvic fluid or with symptoms related to pelvic fluid.

On the standard radiograph this fluid can be recognized because it displaces mesenteric fat away from the bladder (Fig. 32-1). The normal pelvis radiograph (Fig. 32-1a) shows the water-density bladder surrounded by more radiolucent fat. When fluid accumulates in the pelvis, the mesenteric fat (being lighter) floats away, leaving the bladder and fluid to fill the pelvis. This increased pelvic radiodensity can be confirmed as free fluid filling the pelvis, rather than contained fluid in a large bladder, by the identification of a thin layer of fat on the serosal surface of the bladder (Fig. 32-1b). In the presence of free fluid, the bladder, the line of serosal fat, and fluid around the bladder can each be recognized. This pattern can be simulated by fluid-filled bowel loops adjacent to the bladder (Fig. 32-2), though in this case, the serosal fat line is often wider because of the

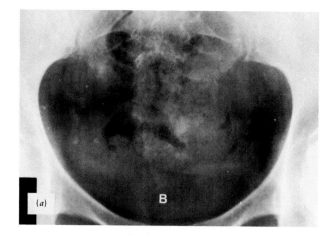

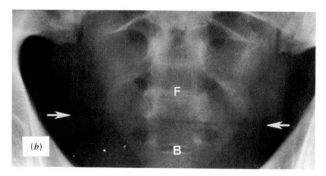

Figure 32-1. (*a*) Normal male pelvis. The fluid-filled bladder (B) can be seen with mixed radiolucency and radiodensity surrounding it. The fat margin of the bladder is not visible. (*b*) The male pelvis with ascites. There is fluid radiodensity (the ascites) (F) just superior to the bladder (B). A thin layer of bladder serosal fat (arrows) separates the two fluid collections. This patient had a ruptured spleen with peritoneal blood (Courtesy M. Toxopeus, M.D.)

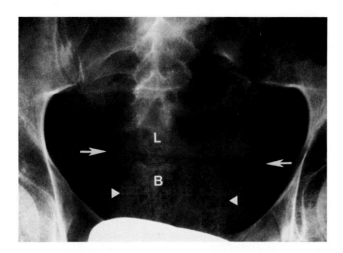

Figure 32-2. Fluid-filled bowel loops (L) lie superior to the bladder (B). The band of fat (arrows) separating the two fluid collections is thicker than seen with ascites because it represents a combination of bladder serosal fat and small bowel mesenteric fat. This patient had a partial small bowel obstruction. The mottled radiolucency superimposd on the bladder (arrowheads) is feces in the rectum.

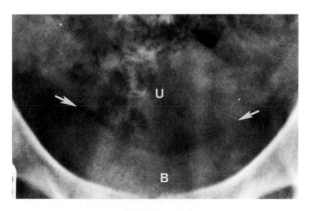

Figure 32-3. Normal female pelvis. The ovoid uterus (U) lies superior to the bladder (B), separated from it by a band of fat (arrows). The superior margin of the uterus is indistinct because mesenteric fat and bowel loops, rather than ascitic fluid, lie adjacent to it.

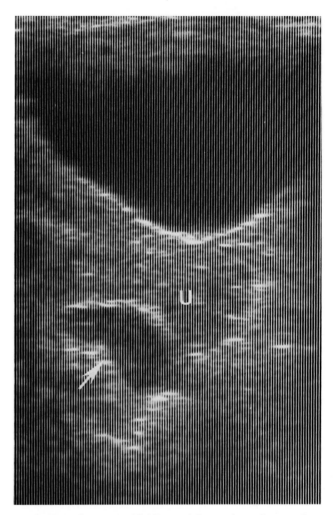

Figure 32-4. Sonogram of fluid in a cul-de-sac. A sonolucent collection of fluid (arrow) lies just posterior to the uterus (U). The patient has ascites. (Courtesy E. Blum, M.D.)

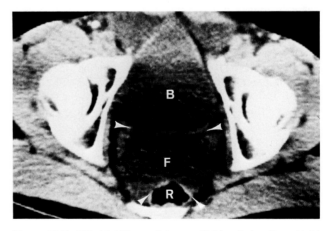

Figure 32-5. CT of fluid in a cul-de-sac. Fluid radiodensity material (F) lies between the bladder (B) and the rectum (R) in this male patient with lymphoma. The walls of the bladder and rectum are marked by arrowheads. (Courtesy N. Whitley, M.D., University of Maryland Hospital.)

presence of mesenteric fat in the margin of the fluid-filled loop of bowel.

In a woman, this sign of ascites is harder to identify because the uterus lies adjacent to the superior margin of the bladder and is separated from it by a thin layer of fat (Fig. 32-3). Fluid will displace the mesenteric fat around the uterus, but if the uterus is large, this may not be visible.

Free intraperitoneal fluid is identifiable on the sonogram as an echo-free region between the bladder and the rectum (Fig. 32-4). A small amount of fluid can be found in the pelvis of normal women by this technique.

Free fluid can be identified in the pelvis on CT as a homogeneous shadow lying behind the bladder and above the rectum (Fig. 32-5). It is often difficult to differentiate this fluid from a mass in the same location. When there is uncertainty of interpretation, the computed tomographic view can be repeated with the patient prone or on his or her side. Fluid will shift to a new site or disappear; masses shift less.

Keynotes

- *The physical examination techniques for detecting a fluid wave or shifting dullness are useful when large amounts of intraperitoneal fluid are present.*
- *The most dependent portion of the peritoneal cavitiy is in the pelvis.*
- *Ascitic fluid displaces the mesenteric fat from the dome of the bladder.*

Case 32-1

The radiograph in Figure 32-6*a* is that of a 28-year-old man. Figure 32-6*b* is a closeup of his pelvis. What do you see?

There are several findings. The urine in the bladder is separated from the remainder of the peritoneal cavity by a thin layer of fat, above which there is more water-density material. In addition, there is no bowel gas in the right upper quadrant of the abdomen. What do you think is going on?

The thin fat stripe surrounding the bladder indicates the presence of ascites. The bowel is displaced by a large liver. A slightly radiodense curved structure in the upper abdomen is the stomach filled with a slightly radiodense food (milk or antacid).

What might be causing this patient's ascites? Table 32-1 lists causes associated with both ascites and a large liver in italics and those associated only with ascites in roman type. As you can see, the causes of ascites are quite varied. This list is organized according to pathophysiology by following Starling's law of fluid transport, but a list by mechanisms of disease (as in Table 32-2) is also acceptable.

This patient had alcoholic liver disease.

SPREAD OF INTRAPERITONEAL FLUID

Case 32-2

KA is a 21-year-old woman who suddenly felt faint, lay down, and developed shoulder pain. She had missed a period, and her pregnancy test was positive. Figure 32-7 is a series of two sonographic views of her pelvis (Fig. 32-8 is a normal view of the same region). What do you see?

Figure 32-7*a* shows the uterus (white arrow) and a small sonolucent area in the cul de sac (black arrow). Although the patient's pregnancy test is positive, the thin line of the uterine cavity (faint open arrows) does not contain a pregnancy. Figure 32-7*b* demonstrates a gestational sac (arrow) with a small fetal pole lying behind the bladder but not within the uterus. Figure

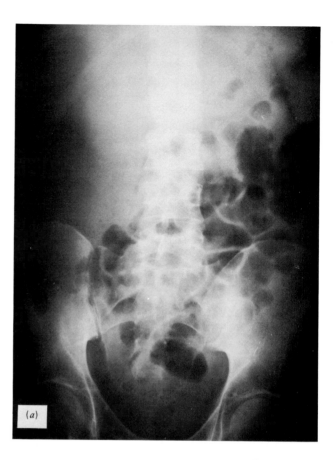

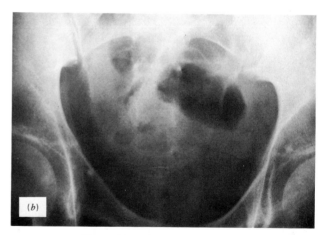

Figure 32-6. Case example 32-1.

32-8 demonstrates a normal pregnancy at a similar gestational age. (Chapter 47 describes in greater detail the sonographic appearance of a normal pregnancy.)

What do you think is going on?

Despite the history of a missed period and the positive pregnancy test, the uterus shows no fetus. The sonolucent region in the cul de sac is ascites.

The diagnosis is a ruptured ectopic (tubal) pregnancy. Why did the patient develop shoulder pain?

TABLE 32-1. CAUSES OF ASCITES

Hydrostatic Pressure	Decreased Colloid (Oncotic) Pressure	Changes in Capillary Permeability	Extravasation
Congestive heart failure	*Liver failure*	Peritonitis	From gut
Hepatic vein obstruction	Starvation	*Metastatic disease*	From vessels
Inferior vena cava obstruction	Catabolic states	Pancreatitis	Arteries
Constrictive pericarditis	Wide-spread cancer	Connective tissue disease	Veins
	Renal failure	Ischemia	Lymphatics
	Protein loss		
	Protein-losing enteropathies		
	Lymphatic fistula		
	Malabsorption from gut		

TABLE 32-2. CAUSES OF ASCITES

Congenital	Infectious	Neoplastic	Traumatic	Metabolic	Allergic	Vascular Extravasation
Erythroblastosis fetalis	Peritonitis	*Metastatic disease*	Ruptured spleen	*Alcoholic liver disease*	Connective tissue diseases	From vessels
Intestinal lymphagiectasia	Tuberculous	*Rupture of hepatic adenoma*		Starvation		Arteries
	Nontuberculous			Hypothyroidism		Veins
	Hepatitis			Renal failure		Lymphatics

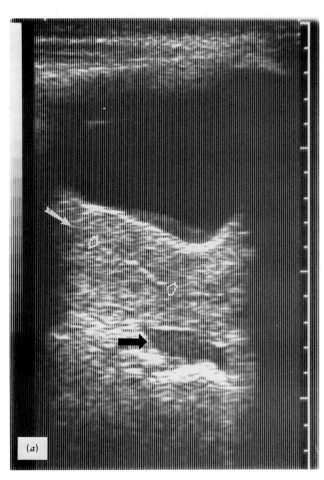
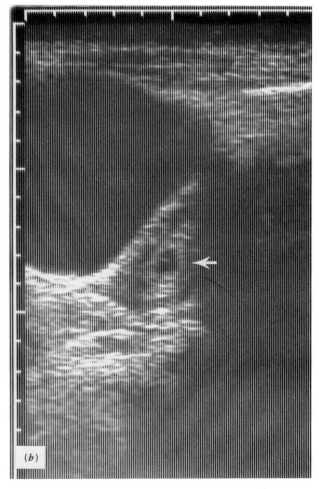

Figure 32-7. Case example 32-2.

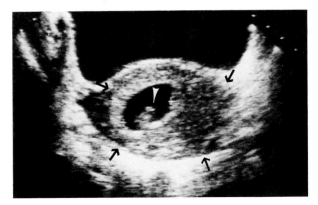

Figure 32-8. Normal early intrauterine pregnancy, sonographic appearance. The uterus (arrows) contains a small gestational sac containing a small fetus (called a fetal pole) (arrowhead). (Courtesy E. Blum, M.D.)

When fluid overflows the confines of the pelvis, it runs up the lateral abdominal gutters until it reaches the subhepatic space on the right and the subdiaphragmatic space on the left. Blood can then irritate the left hemidiaphragm and cause pain that is then referred in the distribution of the cervical root from which the phrenic nerve comes.

Keynote

- *Though the signs are not always present, the classic history of a patient with a ruptured ectopic pregnancy is that she felt severe pelvic pain, felt faint, lay down or fainted, and felt pain in her left shoulder. A menstrual period may or may not have been missed; the pregnancy test may be positive or negative but is frequently positive if a radioimmunoassay is used.*

Case 32-3

The transperitoneal spread of fluid processes in the abdomen and the movement of fluid from one portion of the abdomen to another is an important manner of spread of infections and tumors within the peritoneal cavity. Figure 32-9 is the ^{67}Ga scan of a 19-year-old patient who felt nauseated, with periumbilical pain. The pain eventually shifted to the right lower quadrant of the abdomen. He continued to feel ill, with a low-grade fever, and only after a week of home treatment in bed did he seek medical attention. What does his ^{67}Ga scan show?

There is activity below the right lobe of the liver. With his clinical history this is probably a

Subhepatic abscess caused by . . . ?

A ruptured appendix.

Fluid processes starting anywhere within the abdomen will initially flow into the pelvis, manifesting pelvic symptoms and findings. With more fluid, the processes will collect in the subhepatic and subdiaphragmatic spaces. How many syndromes can you relate to these pathways of fluid

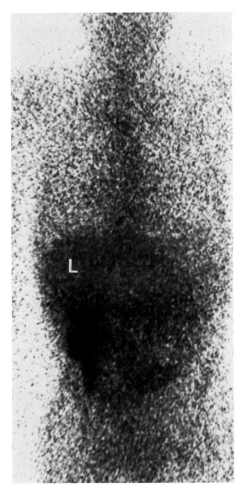

Figure 32-9. Case example 32-3. (Courtesy M. Vaccaro, M.D.)

spread? Your list should include infectious, chemical, neoplastic, and hemorrhagic processes. Compare your list to this one:

Fluid to the Pelvis

Neoplastic

Krukenberg tumor: A Krukenberg tumor is a metastasis from gastric cancer to one or both ovaries; detected as an ovarian mass. How did it get there? By transperitoneal spread.

Blumer's shelf: A Blumer's shelf is a hard tumor mass in the retrovesical space, palpable on rectal exam anterior to the rectum. The tumor may arise in the stomach or pancreas.

Infectious

Appendiceal abscess: A ruptured appendix will have a local abscess, but often a pelvic abscess or a subhepatic abscess will also be present.

Chemical

Passage of gastric or pancreatic juice into the pelvis. The patient with a ruptured gastric or duodenal ulcer or with pancreatitis can have symptoms in the right lower quadrant of the abdomen or in the pelvis as a result of the passage of inflammatory fluid down the right gutter to the pelvis. The right-lower-quadrant pain and tenderness can simulate appendicitis. Tenderness can be elicited on rectal examination.

Fluid to the Subhepatic or Subdiaphragmatic Space

Infectious

Fitz-Hugh and Curtis syndrome: A woman with gonococcal pelvic inflammatory disease may also have right-upper-quadrant pain and tenderness simulating mild hepatitis. In some patients, this is the main symptom. This is due to spread of the gonococcal infection from the pelvis to surround the liver, causing perihepatitis.

Neoplastic

Ovarian cancer sometimes spreads from the pelvis to the perihepatic space, with metastases lodging on the surface of the liver or, less commonly, with metastases encasing the liver. Because these metastases are not infiltrating the liver tissue, the enzyme test for metastases to liver (the alkaline phosphatase test) will be normal, and the common imaging test for hepatic metastases (the nuclear medicine imaging liver scan) will be normal. A sonogram or computed tomography will sometimes, but not always, demonstrate these metastases.

Blood

Blood from anywhere in the peritoneal cavity will usually collect in the pelvis. In a woman, a simple procedure, the *culdocentesis* (needle aspiration through the posterior fornix of the vaginia), will easily demonstrate the presence of blood. In a bleeding (ruptured) ectopic (tubal) pregnancy, the blood will ascend to the diaphragm, and the patient may have shoulder pain from diaphragmatic irritation.

Understanding the pathways of fluid spread makes the analysis of confusing clinical findings and the memorization of bizarre-sounding syndromes easier.

Keynote

• *Fluid processes starting anywhere within the abdominal cavity will usually flow initially into the pelvis and then into the subhepatic or subphrenic space. In some patients, the pelvic brim functions as a continental divide, directing the flow of fluid above it into the subhepatic and subphrenic spaces and the flow below it into the pelvis.*

LARGE AMOUNTS OF FLUID

Figure 32-10*a* is the abdominal radiograph of a 47-year-old woman. Figure 32-10*b* is the abdominal radiograph of an infant. What do you see?

The films have a gray cast to them, and all the bowel loops appear to be centrally located within the abdomen. This is the appearance of marked ascites. The bowel loops are central because, in a patient with marked ascites, the abdomen is football shaped. The bowel loops containing air float to the top of the abdominal cavity, and because of the football-like shape, the top on a film taken supine is also the center. The fixation of the mesentery to the central portion of the posterior abdominal wall also causes floating bowel loops to be central.

Figure 32-11*a* is the computed tomographic scan of a patient with marked ascites. The central location of the bowel loops, their flotation, and their attachment to the mesentery are all demonstrated, helping to explain the appearance of ascites on the plain abdominal film. Marked ascites can also be demonstrated as a fluid collection between the liver and the abdominal wall. This can be seen with ultrasonography and CT (Fig. 32-11*b*).

Figure 32-12 demonstrates the sonographic appearance of moderate and marked ascites. In Figure 32-12*a*, the ascitic fluid lies in the pouch of Douglas, posterior to the uterus. In Figure 32-12*b*, ascitic fluid appears as a thin sonolucent separation between the inferior portion of the liver and the right kidney. In Figure 32-12*c*, marked ascites results in a wider echo-free space between the liver and kidney.

In general, radiographs are not needed for the diagnosis of large amounts of ascites. They are easily recognizable on physical examination by testing for shifting dullness or a fluid wave.

Keynote

• *The bowel loops float to the central portion of the abdomen, both because this is the highest portion and because of their central mesenteric attachment.*

SMALL AMOUNTS OF FLUID

How would you attempt to find small amounts of peritoneal fluid? What would you do if you were looking for small amounts of blood, evidence of peritoneal infection, or fluid that might contain neoplastic cells?

For small amounts of blood in women, culdocentesis is the procedure. In men or women, peritoneal lavage or a four-quadrant tap is sufficient. With peritoneal lavage, 500 cc of normal saline is run through a catheter into the peritoneal cavity and then aspirated. Bloody fluid indicates blood in the peritoneal cavity. The *four-quadrant tap* is needle aspiration from each quadrant of the abdomen, done lateral to the rectus abdominis muscle. Nonclotting blood obtained in any quadrant is indicative of intraperitoneal bleeding.

Small amounts of pus or other ascites are probably best found by sonographic evaluation. Sonography can occasionally detect as little as 15 cc of intraperitoneal fluid. Several hundred cubic centimeters of fluid must be pres-

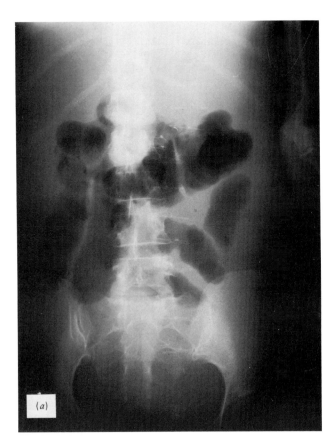

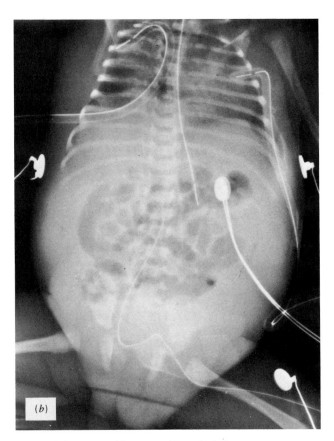

Figure 32-10. Radiographic appearance of marked ascites. (*a*) A 47-year-old woman with metastatic ovarian carcinoma. The abdomen has a gray cast to it, and the bowel loops are central. (*b*) A 1-week-old infant with posterior uretral valves and bladder rupture. There is a gray cast to the bladder, and the bowel loops are central, signs of marked ascites. Many tubes are present in this sick infant. (Courtesy M. Vaccaro, M.D.)

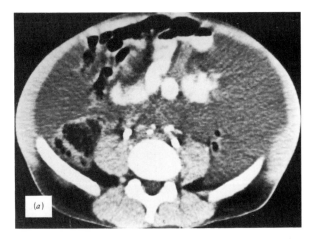

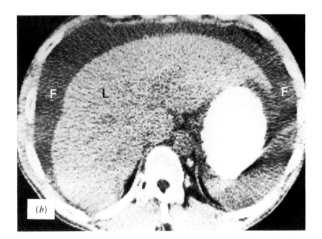

Figure 32-11. CT appearance of marked ascites. (*a*) Midabdominal CT. Most of the air- and contrast-filled bowel loops are in the mid and upper portion of this section, pulled there by the buoyancy of the air within them relative to the ascitic fluid surrounding them. (*b*) Upper abdominal CT in this same patient (also shown in Fig. 32-5). Fluid (F) surrounds the liver (L) and the contrast-filled stomach. This man had widespread lymphoma. (Courtesy of N. Whitley, M.D., University of Maryland Hospital.)

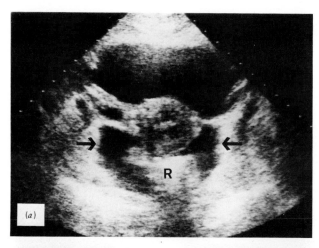

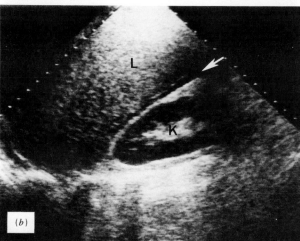

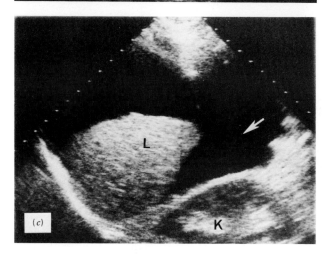

Figure 32-12. Sonographic appearance of moderate and marked ascites. (a) This transverse sonographic image of the pelvis demonstrates the sonolucent ascitic fluid (arrows) in the pouch of Douglas, posterior and lateral to the uterus. The echogenic (white) area behind the uterus with poor through transmission of sound and shadowing is the rectum (R). (b) The thin sonolucent band (arrow) between the liver (L) and the kidney (K) represents fluid in the hepatorenal fossa (Morison's pouch). (c) The large sonolucent area (arrow) between the liver (L) and kidney (K) is due to marked ascites. (All courtesy E. Blum, M.D.)

ent within the abdomen before it can be detected on the radiograph.

Keynotes

- *Culdocentesis, the needle aspiration of the peritoneal cavity through the posterior fornix of the vagina, is a sensitive method of detecting intraperitoneal blood.*
- *Peritoneal lavage and the four-quadrant abdominal tap are sensitive methods of detecting free intraperitoneal blood.*

SUMMARY

Diseases affecting the peritoneum are common and are usually manifest by abdominal guarding, rebound tenderness, rigidity, or the presence of free intraperitoneal fluid. The first three signs are evaluated by physical examination. Although large amounts of peritoneal fluid can be detected by physical examination, small amounts are best detected by the imaging techniques.

Free intraperitoneal fluid can be detected by sonography, radiography, and CT. When the fluid is infected, or infected and localized in an abscess, scanning with gallium citrate Ga 67 may identify the site of infection. Small amounts of blood are usually best detected by culdocentesis (in women), a four-quadrant needle aspiration of the abdomen, or peritoneal lavage.

Because of the pathways by which fluid spreads through the abdominal cavity, disease in or adjacent to the peritoneum may be manifested in symptoms or signs distal to the initial locus of the disease. It is common for diseases that originate anywhere within the peritoneal cavity to spread to the retrovesical space, pouch of Douglas, or subhepatic or subphrenic spaces.

REVIEW QUESTIONS

1. What are the symptoms of a ruptured ectopic pregnancy? What tests can be done to confirm the diagnosis when it is clinically suspected?
2. What are the symptoms of a lesser sac abscess? Of a greater sac abscess? Of a pelvic abscess?
3. What are the physical examination findings of ascites?
4. What is the most dependent portion of the peritoneal cavity when a person is supine? What is the second most dependent portion?
5. What are the radiographic findings in ascites? The sonographic findings? The transmission computed tomographic findings?
6. List the major causes of ascites.
7. Give five examples of the clinical syndromes, symptoms, or signs resulting from the transperitoneal spread of disease.
8. If you clinically suspect that a patient may have blood in his or her peritoneal cavity, how would you confirm its presence?

VOCABULARY

Blumer's shelf

culdocentesis

Fitz-Hugh and Curtis syndrome

fluid wave

greater peritoneal sac

Krukenberg tumor

lesser peritoneal sac

Morison's pouch

pouch of Douglas

ruptured ectopic (tubal) pregnancy

shifting dullness

SUGGESTIONS FOR FURTHER READING

Mark E. Baker, Russell Alan Blinder, Reed P. Rice. Diagnostic imaging of abdominal fluid collections and abscesses. *CRC Critical Reviews in Diagnostic Imaging*, **25**:232–278, 1986.

Robert A. Halvorsen et al. Ascites or pleural effusion? CT differentiation: Four useful criteria. *RadioGraphics*, **6**:135–149, 1986.

For additional suggested reading see Chapter 26.

33

DISEASES WITH BOWEL DISTENSION

KEY CONCEPTS

Radiological

The patterns seen in the bowel on imaging studies can be classified into four different categories: normal bowel pattern, aerophagia (air swallowing), obstruction, and adynamic ileus. The classification depends on determining which bowel loops have air, fluid, or fecal contents and which are distended. The normal pattern consists of air and feces in the colon and perhaps minimal air in the small bowel, but without distension.

With *aerophagia,* more bowel air is seen, both in the small and large bowel; distension is not present, however.

Obstruction can be recognized because there will be distended bowel proximal to some point or points in the bowel, with a lack of distension distal to that point or points.

Adynamic ileus is the distension of nonpropulsive bowel. With a total adynamic ileus, both the colon and small bowel are dilated.

Bowel abnormalities with distension can be detected by conventional radiography and CT. When plain radiography is used, a combination of supine and upright radiographs is desirable at the time of initial evaluation.

Clinical

Aerophagia is a common cause of abnormal radiographs and patient symptoms. It can result in complaints of left-upper-quadrant abdominal pain, distension, belching, passing of flatus, and noisy bowel sounds.

Bowel obstruction can result in constipation, diarrhea, intermittent abdominal pain, and abdominal distension. The common causes of bowel obstruction are adhesions from previous surgery or pelvic infection, metastatic carcinoma, and hernias.

Adynamic ileus results in complaints of abdominal distension. The causes of the adynamic ileus may result in additional symptoms, such as fever or abdominal pain. The common causes include recent abdominal surgery, infection in the abdomen or retroperitoneum, retroperitoneal hemorrhage, and metabolic disturbances.

OBJECTIVES

When you complete this chapter you will be able to

1. Describe the radiographic and CT findings in aerophagia, obstruction, and adynamic ileus.
2. Correctly diagnose selected radiographic and CT examples of aerophagia, obstruction, and adynamic ileus.
3. Correctly classify selected loops of bowel on radiographs, indicating the region of bowel shown and whether or not it is distended.
4. List four symptoms resulting from aerophagia.
5. List four symptoms and the three main causes of small bowel obstruction.
6. List two main symptoms and four causes of a total adynamic ileus.

The interpretation of radiographs of the abdomen taken supine and upright is the main method of evaluating the significance of air collections within the bowel. Air within the bowel can be normal, the result of excess air swallowing (aerophagia), associated with bowel obstruction, or secondary to conditions that limit the motor activity of bowel.

BASIC PATTERNS OF BOWEL

Normal Bowel

The normal patient has minimal-to-moderate air within the colon, often with identifiable feces. Air may be seen in

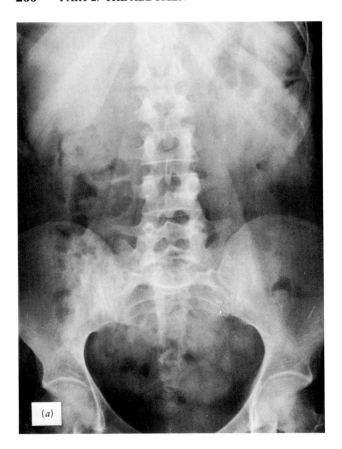

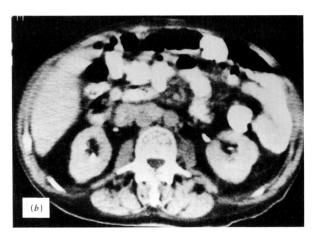

Figure 33-1. (*a*) Abdominal radiograph with normal bowel pattern. (*b*) Abdominal CT with normal bowel pattern. Multiple loops of bowel contain air and swallowed contrast medium. (There is minimal retroperitoneal adenopathy near the vena cava.)

one or two small bowel loops in transit to the colon. The bowel should not be distended (Figure 33-1).

Aerophagia

The patient with aerophagia will be swallowing excess air; more air will therefore be present within the bowel. Many small bowel loops will be identifiable because of the air within them. The colon will contain a moderate amount of air. Distension of bowel is usually absent. In the patient with marked aerophagia, minimal distension of the small bowel may be seen; often there is distension of the splenic flexure of the colon (Fig. 33-2).

Obstruction

The hallmark of bowel obstruction is the presence of distension of the bowel proximal to the obstruction (Fig. 33-3). The amount of air present is variable, and air will occasionally be absent, making recognition of the bowel distension difficult and occasionally impossible.

Adynamic Ileus

The patient with total adynamic ileus (also known as *paralytic ileus* and nonpropulsive ileus) has distension of all the bowel (small bowel and colon) (Figs. 33-4 and 33-5).

Keynotes

- *Normal bowel has a minimal-to-moderate amount of air in the colon, often with identifiable feces. Air may be seen in one or two small bowel loops.*

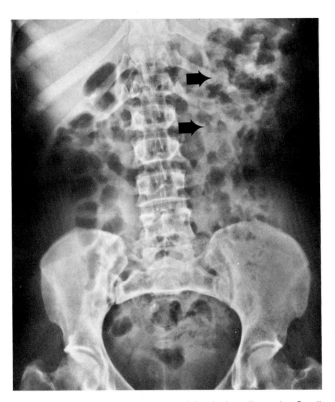

Figure 33-2. Aerophagia, supine abdominal radiograph. Small amounts of air are scattered through the small bowel and colon. The bowel loops are not distended. The arrows mark the appearance of minimal air in the jejunum: note the mottled, irregular pattern.

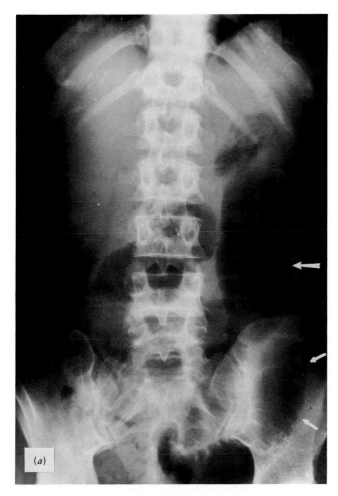 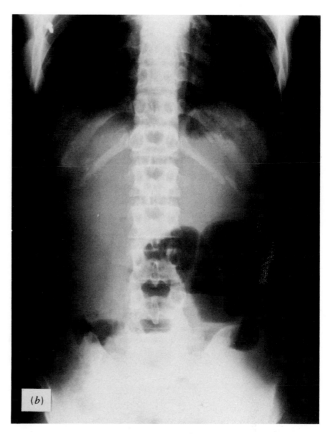

Figure 33-3. Small bowel obstruction. (*a*) Supine view. The air-containing bowel loops are preponderantly jejunum. The small arrows mark a moderately distended loop in which the valvulae conniventes are thinned, stretched and partially effaced; the large arrow marks a markedly distended loop of jejunum in which the valvulae conniventes are effaced. (*b*) Upright view. There are multiple air-fluid levels in the compactly coiled small bowel loops.

- *When the patient is swallowing excessive air, more air will be seen in the bowel, but without distension.*
- *Obstructed bowel shows distension proximal to the level of the obstruction.*
- *Adynamic bowel is dilated.*

KEY TO INTERPRETATION

The key to whether the bowel is abnormal and the type of abnormality is the deciphering of what each bowel loop seen on the radiograph is and whether it is distended. Three main criteria are used in this determination: location, shape, and size.

Location. The jejunum is in the left upper quadrant of the abdomen, the ileum in the right lower quadrant. Most of the colon is at the periphery of the abdominal cavity. Location can guide you when the internal markings of bowel are indistinct.

Shape and size. The shape of the bowel differs in the jejunum, ileum, and colon, and it changes with different degrees of distension. There are multiple patterns to be learned, but in part, they can be remembered by a simple analogy. Consider a circus balloon, one of the long, narrow ones with many curved indentations. Unfilled by air, it is difficult to determine its shape. With minimal filling, the curved shape becomes identifiable. As the balloon is more and more distended, the indentations become flatter and flatter. With marked distension, the balloon becomes a hollow cylinder, and with more distension, it bursts. Bowel is similar: unfilled, its shape and mucosal pattern may be difficult to evaluate; with a little filling, its morphology becomes distinct; the more distended it becomes, the less indented the mucosal markings become; with marked distension, it becomes a hollow cylinder; with more distension, it too will burst. Because of the change of shape seen with progressive distension (increase in size), it is necessary to learn several appearances for each type of bowel. Once

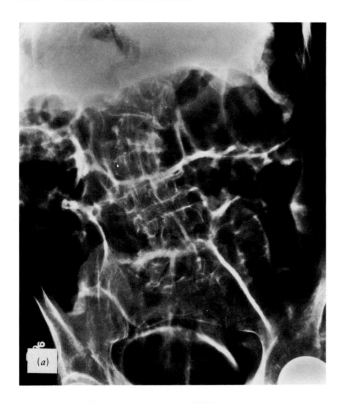

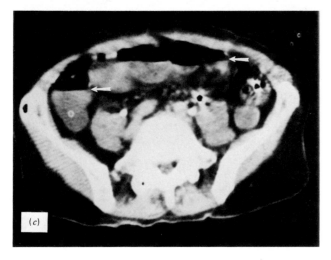

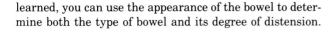

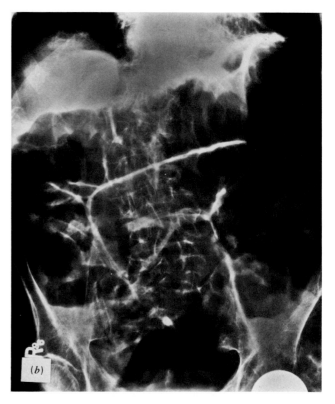

Figure 33-4. Adynamic ileus associated with pneumonia. (a) Supine view. (b) Upright view. Marked distension of the colon is present. Superimposed on the colonic loops, several dilated loops of jejunum can be seen in the left midabdomen. Air-fluid levels are seen in this view. (c) Abdominal CT view. A large amount of fluid is seen in the bowel loops (arrows), with long air-fluid levels.

learned, you can use the appearance of the bowel to determine both the type of bowel and its degree of distension.

Duodenum

The duodenum is rarely seen dilated on the plain film of the abdomen, and its appearance with distension need not be discussed.

Jejunum

The jejunum is the uppermost portion of the small bowel, which is on a mesentery. It is approximately 8 ft long. Its

muscular wall may show circular indentations representing peristaltic contractions, but its major morphological feature is its mucosal shape, which is called by two names: the *plicae circulares* or the *valvulae conniventes*.

When the bowel is unfilled, its mucosal pattern is usually invisible. This is because there is usually no air within the small bowel lumen to outline the mucosa. In the occasional patient in whom a small amount of air permits visualization of the collapsed jejunum, the mucosa has a complex pattern, with plica oriented in a seemingly random pattern (see Fig. 33-2, the left upper quadrant of the abdomen).

With minimal distension, the valvulae appear as a series of parallel lines or as a closely spaced spiral (Fig. 33-

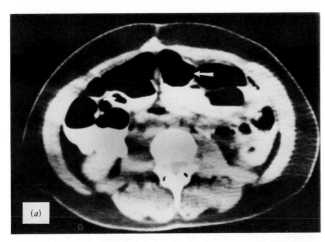 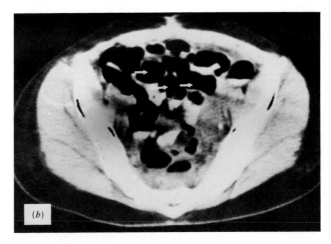

Figure 33-5. Adynamic ileus on CT. (*a*) Midabdominal view. (*b*) Midpelvic section. Multiple loops of both large bowel (large arrow on *a*) and small bowel (small arrows on *b*) contain air, some with air-fluid levels. Although CT is not used to establish the presence or severity of an adynamic ileus, it is frequently used to search for an abscess in a patient with a prolonged adynamic ileus after abdominal surgery.

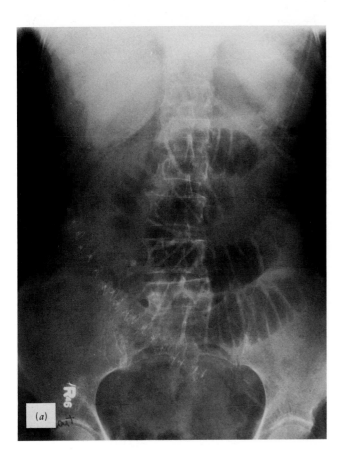

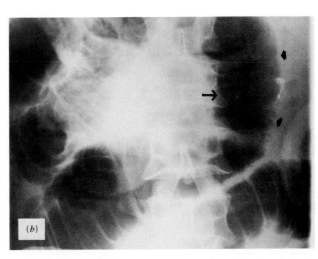

Figure 33-6. Patterns of jejunal distension. (*a*) Small bowel obstruction. The loops of bowel in the midabdomen are jejunal loops, minimally distended. The valvulae conniventes stretched and crossing the lumen appear as parallel lines. (*b*) Moderate distension of the jejunum in a patient with a postoperative adynamic ileus. The valvulae in the left upper loop (long arrow) are effaced, showing only minimal indentation (short arrows) into the lumen. Other loops, less distended, appear with valvulae crossing the lumen.

6*a*). The normal valvulae are less than 1 mm thick and, in the upper jejunum, lie several millimeters apart. Increasing distension stretches the valvulae so that they protrude less and less into the lumen of the bowel (Fig. 33-6*b*). As they project less and less into the lumen, they cast less and less of a roentgen shadow.

Geometrically, the valvulae at the edge of the lumen intersect more of the x-ray photons than those projected over the center of the lumen, and thus they tend to be more visible. With moderate distension, it is often possible to identify the valvulae only along the edge of the bowel, not near its center. With marked distension, even these peripherally projected valvulae become so flattened that they are indistinct and the tube appears to be without markings (Fig. 33-3).

This discussion purposely avoids size measurements in evaluating degree of distension. It is preferable to use internal markers that reflect the disease, rather than measurements that must vary with the size and build of the patient.

Distal Jejunum. Valvulae conniventes are most closely spaced in the upper jejunum. They become progressively less closely spaced in the more distal jejunum.

Ileum

The ileum, like the jejunum, normally contains little or no air and thus, when relaxed, usually cannot be seen. When there is minimal air in the ileum, it resembles a string of small sausages of unequal lengths (Fig. 33-7a). Scattered among the loops, an occasional valvula connivens can be seen. The ileal valvulae conniventes usually extend only part way across the lumen and are spaced widely apart.

With minimal distension of the ileum, the sausage shape begins to disappear and the ileum resembles a cylinder, except where it is folded upon itself. Its valvulae conniventes are widely spaced and scattered. With moderate distension, the valvulae conniventes become indistinct and then disappear, and the ileum looks like an unindented cylinder (Fig. 33-7b). With sufficient distension, jejunum and ileum appear the same.

Colon

Normal Colon. The morphology of the colon differs from the small bowel in several ways (Fig. 33-8). First, its normal diameter is greater, usually measuring more than 4 cm. Second, its indentations, the *haustral folds,* consist of the tissues of the entire colonic wall. This makes the folds thicker than the mucosal folds of the small bowel. Third, a sacculated appearance results from the relative shortness of the three longitudinal muscles, the *teniae coli,* compared with the length of the colonic wall. It is these three anatomic features that permit the identification of the colon on the radiograph.

Differentiation of Haustral Folds from Valvulae Conniventes. Some observers have difficulty differentiating haustral folds from valvulae conniventes. There are two main features that usually permit their differentiation. First, colonic folds are thicker than valvulae conniventes, and second, at the normal 4- to 5-cm diameter of the colonic lumen, the small bowel would be moderately distended, effacing the mucosal valvulae conniventes.

Recognition of Colonic Distension. Recognition of colonic distension is often difficult. The diameter of the colon differs in different people and in the different portions of the colon. The cecum and the rectum are often the most dilated

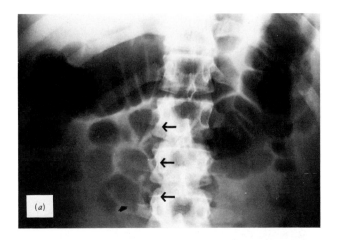

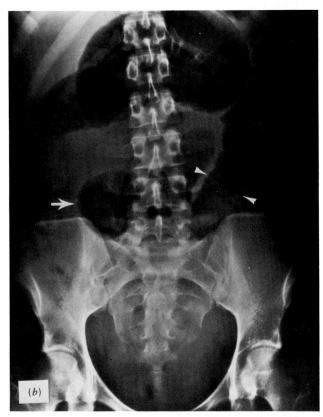

Figure 33-7. (*a*) Ileal loops (long arrows), normal-to-minimally distended, are short sausage- or cuboidal-shaped air collections. A short arrow marks the one valvula that can be identified. The transverse colon (top) is minimally distended with regular haustral folds. This patient has minimal findings of an early adynamic ileus caused by splenic rupture. (*b*) A markedly distended ileal loop (arrow) is present in the right lower quadrant. The remaining bowel loops are jejunum. The folds are effaced in the upper jejunal loop and minimally indent the vertical jejunal loop (arrowheads) in the left midabdomen.

portions of the bowel, and when there is colonic distension, these portions often dilate disproportionately.

In nondistended colon, the haustral folds are usually irregularly spaced, and the haustral sacculations are eas-

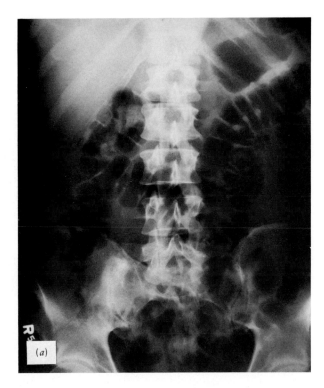

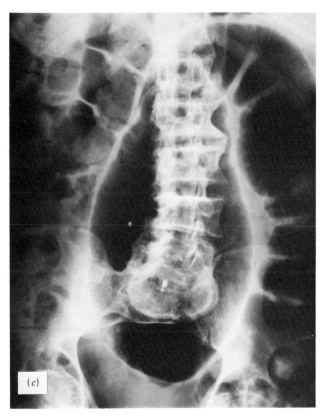

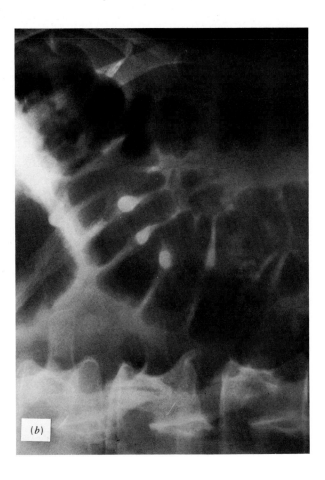

Figure 33-8. (*a*) Radiograph of a normal abdomen with air and feces in the colon. Normal haustral folds are seen, many of which have a rounded tip. The haustral sacculations (or outpouchings) can be seen in some loops. (*b*) Focal view of the normal colonic haustral folds. (*c*) Moderately and markedly distended loops of colon. The sigmoid colon, in the middle, is markedly distended; no haustral folds can be seen. The remainder of the colon is moderately distended. The walls of the colon are parallel, and haustral sacculations (outpouchings) are not seen.

ily seen (Fig. 33-8). With moderate distension, the haustral folds tend to become more regularly spaced, and the sacculations become shallower (Fig. 33-7*a*). With marked distension, the haustral folds become flattened and almost effaced (Fig. 33-8*c*). When the colon exceeds 13 cm, it is likely to burst.

Keynotes

- *The evaluation of bowel depends on its location, shape, and size.*
- *The markings of bowel indent the bowel less with increasing distension.*
- *The plicae circulares, also called valvulae conniventes, are the mucosal indentations of small bowel.*
- *The luminal indentations in the colon are the haustral folds.*
- *Thirteen is an unlucky number: when the colon has dilated 13 cm, it is likely to burst.*

PATTERN DIFFERENTIATION ON THE PLAIN RADIOGRAPH

Once you can tell what loop you are looking at and how distended it is, you can start to assemble the information into a diagnosis. When only a few loops are filled with air, each should be categorized. When there are many, some sampling is necessary to save time. Looking for jejunal and ileal loops and sampling portions of the right, transverse, descending, and sigmoid colon is sufficient most of the time; but if you sample, you should look for the loops most likely to be distended, rather than those that are likely to be normal.

PATTERNS OF DISEASE

Normal Bowel

The normal person has minimal-to-moderate air within the colon, often with identifiable feces. Air may be seen in one or two small bowel loops in transit to the colon. The bowel should not be distended.

Aerophagia

Aerophagia is a common condition in which patients swallow excessive air, which can be identified within the bowel both on physical examination and on radiographs. The abdominal radiograph in a patient with aerophagia will demonstrate many loops of small bowel with air within them. The colon will contain a moderate amount of air. Distension of the bowel is usually absent, but minimal distension can be present with marked aerophagia. Some patients with aerophagia have distension of the splenic flexure of the colon.

Case 33-1

This 34-year-old woman was quite anxious during an intravenous urogram. The initial film and radiograph obtained 15 minutes after the start of the intravenous urogram are shown in Figure 33-9. What do you see?

On the first study, there is some air in the colon, mainly in the cecum and sigmoid colon. On the second film, there is much more air within the bowel, mainly in the central portion of the abdomen. These loops of bowel show no specific mucosal detail, but loops of air-containing bowel found in the midabdomen are usually loops of small bowel. The collecting system of the kidney is also seen on the second film and is normal.

This patient had active aerophagia during the study. Aerophagia occurring acutely is often the result of anxiety. It is common to find increased air within the bowel of many patients seeking emergency care, resulting from the patient's anxiety. It is important not to confuse this air resulting from anxiety with air accumulating from bowel obstruction or adynamic bowel. The major differentiating sign is the lack of more than a minimal amount of bowel distension.

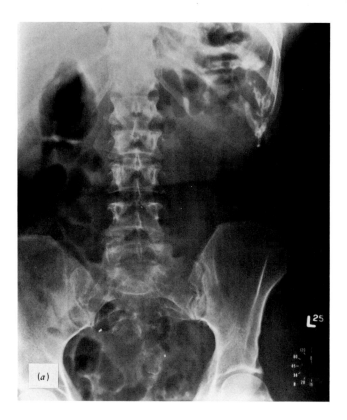

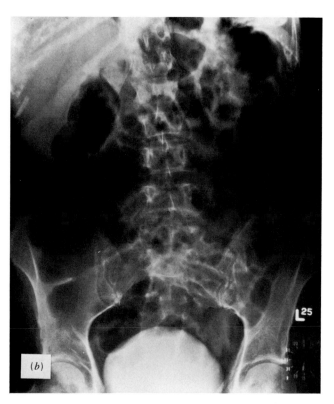

Figure 33-9. Case 33-1. Two films from an intravenous urogram. (a) Preinjection scout film. (b) 15 minutes into the study.

What kind of symptoms would a patient with chronic intermittent aerophagia complain of? Patients with aerophagia often have symptoms of

Bloating.

Belching.

Passage of flatus per rectum.

Audible bowel sounds.

Crampy abdominal pain, often relieved by passage of flatus.

The splenic flexure syndrome: pain in lower left part of the chest, sometimes referred to the left shoulder. The pain is often misinterpreted by the patient as being angina pectoris, and this fear of cardiac pain often makes the aerophagia and its symptoms worse. Some patients give a characteristic history of recurrent bouts of angina relieved by the passage of flatus.

The symptoms of aerophagia are common, and primary care practitioners frequently hear complaints related to it. What would you do for a patient who complains of bloating, audible bowel sounds, or other symptoms of aerophagia? Make a list and compare it to the one that follows. Bowel gas is increased by

Increased swallowing of air

Decreased expulsion of air

Increased fermentation within the bowel

Uncertain cause related to specific foods

broken down more specifically as follows:

Increased swallowing of air, from
  Loose dentures
  Chewing with mouth open
  Talking while chewing
  Eating foods that trap air, for example, salads
  Drinking carbonated beverages
  Chewing gum or tobacco
  Swallowing saliva (control with a mild atropinic drug, only if necessary)
  Saliva from mouth breathing (check for nasal obstruction)
Decreased expulsion of air, from
  Increased colonic transit time (treat with increase in dietary bulk, increase in exercise)
Increased fermentation within the bowel, from
  Nondigestible dissacharides
  Beans
  Peas
  Lactase deficiency with lactose breakdown in the colon
  Slowed bowel transit time
  Partial small bowel obstruction
  Nontropical sprue
  Scleroderma

Other foods related to increased gas:
  Cabbage
  Onions (in some people)

Some patients with aerophagia can be helped by remembering to empty the mouth of air before swallowing saliva. A useful technique for reminding them is to have them keep an object (pencil, pipe, etc.) between their teeth. It is difficult to swallow with the teeth separated, and removing the pipe or pencil can remind the person to empty the mouth of air.

Keynotes

• *Aerophagia often results from anxiety.*

• *The splenic flexure syndrome results from air distending the flexure of the colon. The patient often mistakes chest pain on the lower left side, referred to the left shoulder, for cardiac angina.*

Obstruction

The hallmark of bowel obstruction is the presence of distension of the bowel proximal to an obstruction and nondistension of the bowel distal to the obstruction. Large amounts of fluid are usually present proximal to the obstruction. The amount of air present is variable, and air will occasionally be absent. When air is limited or absent, recognition of the bowel distension is difficult and occasionally impossible. An airless abdomen is worrisome and cannot be considered normal. Airlessness is a nonspecific finding in that it does not indicate which abnormality is present but only that the abdomen is probably diseased.

Several variants of bowel obstruction can be seen. In some patients the bowel distal to the obstruction has been emptied by the increased peristalsis induced by the obstruction. Usually some air persists distal to the obstruction. This air (usually limited to the colon) may persist because the increased peristalsis may be insufficient to empty it. Air may also be seen distal to the obstruction early in its course or because the obstruction is partial.

Case 33-2

PD is a 46-year-old woman with 2 days of intermittent crampy abdominal pain, nausea, and vomiting. Seven years previously, she had a hysterectomy for menometrorrhagia. She has otherwise been healthy. Physical examination reveals peristalsis, which can be seen through the abdominal wall; a healed lower abdominal incision; and easily audible bowel sounds. No tenderness is elicited. The radiographs are obtained (Fig. 33-10). What do you see?

There are multiple loops of distended bowel in the midabdomen. Markings along the margins of some of these loops are indicative of partial effacement of the plicae circulares and due to moderate distension of the small bowel. The upright film demonstrates multiple air fluid levels. What do you think is going on?

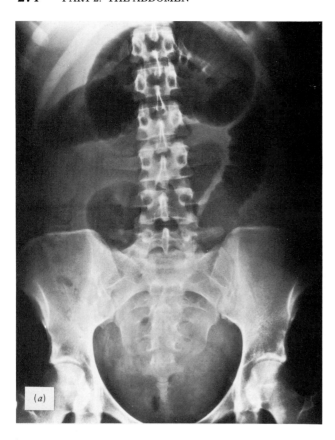

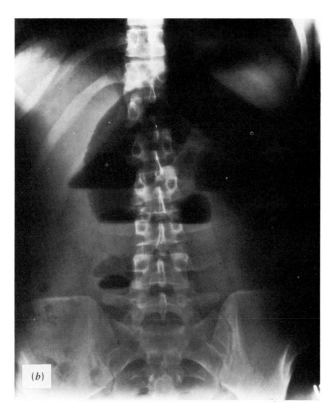

Figure 33-10. Case example 33-2.

History, physical examination, and radiographs all support the diagnosis of small bowel obstruction. What do you think caused it?

Probably an adhesion from the prior surgery. What are the other common causes of small bowel obstruction?

Metastatic disease, adhesions from prior surgery or from pelvic inflammatory disease, and hernias are the major causes of small bowel obstruction. Less common causes include gallstone ileus (the gallstone can sometimes be identified; air can sometimes be seen in the gallbladder), volvulus (abnormal position of the bowel can sometimes be inferred), primary bowel tumors, appendicitis, Crohn's disease, and intussusception.

What is the significance of the air-fluid levels on the upright film?

The main significance of air-fluid levels is that they should remind you that the patient has a large amount of fluid that was extracellular fluid and is now sequestered within the bowel. Replacement of the lost fluid and electrolytes (especially the lost potassium) is of prime importance. Anesthesia induced before the replacement of fluid and electrolytes could kill the patient. Anesthesia would induce vasodilation; the patient's decreased blood volume would be unable to compensate, and the patient would go into shock.

Some people say that the air-fluid levels are important because they signify active peristalsis. They believe that air-fluid levels at different heights within the same air-filled loop indicate motor activity pushing the fluid from one loop to another. If you take bowel removed at autopsy and place fluid and air within it and position it so that multiple loops are formed, differential air-fluid levels will usually form. This is because fluid seeks its own level, but the air does not seek its own level, and thus, even with dead bowel, the air-fluid levels will be at different heights in each air-filled loop. The tightness of the curve of the bowel loop is, however, an important sign of small bowel distension with active peristalsis. Atonic bowel does not assume such hairpin-like curves. When bowel is adynamic, the air-fluid levels are longer (Fig. 33-11), and the bowel loops are less tightly curved.

Colonic Obstruction. Three different patterns are seen in the patient with colonic obstruction: colonic distension with a competent ileocecal valve, colonic distension with an incompetent ileocecal valve, and closed-loop obstruction (volvulus). The ileocecal valve normally permits small bowel contents to pass into the colon but prevents colonic contents from passing into the small bowel. When it acts in this way, the ileocecal valve is competent. Obstruction of the colon occurring with a competent ileocecal valve results in marked and usually rapid distension of the colon (Fig. 33-12).

When the ileocecal valve is incompetent, small bowel material can still flow into the colon, but colonic contents can reflux freely into the small bowel. With colonic obstruction and an incompetent ileocecal valve, both the colon and distal ileum become distended, and the colonic

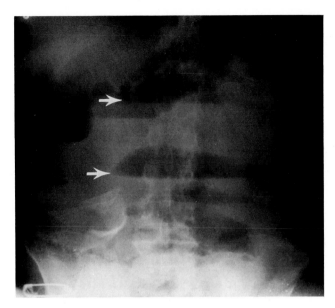

Figure 33-11. Upright abdominal radiograph in a patient with a postoperative adynamic ileus. The small bowel loops have long air-fluid levels (arrows) indicative of their lack of dynamic motion.

distension that occurs tends to be less marked than when the ileocecal valve is competent.

Closed-loop obstructions in the colon are usually due to colonic volvulus and can affect the sigmoid colon, cecum, and uncommonly, the transverse colon. With a closed-loop obstruction, colonic contents can enter the obstructed loop of bowel but cannot pass from it either in a forward or backward direction. The loop therefore distends rapidly.

The common causes of colonic obstruction are colon cancer, diverticulitis, and volvulus.

Case 33-3

This 62-year-old man came to the emergency room complaining that for several days he had had crampy abdominal pain, had been unable to pass a stool, and had noted his abdomen becoming progressively more distended.

The results of a rectal exam were normal except that no feces could be felt in the rectum. His abdominal radiograph is shown in Figure 33-13. What do you see?

There is a large, pear-shaped loop of bowel in the midabdomen. It is sufficiently distended that no inter-

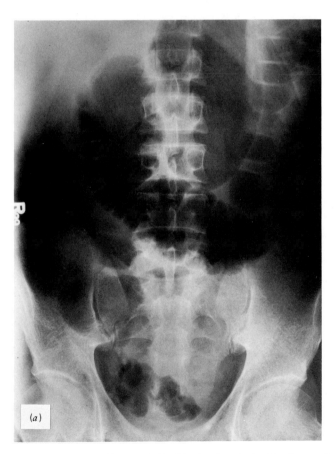

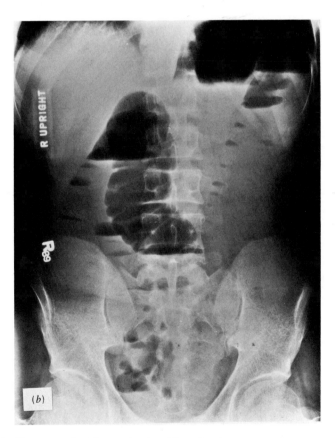

Figure 33-12. Distal colon obstruction in a patient with a competent ileocecal valve. The colon is moderately distended, and on the upright view (*b*), colonic air-fluid levels are seen. The patient had a distal sigmoid colon cancer.

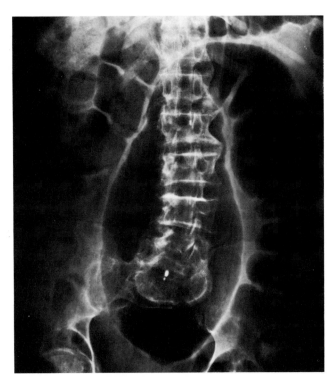

Figure 33-13. Case example 33-3.

nal markings can be identified. With its diameter, it is likely that it is colon, because small bowel would usually burst before reaching that size. What is your diagnosis?

The patient has a sigmoid colon volvulus. What should you do to confirm the diagnosis and treat the patient?

A gentle sigmoidoscopy should be performed, and an attempt should be made to pass a soft rectal tube into the dilated colon. Care is necessary because a rough approach could perforate the colon, and a lack of care by the sigmoidoscopist could result in an explosive decompression of the colonic contents into the sigmoidoscopist's face.

When the diagnosis is uncertain, a gentle barium enema can be used to establish the diagnosis and the level of obstruction. Uncommonly, the barium enema will result in relief of the obstruction.

Keynotes

- *The recognition of bowel distension usually depends on seeing the air in the distended bowel loop. An airless abdomen may conceal distended bowel.*
- *Metastatic disease, adhesions, and hernias are the common causes of small bowel obstruction.*
- *A volvulus is a twisting of the bowel on itself. This twisting often results in bowel obstruction.*
- *The common causes of colon obstruction are colon cancer, diverticulitis, and volvulus.*

Adynamic Ileus

Classic Adynamic Ileus. The classic adynamic ileus has adynamic bowel throughout the small bowel and colon (Fig. 33-4). This lack of forward propulsion results in progressive distension of the entire bowel. Several variants of adynamic ileus occur, and atypical patterns are common (Figure 33-14).

Colonic Adynamic Ileus. Colon adynamic ileus is an adynamic ileus limited to the colon. The colon becomes distended, sometimes markedly distended, but only rarely will it perforate. Because of the marked colonic distension, it resembles an obstruction of the distal colon with a competent ileocecal valve. Colonic adynamic ileus is usually found in patients with one of several predisposing conditions:

1. Motor activity of abdominal wall decreased as a result of being bedridden and institutionalized
2. Hypothyroidism, marked
3. Parkinsonism and drugs with a Parkinsonian side effect (especially the phenothiazines)

The patient with a colonic adynamic ileus usually has progressive abdominal distension and constipation. If the rectosigmoid colon is distended, sigmoidoscopy is the best method of excluding obstruction as the etiology. History is often helpful because these patients usually have recurrent episodes of colonic distension.

Bowel Distension with Superior Mesenteric Artery Ischemia. An adynamic ileus with distension limited to the small bowel and the right and transverse colon may be due to ischemia in the distribution of the superior mesenteric artery (Fig. 33-15). Though this is true, this pattern is more commonly due to the effect of treatment of a total adynamic ileus by rectal tubes or rectal suppositories with emptying of the distal colon.

Superior mesenteric artery ischemia results in recurrent episodes of abdominal pain after meals (*abdominal angina*) or causes nausea, vomiting, or anorexia associated with moderate-to-severe abdominal pain. Some patients who develop this later syndrome of preinfarction are on digitalis glycosides. It is important that any patient suspected of having this syndrome have an arteriogram of the superior mesenteric artery (Fig. 33-15*b* and *c*). The adynamic ileus limited to the distribution of the superior mesenteric artery is a late finding and usually indicates that the bowel is infarcted—that it is too late to save the patient's bowel and, therefore, too late to save her or his life.

Focal Adynamic Ileus, or Sentinal Loop. Inflammation adjacent to the bowel first results in spasm and then in lack of motor activity. The distended loop of bowel (or *sentinal loop*) can be identified on a radiograph and is

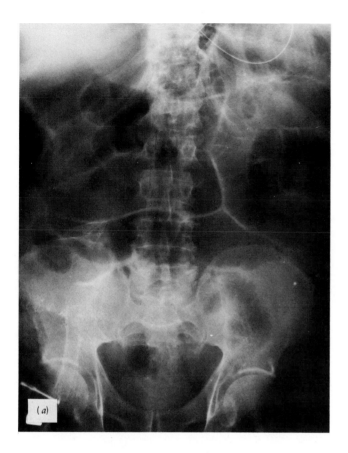

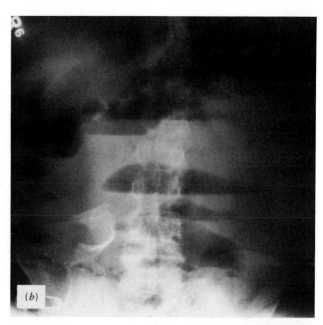

Figure 33-14. Postoperative adynamic ileus. Many distended loops of bowel are seen in the abdomen. These are preponderantly small bowel loops, as shown by the faint valvulae conniventes in the left midabdomen and by the absence of bowel markings in the mid and lower abdomen. Relatively little colonic air is present. (*a*) Supine view. (*b*) Upright view. The long air-fluid levels indicate that this is an adynamic ileus despite the relative lack of colonic air.

indicative of an inflammatory process in the region of the dilated loop or at the site of origin of its mesentery from the posterior abdominal wall (Fig. 33-16). A focal adynamic ileus can affect two adjacent loops of bowel, even if they are not continuous; it is the identification of two discontinuous loops of bowel that points strongly toward this diagnosis.

Appendicitis can result in a dilated loop in the right lower quadrant; acute cholecystitis in a dilated loop in the right upper quadrant; pancreatitis in a dilated loop in the left upper or mid abdomen; and diverticulitis in bowel distension in the left lower quadrant. Pyelonephritis and psoas abscess can occasionally result in focal bowel dilation localized to the site of the acute inflammation.

Total Adynamic Ileus. An example of a total adynamic ileus has been shown in Figure 33-4. There are a large number of processes that can result in a total adynamic ileus:

Traumatic
    After abdominal surgery
    After blunt abdominal trauma
Metabolic
    Hypokalemia
    Diabetic ketoacidosis
    Marked hypercalcemia

Neurological
    Spinal shock
    Postvagotomy
    Diabetic neuropathy
Infectious
    Peritonitis
        Tuberculous
        Pneumococcal
        Mixed
    Intraperitoneal abscess
    Associated with
        Pneumonia
        Pyelonephritis
        Retroperitoneal abscess
Inflammatory
    Systemic lupus erythematosis
Vascular
    Shock
    Infarction
        Superior mesenteric artery
        Associated with sickle cell disease
    Hemorrhage
        Interperitoneal
        Retroperitoneal
Muscular
    Scleroderma

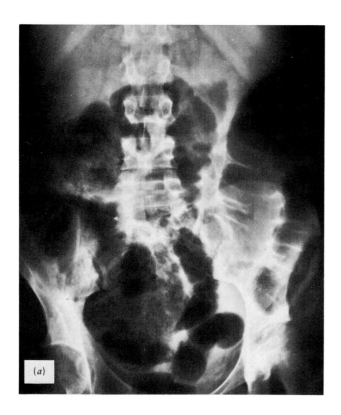

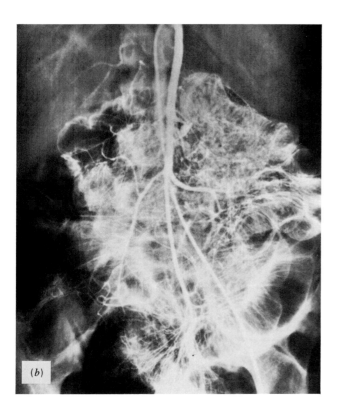

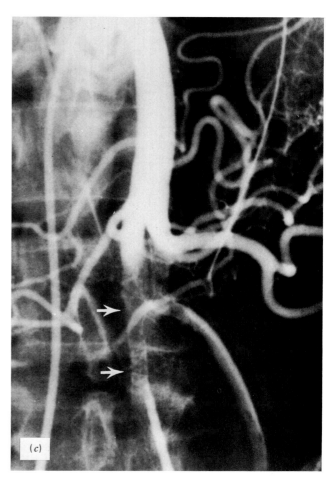

Figure 33-15. Superior mesenteric artery–induced bowel ischemia. (a) The abdominal film in this patient with mesenteric artery ischemia demonstrates marked distension of many loops of small bowel and of the ascending, transverse, and splenic flexure of the colon. Although air is seen in the rectum and sigmoid colon, these portions of the colon are not distended. Distension of the bowel in a patient with mesenteric ischemia is a bad prognostic sign. This patient died 2 days after this film was taken. (b) A superior mesenteric arteriogram in this same patient demonstrates a narrow artery with no focal occlusion, indicating that the ischemia is due to a low flow state or spasm. (c) In another patient with superior mesenteric artery ischemia, a thrombus (arrows) is seen partially filling the superior mesenteric artery. In this patient, the thrombus was successfully removed at the time of surgery, and the bowel and the patient were saved. The abdominal radiograph in the patient was normal.

The most common conditions are

    After surgery
    Peritonitis
    Intraperitoneal abscess
    Hypokalemia

How should you treat an adynamic ileus? Find the cause. Let the air-fluid levels in the bowel remind you to replace fluid and electrolytes.

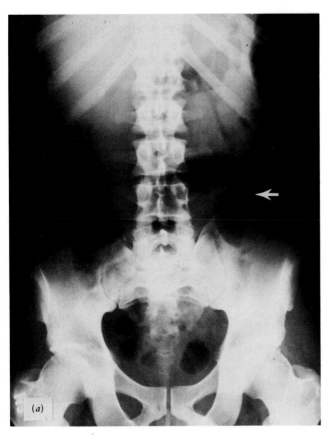 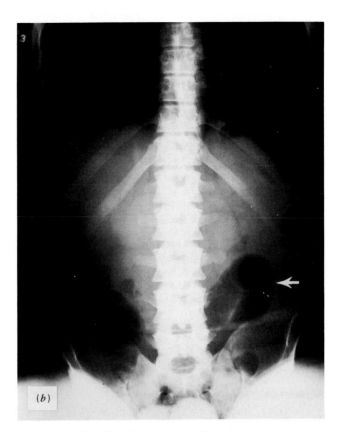

Figure 33-16. A sentinel loop in a patient with pancreatitis. A single dilated loop (arrows) of small bowel is seen on both supine (*a*) and upright (*b*) views.

Keynotes

- *In an adynamic ileus, the bowel lacks propulsive muscular contractions, and all muscular contraction is limited.*
- *A colonic adynamic ileus is an adynamic ileus limited to the colon.*
- *Abdominal angina is the syndrome of recurrent abdominal pain after meals, as a result of vascular insufficiency of the bowel.*
- *When the bowel in superior mesenteric artery ischemia is still alive, the abdominal radiograph is usually still normal. When the bowel dies, recognizable bowel distension occurs. To save the patient's life, diagnosis is best made when the abdominal radiograph is still normal.*
- *A sentinal loop (also called a focal adynamic ileus) is a spastic or dilated loop of bowel adjacent to a focal area of inflammation.*

SUMMARY

The basis for deciding among the four possible bowel patterns—normal bowel, aerophagia, obstruction, and adynamic ileus—is the identification of bowel loops and the determination of their degree of distension. Loops are identified by shape and internal markings. Distension is evaluated by noting the type of change in the internal markings and judging the diameter of the loop.

Aerophagia (air swallowing) results in a common symptom complex of bloating, belching, passing flatus, and audible bowels sounds. It can be caused by increased air swallowing, decreased evacuation of air, or increased fermentation in the bowel.

Obstruction usually results in anorexia, intermittent spasms of abdominal pain, and diarrhea or constipation. In the small bowel it is most commonly due to adhesions, hernias, and metastatic cancer. In the large bowel it is most commonly due to colon cancer, diverticulitis, and sigmoid volvulus.

Adynamic ileus can be localized or diffuse. In the diffuse form, the main symptoms are anorexia and a sense of abdominal fullness or distension. It is most commonly due to abdominal surgery, hypokalemia, or infection in or adjacent to the peritoneum. The focal form usually manifests in the symptoms of the disease that has caused it. It can be associated with appendicitis, pancreatitis, mesenteric ischemia, and localized abscesses.

REVIEW QUESTIONS

1. On an abdominal radiograph, where might you find bowel gas in a normal person?

2. What is aerophagia? What are its symptoms? What might you find on abdominal radiographs? What are its causes? How can you treat it?

3. What is the basic radiographic change in a patient with bowel obstruction?

4. Under what circumstances might a bowel obstruction not be identifiable on an abdominal radiograph?

5. What is an adynamic ileus? What are its common causes? What is its radiographic appearance?

6. What are the common causes of a small bowel obstruction?

7. What are the common causes of a large bowel obstruction?

8. What is the location of the bowel within the abdominal cavity?

9. Describe the appearance of the jejunum, ileum, and colon with different degrees of distension.

10. What are the symptoms of a sigmoid colon volvulus? What is its radiographic appearance?

VOCABULARY

abdominal angina

adynamic ileus

aerophagia
haustral folds

paralytic ileus

plicae circulares

sentinal loop

splenic flexure syndrome

superior mesenteric artery
ischemia

teniae coli

valvulae conniventes

SUGGESTIONS FOR FURTHER READING

For suggested reading see Chapter 26.

SECTION B

THE GASTROINTESTINAL TRACT: CONTRAST STUDIES

The next 10 chapters discuss the appearance of abnormalities of the gastrointestinal tract on radiographic studies in which the bowel has been opacified with contrast media.

Chapter 34 consists of illustrations from normal studies. Chapter 35 discusses the methods used for contrast examinations and basic principles of interpretation.

Chapters 36 through 39 discuss the basic patterns of abnormality seen on contrast studies of the gastrointestinal tract: masses, areas of narrowing, outpouchings, and others. Chapters 40 through 43 discuss, sequentially, the esophagus, stomach, duodenum, and colon.

34

THE NORMAL GASTROINTESTINAL TRACT

This chapter consists of illustrations from normal upper GI tract and colon examinations. It demonstrates the normal patterns seen with both the single- and double-contrast techniques, and it will make the abnormalities discussed in Chapters 35 through 43 more understandable. The student should turn back and forth as necessary between the normal examples in this chapter and the abnormal examples in the subsequent chapters.

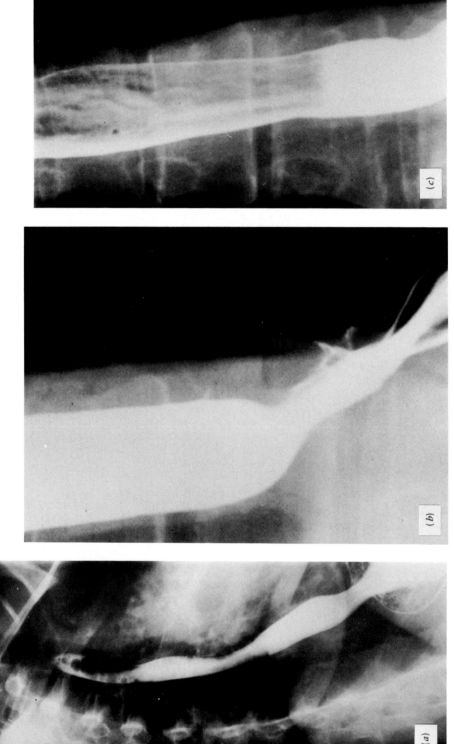

Figure 34-1. Views of the normal esophagus. (a) Single-contrast study. (b) Single-contrast study of the lower portion of the esophagus and the lower esophageal sphincter. (c) Double-contrast air-barium study of the midesophagus.

284

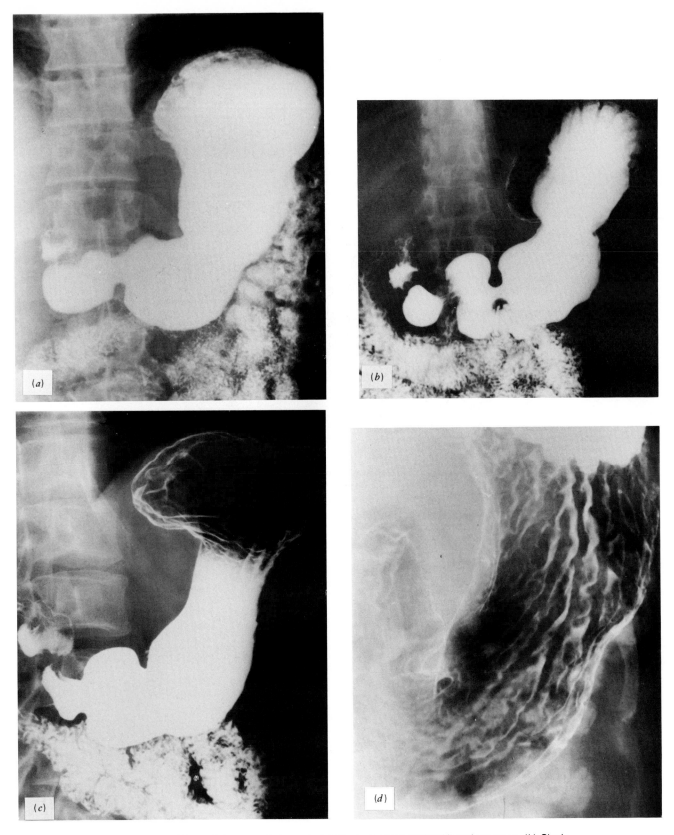

Figure 34-2. Views of the normal stomach. (*a*) Single-contrast study with patient prone. (*b*) Single-contrast study obtained prone. (*c*) Single-contrast study obtained with patient upright. The indentations on the stomach on these views represent peristaltic waves. (*d*) Double-contrast air-barium study demonstrating rugal folds).

285

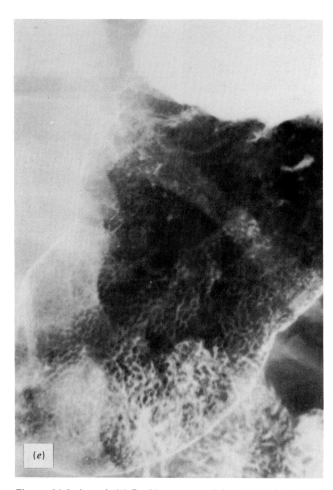

Figure 34-2. (cont.) (e) Double-contrast air-barium study demonstrating finer mucosal markings, called *area gastrica*.

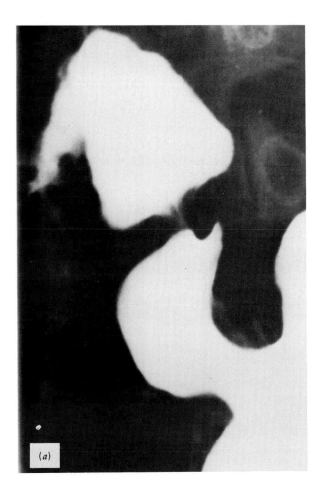

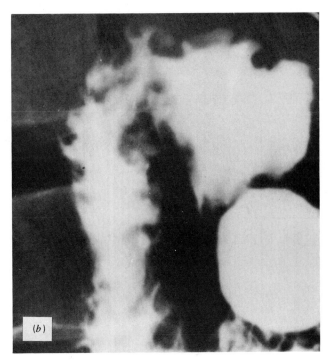

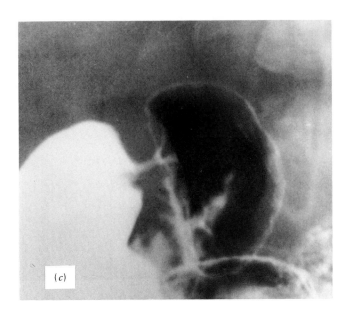

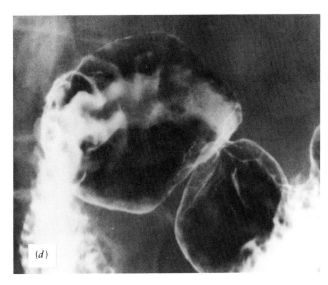

Figure 34-3. Views of the normal duodenal bulb. (*a*) Single-contrast study demonstrating smooth contours of the duodenal bulb. (*b*) Single-contrast study demonstrating mucosal folds. (*c*) Double-contrast study demonstrating smooth contours of the duodenal bulb. (*d*) Double-contrast study demonstrating the mucosal folds of the duodenal bulb.

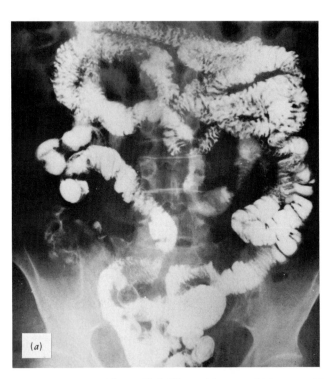

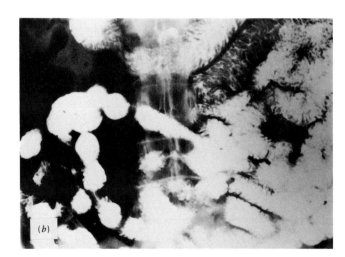

Figure 34-4. Views of the normal jejunum and ileum. The jejunum is to the reader's right, the ileum to the reader's left. (*a*) Normal pattern. (*b*) Normal pattern, focal view.

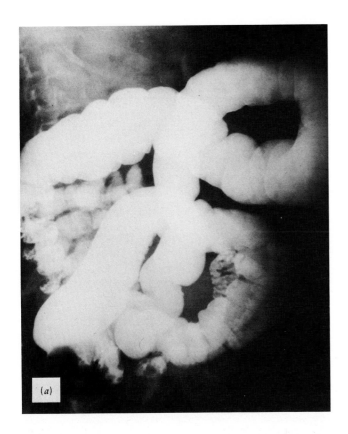

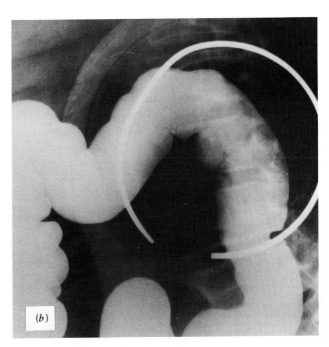

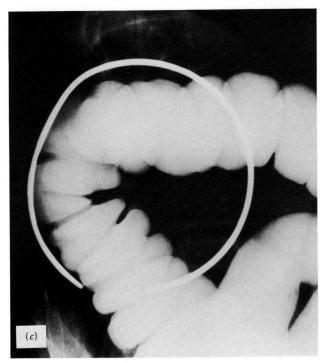

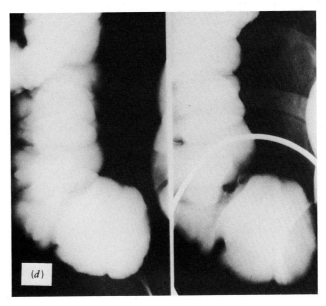

Figure 34-5. Normal single-contrast barium enema. (*a*) Film of the filled colon. (*b*) Compression view of the splenic flexure. (The rounded wire is the marker for the compression device.) (*c*) Compression view of the hepatic flexure. (*d*) Two views of the cecum, one with compression. (*e*) Lateral view of the rectum. (*f*) Angled view of the rectosigmoid colon. (*g*) View obtained after evacuation of most of the barium.

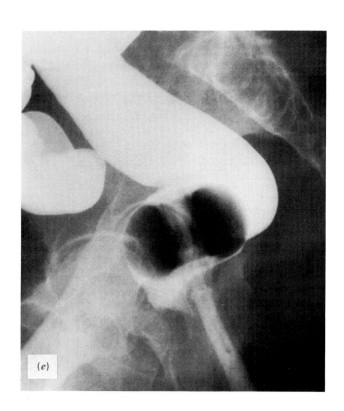

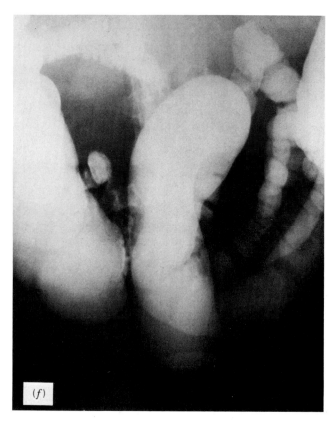

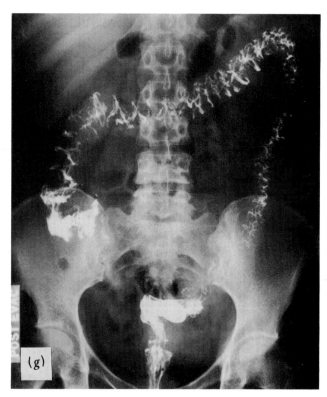

Figure 34-5. (cont.) (*e*) Lateral view of the rectum. (*f*) Angled view of the rectosigmoid colon. (*g*) View obtained after evacuation of most of the barium.

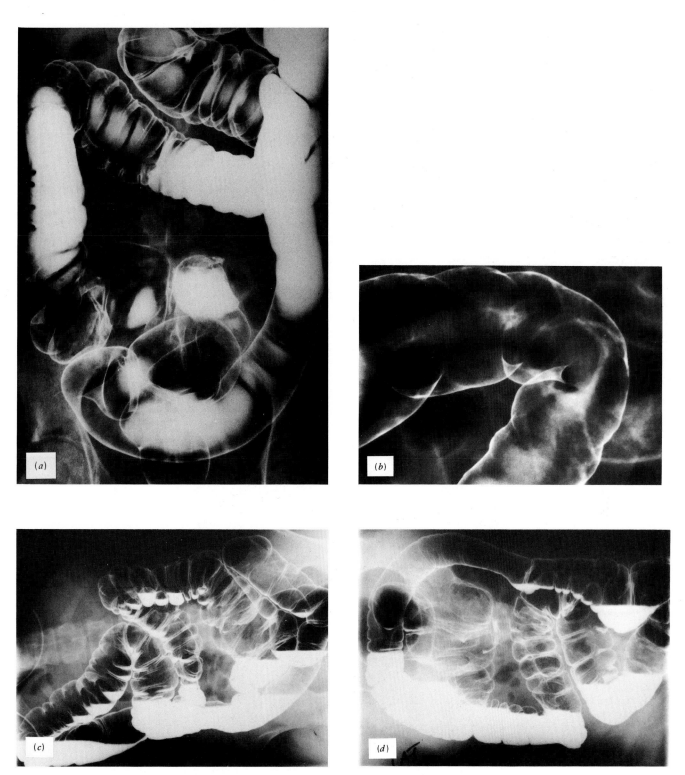

Figure 34-6. Normal air-barium double-contrast enema. (*a*) Prone view. (*b*) Focal view of the splenic flexure. (*c*) and (*d*) Lateral decubitus views.

35

INTRODUCTION TO IMAGING
OF THE GASTROINTESTINAL TRACT

KEY CONCEPTS

Radiological

The hollow tube of the GI tract shows repetitive patterns throughout its course. The interpretation of a pattern is likely to be the same whether the pattern is seen in the esophagus or the colon. The main means of evaluating this hollow tube is to fill it with contrast medium and use the pattern seen in the lumen of the tube to evaluate the entire structure of the disease affecting the tube.

There are two methods: the single-contrast study, in which the bowel is filled with radiopaque contrast, and (2) the double-contrast method, in which the wall is coated with a radiopaque contrast and the lumen then distended with a more radiolucent contrast, such as air. The usual radiopaque contrast used is barium sulfate. Iodinated contrast medium is used less often because of its increased cost and hyperosmolality.

Radiographic studies of the GI tract often use many films. One of the challenges faced by the student is the surveying of the many films obtained in a study. The simplest approach for the student is to look at each area of the gut sequentially on all films that demonstrate it; for example, first look at the esophagus on all films, then the stomach, and so on. Your analysis of each part of the gut should include a statement of the adequacy of its examination and whether it is normal or abnormal.

OBJECTIVES

When you complete this chapter you will be able to

1. Describe and differentiate the single- and double-contrast studies of the GI tract.
2. List two advantages and two disadvantages of the single-contrast study.

3. List three radiographic methods of limiting the disadvantages of the single-contrast study.
4. List two advantages and two disadvantages of the double-contrast examination.

The GI tract (the gut) is a hollow tube extending from the mouth to the anus. Although there are slight differences in the structure of the wall and mucosa of the gut, it is easiest initially to look for the similarities in pattern throughout the gut, rather than at the localized differences. Patterns of normality and abnormality are repeated throughout this hollow tube of gut, permitting the viewer to ascribe the same meaning to the same pattern whether it occurs in the esophagus, stomach, duodenum, small bowel, or colon (Figs. 35-1 and 35-2). An understanding, therefore, of these basic patterns simplifies the task of learning the many manifestations of GI disease.

Keynote

- *The patterns of normality and abnormality are repeated throughout the gut.*

METHODS OF STUDY

Two different radiological methods of evaluating the hollow tube of gut have evolved. The skilled radiologist will often switch from one to the other as need arises and may combine both in the same patient examination; it is easiest, however, for the student to consider these techniques

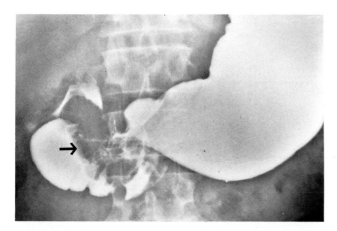

Figure 35-1. Villous adenocarcinoma of the stomach. The irregular-area of barium filling in the distal antrum (arrow) is a large carcinoma of the stomach.

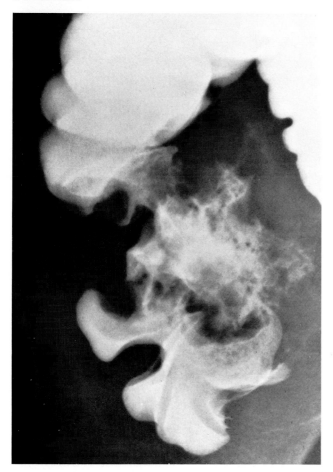

Figure 35-2. Villous adenocarcinoma of the cecum. Note the similarity of its appearance to the gastric cancer shown in Figure 35-1.

as distinct. The two methods are the *single-contrast study,* using a radiopaque medium (usually barium sulfate) to fill the lumen, and the *double-contrast study,* using barium sulfate to coat the mucosa and air to distend the lumen of the hollow tube.

Single Contrast

In the single-contrast method of study, the lumen of the gut is filled with barium sulfate (or uncommonly, with an iodine-containing contrast medium).

Upper GI Series (Barium Meal). The pharynx, esophagus, stomach, duodenum, and small bowel are filled from above, usually by having the patient swallow the contrast medium (Fig. 35-3). Peristalsis then carries the contrast medium to the region of interest. If the patient cannot swallow, the contrast medium can be injected through a catheter.

Barium Enema. Single-contrast studies of the colon and distal ileum are done by filling the colon with barium by enema (Fig. 35-4*a*). It is possible to study the entire small bowel by an enema technique, but the small bowel is usually studied with swallowed barium.

Properties of the Single-Contrast Examination. Barium is very radiopaque and usually appears white on the radiographs. With the lumen filled and distended, the radiopacity of the barium often limits the evaluation of the gut to an analysis of its margin. In the central position of the lumen, the barium is sufficiently radiodense that small defects may be invisible, and only large defects within the lumen can be seen. For this reason, multiple views are obtained to profile as much of the margin of the gut as practical.

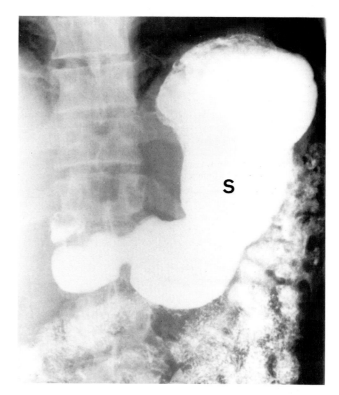

Figure 35-3. Single-contrast upper GI study. The stomach (S) is filled with barium. Barium is also in the duodenum and small bowel.

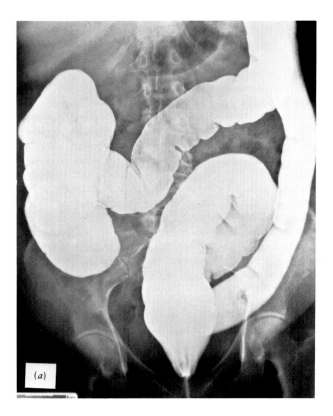

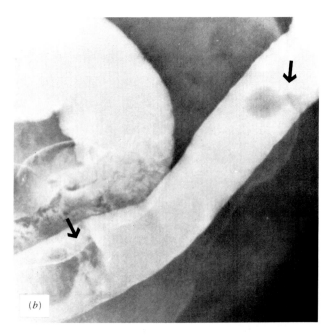

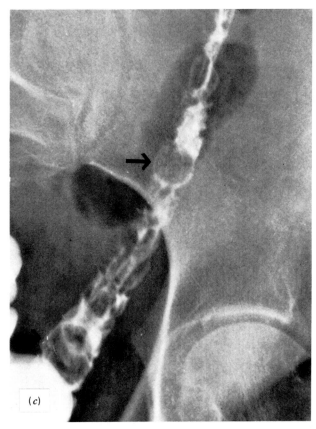

Figure 35-4. (a) One film from a single-contrast study of the colon: a barium enema. This is a single film selected from the 11 taken as part of the barium enema. (b) A film taken early in the study, with the colon less distended, demonstrates two polyps with their stalks (arrows) within the lumen. These are just visible on the larger, better filled film. (c) On the film taken after evacuation of the barium, the two polyps (arrows) can be seen as rounded defects within and slightly distending the lumen. These proved to be benign adenomatous polyps.

This limited visibility of structures superimposed on the center of the barium-filled lumen is the major limitation of single-contrast studies. Because of this limitation, several special methods are used to see within the central portion of the barium-filled lumen; each depends on having less barium in the path of the x-ray beam. Films can be taken early, during the filling of the lumen: with less bar-

ium present, lesions can be seen through it (Fig. 35-4b). Films can be exposed after much of the barium has left the lumen: after evacuation of the colon or emptying of the esophagus or stomach, mucosal detail may be better delineated (Fig. 35-4c). External pressure may be used to flatten the lumen: compression can displace the barium from a site of interest, decreasing the amount in the path of the x-ray beam, thus permitting lesions to be seen within the central portion of the gut lumen. Thus, the single-contrast study of the gut usually uses a combination of filled, partially filled, and compression views.

Double Contrast

The double-contrast study of the gut uses an especially radiodense and adherent barium to coat the mucosa of the gut and gas to distend the lumen (Fig. 35-5). Barium used to study the esophagus, stomach, and duodenum is usually swallowed. In most cases, effervescent granules or powder

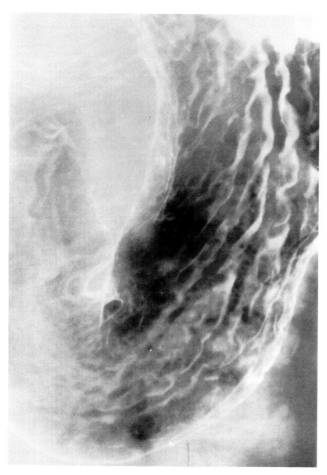

Figure 35-5. A single film from a double-contrast study of the stomach. The rugal folds are well seen.

are swallowed to provide the gas for luminal distention; in some cases, a catheter is used to administer the gas.

Studies of the colon are performed by enema. Especially radiodense and adherent barium is instilled through a catheter into the colon until the barium reaches the splenic flexure of the colon. Air is then injected into the catheter, and with careful positioning of the patient, the injected air will push the barium in front of it, allowing the barium to coat the mucosa and the air to distend the lumen. Multiple radiographs in different positions are then obtained.

The double-contrast study of the gut permits a more detailed evaluation of mucosal detail. Because the lumen is not filled with radiopaque material, lesions can be seen within the central portion of the lumen more easily than with the single-contrast study. Two major problems arise with the double-contrast method: it can be difficult to decide if an abnormality is a polyp lying within the lumen or a diverticulum extending from it (Fig. 35-6), and incomplete distension may permit even large lesions to be overlooked among convoluted loops of gut (Fig. 35-7).

Structures along the dependent and nondependent walls of the gut will have different appearances on double-contrast studies. Because there is usually a puddle of barium lying along the dependent margin of the gut, structures along that margin will often be outlined by the barium, showing as less radiodense structures within a slightly more radiodense region (Fig. 35-8a). Structures on the nondependent margin of the gut will have their surface outlined with thin radiodense lines along their margins (Fig. 35-8b).

Radiodense barium also can hang droplets from the nondependent mucosal surface, resulting in focal dots of radiodensity (the *stalactite phenomenon* simulating ulceration (Fig. 35-9).

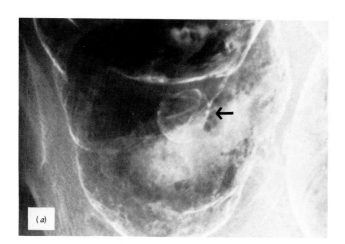

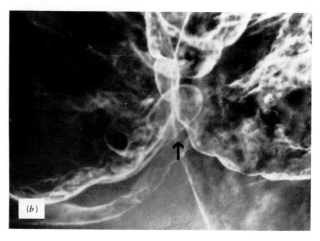

Figure 35-6. Is this a polyp or a diverticulum of the cecum? (a) AP view of the cecum. An arrow indicates the lesion. (b) An oblique view demonstrates that the structure hangs partially outside the lumen (arrow), indicating that it is a diverticulum. (Courtesy M. Vaccaro, M.D.)

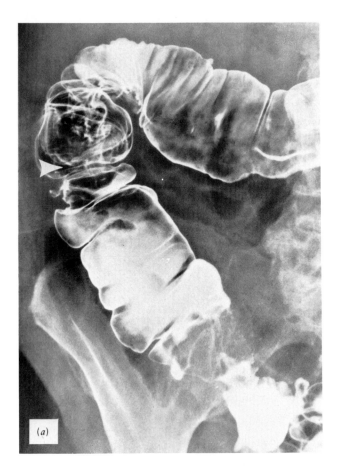

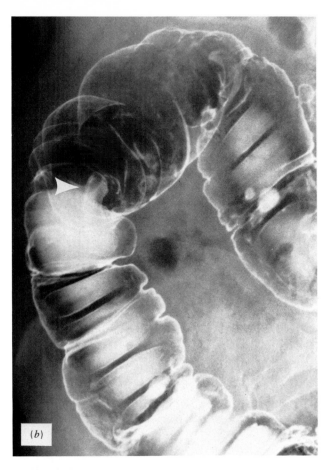

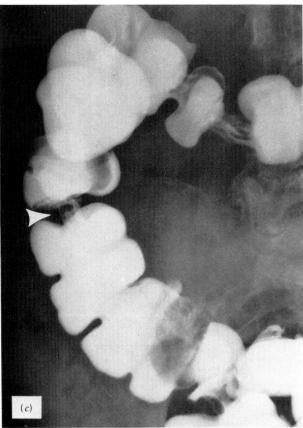

Figure 35-7. Colon cancer almost hidden by incomplete distension of the colon during a double-contrast barium enema. (*a*) Incomplete distension almost hides the lesion (arrowhead). (*b*) Another view demonstrates the narrow tubular lumen (arrowhead) left within the center of the colon cancer. (*c*) On the filled-colon film, the short apple-core lesion (arrowhead) can be seen.

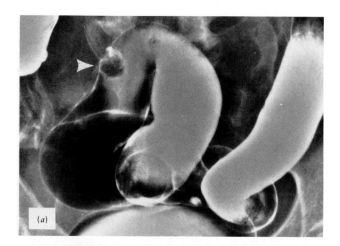

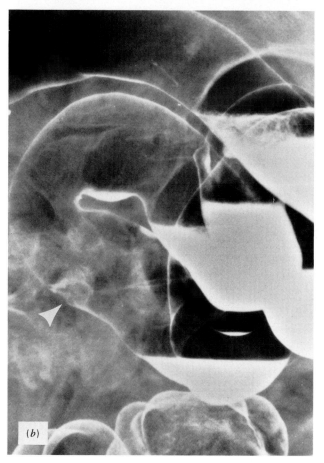

Figure 35-8. Small sessile polypoid carcinoma of the sigmoid colon seen on double-contrast barium enema. (*a*) The cancer (arrowhead) lies in the barium puddle (or pool), showing as a defect within the barium. (*b*) Seen in another view, the cancer (arrowhead) is surrounded by air and has a thin layer of barium on its surface, outlining it.

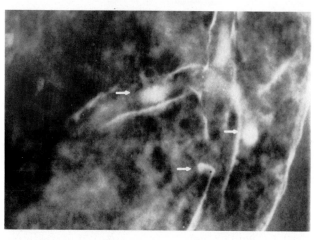

Figure 35-9. The stalactite phenomenon. Several drops of barium (arrows) hang from gastric rugal folds. These partially simulate ulcers because they are focal collections of barium. The lack of edema around them and presence of normal-appearing folds near them make the diagnosis of ulcer less likely.

Keynotes

- *There are two methods of evaluating the gut using contrast media: the single-contrast study and the double-contrast study.*
- *In the single-contrast study, the lumen is filled, usually with barium sulfate.*

  The radiopacity of barium sulfate frequently limits the evaluation of gut to a study of its margin.

  Methods used to aid in seeing through the radiodense barium are
  Early films taken with minimal filling
  Postemptying films
  Films taken as external compression thins the gut
- *In the double-contrast study, the mucosa is coated with barium, and the lumen is distended with air.*

PROBLEMS OF MANY FILMS

Studies of the gut use many radiographs to be certain that all portions have been adequately examined. In viewing the many films, the student may feel overwhelmed by the number and rush through them, missing important findings. A systematic approach is necessary to be sure that nothing is overlooked and that the films are adquate. Two different methods of review can be used.

The first is the method that most students find easiest to use. Each region of the gut is studied, using every film that shows it. For example, an upper GI tract series may have no films showing the pharynx, two showing the esophagus, four of the esophagogastric junction, two of the gastic fundus, four showing the body of the stomach, two of the antrum, four of the pylorus and duodenal bulb, and two films of the duodenal sweep. In such a series of films, the viewer first looks for films of the pharynx. Finding none, she or he notes this mentally and looks at the esophagus. Two radiographs show the esophagus. These are studied first to decide whether the esophagus has been adequately studied and then to search for abnormalities. The four views of the esophagogastric junction are then studied: Are they adequate? Are they normal? This procedure is continued throughout the portion of the gut visualized on the study.

The results of this regional review are then summarized, for example, as follows: "Upper one-third esophagus incompletely studied. Gastric fundus incompletely distended. Duodenal sweep seen only during peristaltic contraction" (this describes the adequacy of study). "Small pyloric channel ulcer with no obstruction, thickened mucosal folds, duodenal bulb compatible with duodenitis" (the recognized abnormality). The summary statement discusses both any sites inadequately studied and the abnormalities seen.

The second method is the one more often used by radiologists, but it is harder for the student to master. Each radiograph is studied in turn, no matter which portion of the gut is shown on it. The viewer depends on his or her memory for what he or she has seen adequately, what not, and what abnormalities are present. For example: Film 1: view of esophagogastric junction: adequate, normal. Film 2: two views of duodenal sweep: sweep contracted by peristalsis; no abnormality seen; inadequate visualization. Film 3: view of antrum of stomach: adequate visualization; possible pyloric channel ulcer. Film 4: view of pylorus and antrum: adequate; pyloric chanel ulcer; no obstruction. This method relies on the viewer's ability to remember and add up his or her interpretation of each film to yield a summary statement.

Keynotes

- *First technique: Study each portion of the gut sequentially on every film that shows it.*
- *Second technique: Look at each film sequentially, remembering what has and has not been adequately seen, and remembering abnormalities.*
- *The summary statement should include a statement of any sites inadequately seen and the abnormalities seen.*

SUMMARY

Two different methods are available for studying the detailed structure of the gut: the single-contrast and the double-contrast methods. Each must be learned because the usual examination of the gut often combines portions of each technique in the same study.

The abnormalities of the gut show as a limited number of patterns, which are of the same significance in the esophagus, stomach, small bowel, and colon. These basic patterns are discussed in the next few chapters.

REVIEW QUESTIONS

1. Describe the single-contrast study of the gut. What are its disadvantages? What methods are used to overcome partially its disadvantages?
2. Describe the double-contrast study of the gut. What are its advantages and disadvantages?
3. Describe two different methods of evaluating the many films used in a contrast study of the gut.
4. Your description of a contrast study of the gut should include two types of statements. What are they?

VOCABULARY

barium enema	single-contrast study
barium meal	stalactite phenomenon
colon exam	upper GI series
double-contrast study	

SUGGESTIONS FOR FURTHER READING FOR CHAPTERS 35 TO 43

Ronald L. Eisenberg. *Gastrointestinal Radiology.* J.B. Lippincott: Philadelphia. 1983. (A fine introductory text)

Alexander R. Margulis, H. Joachim Burhenne. *Alimentary Tract Radiology.* C.V. Mosby: St. Louis. 1983 (An excellent reference text)

Igor Laufer. *Double Contrast Gastrointestinal Radiology.* W.B. Saunders: Philadelphia. 1979. (An excellent text on the double-contrast technique)

36

MASSES AFFECTING
THE GASTROINTESTINAL TRACT

KEY CONCEPTS

Radiological

Masses affecting the GI tract can be divided into three types: extrinsic, intrinsic mucosal, and intrinsic nonmucosal. Extrinsic masses both displace bowel and indent it from one side. When the affected bowel is freely movable, displacement is the predominant finding. When the bowel is relatively fixed in position, the major effect is asymmetric or eccentric compression of the bowel.

Intrinsic mucosal masses can be flat or raised areas of mucosa or polyps on a stalk. The surface of the flat (or sessile) polyps can be smooth, irregular, or nodular. Many sessile polyps are malignant or premalignant. Polyps on a stalk can be benign or malignant. The shorter and thicker the stalk, and the larger the polyp, the greater the chance of malignancy.

Intrinsic nonmucosal lesions arise from the tissues of the wall but are usually covered by normal mucosa. They usually demonstrate an abrupt transition from the normal wall adjacent to them to the stiff and protruding wall at the site of the tumor. Most lesions are caused by metastases; in those that are not, the larger the size, the greater the chance of malignancy.

Clinical

Extrinsic masses may be asymptomatic, may be found on abdominal palpation, may be sensed as a heaviness or fullness, or may result in localized pain. They can be caused by enlargement of an organ from neoplasm, infection, inflammation, hematoma, or cyst. Masses can also occur outside of the major organs and can be caused by peritoneal or retroperitoneal abscesses, hematomas, and neoplasms.

Mucosal masses often result in intermittent blood loss, which might be detected by finding a small or large amount of blood in the stool or by finding iron deficiency anemia. Mucosal masses

may have symptoms resulting from their metastases or from luminal narrowing or obstruction.

Intrinsic nonmucosal masses are often asymptomatic. Sometimes the mucosa over the mass ulcerates, resulting in bleeding. Occasionally, they can cause abdominal pain from obstruction. Sometimes they have symptoms caused by their metastases.

OBJECTIVES

When you complete this chapter you will be able to

1. List the three main types of masses affecting the GI tract.
2. List, for each of the three main types of mass, the major symptoms.
3. Describe the radiographic findings of each of the main types of mass.
4. Correctly detect and classify masses affecting the esophagus, stomach, and colon on selected radiographs.
5. Match the symptoms of anemia, anorexia, depression, thrombophlebitis, abdominal heaviness, colicky pain, blood in stool, constipation, and a sense of early filling of the stomach to the type(s) of mass that can cause each symptom.

Masses affecting the GI tract can be divided into three types: extrinsic, intrinsic mucosal, and intrinsic nonmucosal. Each type is associated with specific clinical symptoms and has a limited range of pathology and its own identifying radiographic characteristics. The major differential features are the shape of the junction between normal and abnormal sites, the presence or absence of luminal narrowing or displacement, and the appearance of the mucosa.

EXTRINSIC MASSES

Extrinsic masses are those that arise from structures outside the gut. They affect the gut by pressure. These masses may be asymptomatic, may be found on abdominal palpation, may be sensed by the patient as a localized heaviness or bulge, or may result in localized pain. When the result of malignant neoplasms, they may be accompanied by a paraneoplastic syndrome or weight loss. In most cases there will not be occult blood loss in the stool. Anorexia can occur with hepatic or pancreatic masses but is uncommon with other extrinsic masses. Thrombophlebitis and depression can occur with pancreatic masses.

Extrinsic masses can have several etiologies. The enlargement of abdominal and retroperitoneal organs can displace gut. Organ enlargement can be due to neoplasm, infection, inflammation, hematoma, or cyst. Nuclear medicine imaging, sonography, and CT can be useful in determining the cause of organ enlargement. Masses within the mesentery, omentum, and peritoneal and retroperitoneal spaces can be due to abcesses, hematomas, lymphomas, and metastases. Evaluation of these masses can be complex, and a careful history and physical exam is usually the best guide for directing further work-up.

The radiographic pattern seen with extrinsic masses depends on whether the mass lies adjacent to gut that is fixed or adjacent to gut that is mobile. Masses extrinsic to mobile portions of gut tend to displace the gut (Fig. 36-1). These masses are analyzed by the direction in which the bowel is displaced. The site of origin of the mass can often be deduced, and this knowledge often permits the type of mass to be inferred.

When the mass adjacent to a mobile portion of gut is large, it tends both to displace and to narrow the gut. The regions of narrowing tend to be eccentric (i.e., more on one side of the lumen than on the other) and usually have a tapered transition from normal to narrowed lumen (Fig. 36-2).

When the extrinsic mass is adjacent to a portion of the gut that is relatively fixed, such as the duodenum or rectum, even a relatively small extrinsic mass can narrow the lumen (Fig. 36-3). Such narrowing may indent either a small or a long segment of bowel. The transition from the normal to a narrowed region is usually tapered, but the transition is usually more abrupt than the transition seen in mobile portions of gut.

When the narrowing of the lumen of gut is due to pressure from an extrinsic mass, it is usually possible to show that the wall of the gut is flexible as peristaltic waves pass through it.

Keynotes

- *An extrinsic mass may have no symptoms or may result in a sense of fullness, local pain, or anorexia. Sometimes, a paraneoplastic syndrome occurs.*
- *Extrinsic masses can be due to organ enlargement, neoplasm, infection, inflammation, hematoma, or cyst.*
- *Extrinsic masses can be detected on barium studies when they displace the gut.*
- *The gut pressed on by an extrinsic mass will show displacement; eccentric narrowing; a smooth, tapered transition from the narrowed to the normal portion; and usually, flexible walls.*

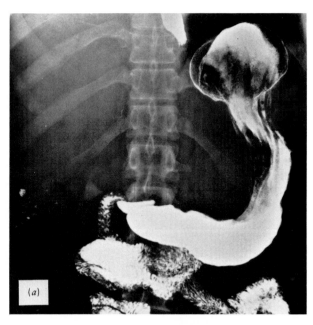
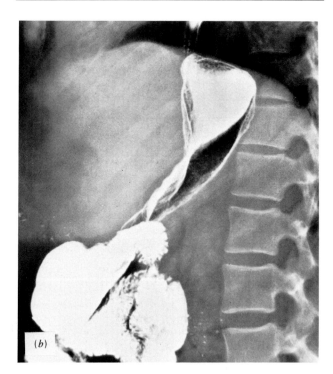

Figure 36-1. Marked enlargement of the liver from metastatic cancer. The enlarged liver presses on, indents, and displaces the barium-filled stomach. Compare the appearance with Figure 34-2a–d. (a) AP view. (b) Lateral view.

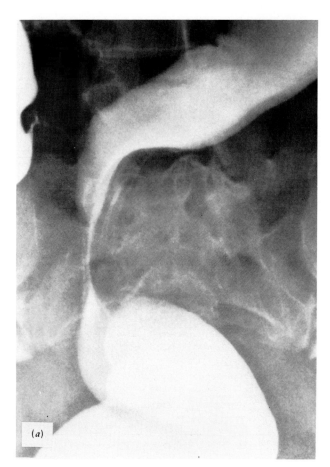
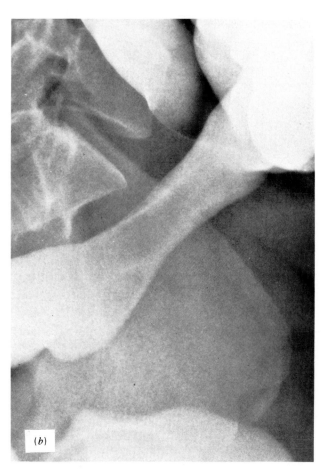

Figure 36-2. A large fibroid uterus both displaces and asymmetrically indents the sigmoid colon. While the sigmoid colon is mobile, the mass is relatively large and still compresses it. Note the tapered transition from compressed to normal colon. (*a*) AP view. (*b*) Lateral view.

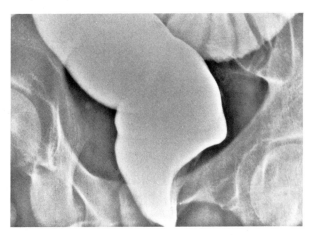

Figure 36-3. A small ischial-rectal abscess markedly indents the rectum. Although the mass is small, the rectum is relatively fixed. Note the more abrupt transition from the indented to the normal colon. (Courtesy E. McCrea, M.D.)

INTRINSIC MUCOSAL MASSES

Intrinsic mucosal masses, benign or malignant, usually result in intermittent minimal blood loss. This may be detected by the finding of a small amount of blood in the stools or by the detection of iron deficiency anemia. Some patients will experience the fatigue and exertional dyspnea of anemia, but most will be asymptomatic. Malignant mucosal lesions may cause symptoms of metastatic disease, and large mucosal lesions may cause luminal obstruction or symptomatic decreased luminal capacity. Obstruction in the upper portion of the gut often causes regurgitation or vomiting and can cause intermittent pain. Obstruction of the small bowel or colon can cause intermittent colicky pain with diarrhea or constipation. Decreased capacity of the stomach can result in anorexia or a sense that the stomach is full after only a litle food has been eaten.

Mucosal masses that narrow the gut lumen are discussed in Chapter 37. Small intrinsic mucosal masses, discussed here, show one of two radiographic patterns: the polyp on a stalk and the sessile polyp.

Polyps on a Stalk

Polyps on a stalk (*pedunculated polyps*) are usually round lesions at the end of a long, narrow stalk (Fig. 36-4). The bulbous end is usually smooth but can be convoluted or irregular. Polyps smaller than 1 cm are usually benign, and solitary polyps less than 0.5 cm are usually hyperplastic rather than adenomatous and can be safely ignored. Polyps 1 cm and larger can be malignant; increased size correlates with an increased chance of malignancy (Figs. 36-5 and 36-6). Even when the identified polyp is benign, the presence of polyps demonstrates reactive mucosa. Careful attention to mucosal detail is necessary to look for cancer elsewhere within the same organ. It is necessary to distinguish stalk polyps from debris, feces, and foreign matter. This is done by the identification of the stalk, by the limited excursion polyps have when barium flows past (the stalk limits the position of the polyp, holding it within a 10-cm excursion), and by persistence within the lumen after the barium has emptied.

Sessile Polyps

The flat, *sessile,* or broad-based *polyp* is a mass arising from the mucosa (Figs. 36-6 and 36-7). It is often raised above the height of the adjacent mucosa, has an abrupt transition from the adjacent normal mucosa, and usually

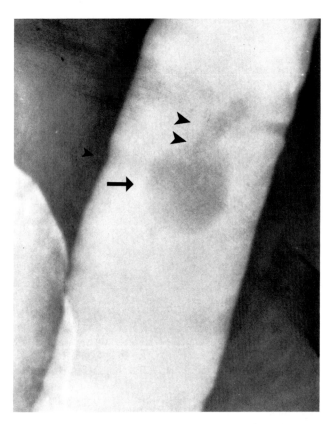

Figure 36-4. Adenomatous colon polyp. The polyp (arrow) and its stalk (arrowheads) can be seen as a defect in the barium in the colon lumen.

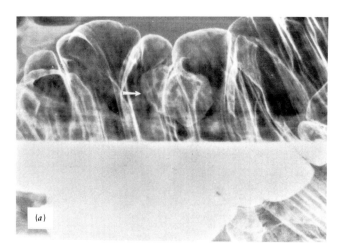

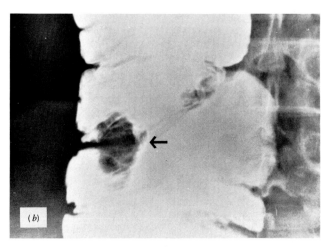

Figure 36-5. Polypoid adenocarcinoma (arrows) is seen on this double-contrast barium enema surrounded by air (*a*) and barium (*b*). The polyp measures approximately 1.5 cm, is irregular, and is on a short stalk. Each of these is a sign that suggests possible malignancy in a polyp.

shows a different surface appearance from the adjacent normal mucosa. In some polyps, the surface is smoother than normal, in some it is rough and irregular, and in some it is nodular. Some broad-based polyps do not project into the lumen; others protrude extensively, narrowing the lumen. In the stomach, the polyp may be a flattened, depressed area of abnormal mucosa.

Keynotes

- *Intrinsic mucosal masses often result in intermittent minimal blood loss.*
- *Malignant mucosal masses may cause symptoms of metastatic disease, anemia, or luminal obstruction.*
- *The chance of malignancy in a polyp on a stalk increases with increasing size of the polyp.*
- *Most sessile polyps are malignant or premalignant.*

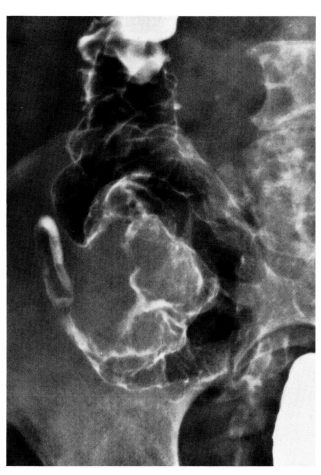

Figure 36-6. A large polypoid carcinoma partially fills the cecum. Its broad base where it joins the colon wall and its large size indicate that it is probably a carcinoma.

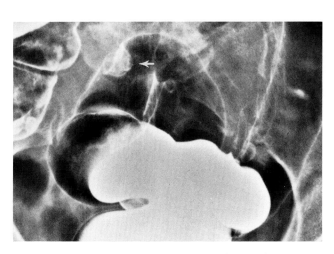

Figure 36-7. A small sessile polyp (arrow) of the sigmoid colon proved, on biopsy, to be a small adenocarcinoma. All sessile polyps should be suspected of being carcinoma.

INTRINSIC NONMUCOSAL LESIONS

The intrinsic nonmucosal lesion (the mural or wall lesion) arises from the tissues of the wall but is covered by initially normal mucosa. These masses are usually asymptomatic and are detected as an incidental finding during barium studies done for some other reason. When the mass is located in a narrow-lumen portion of the gut (such as the small bowel), it may serve as the *nidus* (lead point) for an intussusception, causing colicky abdominal pain and rectal bleeding. In the stomach, the mucosa stretched over the mass can ulcerate, and the patient may bleed massively or occultly. Some of these masses are neoplastic and appear with symptomatic metastases.

Intrinsic nonmucosal lesions often grow as spheres, and this spherical growth is the main radiographic criterion used to diagnose them (Figs. 36-8 and 36-9). The transition zone is abrupt, and the junction of the mass with the normal gut wall usually forms an angle of 90°. The impression on the lumen is usually hemispherical, and if the center of rotation of the sphere is estimated, it will usually lie at about the position one would expect the gut wall to

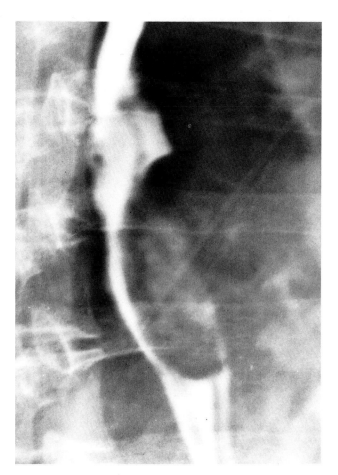

Figure 36-8. This intrinsic nonmucosal lesion of the esophagus is smoothly margined, with an abrupt transition from the normal esophagus. It has the appearance of a lesion arising from the tissues of the wall of the esophagus and proved on biopsy to be a leiomyoma.

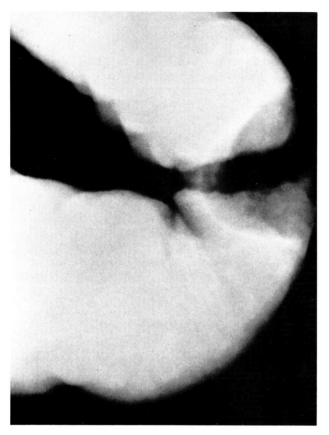

Figure 36-9. This sharply demarcated, smooth-surfaced mass of the sigmoid colon proved to be a lipoma on biopsy.

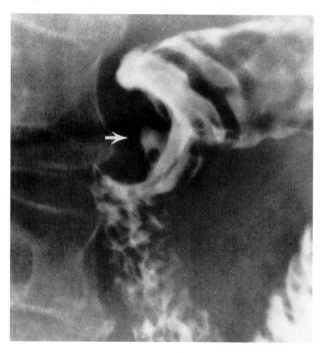

Figure 36-10. This leiomyoma of the duodenum demonstrates the abrupt junction of the mass with the duodenal wall and has a smooth surface except for a focal depression (arrow) that represents an ulcer.

lie. The mucosa over the mass is usually stretched and smooth, but it may be ulcerated (Fig. 36-10). Large masses may appear to be composed of many conglomerate spheres.

Most mural masses have the described appearance. An uncommon variant is for the mass to grow largely extrinsic to the lumen. In such cases, the shape appears to be that of a sphere, but the center of rotation of the sphere lies outside the lumen and the angle formed by the junction of the mass and the normal wall is more than 90°. Uncommonly, too, an extrinsic mass resulting from an abscess or a neoplasm may adhere to the wall of the gut and then begin to expand as a mural lesion, showing many of the same radiographic patterns.

Intrinsic nonmucosal masses can be due to metastases or primary tumors arising from any of the tissues in the wall of the gut. Metastases are most common. Of the primary lesions, smooth muscle tumors are most frequent, but tumors of fat, nerve, lymphatic, and fibrous tissue also occur. Lesions larger than 5 cm are usually malignant sarcomas, smaller lesions may be benign or malignant, and an excisional biopsy is usually necessary to establish the diagnosis.

Keynotes

- *Most intrinsic nonmucosal masses are asymptomatic. Ulceration with bleeding or intussusception can cause symptoms with these masses.*

- *An intussusception is the infolding of one portion of the gut into the lumen of an adjacent portion. It usually occurs because peristalsis pulls a focally enlarged portion of the gut wall through the lumen as though it were a piece of food. Under the age of 2 years, intussusceptions are usually due to enlargement of lymphoid tissues, probably as a result of viral infection. Over the age of 4 years, there is usually a lead point—either a polyp, a submucosal mass, or a carcinoma.*

- *Intrinsic nonmucosal masses are often spherical, have an abrupt transition with the adjacent normal lumen, and may be ulcerated or may appear to be composed of many conglomerate spheres.*

- *Intrinsic nonmucosal masses are usually due to metastases, smooth muscle tumors, tumors of fat, or hematomas.*

SUMMARY

Masses affecting the gut are of three types:

    Extrinsic
    Intrinsic mucosal
    Intrinsic mural, or nonmucosal

Each has its own group of clinical symptoms:

    Extrinsic
      None
      Sense of fullness
      Local pain

Paraneoplastic
   Anorexia
Intrinsic mucosal
   Blood loss
   Anemia
   Intussusception
   Obstruction
Intrinsic nonmucosal
   None
   Intussusception
   Blood loss

Each also has specific radiographic features:

Extrinsic
   Usually:
      Gut displacement
      Extrinsic gut luminal narrowing
Intrinsic mucosal
   Polyp on stalk
   Raised or flat area of:
      Mucosa
      More irregular tissue than surrounding mucosa
      More smooth tissue than surrounding mucosa
Intrinsic nonmucosal
   Abrupt transition, usually 90°
   Portion of a sphere

REVIEW QUESTIONS

1. What are the three types of gut masses?
2. What are the symptoms and radiographic findings of each kind?
3. What are the common causes of extrinsic masses? Intrinsic mucosal masses? Intrinsic nonmucosal masses?
4. What is the significance of finding blood in the stool?
5. How can a polyp on a stalk be differentiated from fecal material?
6. What is the difference between sessile polyps and polyps on a stalk?

VOCABULARY

anorexia

colic

intussusception

nidus

paraneoplastic syndrome

pendunculated polyp

sessile polyp

thrombophlebitis

transition zone

SUGGESTIONS FOR FURTHER READING

William F. Coscina et. al. Gastrointestinal tract focal mass lesions: Role of CT and barium evaluations. *Radiology,* **158:581–587, 1986.**

For additional suggested reading see Chapter 35.

37

AREAS OF NARROWING

KEY CONCEPTS

Radiological

Areas of narrowing of the GI tract are common and can be normal (physiological) or abnormal. The normal areas of narrowing are caused by peristalsis and sphincters. The abnormal ones can be due to abnormal peristalsis, strictures, spasm, and masses.

Normal peristalsis is of three types: primary, secondary, and tertiary. In different portions of the GI tract, the proportions of these three types of peristalsis vary. *Primary peristalsis* is a wave of contraction starting at one end of an organ and sweeping to the other end. *Secondary peristalsis* starts in the middle of an organ and progresses toward its end. *Tertiary peristalsis* consists of contractions that tend to mix the contents of the gut rather than move the contents along the bowel.

Sphincters are regions of the gut that are normally contracted at rest and that relax as the waves of peristalsis reach them. Excessive relaxation or failure of a sphincter to relax are pathological changes in sphincters.

With acute inflammatory narrowings, the wall of the gut is stiff and the mucosa irregular. With strictures, the wall of the gut is usually flexible and can contract. Expansion of the lumen is limited to less than the normal luminal diameter.

Extrinsic masses usually cause an asymmetric narrowing of the lumen. Intrinsic masses can result in concentric or eccentric narrowing of the lumen. The mucosa can be irregular.

OBJECTIVES

When you complete this chapter you will be able to

1. Classify regions of narrowing on selected radiographs into physiological and pathological categories and subclassify them into the type of narrowing represented.

2. Describe primary, secondary, and tertiary peristalsis and name the organs in which each is normally found.
3. Describe a sphincter and list the three types of sphincter abnormalities.
4. List the causes of acute inflammatory narrowings.

There are two main types of narrowings, the physiological and the pathological. The physiological narrowings are the result of peristalsis and sphincters; the pathological narrowings include abnormal peristalsis, spasm, strictures, narrowings by mass, and areas of atresia.

PHYSIOLOGICAL NARROWINGS

The hollow tube that constitutes the GI tract is enveloped by circular and longitudinal muscle. In most portions of the hollow tube, the muscle is relaxed unless stimulated by nerve activity. In several selected portions, however, the muscle is contracted at rest and relaxes in response to nerve activity. The portions contracted at rest are sphincters. Peristaltic waves are usually stopped at sphincters and must originate anew beyond each one.

Normal Peristalsis

Almost all portions of the GI tract show the rhythmic or sequential contractions and dilations that constitute peristalsis. As a normal physiological activity, these contractions have two functions: they serve both to move material from one portion of the hollow tube to another and to mix the contents of the lumen to aid in digestion or absorption. As rhythmic or sequential contractions and dilations, the main key to recognizing them on imaging studies is their continuously changing appearance: areas of contraction will dilate and regions of dilatation will contract (Fig. 37-1).

Types of Peristalsis. There are three different physiological types of peristalsis, called primary, secondary, and tertiary. Primary peristalsis consists of waves of sequential propulsive contraction starting at the top end of an organ and progressing to its distal end. Primary peristalsis of the esophagus, for example, starts at the upper esophageal sphincter and progresses as a wave of contraction to the lower esophageal sphincter.

Secondary peristalsis is peristalsis that starts somewhere in the midportion of an organ and proceeds distally for a variable length, possibly only part way or all the way to the distal end of the organ. Tertiary peristalsis consists of segmental contractions of circular muscle enveloping a portion of an organ; it is nonpropulsive and serves primarily to mix the luminal contents. Different organs have different proportions of primary, secondary, and tertiary peristalsis.

Spasm is an exaggerated and sustained abnormal contraction of the circular muscles within an organ; it is often an exaggeration of the normal tertiary peristalsis (Fig. 37-2).

Sphincters

Sphincters are foci of normal physiological narrowing. Most sphincters are regions of circular muscle that are contracted without nerve activity and relax with nerve activity (Fig. 37-3). They are relatively short regions of luminal narrowing that occur at predictable sites: the upper and lower ends of the esophagus, the distal end of the stomach, the distal end of the pancreatic duct, the ileocecal junction, and the anus. As peristaltic waves reach them, they open in response and then contract again. They usually do not open quite as wide as the lumen on either side of them.

Keynotes

- *In most of the gut, the muscle is relaxed unless stimulated by nerve activity. Areas contracted at rest that relax in response to nerve stimulation are sphincters.*

- *Peristalsis is the sequential or rhythmic contraction of the smooth muscle surrounding the lumen of the gut or ureter.*

- *Peristalsis serves either to move luminal material from one portion of the hollow tube to another or to mix the luminal contents.*

- *Primary peristalsis is a propulsive peristalsis starting at the upper end of an organ and progressing to its distal end.*

- *Secondary peristalsis is peristalsis that propels the luminal contents through a limited portion of the organ.*

- *Tertiary peristalsis is nonpropulsive peristalsis. Physiologically, it serves to mix the luminal contents.*

- *Sphincters are short regions of luminal narrowing from muscle contraction. At sphincters, the muscles are contracted without nerve activity and dilate in response to nerve activity.*

PATHOLOGICAL NARROWINGS

Abnormalities of Peristalsis

Abnormalities of peristalsis are of three types: incorrect proportions of primary, secondary, and tertiary contractions; ineffective or weak contractions; and spasm. Each organ has its own proportion of the types of peristaltic waves, and changes in the relative frequency of these can be used to diagnose abnormalities. This subject is dicussed further in the chapters on each portion of the gut.

Abnormalities of Sphincters

The normal sphincter is a focal region of narrowing of the lumen of the hollow tube; contracted by active muscular contraction in the absence of innervation, it relaxes in response to nerve simulation. Abnormalities of sphincters are of three types: failure of muscle contraction to close off the lumen at rest, delay in relaxation of the sphincter, and failure of relaxation of the sphincter in response to an approaching peristaltic waves. Of these, lack of effective contraction is most common.

Inappropriate Relaxation of a Sphincter. Sphincters normally function to control the movement of the contents of one portion of the GI tract to another. The pylorus serves to limit the rate of movement of gastric contents into the duodenum; the anus controls emptying of the colon. The upper esophageal sphincter helps prevent air from entering the esophagus during breathing. The other sphincters function mainly to prevent reflux of material: the upper esophageal sphincter helps prevent regurgitation from the esophagus into the mouth, the lower esophageal sphincter helps prevent gastroesophageal reflux and heartburn, and the ileocecal valve limits reflux from the colon into the ileum. Lack of adequate contraction of the sphinters, *chalasia,* can result in specific symptoms. Those of common clinical importance are discussed in the chapters on specific organs.

Failure of Relaxation of a Sphincter. Failure of relaxation of a sphincter in response to a peristaltic wave is the second identifiable abnormality of sphincters. Two different types of relaxation failure are seen: a brief, momentary delay and a prolonged or constant delay.

Brief Delay in Sphincter Opening. A brief delay in sphincter opening can result in increased pressure within the lumen proximal to the sphincter. This is of clinical importance in the pharynx and esophagus, where this failure of relaxation can result in diverticula (see Chapter 38) just proximal to the sphincter, for example, Zenker's diverticulum of the lower pharynx (Fig. 37-4). Even in those patients who do not develop a diverticulum, the slight delay in sphincter opening can be recognized in the pharynx as a tightness or the sensation of a lump in the throat.

Prolonged Delay in Sphincter Opening. Prolonged failure of opening of a sphincter can cause pharyngeal or esopha-

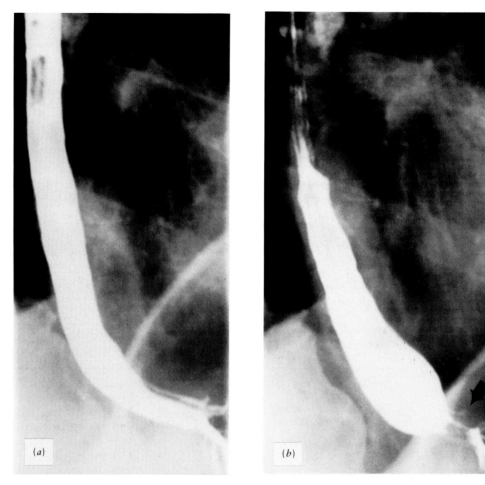

Figure 37-1. Esophageal peristalsis. (*a*) The esophagus is filled with barium, which then flows into the stomach. (*b*) A peristaltic wave is starting to strip the barium from the midesophagus. Because the lower esophageal sphincter (arrow) has partially closed, the lower esophagus is more dilated than it was in (*a*). (*c*) The lower esophageal sphincter has relaxed, and peristalsis has continued to empty the esophagus. (*d*) Only the lower esophagus now contains barium. The remainder of the barium has been pushed into the stomach by the peristalsis.

geal symptoms. In the pharynx, myotonia can result in prolonged contraction of the pharyngeal musculature. In the lower esophagus, failure of relaxation of the lower esophageal sphincter in response to peristalsis is called *achalasia,* a disease in which progressive dilation of the esophagus develops (Fig. 37-5).

Keynotes

- *The inappropriate relaxation of sphincters permits luminal contents to pass freely from one portion of the gut to another.*
- *A brief delay in the opening of a sphincter can cause a diverticulum to be pushed out (a pulsion diverticulum). It can cause the sensation of a lump in the throat.*
- *Prolonged failure to open of the lower esophageal sphincter is called* achalasia. *It results in retrosternal pain, regurgitation, aspiration, pneumonia, and weight loss.*

Acute Inflammatory Narrowings

Acute inflammation can result in narrowing of the tube from a combination of spasm and mucosal edema (Fig. 37-6). The inflammation can be due to infection (moniliasis, amebiasis, diverticulitis), chemical irritations (ingested lye or acid burns, pancreatitis), or idiopathic disease (Crohn's disease). Each of these processes results in mucosal edema, mucosal destruction, and spasm. Each is reversible to differing degrees. The main method of recognition is to note the thickening and, in some cases, the irregularity of the mucosa combined with the luminal narrowing. Often the luminal shape does not change during the study, demonstrating that the wall is stiffened. Because of the combination of mucosal damage and wall stiffness, acute inflammatory narrowings can be confused with mucosal neoplastic processes, and the radiological differentiation may be difficult.

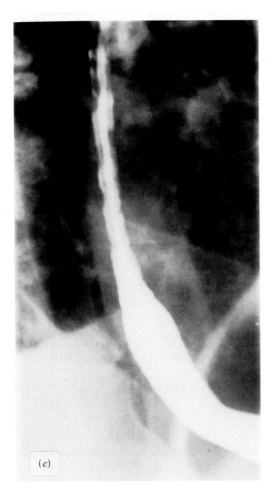

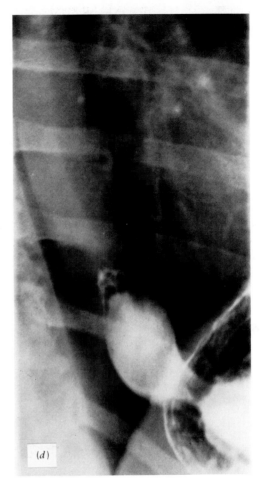

Figure 37.1. (Continued)

Strictures

In most *strictures,* the wall is not stiff; instead, a stricture functions as a limit to the expansion of the lumen. Peristaltic waves can pass through it, narrowing it further, but at the site of stricture, complete distention of the lumen does not occur (Fig. 37-7). Most strictures have long, tapered ends so that a moderately gentle narrowing occurs over a long segment of the bowel. An occasional stricture is short, with an abrupt transition, but these are less common.

Narrowings by Mass

Masses that narrow the GI tract can be of three types: intrinsic mucosal masses, intrinsic nonmucosal masses, and extrinsic masses. Each of these have specific features more fully dicussed in Chapter 36.

Intrinsic Mucosal Masses

Apple-Core Pattern. Mucosal masses that narrow the lumen share three properties: the wall is stiff, the transition from the adjacent normal mucosa is abrupt, and the mucosa usually looks irregular or destroyed (Fig. 37-8). This fixed pattern is usually called an *apple-core* pattern because it looks like the chewed-upon core of an apple. Most mucosal masses that look like apple cores are malignant masses, though occasionally colonic diverticulosis with an extrinsic mass from an abscess can simulate this appearance.

Some narrowings caused by cancer can simulate the tapered transition zone of benign strictures (Fig. 37-9). This occurs in the colon, either in young patients or in patients with ulcerative colitis.

Overhanging Edges. One of the signs indicative of the abrupt transition at the junction of normal mucosa and

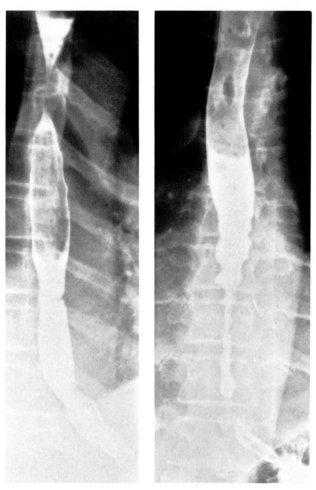

Figure 37-2. Esophageal spasm in a patient with peptic esophagitis. The marked irregular narrowing of the lower esophagus reflects the spasm induced by iced barium. The diagnosis of peptic esophagitis can be confirmed by demonstrating that acidified barium will induce esophageal spasm whereas nonacidified barium will not. The iced barium used in this case is less specific.

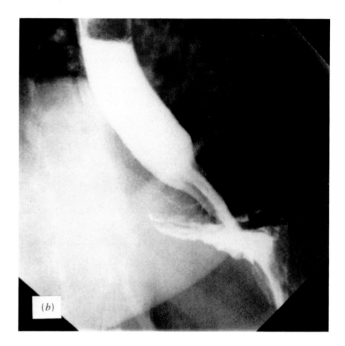

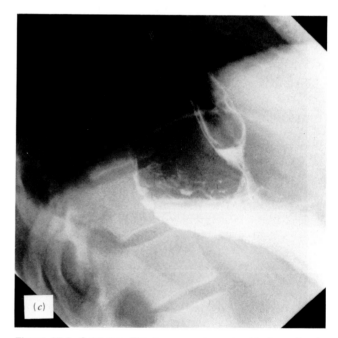

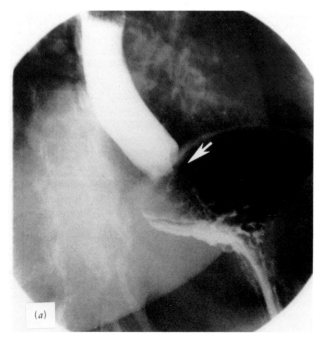

Figure 37-3. Sphincter. The lower esophageal sphincter action is demonstrated. (*a*) The esophagus contains some barium. The lower esophageal sphincter (arrow) is closed. (*b*) The lower esophageal sphincter is now open. This was the maximal opening demonstrated in this swallow; its luminal diameter is less than that of the esophagus. (*c*) The esophagus is almost empty of barium. The sphincter is narrower than in (*b*).

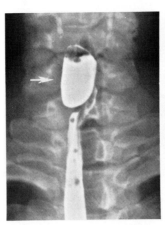
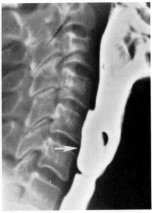

Figure 37-4. A Zenker's diverticulum (arrows). These posterior diverticula occur at the level of the upper esophageal sphincter and are caused by a brief failure of relaxation of this sphincter.

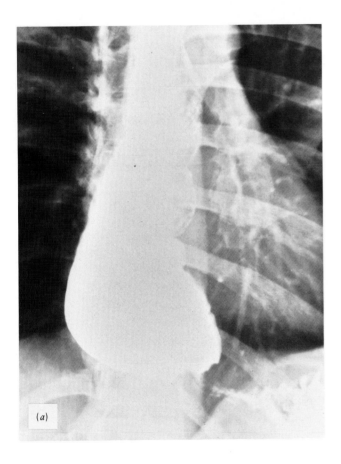

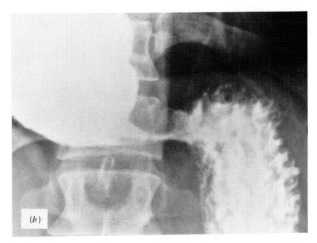

Figure 37-5. Achalasia. (*a*) The prolonged failure of relaxation of the lower esophageal sphincter results in a markedly dilated esophagus. The focal view (*b*) demonstrates the incomplete opening of the sphincter.

the mass is *overhanging edges* (Fig. 37-8). Because the normal wall is flexible, it can be distended by the barium, and the expanded lumen will balloon around the mucosal mass, resulting in overhanging edges.

Intrinsic Nonmucosal Masses. Intrinsic nonmucosal masses, called *mural masses,* usually indent the lumen from one side, rather than envelop it (see Fig. 36-8). Thus

they appear eccentric. The mucosa is usually intact over them, stretched and smooth. The wall at the site of the mass is rigid, and there is an abrupt change from the normal wall to the site of the mass.

Extrinsic Masses. Extrinsic masses usually displace rather than narrow the lumen of the GI tract. Less commonly, fixed portions of gut, such as the duodenal sweep

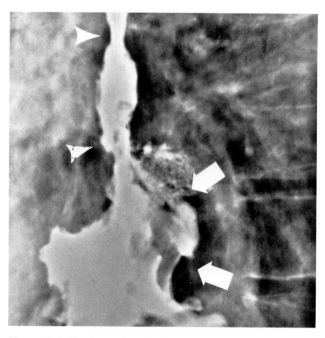

Figure 37-6. Peptic esophagitis. An acute inflammatory stricture (arrowheads) demonstrates irregular narrowing above an area of herniation of the stomach into the chest (a hiatal hernia) (arrows).

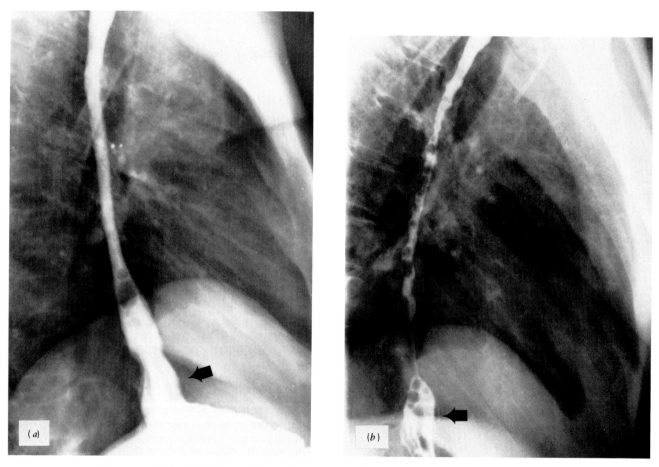

Figure 37-7. Chronic stricture of the esophagus years after a suicide attempt by lye ingestion. The esophagus is narrowed. There is a hiatal hernia (arrows). (a) Maximal distension of the esophagus during swallowing. (b) After passage of the barium, the esophagus is narrower. Despite the marked narrowing seen in (a), the esophagus is even more narrow after most of the barium has passed (b).

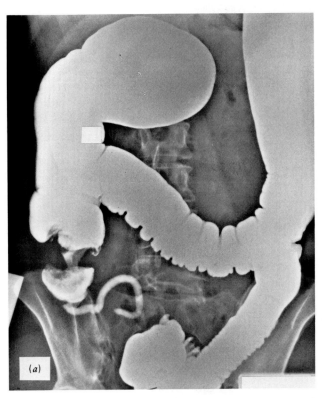

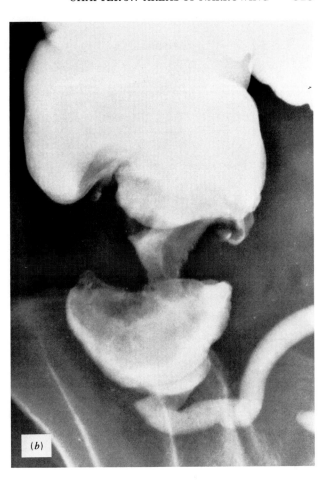

Figure 37-8. Apple-core lesion of the cecum, from colon cancer. (*a*) Full film of the barium-filled colon. (*b*) Focal view of the cecum demonstrates the apple-core lesion. There is marked focal narrowing with an abrupt transition to normal colon both above and below the lesion.

or rectum, may be pressed on by an adjacent mass and narrowed. Uncommonly, an extrinsic mass can envelop a portion of the GI tract, narrowing it (see Fig. 36-2). When narrowing occurs in this last group, the narrowing is usually asymmetrical, and the lumen tapers from normal into the narrowed segment. Peristalsis can pass through the region of narrowing, and for these reasons, the region of narrowing will resemble that from a benign chronic stricture. When there is clinical uncertainty as to whether the narrowing is due to a stricture or an adjacent mass, sonography or transmission CT can be used to demonstrate the presence or absence of a mass.

Keynotes

- *Acute inflammatory narrowing results from a combination of spasm and mucosal edema.*
- *Strictures are regions of fibrosis thickening of the wall of the gut that limit luminal expansion. The margins of a stricture are usually tapered.*
- *Overhanging edges are a sign of the abrupt transition from the normal gut wall to the enveloping mucosal mass.*

SUMMARY

Regions of narrowing are common in the gut. Normal peristalsis repetitively narrows the gut, but as the muscle relaxes, the lumen dilates to normal diameter. Peristalsis is one of three types: primary, secondary, or tertiary. Abnormalities of peristalsis can be abnormal proportions of primary, secondary, and tertiary peristalsis or weak or absent contractions.

Sphincters are portions of the gut in which muscle is contracted at rest, narrowing the lumen. A sphincter dilates as a peristaltic wave reaches it. Abnormalities of sphincters are due to their failure to relax in response to a peristaltic wave or to their failure to contract and occlude the lumen.

Acute inflammation can narrow the lumen, usually by a combination of edema and spasm. The wall is usually stiff, the mucosa irregular. Strictures usually have flexible walls. The lumen is of decreased diameter. Narrowings from mural and extrinsic masses are usually eccentric narrowings. They are discussed more fully in Chapter 36.

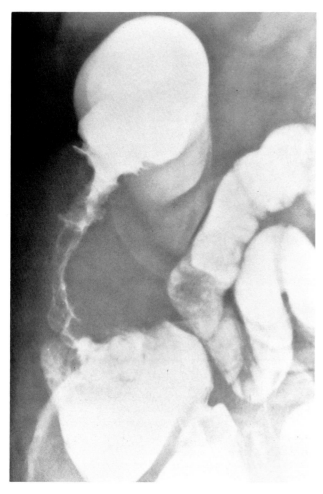

Figure 37-9. A tapered appearance of a colon cancer. In this patient, the transition from the cancer to the normal bowel is more gradual, resulting in the tapered appearance. This is a less common appearance of colon cancer.

REVIEW QUESTIONS

1. What is peristalsis?
2. What are the types of peristalsis?
3. What is a sphincter?
4. What are the three types of abnormalities of sphincters?
5. What are some of the causes of acute inflammatory narrowings?
6. What is the radiographic appearance of acute inflammatory narrowing?
7. What is a stricture? What is its radiographic appearance?
8. What is the radiographic appearance of luminal narrowing from a mass?
9. What is an apple-core lesion?
10. What is the significance of overhanging edges?

VOCABULARY

achalasia	primary peristalsis
apple-core lesion	secondary peristalsis
chalasia	sphincter
Crohn's disease	stricture
overhanging edges	tertiary peristalsis
peristalsis	

SUGGESTIONS FOR FURTHER READING

For suggested reading see Chapter 35.

38

OUTPOUCHINGS

KEY CONCEPTS

Radiological

Outpouchings from the gut can be diverticula, ulcers, or ulcers in neoplasms. The prime differentiating feature is that diverticula have flexible walls, but ulcers and ulcers in neoplasms have fixed walls.

Diverticula are of four types: congential with muscle in their wall; congenital without muscle in the diverticular wall; acquired and caused by traction on the gut; and acquired and caused by pulsion, a pushing out of the gut mucosa.

Benign ulcers are those unassociated with neoplasms. There are several signs of a benign ulcer, but these signs apply mainly to large ulcers. Ulcers of the duodenal bulb are essentially always benign. Ulcers in neoplasms can often be recognized by finding signs of the neoplastic mass in the region adjacent to the ulcer. Most ulcers are small and do not demonstrate signs that would permit accurate differentiation between benign ulceration and ulceration in a neoplasm. Further evaluation of these indeterminate ulcers is usually by endoscopy.

OBJECTIVES

When you complete this chapter you will be able to

1. Differentiate diverticula, benign ulcers, ulcers in neoplasms, and indeterminate ulcers on selected radiographs.
2. List the four types of diverticula.
3. List two characteristics of a benign ulcer.
4. List three criteria of an ulcer in a neoplasm.
5. List the two methods of evaluation of an indeterminate ulcer.

Outpouchings are of three main types: diverticula, benign ulcers, and ulcers in neoplasms. A fourth pattern resembling an outpouching, the pseudodiverticulum, occurs only in the duodenal bulb and is discussed in Chapter 42. The differentiation of a diverticulum from a benign ulcer from an ulcer in a neoplasm depends on three main determinants:

Is the wall flexible or fixed?

Is there a mass?

Does the outpouching extend beyond the expected location of the wall of the gut?

Keynotes

- *The three types of outpouchings are diverticula, benign ulcers, and ulcers in neoplasms.*
- *The criteria used to evaluate outpouchings are wall flexibililty, the presence or absence of a mass, and whether the outpouching extends beyond the outside of the gut wall.*

DIVERTICULA

Diverticula usually have flexible walls and because of this have variable degrees of filling. Most diverticula (all common ones) are outpouchings that extend beyond the expected site of the wall of the gut (Fig. 38-1).

Diverticula are of four types, two congenital and two acquired. The congenital diverticula are divided by whether they have muscle in their wall (like *Meckel's diverticulum*) or no muscle in their wall (like the congenital diverticula of the mid-to-upper esophagus). Diverticula

315

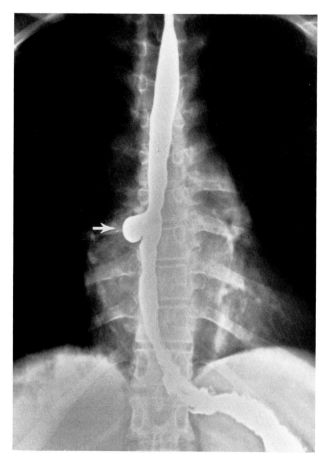

Figure 38-1. A midesophageal diverticulum, probably congenital type. The diverticulum (arrow) extends beyond the expected location of the wall of the esophagus.

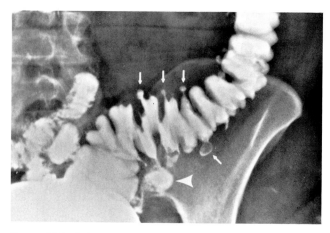

Figure 38-2. Colonic diverticulosis with focal diverticulitis. Several small pulsion diverticula (arrows) are seen in the descending and sigmoid colon in this older man. There is focal communication of one of these diverticula with a small abscess cavity (arrowhead). Some, but not all, patients with diverticulitis will demonstrate communication of a diverticulum with an abscess cavity. Demonstration of this communication is diagnostic of diverticulitis.

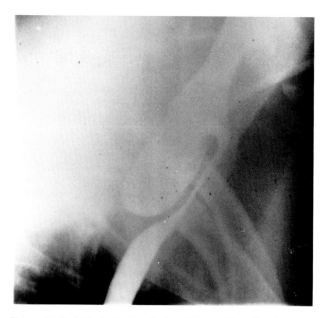

Figure 38-3. A Zenker's diverticulum. This pulsion diverticulum of the upper esophagus occurs at the level of the cricopharyngeus muscle. The diverticulum is pushed out by the muscular contraction of the pharynx pushing against a nonrelaxed cricopharyngeus muscle. The mucosa of the esophagus herniates at a site of relative weakness of the esophageal wall.

with muscle in their wall are often hard to demonstrate with barium because their active peristalsis empties them.

Acquired diverticula may be formed by the wall being pulled out by an adjacent inflammatory scar (*traction diverticula*) or by the mucosa being pushed out because of increased intraluminal pressure (*pulsion diverticula*). Traction diverticula are most often seen in the midesophagus caused by the pull from adjacent subcarinal scarring (though many diverticula of the midesophagus are congential, others are traction diverticula). Traction diverticula are usually asymptomatic.

Pulsion diverticula are mucosal diverticula pushed out because of increased intraluminal pressure. They are most common in the left side of the colon (Fig. 38-2) and also occur in the upper esophagus (Zenker's diverticulum Fig. 38-3). Pulsion diverticula are often associated with symptoms that can result from the increased intraluminal pressure that causes the diverticulum to form, from the diverticulum itself or from rupture of the diverticulum. Pulsion diverticula are discussed more extensively in chapters 40 and 43.

Keynotes

- *Diverticula have flexible walls. They change shape and size.*
- *The Meckel's diverticulum occurs in the distal third of the ileum. It is a remnant of the embryonic yolk stalk.*

• *Traction diverticula occur when the wall of the gut is pulled on by an adjacent inflammatory scar.*
• *Pulsion diverticula are pushed out by increased intraluminal pressure.*

BENIGN ULCERS AND ULCERS IN NEOPLASMS

In most cases it is not possible to use radiological criteria to differentiate benign ulcers from ulcers in neoplasms. Indeed, the major purpose of the barium study of the gut is to find the ulcer; once found, endoscopy is generally used to determine if neoplasm is present.

Methods of Excluding Neoplasms in an Ulcer

Ulcers of the duodenal bulb are essentially always benign. This is because neoplasms of the duodenal bulb are extremely rare, and the few found are usually metastatic, with other foci visible in the gut. Ulcers that penetrate through the wall of the stomach into the adjacent soft tissues are almost always benign, because gastric neoplasms rarely extend directly into the adjacent soft tissue (Fig. 38-4). Several additional signs of benign ulcers can be used, but they are seldom seen.

Methods of Showing an Ulcer Is in a Neoplasm

Radiological techniques are somewhat better at showing that an ulcer is in a neoplasm than they are at showing that an ulcer is benign. Recognizing that an ulcer is in a neoplasm depends upon recognizing the presence of the neoplasm—identifying the irregular mucosal mass and demonstrating ulceration of a portion of it (Fig. 38-5). A nodular mucosa, an irregular mucosa, and thickened mu-

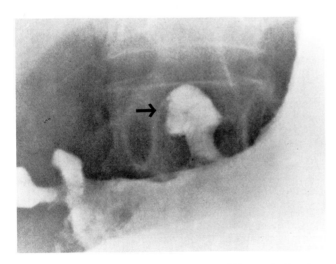

Figure 38-4. Benign penetrating gastric ulcer. This penetrating ulcer (arrow) extends well beyond the expected location of the wall of the stomach. Such penetrating ulcers are almost always nonneoplastic.

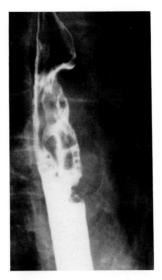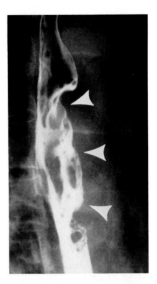

Figure 38-5. Esophageal cancer. This irregular midesophageal mass contains a large ulcer (arrowheads) in its midportion. On biopsy, this 58-year-old man was found to have esophageal cancer.

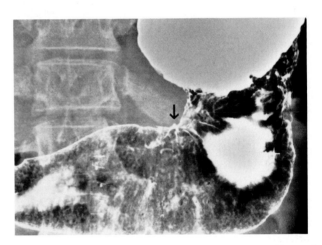

Figure 38-6. Small, ulcerated gastric cancer. Adjacent to this small ulcer (arrow), the mucosa is nodular, indicating the presence of neoplasia. (Courtesy of Jerry Patt, M.D.)

cosal folds can each demonstrate the neoplastic infiltration (Fig. 38-6). This is why the term *ulcer in neoplasm* may be preferable to the term *malignant ulcer:* the first tells you what to look for on the radiograph.

The Indeterminate Ulcer

Most ulcers found within the gut will not demonstrate the specific signs of a benign ulcer (Figs. 38-7 and 38-8), and only a few will demonstrate nodular or irregular mucosa, thickened folds, or a neoplastic mass that permits a confident diagnosis of ulcer in neoplasm. Excluding duodenal bulb ulcers, those ulcers not definitely benign or in neoplasms are *indeterminate ulcers* and must either be fol-

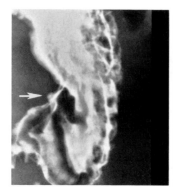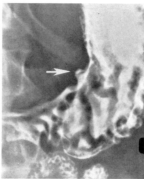

Figure 38-7. This small indeterminate ulcer (arrows) proved to be benign on endoscopic biopsy.

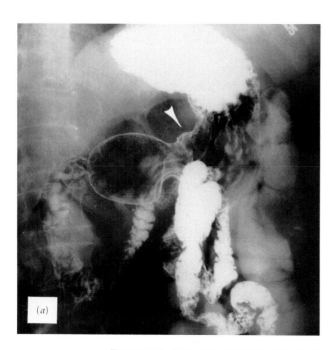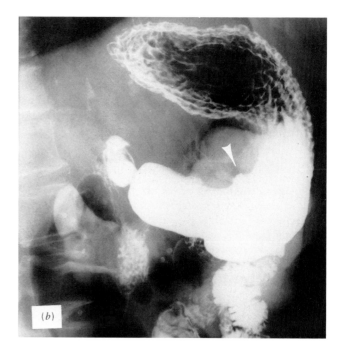

Figure 38-8. This medium-sized gastric ulcer (arrowheads) is slightly more nodular but was considered indeterminate. An endoscopic biopsy specimen demonstrated gastric cancer with ulceration. (*a*) Double-contrast view. (*b*) Single-contrast view.

lowed for evidence of prompt healing after appropriate therapy or, if the patient is in a cancer age group, be studied with endoscopy and an endoscopic biopsy. Only large ulcers can demonstrate the radiographic signs that permit them to be considered definitely benign, so most small ulcers must be classed indeterminate.

The Barrett Ulcer. The esophagus repeatedly exposed to gastric juice from gastroesophageal reflux can develop a mucosal change from squamous to columnar epithelium. At the margin between the normal squamous epithelium and the metaplastic columnar epithelium, ulcers can develop (The Barrett's ulcer in the Barrett's esophagus).

These ulcers often have large amounts of edema surrounding them and can appear to be ulcers in neoplasms (Fig. 38-9).

Keynotes

- *A benign ulcer is an ulcer unassociated with a malignant neoplasm. It may still result in severe symptoms.*
- *The main purpose of the barium study is to find the ulcer, not to tell whether it is associated with neoplasm.*
- *Ulcers of the duodenal bulb are almost always not in a neoplasm.*
- *Penetrating gastric ulcers are almost always unassociated with neoplasm.*

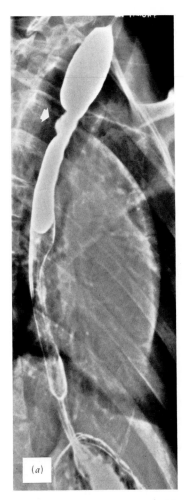 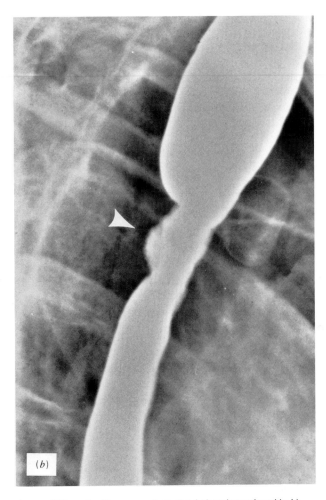

Figure 38-9. Barrett's ulcer of the esophagus. This patient has a medium-sized ulcer (arrowhead in *b*) of the upper esophagus. He had a long history of peptic esophagitis. An endoscopic biopsy specimen excluded malignancy and demonstrated the mucosal changes of Barrett's esophageal mucosal change. (*a*) Oblique view of the esophagus. (*b*) Focal view of the ulcer.

- *A neoplasm associated with an ulcer is recognized because of its mass, irregular mucosa, nodular mucosa, or thickened mucosal folds.*
- *A "malignant ulcer" is an ulcer associated with neoplasm. The ulcer itself is not neoplastic. The term ulcer in neoplasm is preferred.*
- *Those ulcers not definitely benign or associated with neoplasms are classified as indeterminate. They require further evaluation to exclude neoplasm.*

SUMMARY

Outpouchings from the gut can be due to diverticula, benign ulcers, or ulcers in neoplasms. Diverticula have flexible walls. The congenital forms may or may not have muscle in their walls. The acquired diverticula can be due to traction from an adjacent inflammatory process or to pul-

sion, being pushed out by increased or discoordinated muscle contractions of the gut.

Ulcers can be benign or in neoplasms. Small ulcers are usually indeterminate; The radiograph often does not have sufficient information to permit the differentiation of a benign ulcer from an ulcer in a neoplasm. Ulcers in the duodenal bulb are almost always benign. Ulcers that penetrate beyond the outer limit of the gastric wall are usually benign.

An ulcer may be the first sign of neoplasm. The main criterion for determining that the ulcer is in a neoplasm is the presence of signs of neoplasm: irregular mucosa, an irregular mass, or an asymmetric mass around the ulcer.

REVIEW QUESTIONS

1. What are the three types of outpouchings from the gut?
2. Name a congenital diverticulum with muscle in its wall.

3. What is a traction diverticulum?
4. What is a pulsion diverticulum?
5. How can you tell that an ulcer is unassociated with a neoplasm?
6. How can you tell that an ulcer is in a neoplasm?
7. What is an indeterminate ulcer?
8. How should a radiographically indeterminate ulcer be evaluated clinically?

VOCABULARY

benign ulcer	pulsion diverticulum
indeterminate ulcer	traction diverticulum

"malignant ulcer"   ulcer in neoplasm
Meckel's diverticulum

SUGGESTIONS FOR FURTHER READING

For suggested reading see Chapter 35.

39

LUMINAL CONTENTS, MUCOSAL CHANGE, AND CHANGES IN SIZE

KEY CONCEPTS

Luminal Contents: Radiological

The content of the gut lumen is usually of no pathological significance, but it does interfere with the interpretation of contrast studies of the stomach and bowel. Recently swallowed food is the most common stomach content, feces the most common colon content.

Prolonged retention of food in the stomach can result from gastric outlet obstruction or diminished gastric peristalsis. A bezoar is a conglomerate mass of swallowed hair or plant fiber.

Abnormalities of Mucosa: Radiological

Thickened mucosal folds can indicate edema, inflammation, infiltration by tumor, hyperplasia, submucosal venous distension, or submucosal hemorrhage. Absent or shallow folds can be due to atrophy, tumor infiltration or fibrosis. Spiculated folds can be due to infection or inflammation.

Changes in Luminal Size: Radiological

Decreased luminal size is usually due to surgery, less often to stricture. Increased luminal size is usually caused by distal obstruction but can also result from atrophy or from infiltration of gut musculature.

OBJECTIVES

When you complete this chapter you will be able to

1. Identify, on selected radiographs or CT images, gastric contents and feces and differentiate them from polyps and tumor masses.

2. List the three main causes of prolonged retention of gastric contents.
3. List three causes of gastric outlet obstruction and three causes of decreased gastric peristalsis.
4. Identify, on selected radiographs, thickened mucosal folds, absent or shallow mucosal folds, and spiculated mucosal folds and differentiate them from normal.
5. List three causes of thickened mucosal folds.
6. List three causes of absent or shallow folds.
7. List two causes of spiculated folds.
8. List the main cause of increased luminal size.
9. List three causes of decreased luminal size.

This chapter discusses three additional basic patterns of abnormality that can be seen in the GI tract:

1. Luminal contents
2. Mucosal change
3. Changes in size

LUMINAL CONTENTS

There are two types of luminal contents: those of no concern, and those of pathological significance. Recently swallowed food is the most common luminal content of the stomach; feces is the most common luminal content of the colon. Most of the time, the significance of the presence of food or feces is that it may prevent adequate evaluation of the portion of the GI tract under study. Sometimes, however, there is an additional significance implied.

Prolonged Retention of Food in the Stomach

Prolonged retention of food in the stomach is usually an artifact of the patient's concealment of when she or he last ate. When this artifact is excluded, two processes must be considered:

1. Gastric outlet obstruction, usually caused by gastric or pyloric ulcer disease, gastric cancer, or hypertrophic muscle with pyloric obstruction
2. Diminished gastric peristalsis, usually resulting from surgical vagotomy, diabetic gastroenteropathy, or scleroderma.

A *bezoar,* a conglomerate mass of swallowed hair, plant fiber, persimmon fruit, or metal objects, can in some cases be confused with retained food in the stomach.

Appearance of Food in the Stomach. Food in the stomach on a plain film of the abdomen can appear as a mixed pattern of irregular radiolucent areas in the left upper quadrant of the abdomen (Figs. 39-1 and 39-2). Food mixed with barium shows as multiple radiolucencies within the barium (Figs. 39-3 and 39-4). Occasionally, small amounts of food can be confused with polyps but can be differentiated because they are not restricted to one location.

Retained Feces in the Colon

On the plain film of the abdomen, feces may not be visible or they may appear as either a mottled area of air radiolucency (Fig. 39-5) or as moderate-to-large masses within an air-containing portion of the colon (Fig. 39-6). In some patients, the feces contain foci of increased radiodensity; uncommonly, feces are of increased radiodensity.

When the colon is filled with barium, feces show as multiple radiolucent filling defects, large or small, within

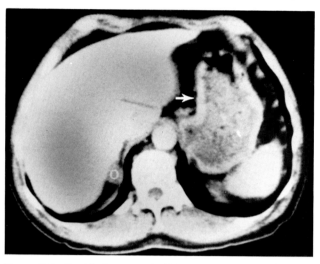

Figure 39-2. Food in the stomach, CT scan appearance. The food in the stomach (arrow) shows a mixed pattern of air within fluid-radiodensity material.

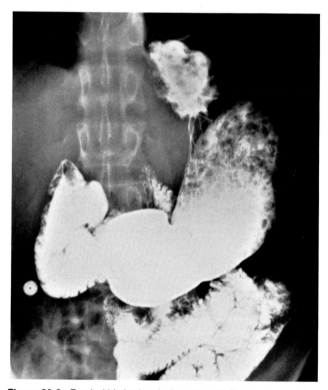

Figure 39-3. Food within barium in the stomach. The irregular radiolucencies within the barium are caused by the presence of food. The importance of not eating the morning of an upper GI series so food will not interfere with the accuracy of diagnosis must be stressed with patients.

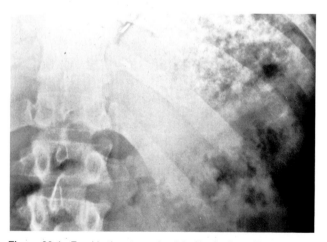

Figure 39-1. Food in the stomach, plain-film findings. There is mottled radiodensity and radiolucency in the left upper quadrant of the abdomen. This is one of the appearances of food in the stomach. Surgical clips, from a previous hiatal hernia repair, can be seen near the spine.

the barium (Fig. 39-7). Most of these scybala are free in the lumen and can be displaced as the barium flows past them. This is the major method of judging, on a single-contrast barium enema film, if a filling defect is indeed feces. On the double-contrast barium enema, the views

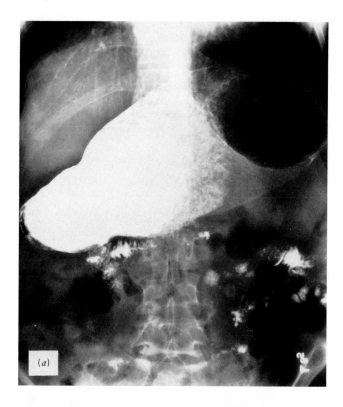

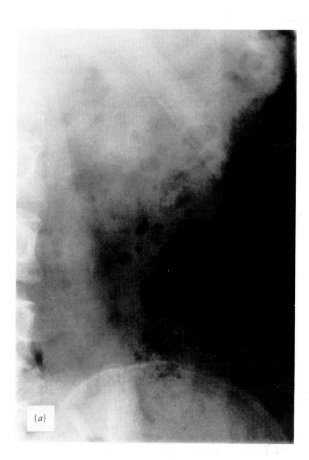

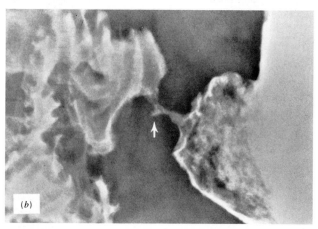

Figure 39-4. Acute gastric retention, with food and secretions mixed with the barium in the stomach. (*a*) The enlarged, filled stomach demonstrates the mixture of radiodense and radiolucent material. (*b*) This focal view of the pylorus demonstrates a pyloric channel ulcer (arrow), which was the cause of the gastric retention. The two main causes of gastric retention in adults are pyloric channel ulcers and distal gastric cancers.

obtained to show air-barium levels (the upright and lateral decubitus views) are the most helpful; feces will stay within the barium, while a true polyp or mass will maintain its relationship to the air-filled portion of the colonic wall.

Adherent Feces. Less commonly, scybala of feces will adhere to the colonic wall and can simulate sessile polypoid

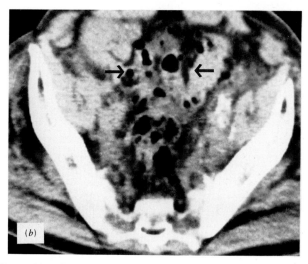

Figure 39-5. Feces in the colon. (*a*) On the plain abdominal film, feces can appear as a mixture of bubbles of air in water-radiodensity feces. Sometimes the feces themselves are of increased radiodensity. The amount of air in feces is variable. (*b*) On the CT exam, feces also appear with bubbles of air (arrows) within the feces. In this case, some of the bowel is faintly opacified by a contrast medium that the patient swallowed hours before.

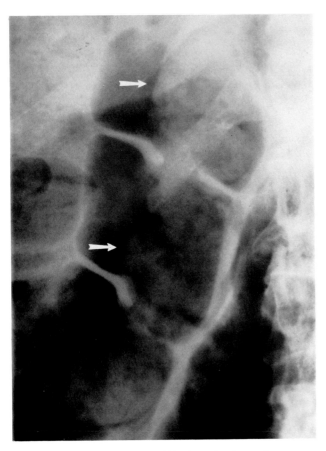

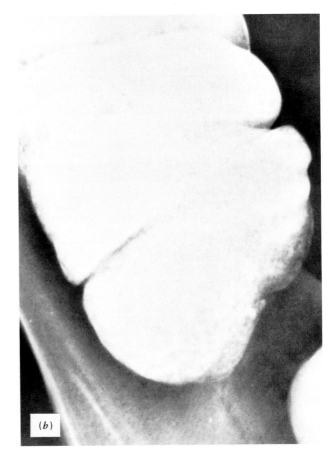

Figure 39-6. Clumps of feces within the colon (arrows) appear as more radiodense areas within the colonic air.

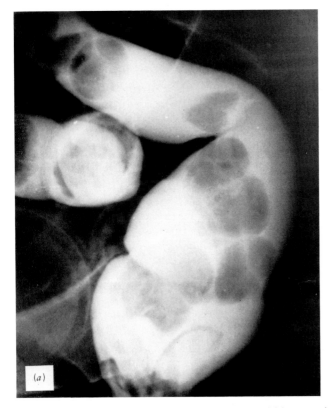

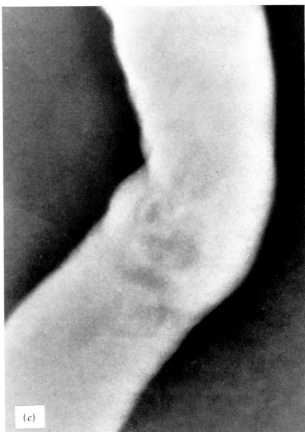

Figure 39-7. Feces within barium. (*a*) Large scybala of feces within barium in the rectosigmoid portion of the colon appear as darker filling defects within the white barium. (*b*) Punctate areas of feces within barium give a granular appearance to the barium in this view of the cecum. (*c*) Intermediate-sized scybala of feces could be confused with a polyp or mass in the descending colon of this patient.

TABLE 39-1. THICKENED FOLDS

	Esophagus	Stomach	Duodenum	Small Bowel	Colon
Common	Varices Esophagitis	Hypertrophic gastritis Lymphoma Varices	Duodenitis (peptic ulcer disease)		Colitis "Spastic" diverticulosis
Uncommon but important	Varicoid carcinoma	Carcinoma Zollinger-Ellison syndrome	Zollinger-Ellison syndrome	Whipple's disease Malabsorption syndromes	Intramural hemorrhage Crohn's disease Adjacent inflammation
Uncommon	Corrosive esophagitis	Ménétrier's disease	Varices Pancreatitis	Hypoalbuminemia Intestinal lymphagiectasia Obstruction Amyloidosis Parasitic disease Giardiasis	Associated with distal obstruction

TABLE 39-2. SHALLOW OR ABSENT FOLDS

	Esophagus	Stomach	Duodenal Bulb	Small Bowel	Colon
			DIFFUSE		
Common	Normal	Atrophic gastritis Pernicious Anemia	Normal		Laxative abuse
Uncommon		Carcinoma	Giant ulcer		Late ulcerative colitis
			FOCAL		
Common	Carcinoma	Carcinoma Scar (prior ulcer) Lymphoma		Lymphoma Carcinoma	Carcinoma Inactive ulcerative colitis

lesions. When the colon is otherwise clean of feces, this is unlikely to occur. When there is other evidence of feces, it may be necessary to confirm the presence of the polyp or mass by repeating the barium enema or by colonoscopy.

The chance of detecting a mucosal abnormality on radiographic colon studies is much increased if the colon is clean. It is most important that the colon-cleaning preparation used in your hospital be closely adhered to for optimal results.

Keynotes

- *Recently swallowed food is the most common luminal content of the stomach; feces is the most common luminal content of the colon.*
- *Prolonged retention of food in the stomach can be due to gastric outlet obstruction or diminished gastric peristalsis.*
- *A bezoar is a conglomerate mass of plant fiber, hair, or metal objects in the stomach.*
- *A scybalum is a hard mass of feces in the lumen of the colon.*
- *Most scybala of feces are free in the lumen and shift position with barium flow. In double-contrast studies, they usually fall to the dependent side of the lumen.*

ABNORMALITIES OF MUCOSA

The mucosal markings can be thicker than normal, shallower than normal, absent, or spiculated. Although there is some organ-to-organ variability, the patterns often reflect the same types of diseases. Thickened folds can indicate edema (often caused by inflammation), infiltration by tumor (often lymphoma as in Fig. 39-8, sometimes carcinoma), hyperplasia (from known or unknown stimulus), submucosal venous distention (Fig. 39-9), or submucosal hemorrhage. Absent or shallow folds can be due to atrophy (Fig. 39-10), tumor infiltration, or fibrosis. Spiculated folds can be due to infection or inflammation (Fig. 39-11) and can be simulated by spasm. Some of the diseases resulting in these changes are summarized in Tables 39-1, 39-2, and 39-3.

CHANGES IN LUMINAL SIZE

Portions of the gut can be diffusely or focally larger or smaller than normal. Increased luminal size is usually due to obstruction or decreased motor activity. Decreased luminal size is most often due to surgery; less often it is

TABLE 39-3. SPICULATED FOLDS

	Esophagus	Stomach	Duodenal Bulb	Colon
Common	Peptic Esophagitis		Peptic ulcer disease	Diverticular disease
Uncommon	Intramural diverticulosis	Erosive gastritis		Ulcerative colitis Granulomatous colitis Amebiasis

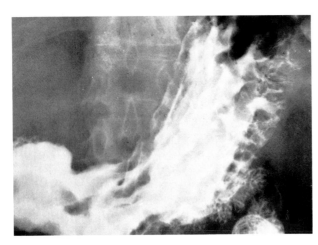

Figure 39-8. Thickened gastric rugal folds can be compared with the normal folds in Figure 34-3b. These thickened folds were caused by infiltration by lymphosarcoma.

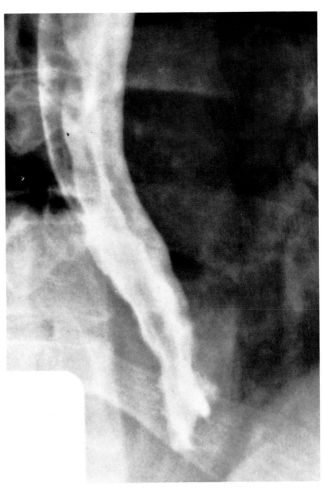

Figure 39-9. Thickened esophageal folds caused by varices. Esophageal varices are usually due to portal venous hypertension from liver disease.

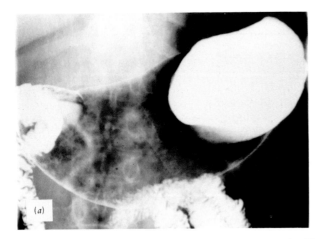

Figure 39-10. The gastric folds in this elderly woman are atrophic and cannot be seen. Not all patients with gastric atrophy demonstrate radiological evidence of gastric atrophy. Gastric mucosal atrophy is associated with aging, pernicious anemia, and gastric cancer. (a) Air-barium double-contrast appearance. (b) Barium-filled appearance. (Both courtesy R. Greyson-Fleg, M.D.)

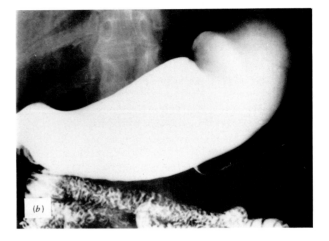

326

TABLE 39-4. CHANGES IN SIZE

	Esophagus	Stomach	Duodenum	Small Bowel	Colon
	LARGER THAN NORMAL: DIFFUSE				
Common	Obstruction (peptic disease) Carcinoma Achalasia	Obstruction (peptic ulcer disease) Hypertrophic pyloric stenosis	Normal variation	Obstruction Adynamic ileus	Obstruction (volvulus, carcinoma) Adynamic ileus Chronic constipation Anal stricture Anal fissure
Uncommon	Lack of contractility Scleroderma	Lack of contractility Postvagotomy Diabetic neuropathy	Giant duodenal ulcer	Scleroderma Malabsorption syndromes Diabetic enteropathy Postvagotomy	Hirschsprung's disease Institutional colon Parkinson's disease Hypothyrodism
	LARGER THAN NORMAL: FOCAL				
Common	Diverticula			Lymphoma	
Uncommon					Diverticula
	SMALLER THAN NORMAL: DIFFUSE				
Common	Stricture (peptic disease, cancer)	Surgery	Scarring (ulcer disease)	Surgery Crohn's disease Lymphoma	Surgery (proximal diversion) Hirschsprung's disease
Uncommon	Stricture (lye ingestion, surgery)	Infiltrative tumor (linitis plastica) Fibrotic scarring, (lye, inflammation, Crohn's disease, TB, syphillis) Starvation			
	SMALLER THAN NORMAL: FOCAL				
	Stricture (peptic, cancer)	Cancer	Peptic ulcer disease	Lymphoma Cancer	Cancer Lymphoma Crohn's disease

due to stricture formation or tumor infiltration. Table 39-4 is a more extensive list of the causes of changes in size.

SUMMARY

Recently swallowed food is the most common luminal content of the stomach. Feces is the most common luminal content of the colon. Prolonged retension of food in the stomach can be due to distal obstruction or to decreased peristalsis.

Mucosa can show thickened folds, decreased folds, or spiculated folds. Thickened folds are most often due to edema but can be from tumor infiltration. Decreased folds can result from mucosal atrophy, tumor infiltration, or fibrosis. Spiculated folds can be due to infection or inflammation and can be simulated by spasm.

Increases in luminal size are usually due to distal obstruction. Decreases in luminal size are usually from surgical resection or stricture. Occasionally, decreased size is from tumor infiltration.

REVIEW QUESTIONS

1. What are the common causes of finding retained food in the stomach on a barium study?
2. How can you differentiate fecal material from a polyp on a barium study?
3. What are the common causes of decreased gastric peristalsis?
4. What materials can be found in bezoars?
5. What are the common causes of thickened mucosal folds?
6. What are the common causes of decreased or absent mucosal folds?

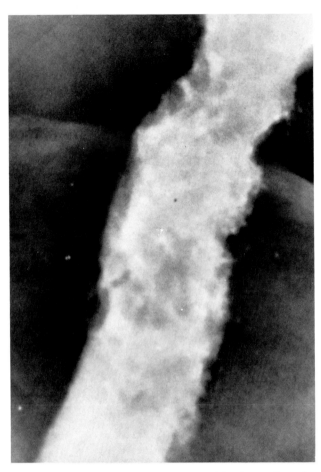

Figure 39-11. The spiculated appearance of the descending colon is caused in this case by ulcerative colitis.

7. What are the common causes of spiculated folds?
8. What are the common causes of increased luminal size in the gut?
9. What are the common causes of decreased luminal size in the gut?

VOCABULARY

bezoar	Ménétrier's disease
Crohn's disease	pernicious anemia
diabetic gastroenteropathy	scleroderma
erosive gastritis	scybala
giardiasis	ulcerative colitis
granulomatous colitis	vagotomy
Hirschsprung's disease	varices
Hypertrophic pyloric stenosis	Zollinger-Ellison syndrome
intestinal lymphangiectasis	

SUGGESTIONS FOR FURTHER READING

For suggested reading see Chapter 35.

40

THE PHARYNX AND ESOPHAGUS

KEY CONCEPTS

Clinical

Patients with pharyngeal and esophageal disease may complain of difficulty swallowing, pain, regurgitation, or bleeding. Complaints of difficulty swallowing should be classified as of pharyngeal or esophageal origin because the methods of evaluation and treatment are different. Symptoms of pharyngeal dysphagia include the entry of food or liquid into the respiratory tract, inability to initiate swallowing, a sense of tightness in the throat, and pain on swallowing.

Esophageal dysphagia can have symptoms of pain, a sense of food sticking, and regurgitation. Esophageal dysphagia can result from abnormalities of esophageal peristalsis, mucosal inflammation, or esophageal obstruction. Regurgitation can result from reflux from the stomach into the esophagus or from esophageal obstruction.

Symptoms and signs of upper GI bleeding can result from bleeding from the nasopharynx, esophagus, stomach, or duodenum. Esophagitis and gastritis, bleeding esophageal or gastric varices, mucosal and submucosal tears, and ulcers. In the acute, actively bleeding case, the patient should be stabilized with blood or blood substitutes and then evaluated with endoscopy. In some patients, radiological intervention will be used to pass a catheter into the bleeding vessel, to clot it off. The patient with a minor degree of upper GI bleeding can be evaluated with radiological barium studies.

Radiological

The patient with pharyngeal dysphagia should be evaluated with a cinepharyngogram or videotape pharyngogram so that the fine muscle coordination of the pharynx can be evaluated. The patient with esophageal symptoms should be evaluated with a barium swallow. It is sometimes helpful to use iced barium if the patient's symptoms suggest thermal sensitivity or acidified barium if the symptoms suggest peptic esophagitis. Both barium studies and nuclear medicine reflux studies can be used to evaluate for gastroesophageal reflux.

OBJECTIVES

When you complete this chapter you will be able to

1. List four symptoms of pharyngeal dysphagia.
2. List four symptoms of esophageal disease.
3. Describe the three types of esophageal peristalsis.
4. List three diseases in which esophageal peristalsis is abnormal.
5. List the stages of evaluation of the condition of the patient with acute upper GI bleeding.

The major symptoms of pharyngeal and esophageal disease are difficulty swallowing (*dysphagia*), pain, regurgitation, and bleeding. An initial clinical differentiation into nasopharygeal and esophageal symptoms will permit the selection of the best imaging study for the evaluation of the symptoms. This chapter discusses dysphagia, esophageal pain, and upper GI bleeding.

PHARYNGEAL DYSPHAGIA

Normal Swallowing

The function of pharyngeal swallowing is to propel a bolus of food or liquid from the mouth to the esophagus without permitting any of it to enter the respiratory system. Swallowing consists of a series of muscular contractions and relaxations that occur so rapidly that they are best evaluated by replaying in slow motion a movie (*cinepharyngogram*) or videotape of a barium swallow. The types of change the movie lets you see are described here.

Initiation of Swallowing. Sequential muscular contraction starts with the tongue pushing the food or medicine bolus into the oropharynx (Fig. 40-1a and b). A tongue painful

from mucosal inflammation may inhibit this starting sequence. Atrophy of the tongue from neuromuscular disease may prevent the swallowing of large amounts of material or may permit a bolus held in the mouth to glide around the tongue into the hypopharynx, resulting in aspiration into the trachea.

Closing of the Nasopharynx. As the material moves into the oropharynx, the soft palate elevates to prevent the

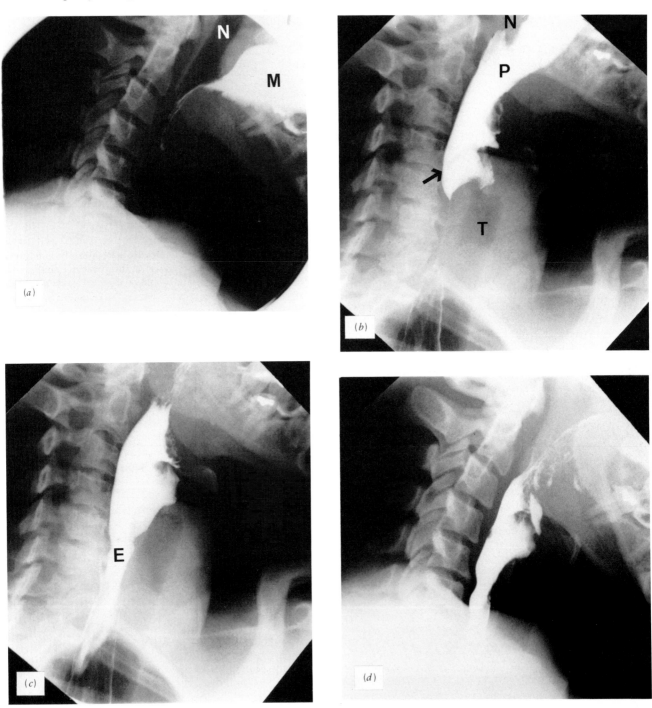

Figure 40-1. Legend on facing page

bolus from entering the nasopharynx (Fig. 40-1b). Nasal regurgitation can occur with failure of the soft palate to elevate and is a sign of pharyngeal dysphagia. Cranial nerve dysfunction and myasthenia gravis can result in nasal regurgitation.

Elevation of the Larynx and Closure of the Vocal Cords. As a bolus passes into the hypopharynx, two actions occur to prevent the bolus from entering the trachea. The larynx elevates, and the vocal cords close (Fig. 40-1b, c, d, and e). Failure of both of these will result in aspiration in most people, but some patients have learned to compensate by hyperextension of the neck or by keeping the vocal cords closed when swallowing.

The larynx may fail to elevate when laryngeal cancer has extended into the adjacent soft tissue or as the result of fibrosis caused by radiotherapy for carcinoma of the larynx. Cranial nerve palsy can result in failure of laryngeal elevation. Vocal cord paralysis can result in aspiration.

Fine Motor Coordinating. In addition to the major features of swallowing just described, there are many subtle sequential changes of muscle contraction and relaxation. These changes require careful study to detect, and this analysis is beyond the scope of this book. It is important to mention them, however, because the major symptom resulting from fine motor discoordination is the sensation of a lump in the throat. It is likely that there is no such disease as "globus hystericus." There is probably always a pathophysiological change in the sequence of swallowing that can explain the sensation. Attention has recently been directed by Heimlich to a swallowing coordination failure that results in severe catastrophe: a bolus of food is abruptly aspirated, obstructs the trachea or larynx, and rapidly results in death if not recognized and treated. In almost all patients with choking episodes, or "*cafe coronaries,*" a pathophysiological change will be found on subsequent cinepharyngography.

Methods of Evaluation

The symptoms of pharyngeal dysphagia result from the entry of the food or liquid bolus into the respiratory tract, causing nasal regurgitation or aspiration; from a sense of tightness or "lump in the throat"; from an inability to initiate swallowing; or from pain on swallowing.

A careful history of all a patient's symptoms should be obtained, with specific attention directed to nasal regurgitation, choking, coughing while eating, and recurrent pneumonias. This should be followed by a physical examination including specific attention to the state of the tongue, the mucosa, and the size and length of the tongue. The ability of the larynx to elevate with swallowing can be observed and palpated externally. Indirect (mirror) laryngoscopy should be used to look at vocal cord movement. After these investigations, a cinepharyngogram and an esophogram should be obtained.

Gastroesophageal Disease and Pharyngeal Dysphagia

Reflux of gastric contents into the esophagus and retrograde peristalsis of the esophagus can result in spasm of the upper esophageal sphincter. This spasm can result in pharyngeal symptoms. Every patient studied for pharyngeal dysphagia should also be evaluated for esophageal disease.

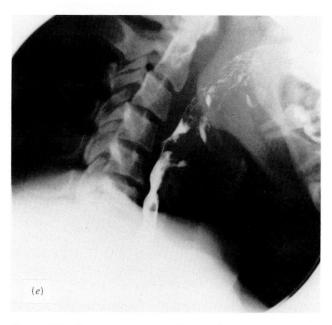

(e)

Figure 40-1. The normal pharyngeal swallowing sequence. (*a*) Barium is seen in the mouth (M). The nasopharynx (N) is open. (*b*) Swallowing has started. The nasopharynx (N) is now closed off. Barium fills the oropharynx (P). The larynx is elevated, as demonstrated by the inverted epiglottis (a faintly seen structure —arrow). No barium is seen in the trachea (T). (*c*) Barium now fills the upper portion of the esophagus (E). (*d*) Barium is now passing from the pharynx. (*e*) Barium is passing from the upper esophagus.

Keynotes

- *Disorders of swallowing can be pharyngeal or esophageal in origin.*
- *A special dynamic study of the pharynx, a cinepharyngogram or videotape pharyngogram, is needed to evaluate pharyngeal dysphagia.*
- *Patients who choke on food should be evaluated for pharyngeal dysphagia. Many patients with acute airway obstruction from food have had milder symptoms of choking first.*
- *Symptoms of pharyngeal dysphagia include aspiration, nasal regurgitation, "lump in the throat," difficulty initiating swallowing, and pain on swallowing.*
- *Gastroesophageal reflux can result in symptoms of pharyngeal dysphagia.*

ESOPHAGEAL DYSPHAGIA

Esophageal dysphagia is different from pharyngeal dysphagia. It can result from three types of abnormality: abnormalities of peristalsis, luminal obstruction, and mucosal inflammation.

Normal Esophageal Peristalsis

Normal esophageal peristalsis consists largely of primary peristaltic waves. These are peristaltic waves that start at the upper esophageal sphincter and continue to the lower esophageal sphincter.

Secondary peristaltic waves normally occur once or twice out of every 10 swallows. They are waves of contraction that start in the midesophagus and continue uninterrupted to the lower esophageal sphincter. Tertiary peristalsis— segmental nonpropulsive contractions—does not occur in the normal esophagus.

Methods of Study

The usual radiographic method of studying the esophagus is the barium swallow. (In selected cases, nuclear medicine imaging techniques can be useful, but they should not be used in the patient whose dysphagia could be due to esophageal cancer.) The barium swallow consists of the visual observation of at least 10 separate swallows of barium. Estimates of the proportion of primary, secondary, and tertiary peristalsis are made. Several films are made to look for contour and mucosal abnormalities and for regions of pathological luminal narrowing. In some cases, barium-air double-contrast studies are done to study the mucosal detail of the esophagus. In some cases, the barium is acidified to see whether the acidified barium will cause esophageal spasm, indicating peptic esophagitis.

Esophageal clearance studies use a radiotracer placed in the esophagus. A gamma camera is used to measure the rate of clearance of the tracer from the esophagus.

Nuclear medicine studies for gastroesophageal reflux are performed by having the patient swallow a radiotracer (usually sodium pertechnetate Tc 99m) in a volume of about 300 cc. This is then washed from the esophagus by having the patient drink water. Serial recordings are then made as an abdominal binder applies a graded increase in pressure to the abdomen. Imaging of the tracer in the esophagus is indicative of gastroesophageal reflux (Fig. 40-2).

Abnormalities of Esophageal Peristalsis

Several processes increase the proportions of secondary peristalsis. The most common of these is reflux of gastric contents into the esophagus. Increased proportions of secondary peristalsis also occur in diseases with muscular weakness, such as early scleroderma.

Tertiary peristalsis occurs in the esophagus in the elderly. Frequently seen in people over the age of 70, the

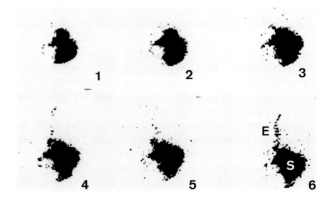

Figure 40-2. Nuclear medicine study for gastroesophageal reflux. Serial images are obtained as an abdominal binder is tightened. The early images demonstrate activity in the stomach (S). The later images demonstrate activity in the esophagus (E), indicating that gastroesophageal reflux is present. (Courtesy D. Moses, M.D.)

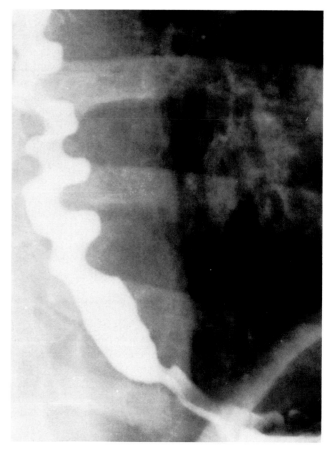

Figure 40-3. Presbyesophagus. The corkscrew appearance of this type of tertiary peristalsis is seen. (Courtesy R. Greyson-Fleg, M.D.)

multiple regions of dilation and narrowing have been called the *corkscrew esophagus* or *presbyesophagus* (Fig. 40-3).

Spasm of the esophagus is exaggerated tertiary peristalsis. It is often painful and can be physiological or pathological. Most of the readers of this book will have occasionally experienced physiological esophageal spasm. This occurs in most people when they drink ice cold soda rapidly on a hot day.

Spasm also occurs in response to gastroesophageal reflux in people with heartburn and can occur as a syndrome of *diffuse esophageal spasm* in type A tense people who develop chest pain on swallowing hot or cold beverages. It is important to question a patient with heartburn or dysphagia about thermal sensitivity because a barium swallow done with room-temperature barium may fail to disclose any abnormality in these people.

Peptic esophagitis is probably the most common cause of esophageal spasm. Relaxation of the lower esophageal sphincter permits the reflux of gastric juice into the esophagus. The acid in gastric contents irritates the esophageal mucosal and can result in burning retrosternal pain and esophageal spasm.

Gastroesophageal reflux or its sequelae can be demonstrated by three different imaging techniques:

1. Barium can be seen, during an upper GI series, to reflux from the stomach into the esophagus.
2. Sodium pertechentate Tc 99m swallowed and then washed out of the esophagus can be monitored with a gamma camera and reflux into the esophagus identified.
3. Peptic esophagitis can be identified by using barium adjusted to a pH of 1.7 with hydrochloric acid. The acid-sensitive esophagus will appear normal with normal barium but will go into spasm with the acidified barium.

Of these methods, only the acidified barium swallow shows that the reflux has resulted in mucosal inflammation. A carefully done air-barium double-contrast esophagram can demonstrate mucosal alteration in the esophagus in some patients with peptic esophagitis.

Case 40-1

GE is a 72-year-old man who has been slowly losing weight for several years. His family complains he seems only to nibble at mealtimes and never eats a substantial meal. The patient tells you that food doesn't taste good anymore. He has no pain on swallowing, but food seems sometimes to get stuck in the lower part of his chest. Films from his barium swallow are shown in Figure 40-4. What do they show?

There are many focal areas of contraction and dilation. What does this mean?

This is the pattern of tertiary peristalsis, in this case from presbyesophagus: "old people's esophagus." Presbyesophagus is a common finding in elderly patients. Usually they will make no complaints from this esophageal abnormality. Questioned carefully, however, many will relate that it does seem to take longer for food to reach the stomach, and some will complain that food occasionally seems to get stuck. The clinical impor-

tance is not these minor symptoms but rather, the effect this process can have on the elderly patient's nutrition. Some of you may have elderly relatives or friends who seem to linger over their meals, eating slowly and slowing up everyone else's meal. Often the elderly person knows that she or he is slowing the meal, keeping the family from its other activities, feels the pressure, and eats less, losing weight and becoming malnourished. When this is occurring, it is important to point out to the family that some elderly people need more time to eat, that it takes more time for the food to get down, and that the family should be patient or provide another way for the patient to have enough time to eat, unpressured.

Depression, loose dentures, a low-salt diet without corrective efforts in spicing food, and slow loss of ability to taste can also affect food intake in the elderly and should be also considered in cases of weight loss.

Case 40-2

BK is a 47-year-old overweight woman who develops such severe burning chest pain when she goes to bed that she now usually goes to sleep in a chair. She has tried antacids, which give her brief relief. Apart from moderate obesity, physical examination is normal. Fasting blood glucose test results suggest mild glucose intolerance and minimal diabetes and is confirmed on a glucose intolerance test. Though it would be acceptable to begin treatment for the diagnosis of presumed peptic esophagitis, confirmation is sought with an acidified barium swallow. Figure 40-5a shows the esophagus with nonacidified barium; Figure 40-5b demonstrates the esophagus with acidified barium. What difference do you see?

The esophagus in Figure 40-5b shows marked irregular contraction from spasm. Because the spasm occurred only with the acidified barium and not with the plain barium, the diagnosis of peptic esophagitis is confirmed.

Keynotes

- *Esophageal dysphagia may cause chest pain, food sticking, or other symptoms of reflux.*
- *Normal esophageal peristalsis consists mainly of primary peristaltic waves.*
- *The usual method of evaluating esophageal dysphagia is the barium swallow.*
- *Gastroesophageal reflux increases the proportion of secondary and tertiary peristalsis.*
- *Tertiary peristalsis is common in the elderly.*
- *Esophageal spasm is exaggerated tertiary peristalsis; it is often painful.*
- *Not all patients with gastroesophageal reflux have symptoms of peptic esophagitis. Reflux can be evaluated by a barium swallow or a nuclear medicine reflux study. Peptic esophagitis can be confirmed by a barium swallow with acidified barium.*
- *Presbyesophagus is only minimally symptomatic but may result in nutritional problems in the elderly.*

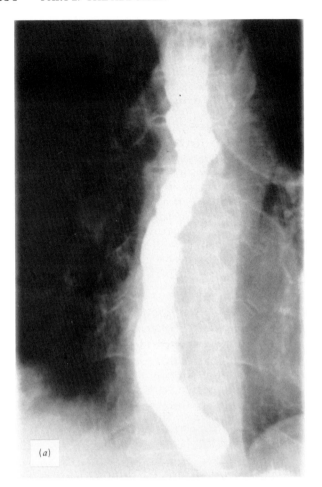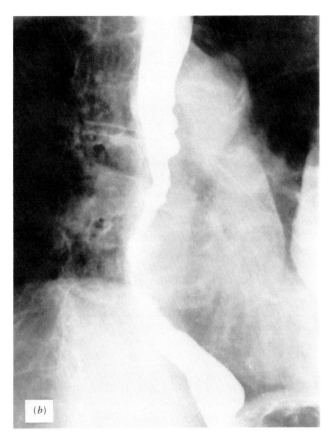

Figure 40-4. Case example 40-1. (Courtesy R. Greyson-Fleg, M.D.)

OTHER DISEASES OF THE ESOPHAGUS

Case 40-3

RB is a 63-year-old man who complains that bread is getting caught in his midchest. He has had no trouble swallowing liquids, but he has had an occasional problem swallowing hamburger. He has smoked for many years and has a chronic cough. He has previously been hospitalized for liver failure and was told by a doctor at the time that he had better stop drinking. On examination, he smells of alcohol; he has lost many of his teeth, and several of those remaining are carious. He appears to have lost weight but tells you he has not. Because of his complaints, a barium swallow is obtained (Fig. 40-6a). What does it show?

There is a short segment of the midesophagus, moderately narrowed. The lumen of the esophagus proximal to this narrowing distends well and shows a normal mucosal pattern. What is your probable diagnosis?

Esophageal cancer is the most likely diagnosis. If this is proved by endoscopic biopsy to be esophageal cancer, what is the patient's prognosis?

Very poor. Esophageal cancer has less than a 5% 5-year survival rate. The patient's CT scan is shown in Figure 40-6b. The amount of tumor (arrowheads) touching the aorta (arrowhead) indicates that the tumor has invaded the aorta and is unresectable.

Case 40-4

RA is a 36-year-old man found unconscious on the street and brought in by the police. On examination, he smells of alcohol and is unkempt, pale, and cold. His pulse is weak and very rapid; his blood pressure 70/?. What would you do? What do you think the patient's problem is?

Clearly the patient is an alcohol abuser, but based on the information above, the patient's main immediate problem is shock. Immediate attention should be directed first to correcting the shock and second to finding the cause.

A venous infusion line is rapidly inserted, with blood drawn, at the same time, to type and crossmatch. Ringer's lactate is infused rapidly, being replaced by plasma when that becomes available. A nasogastric tube is put in place, and coffee ground-like material mixed with some blood is aspirated. What do you do now?

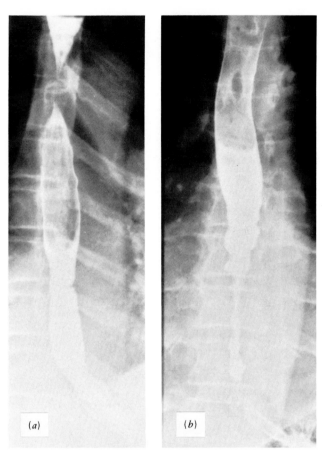

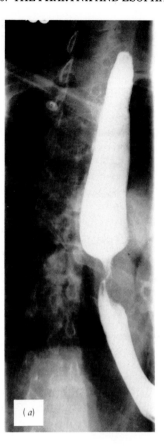

Figure 40-5. Case example 40-2. (*a*) An esophageal study performed with standard barium. (*b*) Study performed with acidified barium.

Add a second intravenous infusion line if the blood pressure is not adequately responding; increase the rate of infusion and start infusing blood when it becomes available.

How would you find the site of the bleeding you discovered in the nasogastric-tube aspirate?

The best method is endoscopy. Esophagoscopy and gastroscopy are the most accurate, rapid methods of finding the cause of upper GI tract hemorrhage. The main problem with endoscopy is that it is not available in all communities. What would you do if endoscopy is not available at your location?

Do your best to stabilize the patient with blood transfusions and then attempt to evacuate him to a hospital where it is available.

How do you evacuate a patient? You don't just send him. You do your best to stabilize his condition using the basic *ABC's of cardiopulmonary resuscitation:* airway, breathing, cardiovascular support. You call the hospital to which you are evacuating the patient to tell them what you about him and to make sure they are ready to receive him. In some states, it is possible to evacuate by helicopter; if the patient is unstable, the most rapid method of transport should be used.

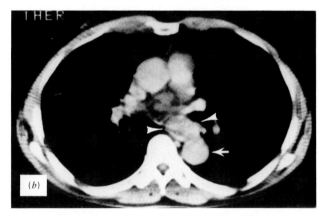

Figure 40-6. Case example 40-3. (*a*) Film from a barium swallow. (*b*) CT scan. The arrow points to the aorta. The arrowheads point to the esophageal mass.

When I was an intern, a patient was evacuated to us with a bullet wound in his head. He had been shot in a bar in Alaska. The medical officer (the only doctor in that community) had never treated a head wound before and decided to evacuate the patient to the closest neurosurgical facility (Seattle). When the patient arrived, I found that the patient had indeed been shot in the head, but on the radiographs that came with him, the bullet was outside the calvaria. The patient's blood pressure was barely measurable, and despite the infusion of volume expanders and blood replacement, he died with infarction of his bowel and abdominal sepsis.

Even if you can't practice neurosurgery, you can still resuscitate a patient with the basic airway, breathing, and cardiovascular support. So, if you decided to send your patient with the upper GI tract bleeding to another doctor or center, provide the basic support first.

In some centers without endoscopy for diagnosis, the Sengstaken-Blakemore tube is used diagnostically to determine the site of bleeding and to treat variceal bleeding.

On your patient, brought in in shock, you are able to have endoscopy done. What are the possible causes of this man's bleeding? Blood can be found in the stomach from nose-bleeds, bleeding from the mouth, esophageal varices, Mallory-Weiss mucosal tears, gastritis, and gastric and duodenal ulcers.

What do you do if endoscopy discloses bleeding from esophageal varices?

Two methods of treatment are available: intravenous infusion of vasopressin and use of the Sengstaken-Blakemore tube.

What do you do if the bleeding is from a tear of the esophagogastric junction (a Mallory-Weiss tear)?

These usually require surgery, but sometimes it is possible to use angiography catheters to cannulate the bleeding vessel and occlude it.

What do you do if the bleeding is from a gastric or duodenal ulcer?

If there is marked bleeding, it is possible to cannulate the bleeding vessel using angiographic technique and to clot off the bleeding vessel.

Gastritis can be treated with blood replacement, gastric washing, and antacids.

The use of barium in the evaluation of current upper GI tract hemorrhage is now seldom done. It is done only in situations in which endoscopy and angiography will not be done, because the barium will prevent these studies from being done for hours or even days. In addition, barium studies are of limited sensitivity in patients with blood clotted in their stomachs.

Patients with minor amounts of bleeding or prior bleeding can be studied with barium. Varices can be identified as curved tubular impressions on the esophageal lumen (see Fig. 40-7). The identification of ulcers has been discussed in Chapter 38.

___

Keynotes

- *The best method for finding the bleeding site of an upper GI tract hemorrhage is endoscopy.*
- *Radiologists can use catheter techniques to stop the bleeding from most, but not all, gastric and duodenal ulcers.*

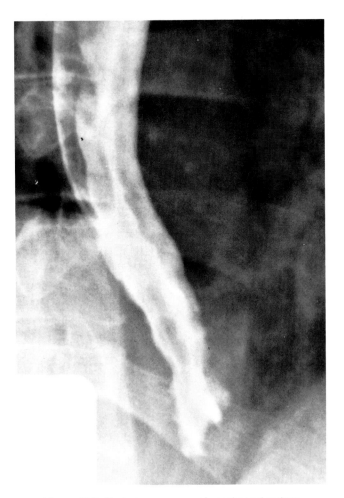

Figure 40-7. Typical appearance of esophageal varices.

SUMMARY

The differentiation of pharyngeal from esophageal symptoms is important in deciding on the type of imaging study a patient needs. Pharyngeal dysphagia should be evaluated by an action recording of pharyngeal swallowing, using either a movie or videotape recording. A frame-by-frame analysis is often necessary to detect minor degrees of incoordination. Symptoms of pharyngeal dysphagia include difficulties in the initiation of swallowing food, a sense of a lump in the throat, and a history of airway obstruction by food.

Esophageal dysphagia results either in a sense of food sticking or in retrosternal chest pain. It is best evaluated initially by a barium swallow, although tracer imaging techniques are quite useful in checking for esophageal clearing and gastroesophageal reflux.

Reflux esophagitis is a common cause of retrosternal chest pain. It is usually treated symptomatically, but when investigation is indicated, several tests are available. The reflux can be demonstrated with a barium swallow or with nuclear medicine imaging studies for gastroesophageal reflux. The actual presence of peptic esophagitis can be confirmed with an acidified barium swallow.

In presbyesophagus, a common abnormality of esophageal peristalsis in the elderly, tertiary peristalsis results in delayed transit of food in the stomach.

The patient with upper GI tract bleeding is best evaluated by endoscopy. Angiographic techniques can be used to occlude bleeding vessels.

REVIEW QUESTIONS

1. What are the symptoms of pharyngeal dysphagia? What are the symptoms of esophageal dysphagia? How do they differ?

2. What is the method of evaluating pharyngeal dysphagia? Esophageal dysphagia?

3. What are the physiological and pathological conditions that result in tertiary peristalsis of the esophagus?

4. What are the symptoms associated with tertiary peristalsis of the esophagus?

5. What symptoms can be associated with gastroesophageal reflux?

6. What symptoms are associated with esophageal cancer?

7. How should the patient with major upper GI tract bleeding be managed?

VOCABULARY

ABC's of cardiopulmonary resuscitation	gastroesophageal reflux
	globus hystericus
cafe coronary	myasthenia gravis
cinepharyngogram	peptic esophagitis
corkscrew esophagus	presbyesophagus
diffuse esophageal spasm	scleroderma
dysphagia	Sengstaken-Blakemore tube
endoscopy	varices

SUGGESTIONS FOR FURTHER READING

Martin W. Donner, George P. Saba, Carlos R. Martinez. Diffuse diseases of the esophagus: A practical approach. *Seminars in Roentgenology,* **16:**198–213, 1981.

William B. Seaman. Pathophysiology of the esophagus. *Seminars in Roentgenology,* **16:**214–227, 1981.

For additional suggested reading see Chapter 35.

41

THE STOMACH

KEY CONCEPTS

Radiological

The main method of evaluating the stomach is with a single- or double-contrast barium upper GI tract series. The stomach can be displaced by masses adjacent to it; it can have intrinsic abnormalities of its wall or mucosa; it can have abnormal intraluminal processes.

Gastric cancer can infiltrate the gastric wall, decreasing the size of the stomach. It can appear as a mass within the stomach or as a flattened or raised area of the gastric wall. It can contain an ulcer.

Clinical

Gastric cancer can result in symptoms of early filling of the stomach, occult or massive blood loss, or symptoms of metastases.

Previous gastric surgery can result in the dumping syndrome, with dizziness, abdominal pain, and sometimes diarrhea. Absorption of vitamin B_{12} and iron can be interfered with. A malabsorption syndrome can result in diarrhea.

Gastric ulcers, even when benign, can result in severe debilitating symptoms that seem to suggest a malignancy.

OBJECTIVES

When you complete this chapter you will be able to

1. List three symptoms of gastric malignancy.
2. Recognize gastric cancer, gastric ulcers, and hiatal hernias on selected radiographs.
3. List four symptoms or signs that can result from gastric surgery.

Radiographs of the barium-filled or barium-and-air-filled stomach can be used to diagnose disease adjacent to the stomach and intrinsic to it. You should compare the images in this chapter with the images of the normal stomach shown in Figure 34-2. The diagnosis of disease adjacent to the stomach depends on the identification of gastric displacement and changes in the gastric contour. The diagnosis of intrinsic gastric abnormalities depends on the recognition of changes in size, shape, mucosal pattern, wall flexibility, and peristalsis and the identification of intraluminal filling defects.

DIAGNOSING DISEASE ADJACENT TO THE STOMACH

The normal stomach lies in the left upper and mid abdomen. Several variants of shape are common, the cascade stomach and the J-shaped stomach being the most common. The stomach lies adjacent to many organs, enlargement of which may result in characteristic changes in the shape and position of the stomach. Enlargement of the liver, spleen (Fig. 41-1), left kidney, and body and tail of the pancreas (Fig. 41-2) can be recognized by their characteristic impressions.

DIAGNOSING ABNORMALITIES INTRINSIC TO THE STOMACH

Case 41-1

This 64-year-old auto mechanic has been feeling nauseated for several months, is eating little, and has been

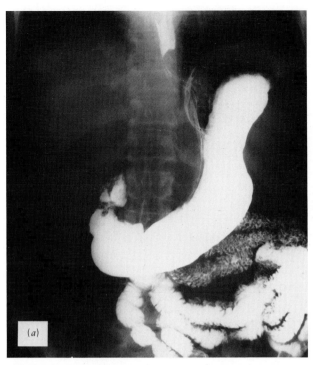

Figure 41-1. Pressure on the stomach from hepatic and splenic enlargement. Compare this appearance with the normal appearances of the stomach shown in Chapter 34. The superomedial wall of the stomach is compressed by the large liver, and the upper lateral wall is compressed by the large spleen. (*a*) AP view. (*b*) Lateral view.

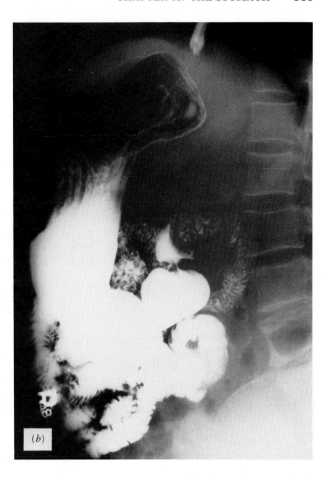

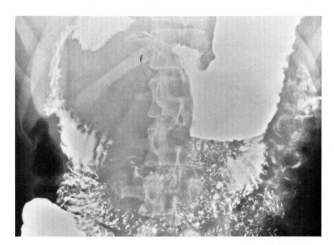

Figure 41-2. Pressure on the gastric antrum and duodenal C loop by a large pancreatic pseudocyst. Compare this image with the normal appearances shown in Chapter 34.

losing weight. When he tries to eat, he rapidly feels full. He is tired and weak. About 20 years ago he had a vagotomy and pyloroplasty for a duodenal ulcer.

Physical examination reveals signs of weight loss. The liver is slightly enlarged. The stool tests guaiac positive. The alkaline phosphatase level is high.

A film from his upper GI series is shown in Figure 41-3. What do you see?

There are surgical clips from his vagotomy adjacent to the esophagogastric junction. There is an irregular narrowing of the body and antrum of the stomach. What do you think this represents?

This is a form of carcinoma of the stomach in which there is extensive submucosal infiltration. It is called *linitis plastica* or *leather-bottle stomach*.

Carcinoma of the stomach this extensive has a very poor prognosis, less than a 5% 5-year survival rate.

Carcinoma of the stomach can also be polypoid, ulcerated (Figure 41-4), or masslike with a smooth or irregular surface (Figure 41-5). Carcinomas of the stomach, when this large, are rarely curable.

Small carcinomas of the stomach are more likely to be curable. They may appear as flat or irregular plaques or as small ulcers (Fig. 41-6).

Keynotes

- *Satiety is the feeling that one has eaten all one cares to.*
- *Early satiety is the feeling of satiety after only a small amount of food has been eaten.*
- *Linitis plastica, the leather-bottle stomach, is a small stomach caused by extensive submucosal infiltration. It results in early sati-*

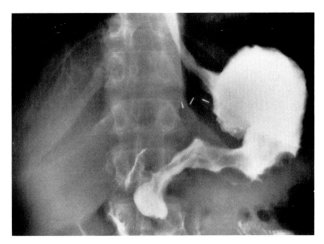

Figure 41-3. Case example 41-1.

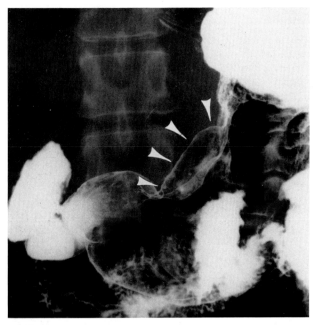

Figure 41-4. Gastric cancer. Arrowheads outline the margin of a large ulcer within the cancer.

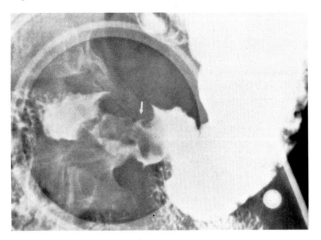

Figure 41-5. Gastric cancer. There is an irregular mass in the distal antrum with a small ulcer (arrow) within it.

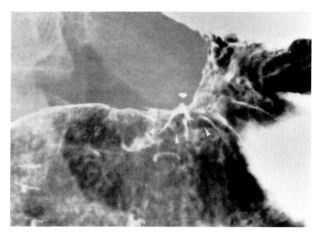

Figure 41-6. Gastric cancer. A small ulcer (arrow) is seen within an area of nodular mucosal change (arrowheads). (Courtesy of Jerry Patt, M.D.)

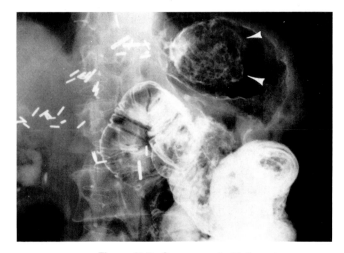

Figure 41-7. Case example 41-2.

ety. *It is usually due to cancer or lymphoma but can occur also from severe inflammation.*

• *Small, curable carcinomas of the stomach most often can be found only on careful air-barium double-contrast studies or endoscopy.*

Case 41-2

Compare the stomach shown in Figure 41-7 with the normal stomach shown in Figure 34-2. What abnormality does this patient have?

His stomach is small, and there is a mass in it (arrowheads). What might this be?

In this case, it is a bezoar from a partial surgical resection of the stomach with a Billroth II anastamosis.

Knowing that the patient has had a partial gastrectomy should lead you to evaluate the patient more fully. You should question actively for the symptoms of the complications of gastric partial resection. What are they?

The symptoms are related to three sequelae of the

surgery: the effect of rapid filling of a small pouch, the effect of slow or rapid emptying, and the effects on digestion and absorption.

Rapid filling of the small gastric remnant can result in early satiety. The patient eats less because his stomach cannot hold as much food. If he is losing weight, smaller but more frequent feedings may help him.

Emptying of the gastric remnant can be too slow or too fast. Too slow emptying can result in obstructive symptoms, with vomiting being the most frequent. Bezoars can form. Too fast emptying of the stomach can result in the *dumping syndrome*. This has two phases, early and late. The early phase is caused by the rapid entry of hyperosmolar fluid into the small bowel, resulting in transient hypovolemia, dizziness, nausea, and sometimes diarrhea. The late phase results from relative hyperinsulinemia with hypoglycemia.

Gastric surgery can also have an effect on the absorption and digestion of food. If much of the antrum is resected, the production of intrinsic factor may become insufficient, resulting in inadequate absorption of vitamin B_{12}. Lack of gastric acidity may prevent the oxidation of iron into its absorbable form, resulting in iron deficiency anemia. Bacterial production in a blind small bowel loop may result in diarrhea with malabsorption.

Many medical students learn to complete the history form by rote, each thing recorded in its proper place. That may be an appropriate way to learn, but in caring for patients a different technique is used. Each positive response should elicit questions about related or possibly related symptoms. This active searching for symptoms may bring to light aspects of the patient's problem that would otherwise have been missed. You must use a system to be complete, but pursuing positive answers to a review of systems may give you a better picture of what really is bothering the patient.

Keynotes

- *The Billroth I anastomosis includes the attachment of the gastric remnant to the duodenal bulb.*
- *The Billroth II anastomosis includes the attachment of the gastric remnant to the jejunum.*
- *A bezoar is a conglomeration within the stomach of animal or vegetable fiber or, uncommonly, metal objects. Those with animal or vegetable fibers are often the result of abnormalities of digestion, gastric motility, or gastric emptying.*
- *The dumping syndrome results from the too rapid emptying of the gastric contents into the small bowel. Hypovolemia with dizziness, sweating, and palpitations, as well as diarrhea and symptoms of hyperinsulinemia can result.*

Case 41-3

This 56-year-old woman complains that her stomach hurts when she eats. She has been losing weight for the last 3 months and has felt run down. Sometimes after she eats, her stomach burns, sometimes it aches, and sometimes she becomes nauseated after she has eaten a little bit and has to stop eating.

On examination, she looks older than her chronological age. She seems depressed. She is minimally tender in her epigastrium. Her stool tests guaiac positive.

Views from her upper GI tract series are shown in Figure 41-8. What do you see?

The upper image shows a focal outpouching from the medial side of the body of the stomach. The lower image shows an ovoid collection of barium. Your diagnosis?

Gastric ulcer. Benign or malignant?

The ulcer extends slightly beyond the outer limit of the inner wall of the stomach, but the mass surrounding it appears asymmetric. This is an indeterminate ulcer. What should be done?

Endoscopy with biopsy demonstrated no evidence of malignancy. The patient was followed and the ulcer healed.

Keynote

- *The patient with a chronic gastric benign ulcer may have the symptoms and signs of malignancy: weight loss and anorexia. Although the ulcer may be unassociated with malignancy, its effect on the patient is often serious and not benign.*

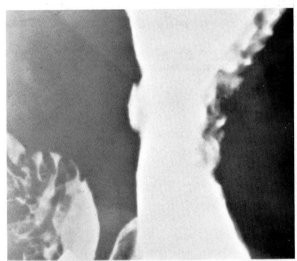

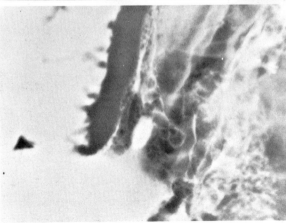

Figure 41-8. Case 41-3.

Hiatal Hernia

Hiatal hernias are hernias of the stomach through the esophageal hiatus of the diaphragm. They are common and in most cases are asymptomatic. They are of two types, the sliding hiatal hernia (Fig. 41-9) and the para-esophageal hiatal hernia (Fig. 41-10). In each, it is the identification of gastric mucosa above the leaflet of the diaphragm that makes the diagnosis.

Keynote

• *Most hiatal hernias are asymptomatic. The symptoms once ascribed to hiatal hernias are actually due to peptic esophagitis secondary to gastroesophageal reflux.*

Gastroesophageal Reflux

Gastroesophageal reflux results in symptoms of heatburn: a retrosternal burning sensation. Reflux of gastric contents into the mouth can also occur. Aspiration of refluxed material can result in coughing spells, particularly when lying down.

Gastroesophageal reflux can be confirmed by placing pH monitors in the esophagus or by detecting reflux of a radiotracer placed in the stomach. Demonstration of reflux during a barium study of the stomach is less reliable.

The symptoms of heartburn from gastroesophageal reflux are due to peptic esophagitis. The diagnosis of peptic esophagitis can be made by a mucosal biopsy of the esopha-

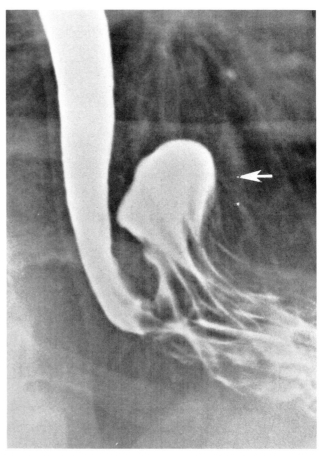

Figure 41-10. Para-esophageal hiatal hernia. The herniated portion (arrow) of the stomach lies alongside the esophagus.

gus, by looking for spasm of the esophagus on an acidified barium swallow, or by the infusion of acid into the esophagus to see if that reproduces the patient's symptoms.

SUMMARY

Imaging studies of the stomach can demonstrate disease intrinsic or adjacent to the stomach. Extensive carcinoma of the stomach can result in weight loss, a sense that the stomach fills early, occult blood loss, or the symptoms of metastatic disease. Extensive carcinoma of the stomach can be encircling (as in linitis plastica), polypoid, or ulcerated.

Early carcinoma of the stomach can be asymptomatic or associated with occult blood loss. It is best detected on air-barium double-contrast studies or endoscopy and can appear as a smooth or irregular mucosal plaque or as a small ulcer.

After partial gastric resection, symptoms can result from a recurrence of the disease (ulcer, cancer, etc.) that led to the initial surgery. A small residual pouch may limit food intake. Slow emptying can result in symptoms of obstruction (nausea, vomiting, anorexia). Rapid empty-

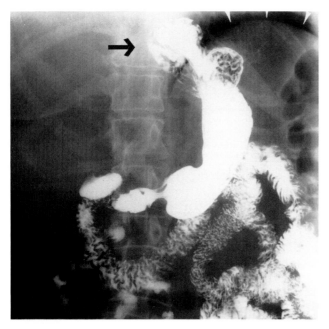

Figure 41-9. Sliding hiatal hernia. Arrows indicate the portion of the stomach that lies above the left hemidiaphragm. Arrowheads mark the location of the hemidiaphragm, which can be identified by noting the air above it.

ing can result in "dumping," with dizziness or diarrhea. The absorption of certain nutrients can be interfered with, especially iron and vitamin B_{12}.

The chronic gastric ulcer of the elderly can result in epigastric pain, anorexia, and weight loss. Endoscopy may be necessary to decide whether the ulcer found is nonneoplastic or in a neoplasm.

There are two types of hiatal hernias: sliding and para-esophageal. They are diagnosed by finding gastric mucosa above the diaphragm. They are usually asymptomatic.

The symptoms often ascribed to hiatal hernias are actually due to gastroesophageal reflux with secondary peptic esophagitis. The reflux is best detected by placing pH probes in the esophagus or by using a radioactive bolus in the stomach. The observation of reflux of barium from the stomach into the esophagus is less reliable. Peptic esophagitis can be diagnosed by seeing the spasm induced by swallowing acidified barium, by noting that the infusion of acid into the esophagus reproduces the patient's pain, or by a biopsy of the mucosa.

REVIEW QUESTIONS

1. What are the symptoms of advanced gastric cancer?
2. What are the radiographic findings in advanced gastric cancer?
3. What is the best method or methods of detecting early gastric cancer?
4. What are the complications of gastric partial resection?
5. What are the symptoms of a chronic gastric benign ulcer?
6. What methods can be used to diagnose gastroesophageal reflux? Peptic esophagitis?

VOCABULARY

dumping syndrome

gastroesophageal reflux

hiatal hernia

para-esophageal hiatal hernia

peptic esophagitis

sliding hiatal hernia

SUGGESTIONS FOR FURTHER READING

For suggested reading see Chapter 35.

42

THE DUODENUM

KEY CONCEPTS

Clinical

The main diseases of the duodenum are related to peptic ulceration: duodenitis and duodenal ulcer. Duodenal ulcers can be detected by endoscopy or upper GI tract series. Symptoms consist of recurrent upper abdominal pain, relieved by eating and recurring several hours after eating.

Radiological

A duodenal ulcer, in an otherwise normal duodenal bulb, can be detected in about 85% of patients with duodenal ulcers. The fixed ulcer crater can be surrounded by a mound of edema. When the duodenal bulb is scarred by previous ulcer disease, an active ulcer is more difficult to detect, and an ulcer scar may simulate an active ulcer.

In some scarred duodenal bulbs, apparent outpouchings, called *pseudodiverticula,* can be seen. These represent more normal areas of duodenum between contracted duodenal scars. Their walls are flexible, and this flexibility is the sign used to differentiate them from ulcers.

In some patients, the gastric mucosa can prolapse through the pylorus, producing a cone-shaped defect in the base of the duodenal bulb.

Diverticula of the duodenum occur almost always beyond the duodenal bulb, while ulceration usually affects the bulb. Duodenal diverticula are usually asymptomatic.

OBJECTIVES

When you complete this chapter you will be able to

1. Correctly identify, on selected radiographs, duodenal ulcers, duodenal diverticula, pseudodiverticula of the duodenal bulb, and prolapsed gastric mucosa.

2. Describe the symptoms of a duodenal ulcer.
3. Discuss why a patient with duodenal ulcer symptoms should or should not have the ulcer proved, either by endoscopy or by an upper GI tract series.

The major disease affecting the duodenal bulb is peptic ulcer disease. The duodenal bulb is evaluated as part of the upper GI tract series. It is usually shown on multiple films, and attempts are made to demonstrate it both with barium and with air-barium double-contrast.

The normal duodenal bulb is triangular (see Fig. 34-3). When distended, its mucosal surface usually is smooth. With muscular contraction, folds can be seen. These folds limit the detection of ulcers.

Ulcers consist of an erosion of the mucosa with surrounding edema. In well-demonstrated cases, both the ulcer crater and the edema can be seen. Sometimes the only indication of the presence of the ulcer is the persistent filling of the ulcer *niche,* or crater, or the persistent ring of the ulcer mouth.

A well-performed study detects more than 85% of all duodenal ulcers. It is difficult, however, to differentiate the acute ulcer from an ulcer scar. Detection of the mound of edema around the ulcer indicates that the ulcer is still active.

Case 42-1

This 44-year-old man has been having recurrent pain in the upper part of his abdomen. The pain, which has been coming and going for several years, is a gnawing pain, like hunger pain. When he eats, the pain goes away, only to recur several hours later. It will often awaken him at night, but after he eats, he rapidly falls back to sleep and sleeps until morning. Because of all the eating, he has gained 15 lb, but every time he tries to diet, the pain comes back.

Physical examination is normal except for minimal right upper quadrant tenderness.

A film from his upper GI tract series is in Figure 42-1. What do you see?

There is an outpouching from the midportion of the duodenal bulb. It is surrounded by an irregular rim of radiolucency, representing a rim of edema.

Your diagnosis?

Duodenal ulcer.

The patient responded rapidly to cimetidine therapy. When this was stopped, the symptoms recurred, and he has required intermittent cimetidine therapy since then.

Keynotes

- *An active duodenal ulcer can be diagnosed when the niche and a surrounding rim of edema are both visualized.*
- *Cimetidine therapy can rapidly relieve the symptoms of duodenal ulcer. It can also mask the early symptoms of gastric cancer, however. Ulcers can recur after the cessation of cimetidine therapy.*

WHEN TO CONFIRM DUODENAL ULCER BY RADIOGRAPHS

There is no generally accepted answer to the question WHEN DO YOU CONFIRM A DUODENAL ULCER BY RADIOGRAPH? Good arguments can be made that the patient with classic symptoms of a duodenal ulcer need not have this ulcer confirmed by an imaging study. Certain patients, however, should have the study:

1. Those whose occupations place themselves, or others, at increased risk, should they develop severe

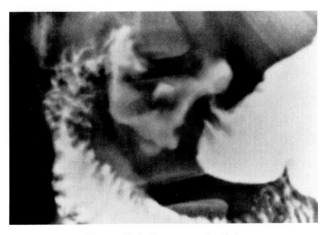

Figure 42-1. Case example 42-1.

bleeding or perforation of the ulcer, such as those working in remote locations, airline pilots, or seamen.
2. Those in the cancer age group, inasmuch as gastric carcinoma occasionally can simulate duodenal ulcer symptoms.
3. Those with major blood loss.
4. Those unresponsive to therapy.
5. Those who require surgery.
6. Those with atypical symptoms that could be due to a gastric ulcer, Zollinger-Ellison syndrome, or gastric cancer.

DIFFICULTIES IN THE DETECTION OF DUODENAL ULCERS

Two common processes in the duodenal bulb can make the detection of ulcers more difficult:

Pseudodiverticula
Prolapsed gastric mucosa

Pseudodiverticula

Pseudodiverticula of the duodenal bulb are common sequelae of healed duodenal ulcer disease. When ulcers heal, they heal with scar formation. The retraction of this scar can result in focal indentations in the margin of the bulb (Fig. 42-2a). The regions of normal bulb between these indentations have acquired the name of pseudodiverticula. They can be differentiated from ulcers because peristalsis will cause them to contract (Fig. 42-2b), but an ulcer, because of the inflammation around it, will not contract.

Ulcers can occur in a scarred duodenal bulb containing pseudodiverticula. Such ulcers often can be identified because of their persistent crater or ring (Fig. 42-3a, b, and c).

Prolapse of Gastric Mucosa into the Duodenal Bulb

Prolapse of gastric mucosa into the duodenal bulb is commonly seen. The gastric mucosa is attached to the gastric wall loosely enough that peristalsis can push it through the pylorus. On the radiograph, the mucosa appears as a cone-shaped defect in the base of the bulb (Fig. 42-4). It can, by covering the mouth of a duodenal ulcer, prevent the demonstration of that ulcer.

Duodenal Diverticula

Duodenal diverticula are common congenital outpouchings occuring distal to the duodenal bulb. They are usually of no clinical signficance. They can be differentiated from ulcers because of their changeable appearance and because the duodenal mucosal folds extend into them (Fig. 42-5).

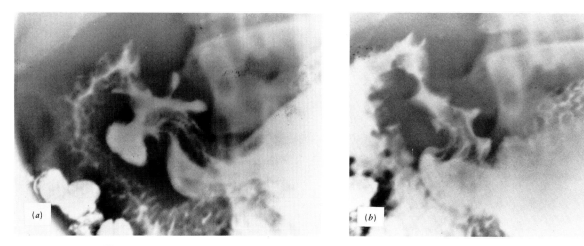

Figure 42-2. Pseudodiverticula of the duodenal bulb. (*a*) Distended view. Multiple outpouchings can be seen. (*b*) Contracted view. The multiple outpouchings have emptied. This is the expected pattern when these outpouchings are due to pseudodiverticula.

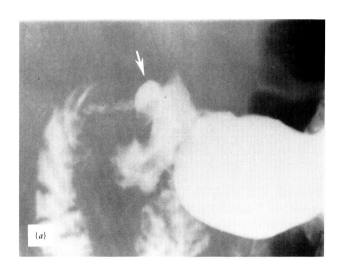

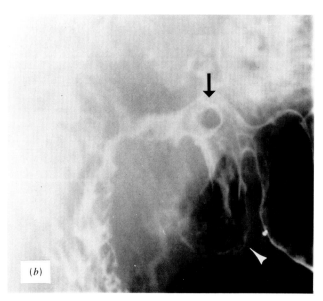

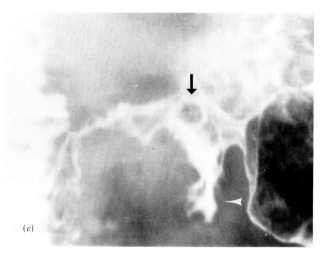

Figure 42-3. Ulcer in a scarred duodenal bulb. (*a*) Filled view. An arrow marks an outpouching that will be shown repeatedly. (*b*) An air-contrast study demonstrates the rounded mouth of the ulcer (arrow). A large pseudodiverticulum (arrowhead) is seen below. (*c*) Air-contrast study. The ring of the mouth of the ulcer is again seen (arrow), but the pseudodiverticulum is now contracted (arrowhead). (All courtesy R. Greyson-Fleg, M.D.)

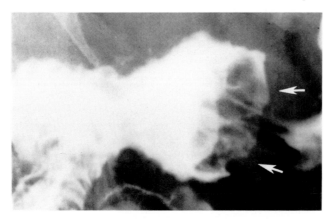

Figure 42-4. Prolapse of gastric mucosa into the duodenal bulb. The lobulated filling defect (arrows) in the base of the duodenal bulb is prolapsed gastric mucosa.

Keynotes

- *Pseudodiverticula are the result of scars of the duodenal bulb from previous ulcer disease. The outpouchings are the unscarred portion of the bulb.*
- *Duodenal diverticula are common and are usually asymptomatic.*

SUMMARY

The patient with an acute duodenal ulcer will have epigastric gnawing pain relieved by food but recurring several hours after eating. When confirmation of the diagnosis is desired, a barium or barium-air study of the duodenal bulb will usually demonstrate the ulcer. It can be difficult to differentiate an acute ulcer from a scar when there has been previous ulcer disease.

Pseudodiverticula of the duodenal bulb are areas of normal duodenal bulb between areas of scar. They extend beyond the areas of scar and can simulate duodenal ulcers. They can be differentiated from duodenal ulcers, however, because the outpouchings contract as peristalsis passes through them.

Prolapse of gastric mucosa can prevent the visualization of a duodenal ulcer.

REVIEW QUESTIONS

1. What are the symptoms of a duodenal ulcer?
2. What are the indications for obtaining a barium study of the

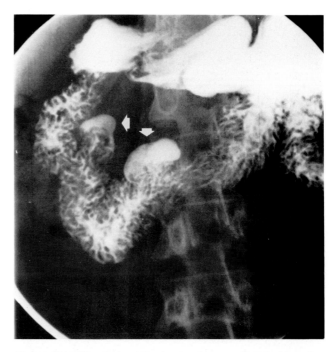

Figure 42-5. Diverticula of the duodenal sweep. Outpouchings (arrows) from the duodenum are commonly seen and are usually not of clinical significance. Duodenal mucosa can be seen extending into the diverticula. (Courtesy B. Friedman, M.D.)

duodenal bulb in a patient suspected of having a duodenal ulcer?
3. How can an ulcer scar be differentiated from an acute duodenal ulcer?
4. How can a pseudodiverticulum of the duodenal bulb be differentiated from a duodenal ulcer?
5. What is prolapsed gastric mucosa?

VOCABULARY

niche	prolapsed gastric mucosa
peptic ulcer disease	pseudodiverticulum

SUGGESTIONS FOR FURTHER READING

David W. Gelfand et al. The radiologic detection of duodenal ulcers: Effects of examiner variability, ulcer size and location, and technique. *American Journal of Roentgenology,* **145**:551–553, 1985.

For additional suggested reading see chapter 35.

43

THE COLON

Radiological

The main radiological method of evaluating the colon is the barium enema (or barium colon examination). This can be performed either with the air-barium double-contrast technique or with the barium single-contrast technique.

Because the bowel preparation and the barium enema can exacerbate an already inflamed colon or increase the amount of leakage from a perforation of the colon, care must be taken not to use the bowel preparation in patients suspected of these conditions.

The barium enema can be used to evaluate unexplained rectal bleeding, guaiac-positive stool tests, bloody diarrhea, suspected colon obstruction, or a change in stool diameter.

Clinical

Colon polyps have an increasing chance of malignancy with increasing size. Colon polyps on a stalk should be removed if they are greater than 1 cm in size and can be reached by a colonoscope. Sessile polyps have a malignant potential whatever their size and should be removed.

The patient with occult blood in the stool, with a normal double-contrast barium enema, and with a normal colonoscopy should have the upper GI tract examined. If the upper GI tract is normal, repeat studies should be obtained at appropriate intervals.

Diverticulosis is a common process in the older patient. Diverticula of the right colon can bleed. Left-colon diverticula can bleed or perforate causing diverticulitis. The patient with diverticulitis can have pain, focal or diffuse abdominal tenderness, and fever.

Inflammatory bowel disease can produce abdominal pain, fever, and diarrhea or bloody diarrhea.

OBJECTIVES

When you complete this chapter you will be able to

1. Identify colon polyps, colon cancer, diverticulosis, diverticulitis, and inflammatory colitis on selected radiographs.
2. List the stages of work-up of the patient with occult blood in stool.
3. List the conditions in which the bowel preparation for a barium enema may be dangerous for the patient.
4. List the conditions in which the barium enema itself may be dangerous for the patient.
5. On selected radiographs, indicate which colon polyps should be resected and which can be safely followed without resection.

METHODS OF EXAMINATION

The colon can be examined by the double-contrast barium-air enema or by the single-contrast enema. In almost all cases, the double-contrast study is the procedure of choice because it can detect smaller polyps, earlier cancer, and the early minor changes of inflammatory bowel disease.

Cleaning the Colon

Cleaning the colon of feces is the most critical part of the study. Feces can be mistaken for polyps or cancer, but most importantly, they can hide small lesions. Different methods of bowel preparation are used. It is important that the method used in your institution be followed accurately. Standard enemas do not clean the colon, nor do mild laxatives.

To clean the colon, many institutions use a 24- to 48-hour preparation that combines a low-residue diet with several oral doses of laxative and a laxative suppository to clean the rectosigmoid colon. Some institutions add to this preparation a cleansing enema. Because of the severity of the multiple laxatives, the bowel preparation may exacerbate preexisting bowel conditions.

When Not to Use the Bowel Preparation

1. In active ulcerative or granulomatous colitis
2. In patients with peritonitis or peritoneal inflammation
3. In active diverticulitis
4. In patients on high-dose steroids, where the signs of peritoneal inflammation can be missed

When Not to Do a Barium Enema

1. In suspected colonic perforation
2. In acute inflammatory colitis
3. Immediately after sigmoidoscopy or colonoscopy (24–48 hours delay being preferred)
4. Within 2 weeks of a colonic biopsy
5. Until colonic surgery has healed

Indications for a Double-Contrast Barium Enema

1. Unexplained rectal bleeding
2. Guaiac- or fecal blood slide test positive stool confirmed on a meat-free diet.
3. Bloody diarrhea, unexplained (do not study if active colitis is suspected)
4. Suspected colonic obstruction
5. Change in stool diameter

Indications for a Single-Contrast Barium Enema

1. If the patient is unable to cooperate for a double-contrast barium enema
2. As an acceptable alternate procedure in children
3. To reduce colonic intussusception in children

Keynote

• In almost all patients, the air-barium double-contrast study of the colon is preferred to the single-contrast study.

DISEASES THAT CAN BE EVALUATED ON BARIUM COLON EXAMINATIONS

Colon Cancer

Case 43-1

This 64-year-old man was found on his annual physical examination to have stool that tested guaiac positive.

The stool exam had been done during diet restriction and was considered reliable. The patient was 20% overweight and had ischemic changes on an exercise electrocardiogram.

How would you evaluate the occult fecal blood?

Both sigmoidoscopy and an air-barium double-contrast colon exam are indicated. Films from the study are shown in Figure 43-1. What do you see?

There is a 1-cm polyp on a stalk showing as a persistent defect in the sigmoid colon. Figure 43-1a is a single contrast view with the polyp (arrow) appearing as a filling defect in the column of barium. Figures 43-1b and c are double contrast studies demonstrating that the polyp (arrow) has a very short stalk. The shortness of the stalk is an indicator of increased risk of malignancy and such polyps on short stalks should be excised. In Figure 43-1c, the view is taken looking down on the polyp and its stalk. This view results in a double ring shadow (arrow), the outer ring representing the polyp and the inner ring representing the stalk. What should be done now?

Fiberoptic flexible sigmoidoscopy to remove the polyp. This was an adenomatous polyp with focal malignancy within it.

All polyps larger than 1 cm in diameter and accessible to the fiberoptic colonoscope should be resected because of the potential that the polyp is adenomatous and could contain cancer.

What would you do if the colonoscope could not reach the polyp?

You would have to compare the operative risk with the relative risk of cancer and make a decision. Cancer risk depends on the size of the polyp. The larger it is, the more likely it is to contain cancer. Medical illnesses affect the operative risk.

Csae 43-2

This 54-year-old woman was found to have stools that tested guaiac positive. Sigmoidoscopy and an air-barium double-contrast enema were both normal. What would you do next?

Assuming that the guaiac test was positive on a restricted diet and that the double-contrast enema was of good quality, then two evaluations are needed: endoscopic colonscopy and double-contrast and endoscopic evaluations of the esophagus and stomach.

What if these studies were all of good quality and normal? What would you do next?

The patient should be followed with repeat studies. The interval between these exams is under active study by the American Cancer Society. Pending the cancer society's final results (but using some of their data), I suggest repeat double-contrast upper GI tract series at 3, 6, and 12 months, then repeat endoscopy at 12 months, and then an upper GI tract series annually for 3 years.

The colon should be reevaluated with both method

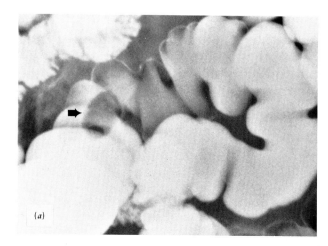

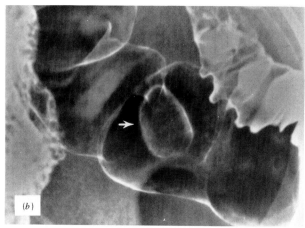

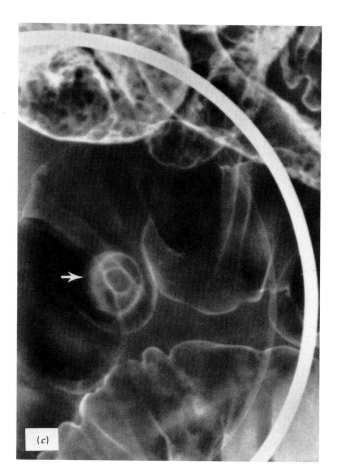

Figure 43-1. Case example 43-1.

at 1 year and then followed every 2 years with both methods.

Case 43-3

This 49-year-old man has had several attacks of crampy lower abdominal pain followed by diarrhea over the last few weeks. He came in frightened because the last two diarrheal stools had been bloody. He was quite anxious, but the remainder of his history was normal.

Physical examination is normal except that his stool tests guaiac positive.

A view from his barium enema is shown in Figure 43-2. This image is from the lower portion of the descending colon. What does it show?

There is a focal area of narrowing of the colonic lumen. The transition to the normal lumen is abrupt. Proximal to the narrowing the mucosa is irregular. What do you think is going on?

This patient has carcinoma of the colon. This is a variant of the apple-core pattern. The irregularity of the mucosa proximal to the obstruction is due to focal colitis; focal colitis is common proximal to colonic obstructions.

Other patterns of colon cancer include polypoid cancer (polyps larger than 1 cm and on stalks may be cancerous). The larger the polyp, the greater the chance of neoplasm. Masses with mucosal irregularity can be cancerous (Fig. 43-3). Figure 43-4 demonstrates a complete obstruction from an apple-core lesion. Only the distal portion of the apple core is demonstrated.

Larger colon cancers can sometimes be identified on CT scans as masses within the lumen of the colon (Fig. 43-5); most masses within the colonic lumen will, however, be feces.

Keynotes

- *A test for blood in the stool should be part of the evaluation of every patient over the age of 40.*
- *All colon polyps larger that 1 cm in diameter should be resected if accessible to the colonoscope.*
- *Patients with a positive stool guaiac test on a meat-free diet should undergo repeated evaluations for colon cancer. In some cases, the colon cancer will be fcund only after 4–6 years of follow-up.*

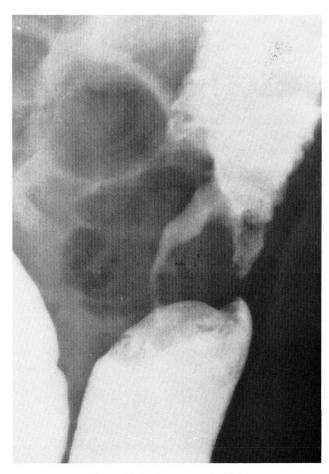

Figure 43-2. Case example 43-3.

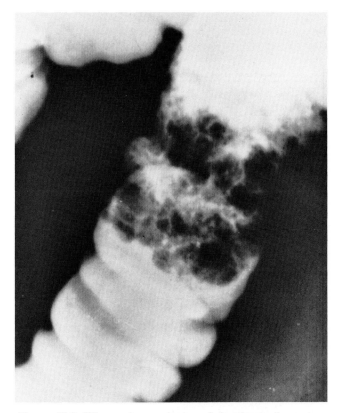

Figure 43-3. Villous adenocarcinoma of the descending colon. Marked irregularity is seen, with many villous adenomas and adenocarcinomas, because the barium can fill the interstices within the fronds of the tumor.

Diverticulosis and Diverticulitis

Colonic diverticula are common abnormalities. They are of two types: congenital and acquired. The congenital diverticula are uncommon and occur primarily in the right side of the colon. They are usually asymptomatic but can bleed massively.

Acquired diverticula of the colon are common (Fig. 43-6). They are most often seen in the sigmoid colon but can occur in any portion. They are seen in 10% of the population over 50 years of age, and their frequency increases with increasing age. They are usually asymptomatic, but they can bleed, sometimes massively; occasionally they perforate, resulting in diverticulitis.

Diverticulosis is easily detected by barium enema. Most patients with *diverticulitis* have the same radiographic pattern as those with diverticulosis. The diagnosis of diverticulitis usually must be made clinically: left lower quadrant pain, fever, and palpable tender tubular mass are the common clinical findings. Occasionally, the barium enema in a patient with diverticulitis will demonstrate communication of the colonic lumen with an abscess cavity (Fig. 43-7). Sometimes the abscess will be seen to press on the colonic lumen, but without a communication being demonstrated.

Keynotes

- *Colon diverticula are common in older patients. Most are asymptomatic, but they can bleed. Occasionally, they perforate, resulting in diverticulitis.*
- *In most patients with diverticulitis, no specific radiological sign of the infection is seen.*

Inflammatory Bowel Disease

Inflammatory bowel disease can be infectious or noninfectious. The infectious forms include shigellosis, salmonellosis, amebiasis, and pseudomembranous colitis; the noninfectious forms are ulcerative colitis and granulomatous enterocolitis (or Crohn's disease). In each of these diseases, the major radiographic finding is mucosal irregularity.

Ulcerative Colitis. The patient with *ulcerative colitis* usually has recurrent episodes of crampy abdominal pain associated with bloody diarrhea or bloody mucoid diarrhea. Diagnosis can be made by sigmoidoscopy because the disease almost always extends to the rectum. A barium enema can be used to evaluate the extent of the disease and to look for the complications of stricture formation and cancer.

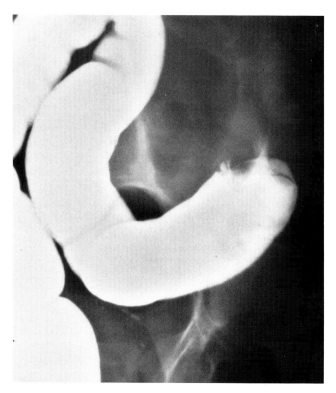

Figure 43-4. Colon cancer with complete obstruction of the lumen. The pattern is similar to the distal portion of the cancer shown in Figure 43-2.

The colon in ulcerative colitis undergoes several sequential changes. Initially, many small ulcers can be seen in the involved areas of the colon (Fig. 43-8). These can deepen and can connect in the submucosa. Spasm is often present. As the disease becomes more chronic, areas of focal mucosal hypertrophy can occur, resulting in multiple pseudopolypoid lesions (Fig. 43-9)

With long-standing disease, the colonic wall becomes fibrotic, the length of the colon shortens, and the wall becomes less flexible (Fig. 43-10). Focal strictures can occur. When the duration of disease exceed 10 years, carcinoma of the colon can occur.

Clinically and radiographically, ulcerative colitis must be differentiated from granulomatous colitis (Crohn's disease), though in many patients symptoms and signs seem to overlap. The radiological findings more suggestive of ulcerative colitis include symmetrical involvement of the entire circumference of the bowel, continuous involvement from the rectum proximal to the limit of the disease, and dilation of the terminal ileum if it is involved by the disease (Table 43-1).

Granulomatous Colitis. Colonic involvement by *Crohn's disease* can be isolated in the colon or can coexist with small bowel involvement. The disease can result in fever and weight loss, or it can be associated with abdominal pain, often crampy; loose stools; and rectal urgency. Fistulae can form, abscesses can occur, and small bowel obstruction is common.

Radiologically, the initial ulcers in *granulomatous enterocolitis* are quite shallow and can be seen only on carefully performed air-barium double-contrast studies. Deep ulcers are often seen within the colon. The involvement of the colon is often asymmetric (Figs. 43-11 and 43-12); there are often uninvolved areas (skip areas) separating abnormal areas. When the disease affects the small bowel,

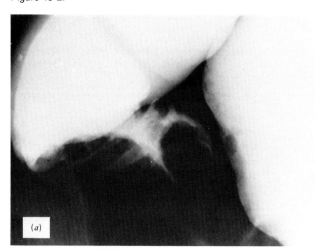

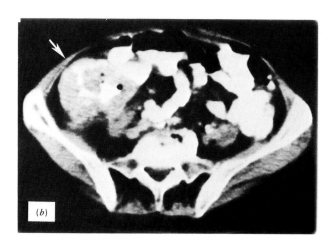

Figure 43-5. Cecal cancer shown on barium enema and CT. (*a*) Appearance on barium enema. A large lobular mass fills the cecum, preventing its filling with barium. The rounded lobules of tumor can be seen impressing on barium. (*b*) Appearance on CT. The bowel has been opacified with swallowed contrast medium, which has filled some of the interstices of the cecal tumor (arrow). In this 74-year-old man, the CT was performed first, looking for an explanation of abdominal pain, and the tumor was found.

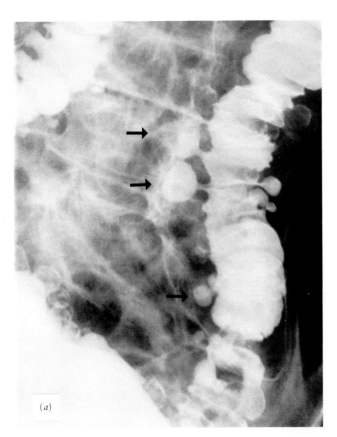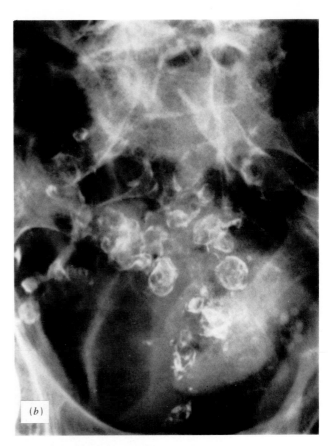

Figure 43-6. Diverticulosis. (*a*) Barium in the descending colon demonstrates multiple diverticula (arrows). (*b*) Barium residua in diverticula. Barium can be retained in colonic diverticula for many weeks, resulting in round or ringlike areas of increased radiodensity.

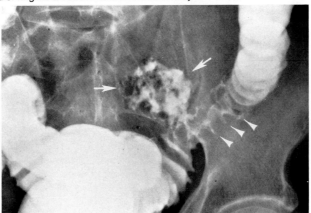

Figure 43-7. Diverticulitis. Small diverticula (arrowheads) of the sigmoid colon are seen. There is a larger irregular pocket of barium adjacent to the colon (arrows) representing the abscess of the diverticulitis.

TABLE 43-1.   RADIOLOGICAL CRITERIA AIDING IN THE DIFFERENTIATION OF ULCERATIVE AND GRANULOMATOUS COLITIS

Ulcerative Colitis	Granulomatous Colitis
Symmetrical involvement	Deep, isolated ulcers
Continuous involvement starting in rectum	No circumferential involvement
Dilation of the terminal ileum if involved by the disease	Fistulae
	Narrowing of the terminal ileum
	Involvement of the more proximal portions of small bowel

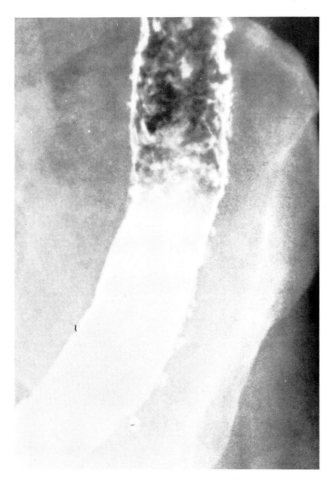

Figure 43-8. Ulcerative colitis. Small ulcers in the mucosa result in the irregularity in the contour of the colon. Multiple small ulcers are filled with barium.

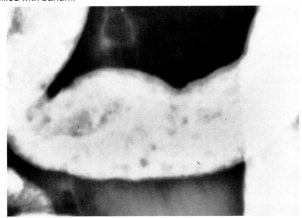

Figure 43-9. Ulcerative colitis. Pseudopolyps (areas of mucosal hypertrophy) appear like filling defects in the barium.

there are often areas of marked narrowing present. The left side of the colon may be uninvolved.

The main radiological findings that support the diagnosis of granulomatous colitis are asymmetric, noncontinu-

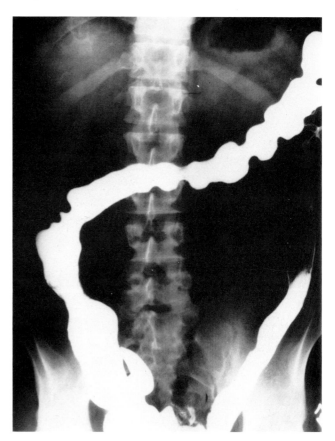

Figure 43-10. Ulcerative colitis, fibrotic phase. The colon is shortened and lacks normal haustral folds.

ous involvement; fistulae (Fig. 43-13); narrowing of the terminal (i.e., most distal) ileum; and involvement of more proximal portions of the small bowel (Table 43-1).

Keynote

• *There is an increased incidence of colon cancer in patients who have had ulcerative colitis for more than 10 years. Careful and repeated screening for these possible cancers is desirable.*

SUMMARY

It is most important that the colon be properly cleaned (prepped) before a barium study. Feces can make the evaluation of the colon most difficult. Certain patients, however, should not receive the bowel preparation. High doses of steroids can mask acute inflammation, and care is necessary in these patients.

A barium enema should not be done in suspected colonic perforation, in acute active colitis, within 2 days of sigmoidoscopy, within 2 weeks of colonic biopsy, or until colon surgery has healed. The barium enema is useful in

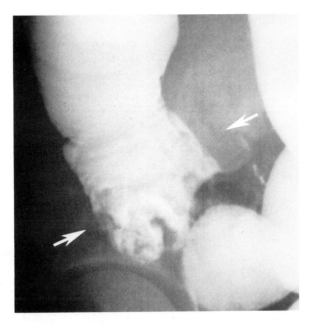

Figure 43-11. Granulomatous colitis (Crohn's disease). The cecum (arrows) demonstrates irregularity of the mucosa caused by deep ulcerations. The diameter of the cecum is decreased. (Courtesy R. Greyson-Fleg, M.D.)

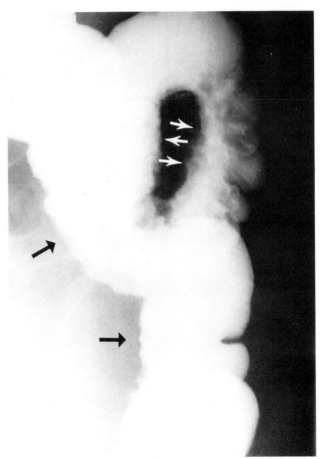

Figure 43-12. Granulomatous colitis. The splenic flexure of the colon and the descending colon demonstrate asymmetric ulcerations (arrows) indicative of Crohn's disease. (Courtesy of R. Greyson-Fleg, M.D.)

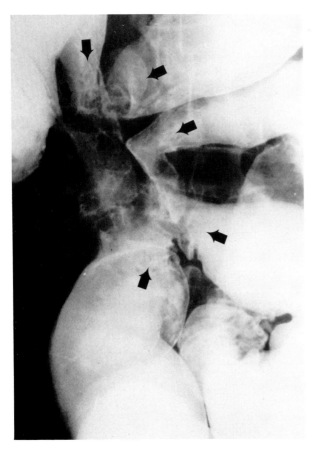

Figure 43-13. Granulomatous enterocolitis with extensive fistularization. Multiple loops of small and large bowel (arrows) interconnect. In Crohn's disease, fistulae can form between bowel loops and between bowel and other structures, such as abscess cavities, the skin, and the bladder. (Courtesy R. Greyson-Fleg, M.D.)

evaluating blood loss or other symptoms of colon cancer and symptoms of nonacute colitis.

Colonic polyps are common, and those over 1 cm in diameter should be removed because of the possibility of cancer. Some polyps are too small to be detected. Occult blood loss should be carefully evaluated, and if no cause is found, the patient should be followed, looking for the cause.

Diverticulosis of the colon is a common finding in the elderly. Perforation of a diverticulum can result in diverticulitis with local pain, fever, and local mass.

Noninfectious causes of colitis are ulcerative colitis and granulomatous colitis. The radiological findings most helpful in differentiating them are listed in Table 43-1.

REVIEW QUESTIONS

1. When might the bowel prep for a barium enema be dangerous to the patient?
2. In which patients might a barium enema be dangerous?
3. What are the indications for obtaining a barium enema?
4. Which colonic polyps should be removed?
5. How should the case of a patient with occult blood in the stool be worked up?
6. What are the symptoms and radiographic findings of diverticulitis?
7. How do the symptoms and radiographic findings of ulcerative and granulomatous colitis differ?

VOCABULARY

Crohn's disease
diverticulitis
diverticulosis

granulomatous enterocolitis
ulcerative colitis

SUGGESTIONS FOR FURTHER READING

Frederick M. Kelvin, R. Kristina Gedgaudas, Radiologic diagnosis of Crohn disease (with emphasis on early manifestations). *CRC Critical Reviews in Diagnostic Imaging,* **16**:43–91, 1981.

For additional suggested reading see Chapter 35.

SECTION C

LIVER AND PANCREATIC IMAGING

The next two chapters discuss the imaging of the liver, biliary tract, and pancreas. There are multiple methods of imaging these organs. With the liver and biliary tract, choosing the best technique is a major challenge. With the pancreas, this book emphasizes the CT examination because it is the easiest for the student to interpret and has the widest use.

44

THE LIVER AND BILIARY TRACT

KEY CONCEPTS

Radiological

The choice among the techniques for imaging the liver and biliary tract depends on the clinical history, physical examination, and patient's presumed disease. The choices:

1. The plain abdominal radiograph has a limited role. It may demonstrate a gallstone or biliary air.
2. The oral cholecystogram can be used to evaluate suspected chronic cholecystitis.
3. The intravenous cholangiogram can demonstrate bile duct stones after cholecystectomy, but is not commonly done.
4. The angiogram can be used to establish the diagnosis of suspected hepatic angiomas.
5. Nuclear medicine scans for Kupffer cell location can be used in the evaluation of hepatic enlargement, looking for hepatic masses, and evaluation of the severity of cirrhosis.
6. Gallium citrate Ga 67 scanning can demonstrate hepatic abscesses and hepatomas.
7. Nuclear medicine scanning of the biliary tract is the method for diagnosing acute cholecystitis and can be used to differentiate obstructive from nonobstructive jaundice.
8. The sonogram can be used to evaluate the patient with suspected chronic cholecystitis, to help differentiate obstructive from nonobstructive jaundice, to differentiate hepatic cysts from solid tumors, and to find biliary stones.
9. Computed tomography is the preferred method for evaluating obstructive jaundice and can be used in place of nuclear medicine scanning in the detection of focal hepatic masses.
10. The transhepatic cholangiogram can be used to diagnose the cause of obstructive jaundice when the CT is not successful and can be extended to provide either internal or external drainage of the biliary tract.

OBJECTIVES

When you complete this chapter you will be able to

1. Indicate the preferred method or methods of evaluating
   a. Acute cholecystitis
   b. Chronic cholecystitis
   c. Hepatomegaly, possibly from a mass
   d. Jaundice, differentiating obstructive and non obstructive forms
   e. Suspected hepatic abscess
2. Describe the method for internal drainage of an obstructed biliary tract.

Many methods are available for imaging the biliary system. The selection of the best techniques for your patient can be complex because there is a preferred imaging technique for each potential hepatobiliary abnormality. For this reason, the initial evaluation of a patient with suspected hepatobiliary disease must consist of a careful history and physical examination followed by an appropriate choice of clinical chemical tests. The imaging techniques are then used to confirm or exclude a suspected diagnosis.

PATTERNS OF ABNORMALITY

Liver and biliary tract disease can result in several different patterns of abnormality:

Changes in size
Presence of a mass or masses

Disorganization of liver architecture

Bile duct dilation, with or without obstruction
  Intrahepatic
  Extrahepatic

Cystic duct obstruction

Gallbladder wall inflammation
  Acute
  Chronic

Stones in
  Gallbladder or bile ducts
    Precholecystectomy or postcholecystectomy
    With or without obstruction

Hepatic vein obstruction

Portal vein dilation
  With or without obstruction

TYPES OF IMAGING TECHNIQUES

The variety of imaging choices is broad. In selected cases, the plain abdominal radiograph, the oral cholecystogram, the intravenous cholangiogram, the angiogram, nuclear medicine imaging studies for Kupffer's cell location, ^{67}Ga tracer imaging, nuclear medicine imaging for biliary tract excretion, the sonogram, the transmission computed tomogram, the percutaneous transhepatic cholangiogram, or the endoscopic retrograde cholangiogram can be performed. Each study yields specific types of information about the liver and biliary tract. This chapter attempts to guide you toward the proper selection.

Keynotes

* *Cholecysto-, pertaining to the gallbladder.*
* *Kupffer's cells are phagocytic cells (cells that ingest particulate matter) in the hepatic parenchyma.*
* *Cholangio-, pertaining to the bile ducts.*

Plain Abdominal Radiograph

Uses. There is no primary use for the plain abdominal radiograph. When obtained for other purposes the radiograph may demonstrate biliary stones. Approximately 20% of biliary stones contain sufficient calcium to be seen (Fig. 44-1). Occasionally the gallbladder wall itself is calcified (Fig. 44-2).

Patterns of Abnormality

Biliary Air. Air in the biliary tract is most often due to prior common duct surgery. It can be due to biliary fistulae or the recent passage of a gallstone.

Air in the wall of the gallbladder (Fig. 44-3) is rare, but it is a sign of acute cholecystitis. Air within the gallbladder is usually due to acute cholecystitis but uncommonly to the passage of a gallstone directly from the gallbladder into the bowel or to a biliary fistula to the bowel.

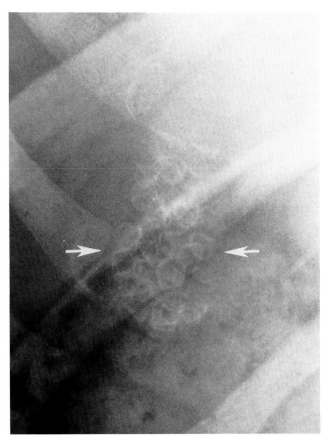

Figure 44-1. Multiple small calcified gallstones (arrows) are seen in this focal view of the right upper quadrant of the abdomen.

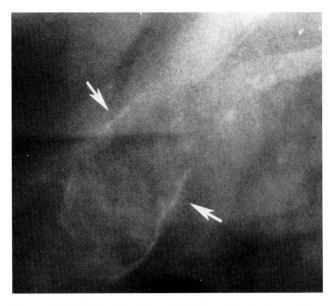

Figure 44-2. Calcification of the wall of the gallbladder (arrows) is a sign of chronic cholecystitis.

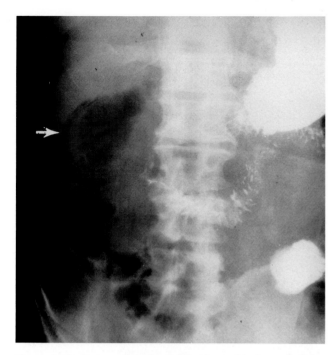

Figure 44-3. Air is seen in the gallbladder and in the wall of the gallbladder (arrow). When this is due to infection, as in this case, the process is called emphysematous cholecystitis. (Courtesy M. Vaccaro, M.D.)

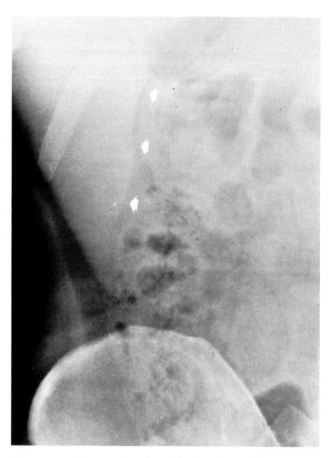

Figure 44-4. The posterior edge of the liver (arrows) is outlined by retroperitoneal fat. When this posterior edge lies below the iliac crest on a supine radiograph, the liver is usually enlarged.

Air in the hepatic veins is usually from a bowel infarction.

Enlargement. only the posterior margin of the liver is outlined by fat (Fig. 44-4). Marked hepatomegaly can be judged by whether the lower margin of the liver overlaps the iliac crest on a radiograph done with the patient supine.

Keynote

- *The plain abdominal film can demonstrate marked hepatomegaly, 20% of gallstones, and biliary air.*

Oral Cholecystogram

The normal appearance of the gallbladder on oral cholecystograms is shown in Figures 44-5 and 44-6.

Uses. The oral cholecystogram competes with ultrasonography in

1. The diagnosis of chronic cholecystitis and the cholecystoses
2. The detection of gallstones (Figs. 44-7 and 44-8)

Limitations and Cautions. Oral cholecystography

1. Works best if bilirubin is less that 5 mg%
2. Can cause idiosyncratic, allergylike reactions
3. Should not be performed in the presence of renal failure.

Technique. After eating a meal containing fat, the patient is placed on a fat-free diet. The evening before the examination, the patient takes six tablets of an oral cholecystographic agent. These should be taken 30 minutes apart to avoid nausea. The next morning, radiographs of the right upper quadrant of the abdomen are taken. If the contrast medium has concentrated in the gallbladder, multiple views are taken to look for gallstones. If these views are normal, the patient is then given a fatty meal to eat (or cholecystokinin is injected) to evaluate gallbladder contraction.

If the gallbladder has not concentrated the contrast sufficiently to decide whether stones are present, two different techniques can be followed. In the classical technique, the patient is maintained on a fat-free diet and is asked to take an additional six tablets that evening and return for

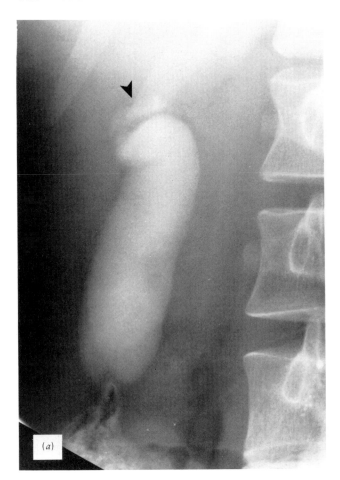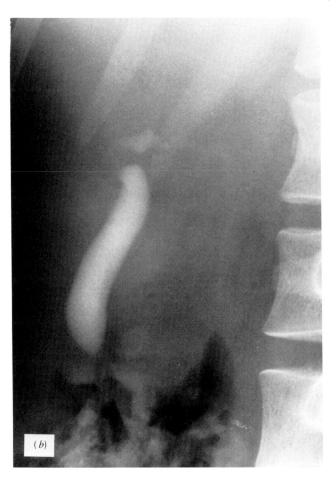

Figure 44-5. Normal appearance of the gallbladder visualized by oral cholecystography. (*a*) Filled view. (*b*) View after a fatty meal. An arrowhead marks the cystic duct.

additional radiographs the next morning. This second dose (often incorrectly called a "double dose") will, with 98% accuracy, differentiate chronic cholecystitis from a normal gallbladder. In chronic cholecystitis, either the gallbladder will not opacify on the second day or gallstones will be demonstrated.

The second technique for evaluating the gallbladder inadequately visualized on the first cholecystographic attempt is to do a sonogram of the gallbladder looking for gallstones. If gallstones are found, chronic cholecystitis is diagnosed, and the patient need not return for a second day of study. If no gallstones are found, the traditional second dose is given because not all gallstones can be detected by sonography and because sonography can fail to detect chronic cholecystitis unaccompanied by stones (acalculous cholecystitis).

Keynotes

- *The oral cholecystogram competes with ultrasonography as the preferred method for the detection of chronic cholecystitis, gallstones, and the cholecystoses.*

- *The cholecystoses are a group of chronic gallbladder processes including cholesterosis (cholesterol polyps) and adenomyomatosis (epithelial proliferation). They are probably unrelated to symptoms.*
- *It is often necessary to give the patient two consecutive daily doses of oral cholecystographic medicine to obtain opacification of the gallbladder. This second-dose study is often incorrectly called a "double-dose" study. Doubling the dose of medicine can result in serious drug toxicity.*
- *Chronic cholecystitis is diagnosed when there*
  - *a. Are gallstones*
  - *b. Is failure of opacification by the second day (if patient is not jaundiced, took the medicine, and did not vomit it up)*

Intravenous Cholangiogram

The normal intravenous cholangiogram study is shown in Figure 44-9.

Use. Intravenous cholangiography is no longer commonly used because of the toxicity of the contrast medium. It still has an occasional use as a method for finding common hepatic and common bile duct stones in patients with

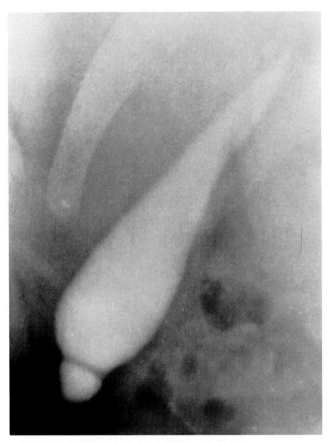

Figure 44-6. Normal variant of gallbladder appearance on an oral cholecystogram. Partial septa and folds are commonly seen.

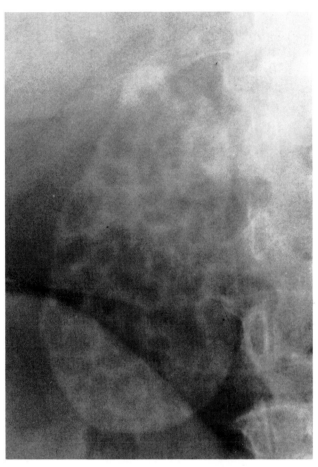

Figure 44-7 Many small gallstones are surrounded by faint gallbladder contrast medium in this oral cholecystogram. The presence of gallstones indicates the presence of chronic cholecystitis.

biliary pain but without jaundice after cholecystectomy. In such patients, sonography is the preferred initial procedure, followed when necessary in many institutions by endoscopic retrograde cholangiography. Should those procedures fail to explain the patient's problem, intravenous cholangiography or percutaneous transhepatic cholangiography can be used.

Limitations and Cautions. Intravenous cholangiography

1. Works best if bilirubin is less than 2 mg%.
2. Will not be successful if bilirubin is more than 4 mg%
2. Can induce severe and fatal idiosyncratic drug reactions
3. Can increase severity of renal failure
4. Can induce renal failure if done within 24 hours of an oral cholecystogram

Technique. Contrast medium is injected intravenously into a fasting patient slowly (over 10–20 minutes). Multiple radiographic tomographic sections are made through the region of the common bile duct every 20 minutes for 1

hour and then each hour for 4 hours unless adequate visualization occurs before that time.

Patterns of Abnormality

1. Stones may be seen in the bile ducts (Fig. 44-10).
2. Filling of bile ducts with nonfilling of gallbladder in 4 hours is diagnostic of acute cholecystitis.
3. Nonvisualization of bile ducts—a nondiagnostic study—can occur in normal or abnormal bile ducts.
4. A dilated common bile duct may be seen. Ducts larger than 11 mm are indicative of current or prior obstruction. Ducts 7–11 mm are suspicious for current or prior obstruction if the patient has not had common duct surgical exploration.

Keynote

• *The intravenous cholangiogram can be used in the of evaluation for common duct stones after cholecystectomy when sonography is indeterminate.*

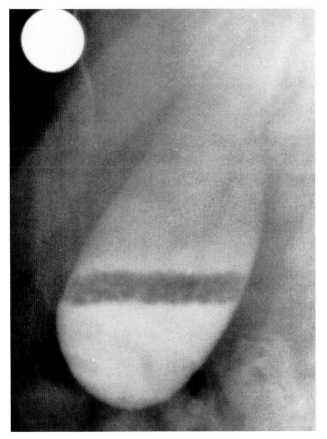

Figure 44-8. Many small gallstones layer in the gallbladder on this upright view.

Angiogram

Uses. There is no primary use for the angiogram in biliary tract imaging. Secondary uses are:

1. For diagnosis of suspect hepatic hemangioma
2. For preoperative evaluation before resection of primary hepatic neoplasms

Nuclear Medicine Imaging for Kupffer's Cell Location

The normal study using nuclear medicine imaging for Kupffer's cell location is shown in Figure 44-11.

Uses. Nuclear medicine imaging for Kupffer's cell location is used to

1. Detect a hepatic mass or masses (Fig. 44-12)
2. Evaluate liver size
3. Evaluate severity of cirrhosis

Limitations and Cautions. With this nuclear imaging technique, there are no limitations or cautions.

Technique. Particles of technetium Tc 99m sulfur colloid of the proper size to be ingested by cells of the reticuloendothelial (R-E) system are injected intravenously. Once ingested by the R-E cells, the radioactivity in these cells can be used to demonstrate the architecture of the liver. Masses larger than 2–3 cm can be identified as focal regions of lack of activity.

Keynote

• *The reticuloendothelial system is composed of those cells that can ingest particulate matter. Major portions of it are in the liver, spleen, bone marrow, and lung.*

Nuclear Medicine Imaging with Gallium Citrate Ga 67

Uses. Nuclear medicine imaging with gallium citrate Ga 67 is useful in the identification of

1. Hepatic abscesses
2. Hepatomas

Hepatomas and abscesses are regions of nonactivity on technetium Tc 99m sulfur colloid imaging studies. Most abscesses and many hepatomas are, however, ^{67}Ga-avid and can be visualized as regions of increased radioactivity within the less diffuse liver activity seen on ^{67}Ga liver images (Fig. 44-13).

Limitations. Gallium 67 must be given 48–72 hours in advance of making the images.

Nuclear Medicine Imaging of the Biliary Tract

The normal study of the biliary tract by nuclear medicine imaging is shown in Figure 44-14. [99m]Tc iminodiacetic acid derivatives (IDA) are processed by the hepatocytes and are excreted into the biliary tract. They pass through the bile ducts into the gallbladder and small bowel.

Uses. Biliary tract imaging by nuclear medicine is

1. A method for differentiation of obstructive from non-obstructive jaundice
2. The method of choice for diagnosis of acute cholecystitis when history and physical examination are equivocal

Limitations. Maximum bilirubin levels for imaging are about 10 mg%.

Technique. The compound is injected intravenously. Serial images of the hepatobiliary region of the abdomen are obtained over a period of 1 hour. In the normal person, filling of the gallbladder and some small bowel excretion will occur within 1 hour (Fig. 44-14).

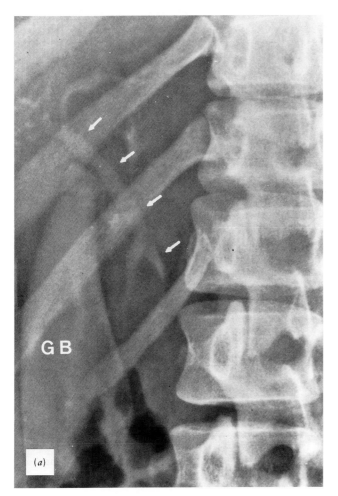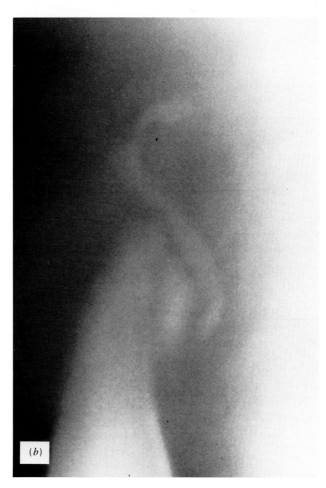

Figure 44-9. Normal intravenous cholangiogram. (*a*) Focal conventional view of the right upper quadrant of the abdomen. (*b*) Tomographic view. The tomogram blurs out the overlying bony structures. The gallbladder (GB) and the common duct (arrows) are well seen.

Patterns of Abnormality.

1. Chronic cholecystitis may show as a delay in filling of the gallbladder up to 2 hours.
2. Biliary tract obstruction may be indicated when no activity seen in small bowel at 1 hour (Fig. 44-14).
3. Acute cholecystitis is suggested by activity in the common bile duct, but no activity in the gallbladder. You must follow the study for a minimum of 2 hours (Fig. 44-16). In some cases a longer study is necessary.

Keynote

- *Iminodiacetic acid (IDA) derivatives are processed by the hepatocytes and excreted into the biliary tract. Tracer imaging with these agents is used in the diagnosis of acute cholecystitis and in identifying biliary tract obstruction.*

Sonogram

The normal sonogram study of the gallbladder is shown in Figure 44-17.

Uses. The sonogram can

1. Identify dilated intrahepatic bile ducts and show that jaundice is probably due to biliary tract obstruction
2. Identify dilated intrahepatic portal veins, often a sign of portal hypertension
3. Detect 95% of gallstones (Figs. 44-18, 44-19, and 44-20)
4. Differentiate hepatic cysts from solid tumors, confirming that an abnormality seen on a technetium Tc 99m sulfur colloid liver scan is due to metastasis

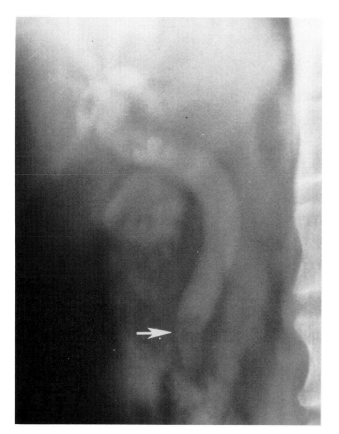

Figure 44-10. Intravenous cholangiogram in a postcholecystectomy patient. The arrow indicates a filling defect in the distal common duct that was due to a stone.

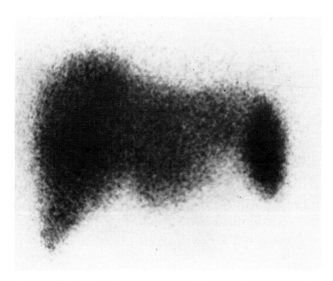

Figure 44-11. Normal liver scan done with technetium Tc 99m sulfur colloid.

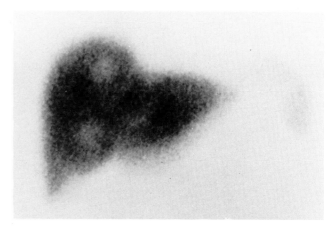

Figure 44-12. Several masses are seen within the liver. These were metastases from pancreatic carcinoma.

5. Diagnose acute cholecystitis, although a biliary excretion scan with ^{99m}Tc IDA derived compound is more sensitive
6. Diagnose perihepatic abscesses
7. Partially substitute for a second day of oral cholecystogram (as already described in the paragraph on the technique for oral cholecystography)

Limitations and Cautions. There are no limitations or cautions with sonography.

Keynote

- *The sonogram can identify*
  - a. *Biliary tract dilation*
  - b. *Portal vein dilation*
  - c. *Gallstones*
  - d. *Possible cystic nature of hepatic masses*
  - e. *Many cases of acute cholecystitis*
  - f. *perihepatic abscesses*

Transmission Computed Tomogram

The normal CT study is shown in Figure 44-21.

Uses. Computed tomography is

1. The preferred method for evaluating painless obstructive jaundice (competes with sonography) (Fig. 44-22)
2. The preferred method of looking for pancreatic and porta hepatis masses causing obstructive jaundice
3. The best imaging method of looking for metastases to the liver surface from transperitoneal seeding, particularly from ovarian lesions (but surgical exploration or laparoscopy are more sensitive)

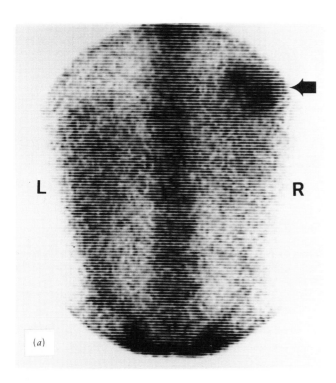

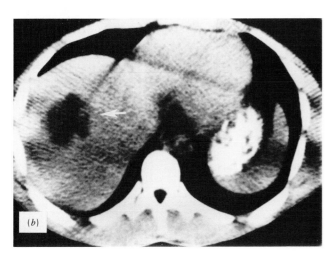

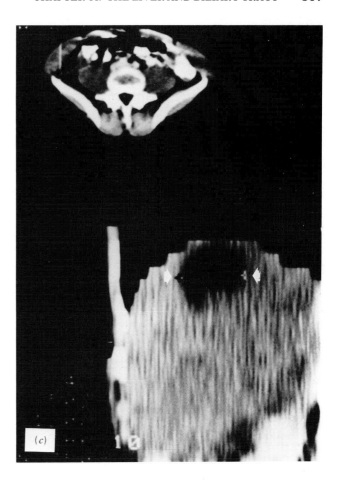

Figure 44-13. This 27-year-old man had been febrile and losing weight for 5–6 weeks. (*a*) A ^{67}Ga scan of the liver, posterior view. The area of increased uptake posteriorly (arrow) was the site of a hepatic abscess. (*b*) A CT section through the area of increased ^{67}Ga activity demonstrated a focal area of radiolucency (arrow). (*c*) A sagittal reconstruction of the CT images again demonstrated the location of the abscess (arrows), which was drained percutaneously by the radiologist. (All courtesy E. Blum, M.D.)

4. Used to diagnose hepatic hemangiomas
5. Used to identify hepatic metastases (Fig. 44-23).

Cautions. Because CT is often used with an intravenous contrast medium, there is a chance of idiosyncratic reactions.

Keynote

* *Computed tomography is of greatest use in demonstrating pancreatic or porta hepatis masses causing obstructive jaundice. It can also demonstrate hepatic metastases.*

Transhepatic Cholangiogram and Transhepatic Drainage

Uses. The transhepatic cholangiogram is useful

1. In suspected obstructive jaundice when transmission computed tomography or sonography fails to reveal the cause of the obstruction
2. In patients with obstructive jaundice who are not candidates for surgical cure of the cause of the obstruction (poor operative risk, unresectable neoplasms) to permit placement of a catheter for internal or external drainage of bile

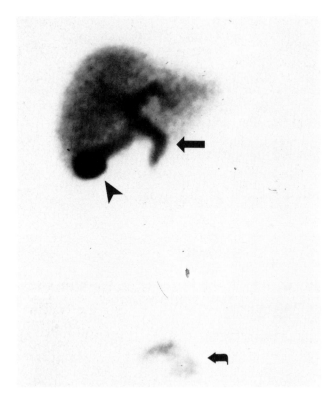

Figure 44-14. Normal biliary tract image using a ^{99m}Tc IDA derivative. The common duct (straight arrow) and the gallbladder (arrowhead) are both seen. Bowel activity (curved arrow) is also present.

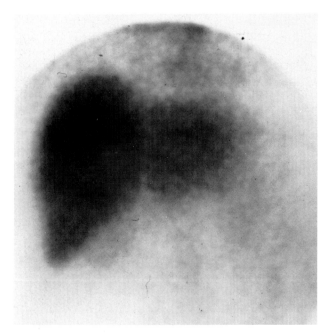

Figure 44-15. Biliary tract obstruction. The liver is opacified, but the duct system is not visualized after 60 minutes. (Study done with a ^{99m}Tc IDA derivative.) (Courtesy M Vaccaro, M.D.)

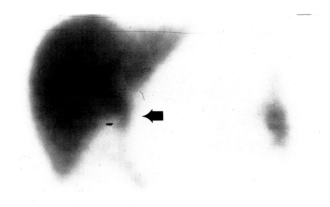

Figure 44-16. Acute cholecystitis. On this ^{99m}Tc IDA derivative study the liver and the common duct (arrow) are opacified, but after 90 minutes, there is still no filling of the gallbladder.

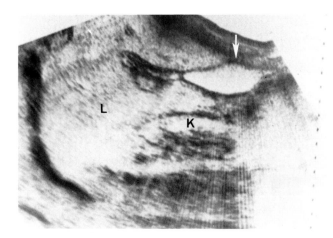

Figure 44-17. Sonogram of the gallbladder, normal study. The gallbladder (arrow), liver (L), and Kidney (K) can be identified.

Limitations and Cautions. When using transhepatic cholangiography or drainage, bear in mind that

1. There is a chance of inducing hemobilia.
2. There is a slight chance of liver laceration.
3. If obstruction is present, some form of drainage is then necessary to prevent bile peritonitis.
4. If bile is infected, there is danger of inducing bacteremia.

Technique

For imaging. A 23-gauge needle is passed through the abdominal wall into the liver. Contrast medium is injected. Multiple placements of the needle are made until a bile duct is entered. When dilated bile ducts are present, opacification of the bile ducts is possible, and the cause of the obstruction can usually be diagnosed (Fig. 44-24a).

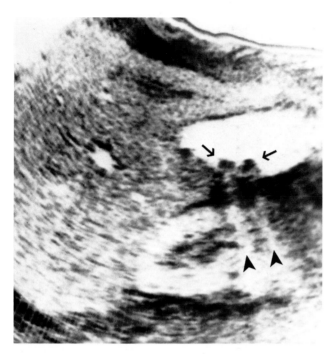

Figure 44-18. Sonogram of the gallbladder. Two gallstones are seen (arrows) with sonic shadowing (arrowheads). (Courtesy R. Sanders, M.D.)

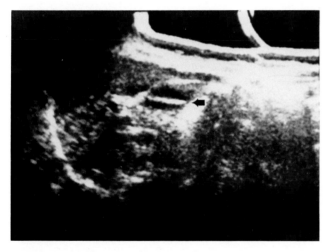

Figure 44-19. Sonogram of the gallbladder. A horizontal band of gallstones (arrow) is seen. Compare this sonographic appearance with the radiographic appearance in Figure 44-8. (Courtesy R. Sanders, M.D.)

For drainage. If the obstruction is due to a nonoperable cancer, a guide wire can usually be manipulated past the obstruction (Fig. 44-24*b*). If the obstruction can be passed, a drainage catheter can be placed over the guide wire, reestablishing continuity of the biliary tract via the catheter (Fig. 44-24*c*). This results in internal drainage of the bile.

If the guide wire cannot be placed through the site of

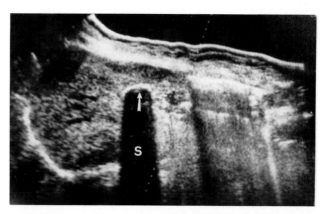

Figure 44-20. Sonogram of the gallbladder with marked sonic shadowing. While the gallbladder itself is not seen, the markedly echogenic gallstones result in an intense area of echogenicity (arrow) with sonic shadowing (S) behind them.

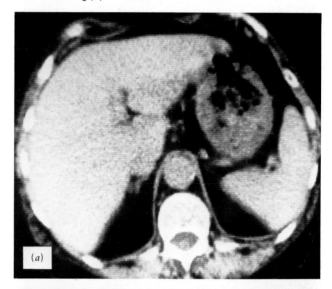

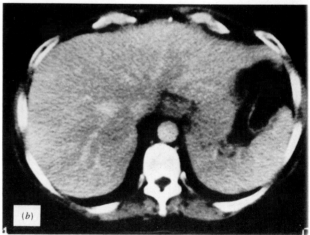

Figure 44-21. Normal CT of the liver. (*a*) The liver has a homogeneous texture. (*b*) During the rapid infusion of contrast medium, the hepatic blood vessels are opacified, appearing as whiter areas within the liver.

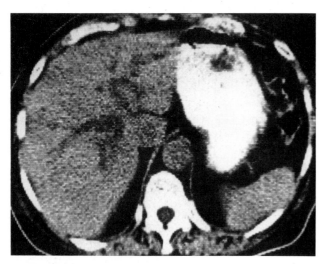

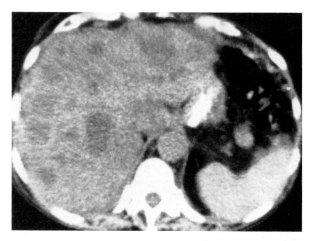

Figure 44-23. CT demonstrating metastases. The multiple rounded radiolucencies in the liver are metastases from pancreatic carcinoma. (Courtesy of N. Whitley, M.D., University of Maryland Hospital.)

Figure 44-22. Biliary duct dilation within the liver. The dilated bile ducts are more radiolucent than the liver parenchyma. When there is a question of whether the radiolucencies are bile ducts in normal liver or blood vessels in radiodense liver, an infusion of contrast medium can be used to opacify the blood vessels.

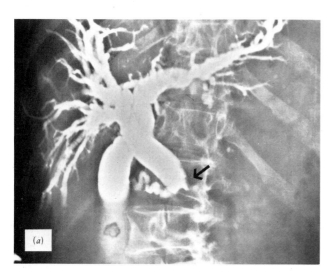

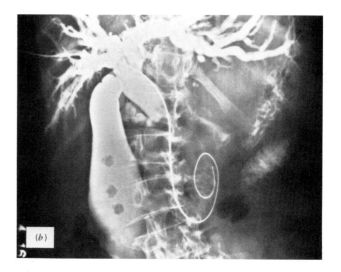

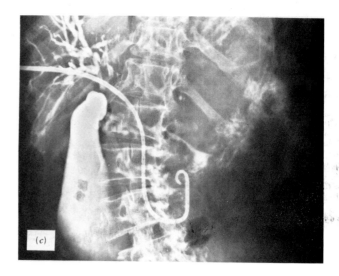

Figure 44-24. Transhepatic cholangiogram with placement of an internal biliary drainage catheter for palliation of pancreatic carcinoma. (a) The transhepatic cholangiogram demonstrates a dilated biliary tract. The tip of the common duct (arrow) demonstrates eccentric narrowing from the enveloping pancreatic carcinoma. The biliary tract has been filled through a catheter. (b) A guide wire has been placed through the catheter, past the cancer, into the duodenum. (c) A drainage catheter has been passed over the guide wire and now allows bile to drain through the catheter into the duodenum. (All courtesy of S. Cisternino, M.D.)

obstruction, a catheter can be placed in the dilated intra-hepatic bile ducts, permitting external drainage through the abdominal wall.

Endoscopic Retrograde Cholangiography

Uses. Endoscopic retrograde cholangiography has two uses. It

1. Is an alternative to percutaneous transhepatic chol-angiography for identifying the cause of biliary ob-struction
2. Permits a sample of bile from the common bile duct to be obtained for analysis from patients with sus-pected chronic cholecystitis but normal oral cholecystograms

Technique. A gastroenterologist passes a fiberoptic gas-troscope into the duodenum and cannulates the common bile duct. Bile samples can be aspirated. Retrograde injec-tion of contrast medium can opacify the biliary system.

CLINICAL CASES

Now that you know something about the techniques of evaluating the liver and biliary tract, you should see how these techniques are used in practice.

Case 44-1

BL is a 62-year-old man who has been losing weight for at least 6 weeks. He has lost his appetite and feels a heaviness in his upper abdomen. On physical examina-tion a large, lumpy mass is felt in the right upper quad-rant. The stool tests guaiac positive. What imaging study do you want to do?

In this case, a liver scan with technetium Tc 99m sulfur colloid is done, and the image is in Figure 44-25a. What do you see?

There are many large masses displacing and distort-ing the liver architecture. What additional imaging study is needed?

With this history, it is unlikely that these masses are anything other than metastases. Sonography could be used to prove they are not cysts, but that is probably a waste of money. With metastases strongly suspected, a search for the primary tumor should be done to aid in offering a prognosis and in the hope (though unlikely) that a specific therapy for the tumor may exist.

With liver metastases, the likely primary tumors are tumors of the colon, stomach, pancreas, or lung, though any tumor could go to the liver. In this case, a barium enema showed an annular lesion with 80% nar-rowing of the ascending colon lumen (fig. 44-25b). What should be done now?

If clinical evaluation suggests that the patient has a life expectancy of more than 3 months, the primary colon cancer should be resected to prevent development of colonic obstruction.

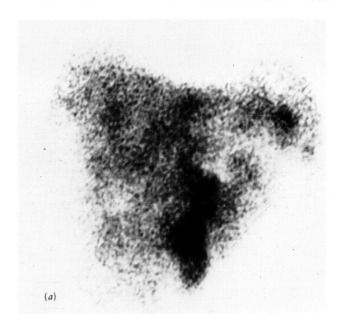

(a)

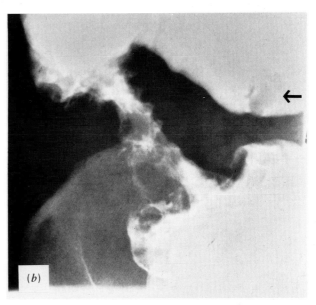

(b)

Figure 44-25. (a) Case example 44-1. (b) The barium enema in this case demonstrated an annular lesion of the ascending colon. The mucosa within the lesion is irregular, and the junction of the normal bowel to the lesion is abrupt. This is a typical appearance of colon cancer. A smaller polypoid cancer (arrow) is also present and lies in the transverse colon. Patients with colon cancer often have polyps and occasionally have cancer elsewhere in the colon.

Once the patient has recovered from the colon sur-gery, what should be done?

Is there any effective therapy for colon cancer meta-static to the liver?

If you are like me, you probably don't know of any specific therapy for metastatic colon cancer; but there are always new experimental therapies being devised. It is appropriate to contact an oncologist to discuss the problem and to get some idea of what the likely effect of any new therapy would be. If it sounds reasonable, then you should discuss your understanding of the therapy with the patient and his family, giving a realistic prognosis. If the patient wants to discuss the treatment with the oncologist, you can refer the patient, but be sure that you indicate to the patient and the patient's family that you will be available to discuss any problems that might arise, no matter how minimal.

What you are likely to find is that the patient will go to the oncologist and, in the initial period of hopefulness, you will not be contacted by the patient. As the patient realizes that the therapy is ineffective, he or his family may return to you for counseling for many types of problems. You should then be available to practice the art of medicine.

Some physicians, when they find a patient has inoperable cancer, send the patient to the oncologist for management and fail to indicate to the family and the patient that they remain available to help. When this is done, the patient and family feel that the physician is abandoning them; he may lose the remainder of the family as patients.

Case 44-2

FB is a 42-year-old woman who was well until 2 days ago, when she felt nauseated and vomited. For the next 2 days she did not feel like eating much. On the night of the second day, she felt nauseated and developed a constant dull right-upper-quadrant pain. This persisted for several hours and she came to the emergency room.

On physical examination, the patient, a heavy woman, is tender in the right upper quadrant with rebound tenderness but no guarding. A possible tender mass is felt in the right upper abdomen. Her leukocyte count is 12,000, with many polymorphonuclear leukocytes.

What diagnosis are you considering? What imaging study would you want to do?

Acute cholecystitis is the probable diagnosis, though appendicitis and pancreatitis are also possible. A ^{99m}Tc IDA nuclear medicine imaging scan would be the most appropriate imaging study. This is done (Fig. 44-26).

The serial images of the ^{99mtc}TC IDA study show good biliary tract excretion. The bile ducts are opacified rapidly, and tracer is present in the small bowel at 20 minutes. Serial images to 2 hours fail to show any tracer in the gallbladder. If the patient has not had a cholecystectomy, the likely diagnosis is acute cholecystitis.

The patient was operated on the next morning, and an inflamed gallbladder was removed.

Case 44-3

JB is a 46-year-old accountant who has had multiple episodes of right-upper-quadrant pain. Most often, these have occurred an hour or two after eating, and the patient believes that fatty foods make the attacks more

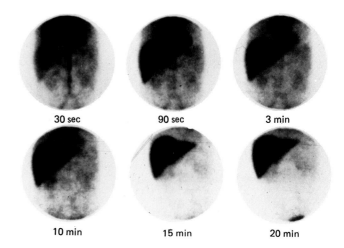

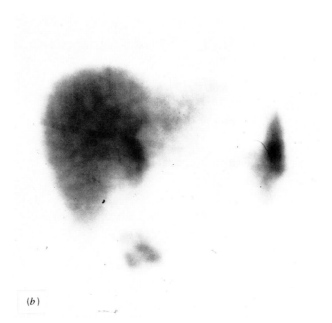

(b)

Figure 44-26. Case example 44-2. (a) Serial images 0–20 minutes. (b) Two-hour image.

frequent. Since he has started to avoid french fries and other fatty foods, the pains have occurred less often, but he wants to know what's wrong.

On physical examination, JB is found to be a little overweight, but no other abnormalities are found.

What do you think is going on? How would you investigate it?

Chronic cholecystitis is a likely cause of these episodes of pain. An oral cholecystogram or a sonogram are the preferred methods for the detection of chronic cholecystitis. JB's oral cholecystogram from the first day is shown in Fig. 44-27. What do you see?

There is no opacification of the gallbladder. The few white flecks in the feces in the colon are contrast me-

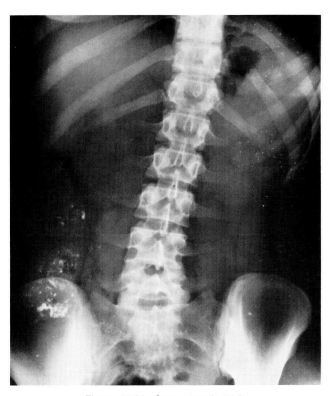

Figure 44-27. Case example 44-3.

dium and indicate that he took the medicine. What should you do now?

There are two choices, a sonogram could be done or the patient could be asked to repeat the dose and to return the next day for additional radiographs. In this case, he takes additional tablets and returns the second day. The radiographs look the same. Again, there is no opacification of the gallbladder. What does this mean?

At this point, you review with the patient how he took the medicine: did he vomit the pills up? You look for evidence of liver disease: is there any evidence of jaundice? If these inquires are negative, there is a 98% chance that the patient has chronic cholecystitis.

Because of his symptoms, surgery was performed and a chronically inflamed and fibrotic gallbladder containing stones was removed.

SUMMARY

The choice of imaging technique in patients with hepatic and biliary tract disease is based on the suspected diagnosis, which in turn is based on the history and physical examination, sometimes supplemented with clinical laboratory tests. The following list, based on the patient's clinical problem, is a guide to imaging test selection.

Changes in liver size:
    Technetium Tc 99m sulfur colloid nuclear medicine scan

Presence of masses:
    Technetium Tc 99m sulfur colloid nuclear medicine scan or CT
Evaluation for etiology of mass:
    Metastasis versus benign cyst(s): sonogram
    Metastasis versus abscess or hepatoma: [67]Ga nuclear medicine scan
Confirmation of cirrhosis:
    Technetium Tc 99m sulfur colloid nuclear medicine scan
Jaundice, differentiating hepatocellular jaundice from obstructive jaundice:
    [99m]Tc IDA derivative nuclear medicine scan or sonogram
Jaundice, obstructive, to find etiology:
    Transmission computed tomography; sonography slightly less useful; percutaneous transhepatic cholangiography if either or both of these fail to find the cause of obstruction
Suspected acute cholecystitis:
    [99m]Tc IDA derivative nuclear medicine study; a sonogram is a secondary (less sensitive) choice
Suspected chronic cholecystitis and suspected biliary calculi:
    Sonogram or oral cholecystogram
Evaluation of biliary-type pain after a cholecystectomy:
    Nonjaundiced patient: sonogram
    If negative, then
    endoscopic retrograde cholangiography or percutaneous transhepatic cholangiography or intravenous cholangiography
If jaundiced: Sonogram if stone is suspected cause; if negative, then CT
    CT if tumor is suspected cause
    if negative, then
    transhepatic cholangiography or endoscopic retrograde cholangiography

REVIEW QUESTIONS

1. What imaging techniques should be used to evaluate the patient with suspected
   a. Acute cholecystitis?
   b. Chronic cholecystitis?
   c. Obstructive jaundice?
   d. Suspected hepatic metastases?
   e. Biliary stone after cholecystectomy?
2. How might you differentiate obstructive from nonobstructive jaundice using clinical information, laboratory values, and imaging techniques?
3. How would you differentiate a hepatic cyst from a solid mass?

VOCABULARY

| acute cholecystitis | oral cholecystogram |
| bile peritonitis | phagocytic |

chronic cholecystitis
endoscopic retrograde cholangiography
jaundice
obstructive jaundice

R-E cell
reticuloendothelial system
second-dose oral cholecystogram
transhepatic cholangiography

SUGGESTIONS FOR FURTHER READING

Roy M. Waller III et al. Computed tomography and sonography of hepatic cirrhosis and portal hypertension. *RadioGraphics,* **4**:677–715, 1984.

45

THE PANCREAS

MORGAN G. DUNNE

KEY CONCEPTS

Radiological

The normal pancreas, lying deep in the abdomen, in the retroperitoneum, is not visible on the plain abdominal radiograph, can be seen partially by ultrasonography, and can be well seen by CT. Nuclear medicine pancreatic imaging is less useful than CT imaging of the pancreas and is not commonly done.

When the pancreas is enlarged, it can be detected by the pressure effect it has on adjacent organs, such as the stomach and transverse colon. Masses of the pancreatic head can be detected by ultrasound, but masses throughout the pancreas can be seen by CT. For this reason, CT is the preferred examination to demonstrate the pancreas.

On CT, the normal pancreatic size is related to the transverse measurement of the adjacent vertebral body, with the AP measurement of the head being between two-thirds and full width of the adjacent vertebra and with the AP measurement of the body of the pancreas being between one-third and two-thirds the width of the adjacent vertebra.

The pancreatic radiodensity is about 50 Hounsfield units. Increased radiodensity occurs with chronic pancreatitis with calcification; decreased radiodensity can occur with normal aging (caused by fatty infiltration), with acute pancreatitis, and focally within pancreatic pseudocysts and pancreatic abscesses. Pancreatic adenocarcinoma is usually of the same radiodensity as the adjacent normal pancreas.

With acute pancreatitis, the gland can appear normal or swollen with decreased radiodensity. The inflammation may obliterate adjacent fat planes and can induce peripancreatic fluid collections. In chronic pancreatitis, the gland can appear irregular in outline, have flecks of calcium within it, and have a dilated pancreatic duct.

Pancreatic pseudocysts can be unilocular or multilocular fluid collections in or near the pancreas. Pancreatic adenocarcinoma is detected as it enlarges the pancreas or bulges outward from the margin of the pancreas.

CT can be used to guide the drainage of pancreatic pseudocysts and the percutaneous biopsy of pancreatic masses.

OBJECTIVES

When you complete this chapter you will be able to

1. Identify the normal pancreas on selected CT sections.
2. Identify acute and chronic pancreatitis on selected CT sections.
3. Identify pancreatic masses on selected CT sections.
4. List the clinical symptoms of acute pancreatitis and pancreatic abscess.

Before the advent of nuclear imaging, ultrasound, and CT, the pancreas, being a soft tissue structure surrounded by tissues of similar radiographic density, could not be imaged directly using standard radiographic techniques. The normal pancreas and most pancreatic diseases are invisible on plain abdominal radiographs. Occasionally, however, pancreatic disease can be inferred because of its effect on adjacent organs. Inflammation can cause a localized ileus with dilation of bowel loops adjacent to the pancreas. The transverse colon's air column as radiographically demonstrated may be abruptly attenuated as it crosses the midline in cases of acute pancreatitis (the so-called colon cut-off sign). Pancreatic masses can be detected when they impinge on adjacent organs, and such impingement on the normal intraluminal air of viscera, such as the stomach, can be seen on plain abdominal radiographs. Only in some patients with chronic calcific pancreatitis can the pancreas be seen on the plain abdominal radiograph (see Fig. 28-9). Chronic calcific pancreatitis may appear as multiple foci of calcification projected over the gland in the upper abdomen (Fig. 28-1).

If a contrast medium such as barium is introduced into the GI tract, rendering it radiographically visible, then pancreatic disease can be inferred if there is deformity of those portions of the GI tract intimately adjacent to the pancreas (Fig. 41-2). Thus an extrinsic impression on the second portion of the duodenum seen on an upper GI tract series would be highly suspicious, suggestive of a mass in the pancreatic head. An impression on the posterior wall of the stomach would be suggestive of a mass in the body or tail of the pancreas. The sensitivity of this method can be enhanced by special techniques. Hypotonic duodenography was developed to improve the visualization of the fine mucosal detail of the duodenal loop. Using this technique, the duodenum is rendered hypotonic or atonic by the administration of a drug such as glucagon or propantheline so that the flaccid medial wall of the contrast-filled duodenum will reflect more exquisitely the impression of the lateral surface of the pancreatic head. Pancreatic masses impressing the posterior wall of the stomach are better seen if the stomach is brought closely to the pancreas by placing the patient in the supine position and taking a cross-table lateral film using a horizontal x-ray beam.

More invasive contrast techniques would include pancreatic arteriography and endoscopic retrograde pancreatography. In pancreatic arteriography, the main arteries supplying the organ are selectively catheterized. Masses can be detected by the deformity and displacement they produce.

Pancreatic disease has variable symptoms and must be included in the differential diagnosis of both acute and chronic abdominal pain. Before the development of modern pancreatic imaging with CT and ultrasound, the diagnosis of pancreatic disease was based on clinical criteria and careful analysis of certain specific serum enzymes such as amylase and lipase. Although a carefully performed barium GI tract series could yield valid information about early disease of the pancreatic head, the remainder of the organ could not be readily evaluated unless the pancreatic disease was severe or advanced.

Currently, CT is the procedure of choice for imaging the pancreas in adults. Since ultrasound and barium GI examination play a limited role in modern pancreatic imaging, this chapter discusses mainly the CT evaluation of the pancreas.

Keynotes

- *Acute pancreatitis will sometimes induce an adynamic ileus in loops of bowel adjacent to the inflamed pancreas.*
- *The calcifications that appear in some patients with chronic pancreatitis can be seen on abdominal radiographs.*
- *An enlarged pancreas or pancreatic mass can press on adjacent structures. The barium-filled stomach or duodenum may demonstrate these impressions.*

- *Pancreatic disease can result in both acute and chronic abdominal pain.*
- *Computed tomography is the imaging procedure of choice for the pancreas; ultrasound, barium GI tract series, and angiography have limited roles.*

PATIENT PREPARATION AND PROCEDURE

Little, if any, patient preparation is necessary before pancreatic CT. Remember that the presence of barium in the GI tract will significantly degrade the CT examination and may render the study useless. Barium, because of its radiographic density, produces marked artifacts on CT images, so it should be cleared from the GI tract before performing an abdominal CT.

The patient does not have to be fasting before CT examination of the pancreas. Usually, the patient will be asked to ingest about 500 cc of a water-soluble contrast material before the study in order to opacify the GI tract on the CT images. This oral contrast medium will usually be administered at least 30 minutes before the examination. On occasion, and at the discretion of the radiologist, it may be necessary to administer 50–100 cc of intravenous contrast medium in order to opacify certain major blood vessels in the vicinity of the pancreas, such as the splenic artery, the splenic vein, and the superior mesenteric vein and artery.

NORMAL ANATOMY

Pancreatic Shape and Position

The pancreas is usually obliquely oriented relative to the transverse or axial plane of the patient, with the tail lying in a more cephalad and the head in a more caudad plane. As serial sections are made moving in a caudad direction from the level of the diaphragm, the tail would be seen first on the more cephalad sections intimately related to the spleen on its lateral aspect (Fig. 45-1*a*), the upper pole of the left kidney on its posterior aspect, and the stomach on its anterior aspect. Lower sections will demonstrate the body of the pancreas with the posterior wall of the stomach lying on its anterior aspect and the mesenteric and splenic vessels related on its posterior aspect. Sections made at a more caudad level will show the pancreatic head with the contrast-filled second portion of the duodenum on its right lateral aspect. The body of the pancreas is related on its posterior aspect to the inferior vena cava, and the uncinate process of the pancreas can usually be seen interposed between the superior mesenteric vessels and the abdominal aorta (Fig. 45-1*b*). On exceptionally high-quality scans, the normal pancreatic duct can be demonstrated traversing the pancreatic body in its long axis. Also, on extremely high-quality studies, the distal common bile duct occasionally can be demonstrated coursing through the pancreatic head. It is, however, more usual to demonstrate the pancreatic and common bile ducts only when they are abnormally di-

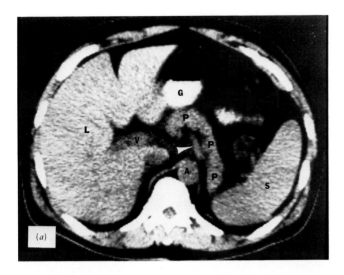

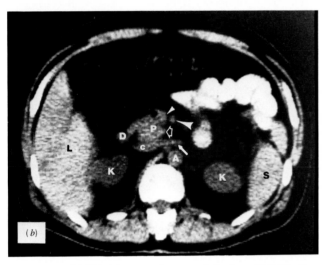

Figure 45-1. (a) CT of the normal pancreatic body and tail (P). Also shown on this section are the liver (L), spleen (S), portal vein (V), contrast-filled gastric antrum (G), aorta (A), and splenic artery (arrowhead). (b) CT of the same patient at a slightly more caudad level, showing normal pancreatic head (P), uncinate process (open arrow), second portion of duodenum (D), superior mesenteric vein (small arrowhead) and artery (large arrowhead), inferior vena cava (c), left renal vein (arrow), aorta (A), kidneys (K), liver (L), and spleen (S).

lated. These structures are not usually seen on normal pancreatic CT scans.

Pancreatic Radiodensity

The normal pancreatic parenchymal radiodensity is greater than that of water and has an attenuation approximating that of normal liver and spleen. The CT image allows one to measure the actual radiographic attenuation of tissues displayed on the scan section using a movable cursor on the screen. The scale used by most machines in operation today ranges from −1,000 to +1,000 Hounsfield units, with air equal to −1,000 Hounsfield units, water equal to 0

Hounsfield units, and dense bone equal to +1,000 Hounsfield units. On this scale, normal pancreatic tissue measures approximately +50 Hounsfield units. The pancreatic parenchymal radiodensity will vary somewhat because the organ may be variably infiltrated with fat, which tends to lower its radiographic attenuation.

Pancreatic Size

The size of the pancreas varies with age. The organ is small in infants and reaches full size in young adults. Later in adult life the organ tends to atrophy and become infiltrated with fat to the extent that in the elderly patient it may be inhomogeneous and even difficult to define on CT amid the retroperitoneal fat (Figs. 45-2). In adult life the normal pancreatic size on CT is as follows: The maximum AP dimension of the pancreatic head should be at least two-thirds of but not greater than the full lateral width of the adjacent lumbar vertebral body; the AP dimension of the pancreatic body should be at least one-third but not greater than two-thirds of the width of the adjacent lumbar vertebral body. Keep in mind that considerable pancreatic size variability exists and that experience will be necessary to determine whether a given organ is or is not enlarged.

Keynotes

- *Serial CT sections are necessary for the complete demonstration of pancreatic anatomy.*
- *Pancreatic radiodensity approximates that of the liver and spleen, approximately +50 Hounsfield units; fatty infiltration, however, is common and can decrease the pancreatic radiodensity.*
- *The normal pancreatic head measures between two-thirds of and the full lateral measurement of the adjacent lumbar vertebra. The body of the pancreas is between one-third and two-thirds of the full lateral measurement of the adjacent vertebra.*

PANCREATIC DISEASE

Acute Pancreatitis

In *acute pancreatitis,* the pancreas may have a normal CT appearance or be enlarged and have decreased radiographic attenuation because of edema. The organ becomes inflamed from the seepage of activated proteolytic enzymes into the parenchymal tissue of the organ. The process may be of varying severity. The organ may become sufficiently swollen from edema to appear enlarged on the CT image, and the radiodensity of the gland may decrease because of increased water content (Fig. 45-3). The CT attenuation value may decrease from a normal value of +50 to less than +10 Hounsfield units.

On occasion, in acute pancreatitis, a sympathetic effusion develops adjacent to the gland in response to the inflammation and this effusion may be demonstrable on CT. It is common in acute pancreatitis of significant degree to be able to demonstrate effusion in the lesser sac of the peri-

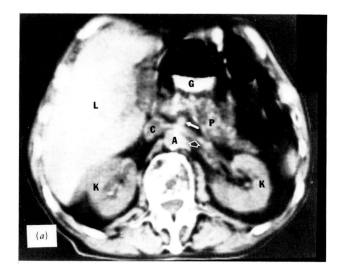

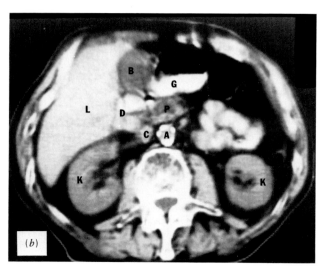

Figure 45-2. (*a*) CT of the pancreas in a normal elderly patient, showing inhomogeneity of body and tail from fatty infiltration (P), contrast-filled gastric antrum (G), inferior vena cava (C), left renal vein (open arrow), superior mesenteric artery (arrow), liver (L), and kidneys (K). (*b*) CT of the same patient at a more caudad level, showing inhomogeneity of the pancreatic head from fatty infiltration (P), contrast-filled second portion of the duodenum (D), gastric antrum (G), inferior vena cava (C), aorta (A), gallbladder (B), liver (L), and kidneys (K).

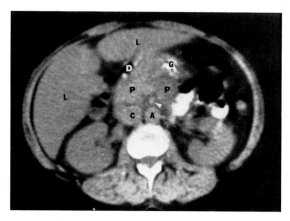

Figure 45-3. CT of mild acute pancreatitis. Note swelling of pancreatic head (P), with impression on the contrast-filled gastric antrum (G) and the second portion of the duodenum (D). The scan also shows the liver (L), inferior vena cava (C), aorta (A), and superior mesenteric artery (arrowhead).

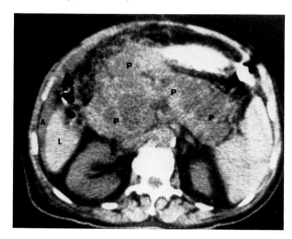

Figure 45-4. CT of severe acute pancreatitis. Note gross swelling, inhomogeneity, and edema of the pancreas (P). A small amount of ascites (A) can be seen lateral to the liver (L).

toneal cavity. Effusions may be present also in the retroperitoneum, specifically in the anterior pararenal space (that space in which the pancreas lies).

The most severe degrees of pancreatitis may appear on CT as gross swelling of the organ with obliteration of the fat planes about the gland and inhomogeneous areas of radiolucency within the parenchyma (Fig. 45-4). Pancreatic pseudocysts may form rapidly in cases of acute pancreatitis and may be demonstrable on the initial acute-phase study (see the following section on pancreatic pseudocyst). In acute pancreatitis there may be considerable localized or even generalized abdominal ileus, and the

adynamic distended loops of intestine characteristic of this entity may be seen on the CT scan. Frequently, you will see a pleural effusion on the left accompanying acute pancreatitis, and this may also be demonstrated on the CT study if present. Pleural effusion on the left is thought to develop as a sympathetic response to inflammation in the pancreatic tail in the left subphrenic area.

Swelling of the pancreatic head in acute pancreatitis is occasionally sufficient to compress the distal common bile duct with resultant extrahepatic biliary obstruction. Dilated bile ducts proximal to the distal common bile duct may be visible on the CT image.

Pancreatitis is often associated with cholelithiasis, and thus it behooves the diligent radiologist to examine the gallbladder carefully on the CT sections obtained while studying the pancreas. While most gallstones are not sufficiently calcified to be visible on plain radiographs, a much greater number will be demonstrable on CT because of the vastly greater tissue contrast possible with CT.

Chronic Pancreatitis

Chronic pancreatitis is frequently the result of repeated bouts of acute pancreatitis and may be demonstrable on CT. The gland will usually have an irregular outline from extensive scarring, and multiple small flecks of calcium may be seen in the parenchyma (Fig. 45-5). This type of dystrophic calcification seen in the pancreas in cases of chronic pancreatitis may be visible on plain abdominal radiographs. The pancreatic duct is frequently dilated in chronic pancreatitis, and this dilation can usually be seen on good-quality CT scans (Fig. 45-5). The CT changes of chronic pancreatitis are often discovered in patients studied for a current bout of acute pancreatitis, so that the patient will have features of both acute and chronic pancreatitis visible on the CT scan. Long-standing cases of chronic pancreatitis may have marked atrophy of the organ and indeed may have symptoms of pancreatic insufficiency (malabsorption syndromes and diabetes mellitus). Pancreatic pseudocysts may be found in both acute and chronic pancreatitis.

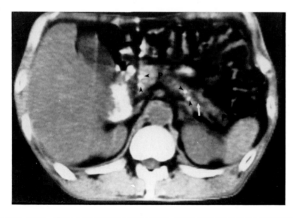

Figure 45-5. CT of chronic pancreatitis. Note atrophy and inhomogeneity of the pancreas (P) with a dilated pancreatic duct (arrow) and scattered calcifications (arrowheads).

Pancreatic Pseudocyst

A pseudocyst is a collection of fluid rich in pancreatic enzymes. The cyst forms as a result of disruption of the pancreatic ductal system so that the intraluminal enzymes are released into the parenchyma of the gland. The cyst is not epithelialized, hence the term *pseudocyst*. A *pancreatic pseudocyst* is an attempt by the body's defense mechanisms to wall off and contain digestive enzymes leaking from the disrupted pancreatic ducts. Pseudocysts usually develop during or after an episode of acute pancreatitis, though they may occur after trauma or pancreatic surgery. Pseudocysts can vary greatly in size and may be unilocular or multilocular. Because the fluid contains proteolytic enzymes, pseudocysts dissect easily along tissue planes and can appear as palpable masses anywhere in the abdomen. On occasion, pseudocysts can dissect into the mediastinum and into the groin.

On CT scans, the pancreatic pseudocyst has a fairly characteristic appearance as a well-defined mass, usually with a CT attenuation value close to that of water (i.e., 0 Hounsfield units) (Fig. 45-6a). Less often, pseudocysts may contain hemorrhage or necrotic debris, which will serve to raise the CT attenuation value higher than that of water. Pseudocysts may compress adjacent viscera with resultant effects, such as partial bowel obstruction, extrahepatic biliary obstruction, and even hydronephrosis. Long-standing pseudocysts may have calcified walls that would be clearly defined on CT images.

Most pancreatic pseudocysts resolve spontaneously by decompression through the pancreatic ductal system or an adjacent viscus (e.g., the stomach). Computed tomography studies can be used to follow pancreatic pseudocysts and ensure their resolution over time. Persistent pseudocysts, especially if they are symptomatic, may be treated by percutaneous catheter drainage (Fig. 45-6b) or creation of a surgical fistula between the cyst and an adjacent bowel loop or the stomach. The latter procedure is termed *marsupialization*.

Pancreatic Abscess

The diagnosis of *pancreatic abscess* is very important because of the high mortality from this condition. Pancreatic abscess is a surgical emergency, and the advent of CT scanning has greatly aided its detection. In pancreatic abscess, the pancreas is not only inflamed but also infected,

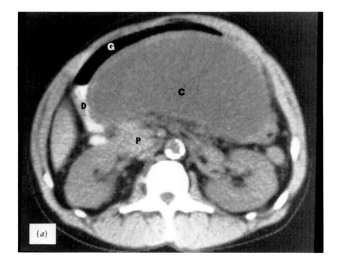

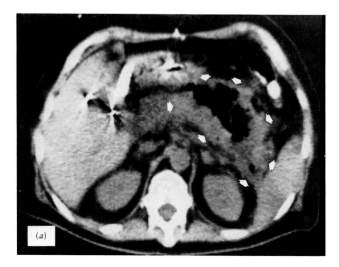

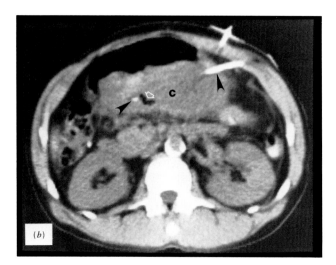

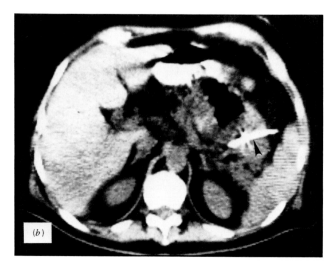

Figure 45-6. (*a*) CT of a large pancreatic pseudocyst. Note the large collection of fluid in the pseudocyst (C), which is displacing the gastric antrum (G) and the second portion of the duodenum (D). The pancreatic head is also visible (P). (*b*) CT of same patient after placement of a percutaneous drainage catheter (arrowheads) into the pseudocyst (C) under CT guidance. A small amount of air (open arrow) has been introduced into the pseudocyst cavity through the catheter.

Figure 45-7. (*a*) CT of a pancreatic abscess. Note the large irregularly shaped collection, involving the pancreatic body and tail, and containing gas, fluid, and necrotic tissue (arrows). (*b*) CT of same patient after placement of a percutaneous drainage catheter (arrowhead) into the abscess cavity, reducing the size of the abscess.

with formation of a purulent collection within the organ. A pancreatic abscess may develop after an episode of acute pancreatitis, especially in those cases where extensive necrosis of pancreatic tissue has occurred. Occasionally, pancreatic abscess may develop as a result of infection of a pancreatic pseudocyst. Whatever the etiology, the classical appearance on CT of a pancreatic abscess is a poorly defined mass in the pancreatic bed with lower CT attenuation values than normal pancreatic tissue but usually not quite as low as those found in pseudocyst fluid. Gas bubbles may be seen within the mass if the infecting organism is a gas producer (Fig. 45-7a). The presence of gas bubbles in a swollen pancreas is strongly indicative of pancreatic abscess. Because of the presence of proteolytic enzymes in

the abscess cavity, the process is capable of dissecting along tissue planes some distance from the pancreatic bed, though most pancreatic abscesses are within the organ or its immediate environs.

The patient is usually extremely toxic and often has a recent history of sepsis. Surgical drainage and antibiotic therapy are necessary. On occasion, drainage can be accomplished by percutaneous catheter placement under CT or ultrasonic guidance (Fig. 45-7b). The mortality from surgically treated pancreatic abscess is 30–50%, whereas in untreated cases it approaches 100%. Any patient with a diagnosis of acute pancreatitis who becomes septic should be evaluated with an emergency CT, for possible pancreatic abscess without delay.

Pancreatic Neoplasia

Computed tomography is the method of choice for imaging suspected pancreatic neoplasia. It is particularly suited to this role because of its ability to display the entire organ, whereas ultrasound and contrast GI examinations have difficulty demonstrating the pancreatic tail. Pancreatic tumors appear on CT as soft tissue masses of CT attenuation similar to the normal-gland parenchyma. Tumors of the pancreas may be of both exocrine and endocrine origin.

Adenocarcinoma. The most common tumor of the pancreas is adenocarcinoma, a tumor of exocrine origin that is now the ninth most frequent visceral malignancy and the fourth most frequent cause of death from cancer in the United States. This neoplasm more common in elderly patients usually causes abdominal or back pain. Its peak incidence is in the eighth decade of life. The prognosis in carcinoma of the pancreas is very poor, most cases being unresectable at the time of discovery. Carcinoma of the pancreas is usually detectable on CT images by the time it is clinically apparent. Occasionally a small, early strategically placed tumor adjacent to the intrapancreatic portion of the distal common bile duct will manifest jaundice (caused by extrahepatic biliary obstruction) before the tumor itself is visible on CT. In order for a CT study of the pancreas to diagnose a tumor, a mass must deform or enlarge the outline of the gland (Fig. 45-8*a*). It is generally not possible to detect a tumor of the pancreas on CT if the lesion is less than 2 cm in diameter. Once a tumor is discovered on CT, possible extrapancreatic spread should be sought in the retroperitoneal and porta hepatis lymph nodes and in the liver. Rarely, calcification and cyst formation can be seen in pancreatic malignancy in the cystadenocarcinoma type of tumor.

Endocrine Tumor. The most common endocrine tumor of the pancreas is an *insulinoma,* a histologically benign but hormonally active tumor that secretes insulin. These tumors are usually quite small and lie deep within the pancreatic parenchyma. Because of this, they are usually not detectable by CT scanning. Rapid injection of intravenous contrast medium during the CT scan will, on occasion, render previously invisible insulinomas visible within the parenchyma of the organ. This is because insulinomas are highly vascular lesions and the circulating intravascular contrast medium makes them denser on the CT image. Selective and superselective pancreatic arteriography is recommended as the method of choice for diagnosis of insulinoma.

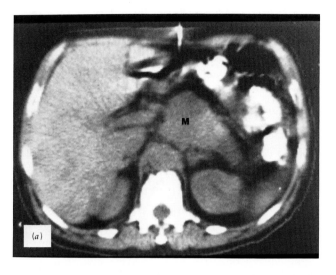

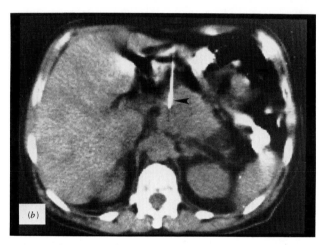

Figure 45-8. (*a*) CT of pancreatic adenocarcinoma. Note the large soft tissue mass (M) in the pancreatic body. (*b*) CT of the same patient, showing placement of a biopsy needle (arrowhead) into the mass. The aspirate yielded adenocarcinoma.

PANCREATIC BIOPSY

Computed tomography scanning is extremely useful for guiding percutaneous needle biopsy procedures on the pancreas (Fig. 45-8*b*). The availability of fine (22– or 23-gauge) flexible needles and rapid, high-resolution CT scanners has enabled the radiologist to place these needles into pancreatic masses safely and accurately and to obtain small tissue samples and cytological material from these lesions. The small diameter and flexibility of these needles makes pancreatic biopsy through overlying viscera, such as the stomach, liver, and colon, an acceptably safe procedure.

Keynote

- *CT can be used to guide the placement of percutaneous biopsy needles.*

SUMMARY

Computed tomography is now the preferred method of imaging the pancreas, with ultrasound and angiography having subsidiary roles. Although the plain abdominal film and the GI tract barium series can demonstrate the effects of pancreatic disease, they do not directly visualize the pancreas.

The pancreas lies obliquely in the retroperitoneum, and therefore, sequential CT sections are needed to demonstrate its entire structure. Pancreatic size is greatest in the young adult. The pancreas tends to atrophy and become infiltrated with fat in the elderly. Pancreatic size can be related proportionately to the adjacent lumbar vertebra, with the AP measurement of the pancreatic head being from two-thirds to equal to the transverse width of the vertebra and the pancreatic body from one-third to two-thirds of the width of the adjacent vertebra. The attenuation of the pancreas is approximately +50 Hounsfield units.

In the patient with acute pancreatitis, the pancreas may appear normal or may be enlarged and have decreased radiographic attenuation from edema. Effusions may form adjacent to the pancreas. Fat planes adjacent to the pancreas may become obliterated, and pseudocysts may form.

In the patient with chronic pancreatitis, the gland will often have an irregular outline, and multiple small flecks of calcium may be seen within the organ. The pancreatic duct is frequently dilated. Acute pancreatitis can coexist with chronic pancreatitis, and the signs of both diseases may be seen concurrently. Pancreatic pseudocysts may be present.

Pancreatic pseudocysts are walled-off collections of pancreatic enzymes and fluid. They can be unilocular or multilocular. They can develop within or adjacent to the pancreas and occasionally some distance from the pancreas. They appear as well-defined masses with a CT attenuation near that of water.

Pancreatic abscesses may or may not demonstrate specific CT findings. Characteristic findings on CT include a poorly defined mass in the pancreatic bed with a CT attenuation lower than normal pancreas but usually not as low as pseudocysts. Gas bubbles may be seen within the mass.

Pancreatic adenocarcinoma is usually undetectable until the mass exceeds 2 cm. When seen, the mass has a similar attenuation to that of normal pancreas and may either enlarge or distort the contour of the pancreas. Pan-

creatic carcinoma is usually incurable by the time it is large enough to be detected by CT scanning.

With occasional exceptions, endocrine tumors of the pancreas are usually too small to be detected by CT scanning.

Computed tomography can be used to guide the placement of catheters for the drainage of pancreatic pseudocysts and selected pancreatic abscesses. It can also be used to guide percutaneous biopsy of pancreatic masses.

REVIEW QUESTIONS

1. What symptoms are associated with pancreatic disease?
2. What patient preparation is necessary for a pancreatic CT?
3. Describe the location of the pancreas. What is its appearance on CT images?
4. How large is the normal pancreas on CT images? How does its size change with age?
5. What is the normal radiodensity of the pancreas, and how is that radiodensity changed by disease?
6. What are the CT findings seen in acute pancreatitis? How does the severity of the disease alter these findings?
7. Where can fluid collect in the patient with acute pancreatitis?
8. What effects can the swollen pancreas have on adjacent organs? What symptoms can result from these effects?
9. What are the common causes of acute pancreatitis? How can the CT examination help you determine the cause of acute pancreatitis?
10. What are the symptoms and CT findings of chronic pancreatitis? What are the nonpancreatic complications of chronic pancreatitis?
11. What is a pancreatic pseudocyst? Why is it a pseudocyst rather than a true cyst?
12. Where can pancreatic pseudocysts be located? What is their natural history?
13. What are the symptoms and potential complications of pancreatic pseudocysts?
14. What is a pancreatic abscess? What are its clinical symptoms and signs? What is its CT appearance? How is it treated?
15. What clinical symptoms are found in the patient with pancreatic adenocarcinoma? What CT findings suggest the presence of pancreatic adenocarcinoma? How can the diagnosis of pancreatic adenocarcinoma be proved?

VOCABULARY

acute pancreatitis
chronic pancreatitis
endocrine tumors
endoscopic retrograde pancreatography

exocrine tumors
insulinoma
pancreatic abscess
pancreatic pseudocyst

SUGGESTIONS FOR FURTHER READING

R. Kristina Gedgaudas, Reed P. Rice. Radiological evaluation of complicated pancreatitis. *CRC Critical Reviews in Diagnostic Imaging,* **15:**319–367, 1981.

PART 3

THE PELVIS: ULTRASOUND IN GYNECOLOGY AND OBSTETRICS

The next two chapters discuss the applications of ultrasound to the evaluation of the female pelvis. Ultrasound is the main imaging method used in the evaluation of obstetric and gynecologic processes. Its use in obstetrics permits the evaluation of the fetus without exposing the fetus to possibly harmful radiation. In both obstetrics and gynecology, the ability to obtain ultrasound images in many different planes aids in the evaluation of complex pelvic processes.

46

ULTRASOUND IN GYNECOLOGY

DAVID GRAHAM

KEY CONCEPTS

Radiological

The ultrasound examination is a major method of evaluating the female pelvis. Using the full bladder as an acoustic window into the pelvis, the uterus, ovaries, and adnexal structures can be visualized and evaluated.

Ultrasound can be used to characterize pelvic masses as cystic, solid, or complex and to determine whether their origin is ovarian, uterine, or other pelvic structures. Uterine fibroids appear as lobular enlargements of the uterus with a nonhomogeneous echo pattern.

Ovarian masses can be small functional cysts that usually disappear after several menstrual cycles, corpus luteum cysts associated with pregnancy, or benign or malignant neoplasms. Sonographic characteristics that suggest a mass is malignant are large amounts of solid tissue in the mass, ascites, and pelvic adenopathy. Dermoid cysts of the ovary may demonstrate areas of shadowing (from calcium deposits) and fat-fluid levels.

Ultrasonography may be useful when a patient has pelvic inflammatory disease that does not respond to therapy. It can demonstrate tubo-ovarian abscesses.

Ultrasonography can be used to demonstrate that an intrauterine device *is* intrauterine.

Ultrasonography can aid in the diagnosis of ectopic pregnancy by demonstrating that the uterine cavity does not contain a pregnancy. If the patient has a positive pregnancy test or an appropriate clinical history for recent pregnancy, an "empty" uterus implies that the pregnancy may be ectopic.

Clinical

It is not uncommon for the string of an intrauterine device to disappear into the uterine cavity. This normal occurrence must be distinguished from the expelling of the device from the uterus as well as from its penetration through the uterine wall into the abdominal cavity. Ultrasonography can demonstrate whether the device is intrauterine, but if it is not, a plain abdominal film must be used to determine whether it has been expelled or has penetrated into the peritoneal cavity.

The patient with an ectopic pregnancy often has lower abdominal pain. In 50% of the patients there is a recent history of amenorrhea, and in 50% an adnexal mass is palpated. Because an ectopic pregnancy can rupture and bleed massively, early diagnosis is important. Ultrasound, by demonstrating the presence or absence of an intrauterine pregnancy, aids in this difficult clinical diagnosis.

OBJECTIVES

When you complete this chapter you will be able to

1. Identity on selected sonographic images
   a. The normal uterus and ovaries
   b. Uterine fibroids
   c. Ovarian cysts
   d. Ovarian neoplasms
   e. Intrauterine devices
2. Describe the clinical symptoms, signs, and ultrasound findings of an ectopic pregnancy.
3. Describe the role of ultrasonic examination in ovulation induction.

Sonography has proven to be of great value in the diagnosis and management of a number of gynecological conditions, for it allows visualization of the uterus, the ovaries, other normal structure of the pelvis, and any additional masses. Optimal examination requires that the patient have a full bladder, which pushes the bowel out of the pelvis, elevates the uterus, and thus creates an *acoustic window* to the pelvic organs. A complete sonographic exam consists of a number of longtitudinal and transverse scans usually spaced at 1-cm intervals. The major purposes of sonography in the female pelvis are

1. Diagnosis of a pelvic mass discovered on physical examination by characterizing it as cystic, solid, or complex and its origin as uterine, ovarian, or other pelvic structure.
2. Assessment of pelvic inflammatory disease
3. Diagnosis and follow-up of endometriosis
4. Localization of an intrauterine device
5. Diagnosis of suspected ectopic pregnancy
6. Diagnosis of congenital uterine anomalies
7. Assessment of infertility
8. Assessment of a gynecologic malignancy, for demonstration of extent of primary disease and determination of metastatic disease
9. Evaluation of postoperative complications such as fever or drop in hematocrit level
10. Evaluation of certain gynecologic urologic problems

NORMAL ANATOMY

In longitudinal sections, the uterus of the patient in the reproductive years may be visualized as an oblong structure immediately posterior to the bladder. In the center of the uterine cavity is a thin echogenic line, representing the endometrial cavity. The cervix and the vagina may also be readily seen, as illustrated in Figure 46-1. On transverse sections, the uterus, ovaries, and muscular structure of the pelvis may also be readily visualized (Fig. 46-2). The bowel may be visualized in the pelvis either as cystic collections when there is fluid within the lumen or as areas of shadowing where the lumen contains air. When there is any doubt whether a visualized mass represents bowel, a water enema may be done to determine whether the "lesion" is indeed bowel. Real-time examination might also demonstrate peristalsis, which would confirm that the "lesion" was indeed bowel.

Keynotes

- *Ultrasound examinations of the pelvis use the full bladder as an acoustic window.*
- *Because fluid-filled bowel loops can simulate a pelvic mass, sometimes a water enema is used to distend a bowel loop or to change its echogenicity, and sometimes real-time imaging is used to demonstrate peristalsis.*

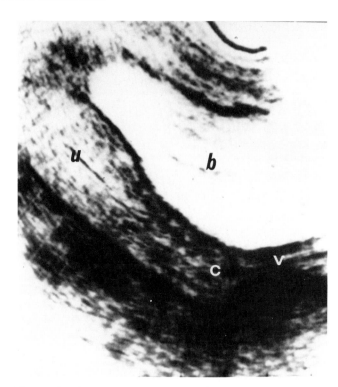

Figure 46-1. Longitudinal section of the female pelvis showing the uterus (u), bladder (b), vagina (v), and cervix (c). The endometrial cavity is seen as a thin black line in the longitudinal axis of the uterus. In this and all other scans in this chapter, the standard nomenclature for labeling scans is followed. In both longitudinal and transverse scans, anterior is at the top of the scan, posterior at the bottom. In longitudinal scans, cephalad is to the left and caudad to the right. In transverse scans, the patient's right is on the left of the picture.

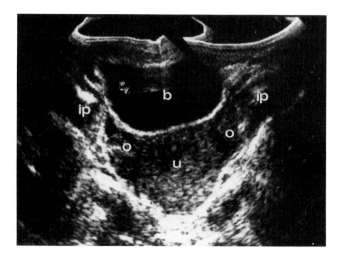

Figure 46-2. Transverse section of a female pelvis showing bladder (b), uterus (u), and ovaries (o). The iliopsoas muscles are also shown (ip).

PELVIC MASSES

Sonography allows characterization of any mass as predominantly cystic, solid, or a complex of both cystic and solid areas. Internal structures, such as septations or solid material, may also be demonstrated. The fluid nature of a cystic mass in certain instances can be determined to be blood or pus rather than serous fluid. Masses may also be characterized as uterine or ovarian or as arising from other pelvic structures.

Uterine Masses

Fibroids. Fibroids, the most common benign tumors of the uterus, are visualized sonographically as an enlarged uterus, usually with a lobulated contour and with nonhomogeneity of the echo texture (Fig. 46-3). Subserosal fibroids may appear to lie adjacent to the uterus, and on occasion it may be difficult to distinguish them from solid adnexal masses. Areas of degeneration within a fibroid may show as cystic areas from necrosis or as areas of increased echogenicity from calcification.

Malignancies. Malignant tumors of the uterine body are most often endometrial carcinoma, which also causes enlargement of the uterus. Sonographically, it may be impossible to distinguish uterine enlargement caused by fibroids from that caused by endometrial cancer. Where the tumor is breaking through to the serosal surface of the uterus, however, it may produce irregularity of outline. Sarcomas are less common neoplasms of the uterus and also produce uterine enlargment, which again may be indistinguishable from fibroids unless there is serosal involvement that produces irregularity of uterine outline.

Carcinoma of the Cervix

Ultrasound is of limited value in the diagnosis and management of carcinoma of the cervix because initial diagnosis is usually by clinical examination together with bi-opsy. Staging of the lesion is also primarily a clinical process. Sonography will, however, confirm clinical findings, and show the extent of a neoplasm and the degree to which it involves parametrial structures, bladder, and ureter. Pelvic adenopathy may also be diagnosed.

Ovarian Masses

Functional Cysts. Several functional (nonneoplastic) cysts may occur in the ovary. Normally, in the preovulatory phase of the menstrual cycle, the developing follicle can be visualized, using good resolution ultrasound equipment, as a cystic structure in one of the ovaries (Fig. 46-4). This cystic structure will gradually increase in size to an average diameter of 2–2.5 cm in the immediate preovulatory phase. After ovulation the follicle markedly decreases in size, filling with echos as the corpus luteum is formed. Occasionally a developing follicle will continue to enlarge and produce a functional ovarian cyst. The natural history of such cysts is that they usually disappear spontaneously when followed clinically through two to three menstrual cycles. They are visualized sonographically as well-defined cystic masses in one or another adnexal area, usually without any internal structure (Fig. 46-5). Where there has been bleeding into such a cyst, internal echos may appear.

The *corpus luteum cyst* in association with pregnancy is also most often visualized sonographically as a simple, well-defined cystic lesion. Because such cysts are human chorionic gonadotropin (HCG) dependent, they usually markedly decrease in size by early in the second trimester (Fig. 46-6).

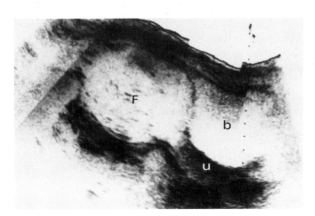

Figure 46-3. Longitudinal section of pelvis showing a large fundal fibroid (F) arising from the uterine body (u); b = bladder.

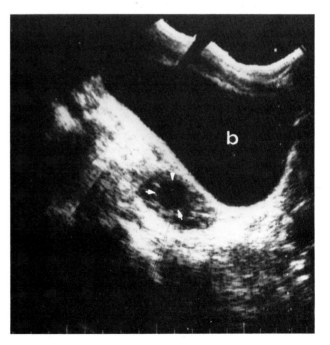

Figure 46-4. Longitudinal scan of the ovary showing a developing ovarian follicle (arrows), measuring 12 mm in diameter; b = bladder.

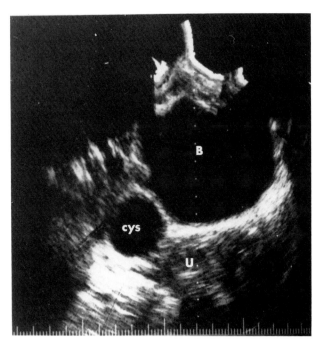

Figure 46-5. Transverse section of the pelvis showing a right adnexal follicular cyst (cys), uterus (U), and bladder (B). The cyst has sharp borders and no internal echos, consistent with a simple cyst.

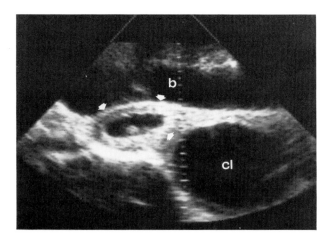

Figure 46-6. Transverse section of the pelvis in pregnancy, showing a left adnexal cyst compatible with a corpus luteum cyst (cl). The uterus with a gestational sac is also visualized (arrows); b = bladder.

Neoplasms. A number of neoplastic tumors of the ovary, both malignant and benign, may occur. Sonographically, the appearances may be nonspecific, allowing only the diagnosis of an ovarian mass. There are, however, occasions on which the sonographic appearances are relatively specific for a particular type of neoplasm or in which malignancy is highly likely. Findings that are more suggestive of malignancy are the presence of large masses of solid tissue within the lesion, coexistent ascites, or pelvic adenopathy (Fig. 46-7). Ovarian malignancies characteristically spread transperitoneally, producing metastatic disease

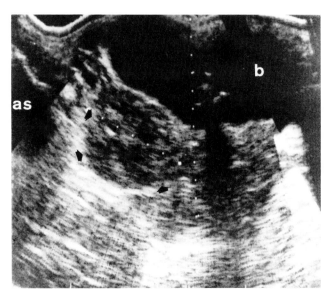

Figure 46-7. Longitudinal section of the abdomen and pelvis (b = bladder) showing a complex pelvic mass (arrows) from an ovarian epithelial tumor. There is marked ascites (as). (Courtesy of Eric Blum, M.D.)

over the surface of the liver, on the under surface of the diaphragm, and on the peritoneum of the abdominal wall.

Several ovarian tumors may be diagnosed sonographically with a fair degree of confidence.

Dermoid Cysts. The dermoid or cystic teratoma is a tumor of all three germinal layers. Benign cystic teratomas usually contain a number of different tissues, including sebaceous material, hair, teeth, and skin. Because of their variable composition, they produce rather a wide spectrum of sonographic findings. These findings are often quite complex, with areas of shadowing from hair or teeth and with fluid-fluid levels in the cystic areas and often in a location superior to the uterus (Fig. 46-8). They are bilateral in approximately 10–15% of patients.

Serous Epithelial Tumors. The serous tumor, the most common benign tumor of the ovary, appears sonographically as cysts, variable in size, usually containing one or more septa. Occuring in groups, one cyst is usually predominant in size.

Mucinous Tumors. Mucinous tumors are slightly less common than the serous variety and have a fairly typical sonographic appearance that is seen as a cystic mass with a number of internal septations (Fig. 46-9). These septations are usually thin, but a considerable amount of solid tissue may be present within.

Keynotes

- *Pelvic masses are characterized as cystic or solid or mixed, as containing blood or pus, as uterine or ovarian.*

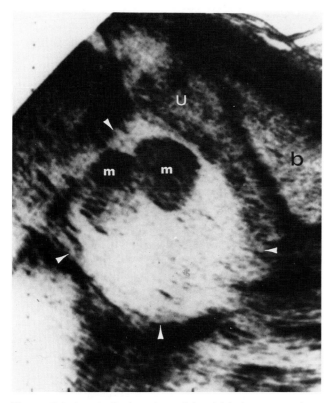

Figure 46-8. Longitudinal sections of the pelvis (u = uterus, b = bladder) showing a demoid cyst (arrowheads). In the superior aspect of the cyst, there are two rounded echo-dense masses (m) that changed position with change in patient position and that represent sebaceous material.

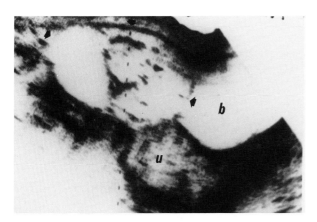

Figure 46-9. Longitudinal section of the pelvis; b = bladder. There is a cystic mass (arrows) with internal septations, superior to the uterus (u); The borders of the lesion are well defined. This is a characteristic sonographic appearance of mucinous cystadenoma.

- *Uterine fibroids usually appear as an enlarged lobular uterus with a nonhomogeneous echo texture.*
- *On sonography uterine carcinoma may be indistinguishable from uterine enlargement caused by uterine fibroids; sometimes irregularity of the outline of the uterus may indicate the presence of uterine carcinoma.*

- *Functional ovarian cysts are usually less that 2.5 cm in diameter, are usually without internal echoes, and usually disappear within two to three menstrual cycles.*
- *The corpus luteum cyst is associated with pregnancy and usually markedly decreases in size by the early second trimester.*
- *Tumors of the ovary usually cannot be differentiated into benign and malignant processes by sonography. Signs suggestive of malignancy are large masses of solid tissue within the lesion, ascites, and pelvic adenopathy.*
- *Dermoid cysts have a wide spectrum of sonographic findings, sometimes including a complex pattern with areas of shadowing and fluid-fluid levels, and they are often superior to the uterus. They are bilateral in 10–15% of patients.*

PELVIC INFLAMMATORY DISEASE

The term *pelvic inflammatory disease* (PID) encompasses a spectrum of clinical presentations ranging from endometritis through tubo-ovarian abscess and peritonitis. Most often the clinical findings are fairly typical, and antibiotic therapy is instituted promptly. As the clinical response is usually fairly rapid, most patients with PID do not require sonography. In those instances in which there is doubt as to the diagnosis or where there is a suboptimal response to the antibiotic therapy, sonography may, however, be indicated. Most often, poor response to appropriate therapy is due to abscess formation, which in PID is usually a tubo-ovarian abscess. A tubo-ovarian abscess is sonographically represented as one or more cystic masses within the pelvis, having slightly irregular walls, and often containing a number of low-level echos. In some instances a fluid-fluid level may be visualized (Fig. 46-10). Because of the inflammatory disease present, the boundaries between normal organs are somewhat obscured. In a number of instances a developing abscess will dissect down the rectovaginal septum, point toward the vagina, and become amenable to transvaginal

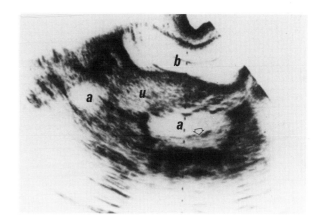

Figure 46-10. Longitudinal scan of the pelvis (b = bladder) showing two abscesses (a), a large abscess posterior to the uterus (u) and a second, smaller, collection adjacent to the uterine fundus. The larger collection has a fluid-fluid level (arrow). Both collections have irregular walls in comparison to the smooth walls of simple cysts.

drainage. Sonography is then of value in localizing those abscesses that are suitable for such drainage, aiding with the placement of a drainage tube, and assessing residual disease after the procedure.

After successful therapy the patient may be left with several residua that may be detected sonographically. A cystic dilatation of the fallopian tube, a *hydrosalpinx*, will usually have a fairly characteristic sonographic appearance, being visualized as a cystic tubular mass adjacent to the uterus, often folded upon itself (Fig. 46-11). Adhesion formation after PID may also result in distortion of normal pelvic anatomy with production of a retroverted uterus and with the ovaries in a position more medial than normal.

Keynotes

- *Patients with pelvic inflammatory disease usually can be treated without sonographic examination. Sonography may be of value for those in whom the diagnosis is in doubt and those in whom there is a suboptimal response to antibiotics.*

- *Tubo-ovarian abscess appears as one or more cystic masses within the pelvis, with slightly irregular walls, and often containing a few echos. A fluid-fluid level may be present.*

- *Sonography can guide the placement of tubes to drain pelvic abscesses.*

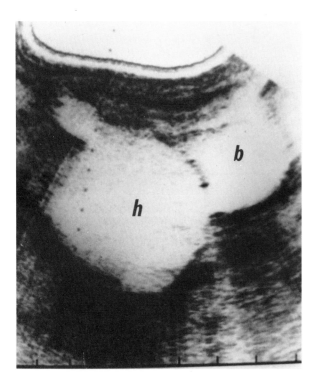

Figure 46-11. Longitudinal section of the pelvis in a patient who had had a hysterectomy 2 years previously. There is a large cystic mass (h), a hydrosalpinx, superior to the vaginal vault and bladder (b), representing the markedly dilated distal tube. The less distended proximal tube is seen as a smaller cystic collection adjacent to this.

ENDOMETRIOSIS

Endometriosis is the occurrence of endometrial tissue outside of its normal location in the endometrial cavity. The most common sites for ectopic occurrence of endometrial tissue are in the cul-de-sac area, on the ovaries, and on the pelvic peritoneum. Endometriosis is associated with a wide variety of symptoms, often out of proportion to the amount of disease present. It may be responsible for abdominal or pelvic pain, dyspareunia, and infertility. Where endometrial tissue is present in an ectopic site, it remains responsive to the hormonal changes of the menstrual cycle and as such will grow and bleed at the appropriate intervals. Recurrent bleeding may lead to the formation of endometrial cysts, which contain altered blood and are referred to as *chocolate cysts*. Sonographically, endometriosis may be visualized as multiple cysts, occasionally containing internal echos because of the blood content (Fig. 46-12). These cysts may be quite large even though the patient's symptoms are minimal. Where there has been fibrosis resulting from recurrent bleeding, there may be distortion of the pelvic architecture, with medial location of the ovaries and with a fixed retroverted uterus. Small desposits of endometrial cysts, the so-called *powder burns*, are usually not visualizable on ultrasound.

Ultrasound is not only of value in the diagnosis of endometriosis but may also be used for following the response of such lesions to hormonal therapy. The patient may be scanned sequentially and the size of the lesions measured.

Keynotes

- *Endometriosis is the occurrence of endometrial tissue outside of its normal location in the endometrial cavity of the uterus.*

- *Only some patients with endometriosis will have sonographic abnormalities. Multiple cysts, some with internal echoes, and distortions of the locations of pelvic structures from fibrosis can be seen.*

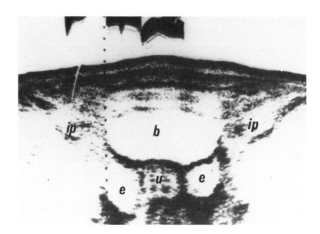

Figure 46-12. Transverse section of the pelvis showing bilateral endometriosal cysts (e). The iliopsoas muscles (ip) and bladder (b) are also demonstrated.

LOCATION OF AN IUD

The IUD remains one of the most common and most efficient forms of contraception used at this time, having a 97–98% effectiveness rate. One of the most common problems patients with an IUD report is their inability to detect the string of the device on examination. This may be the result of perforation of the uterus (most commonly occurring at the time of the insertion of the device), undetected expulsion of the device, or drawing up of the IUD string into the uterine cavity so that it is no longer palpable.

Several methods are available for determining whether a device is or is not intrauterine in location. An AP radiograph of the pelvis will determine that the IUD is indeed somewhere in the pelvis because all IUDs in current use are radiopaque. The plain radiograph will not, however, demonstrate the endometrial cavity and thus will not show the exact relationship of the device to this cavity. The physician may insert a probe or a second intrauterine device into the uterine cavity before obtaining the radiograph, and in this manner the location of any IUD can be assessed in relation to the probe or second device. This assumes, of course, that the second device or probe has been placed inside the endometrial cavity and has not itself passed through a perforation produced by the original insertion. A hysterosalpingogram provides an accurate method of determining the relationship of the IUD to the endometrial cavity, but it is uncomfortable and invasive. Ultrasound provides a safe, reliable, and noninvasive method of IUD localization. It is in fact the only method that simultaneously shows the IUD, the endometrial cavity, and the myometrium.

Intrauterine devices, depending on type, have differing sonographic appearances. The Lippes Loop, in longitudinal sections of the uterus, will be shown as four or five echogenic dots representing cross sections through the transverse limbs of the device (Fig. 46-13). The Copper-7 and Copper-T devices have, wound around their stem, fine copper wire that is quite echogenic, making the devices readily visible on both longitudinal and transverse sec-

tions of the uterus (Fig. 46-14). Other devices, such as the Progestersert, the Dalkon Shield, and the Saf-T-Coil, are also readily visualized sonographically. For maximal efficiency the device should be located near the fundus of the uterus, and this is readily evaluated sonographically.

One of the major disadvantages in the use of ultrasound for evaluation of IUD location is the fact that if the IUD is indeed in an extrauterine location, for example in the peritoneal cavity, then it is unlikely that it will be visualized sonographically because of shadowing by overlying bowel gas. If the device is in fact in the endometrial cavity or in the myometrium or cervix, it should, however, be consistently visualized.

A sonogram should be the first line of imaging investigation because in most instances where there is nonvisualization of the string, the device is indeed in an intrauterine location, and in a percentage of cases there is a coexistent pregnancy (Fig. 46-15). Sonography will not only con-

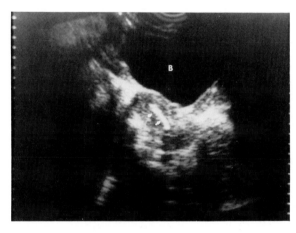

Figure 46-14. Longitudinal section of the pelvis (b = bladder) showing the dense linear echos produced by the copper wound around the stem of a Copper-7 IUD.

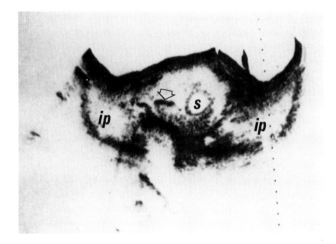

Figure 46-15. Transverse section of the pelvis showing an early intrauterine gestational sac (s). A copper IUD (arrow) is seen in the uterus lateral to the sac. The iliopsoas muscles (ip) are well demonstrated. The bladder is not demonstrated on this section.

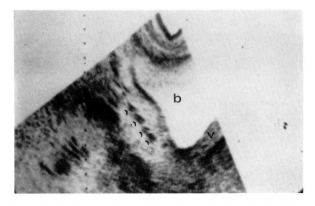

Figure 46-13. Longitudinal section of the pelvis (b = bladder) showing four echogenic areas (arrowheads) produced by the limbs of a Lippes Loop, situated in a satisfactory intrauterine location.

firm the intrauterine location of the device but also avoid exposing an early intrauterine pregnancy to ionizing radiation. Where the device is not visualized and there is no evidence of an intrauterine pregnancy, then a single AP radiograph of the pelvis may detect the IUD in an extrauterine location.

Keynotes

- *A hysterosalpingogram is a radiological study in which a contrast medium is injected through the cervix into the uterine cavity, after which radiographs are taken demonstrating the anatomy of the uterine cavity and the fallopian tubes.*
- *Ultrasonic examination is an effective method for determining that an IUD is in an intrauterine location.*

ECTOPIC PREGNANCY

Ectopic pregnancy is the presence of a pregnancy in a location other than the endometrial cavity. Most often this is a tubal pregnancy. The most common portion of the tube affected is the ampullar portion. The incidence of ectopic pregnancy varies in differing geographic areas; it occurs mainly in those areas where there is a high incidence of PID. Although antibiotic therapy is usually successful in treating PID, in a number of instances it results in the fallopian tubes remaining patent although damaged.

Ectopic pregnancy remains a major clinical problem in gynecology because the symptoms and signs are often varied. Most patients have lower abdominal pain. In about 50% of patients there is a recent history of amenorrhea, and in 50% an adnexal mass is palpated on bimanual examination. A urinary pregnancy test is often negative, but the more sensitive serum radioimmunoassay for HCG is usually positive. Similar symptoms and physical findings may be produced by other disease processes such as a hemorrhagic ovarian cyst, torsion of a cyst, or PID. Uncommonly, the first presentation is shock from hemorrhage from a ruptured tubal pregnancy.

The value of sonography in ectopic pregnancy diagnosis is limited. Its greatest value is in demonstrating the presence or absence of an intrauterine pregnancy. Sonographic demonstration of an intrauterine pregnancy makes a coexistent ectopic pregnancy extremely unlikely. Occasionally the decidual cast produced in the uterus by an ectopic pregnancy will mimic an early gestational sac without a *fetal pole* (a small cluster of echos representing the embryo), causing some confusion (Fig. 46-16). When an intrauterine gestational sac with viable a fetal pole is demonstrated, an ectopic pregnancy is all but excluded. Any other sonographic appearance, including normal, is compatible with ectopic gestation. In a number of instances an adnexal mass may be demonstrated, and the uterus may be seen to be slightly enlarged with increased endometrial echos. Infrequently, a definite extrauterine gestational sac with a fetal pole demonstrating fetal movement and cardiac activity is seen. This is the only sonographic appearance that is specific for ectopic gestation (see Fig. 32-7).

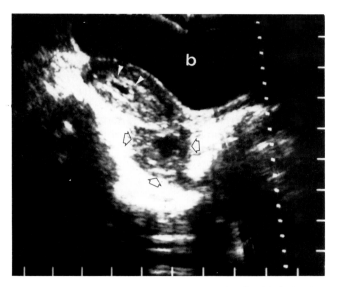

Figure 46-16. Longitudinal scan of the pelvis (b= bladder) showing an intrauterine decidual cast (arrowheads) mimicking an early gestational sac. There is a complex mass (open arrows) in the cul-de-sac, representing an unruptured tubal pregnancy.

Keynotes

- *Ectopic pregnancy is the presence of a pregnancy in a location other than the endometrial cavity of the uterus.*
- *The major value of sonography in a patient with suspected ectopic pregnancy is the demonstration of the presence or absence of an intrauterine pregnancy.*
- *The only specific finding of ectopic pregnancy is the demonstration of a definite gestational sac and a viable fetal pole in an extrauterine location; most patients with an ectopic pregnancy however, will not show this finding. In those, the diagnosis of ectopic pregnancy can be inferred from the absence of an intrauterine pregnancy. In many instances of ectopic pregnancy, the sonogram is normal.*

CONGENITAL UTERINE ANOMALIES

Traditionally, congenital uterine anomalies have been investigated with hysterosalpingography (Fig. 46-17), a procedure that involves the injection of a radiopaque contrast medium through the cervical canal into the endometrial cavity before radiography. This allows demonstration of the shape and size of the endometrial cavity and fallopian tubes. Sonography offers a new technique for evaluation, and in certain ways it provides information not available with conventional hysterograms. With sonography, not only does one visualize the endometrial cavity, but one is able also to visualize the myometrium, which is not seen with hysterography.

The uterus, fallopian tubes, and upper portion of the vagina are formed from the paired müllerian ducts. In embryonic life these ducts come together and fuse, and the intervening septum between them resorbs. The lower one-third of the vagina is formed from the urogenital sinus. Most uterine anomalies are produced because of a failure of this process of fusion. Where this failure is only minor, an arcuate or a mild bicornuate uterus is produced. More severe failure produces a marked bicornuate uterus, and total absence of fusion produces a double uterus with double cervix and duplication of the upper two-thirds of the vagina. Where there has been fusion of the müllerian system but a failure of breakdown of the intervening septum, then a septate uterus is formed, which is different from the bicornate uterus: the external configuration of the septate uterus is normal, whereas that of the bicornuate uterus is abnormal (Fig. 46-18).

Sonography allows visualization of the external configuration of the uterus and also of the shape and orientation of the endometrial cavity. With a bicornuate uterus, the uterus is seen to be widened and may be heart shaped in

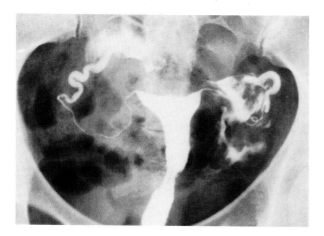

Figure 46-17. Hysterosalpingogram of a normal female pelvis. A cannula has been placed into the cervical canal, and contrast medium has been injected, filling the uterine cavity and fallopian tubes. Some contrast has spilled into the peritoneal cavity, indicating that the tubes are patent.

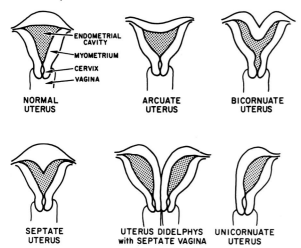

Figure 46-18. Schematic representation of the major uterine anomalies. (Illustrative Services, Art Department, University of Maryland Medical School.)

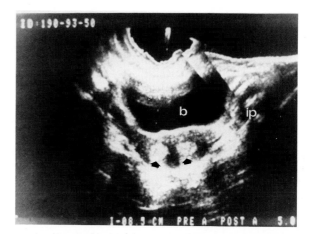

Figure 46-19. Transverse section of the pelvis (b = bladder, ip = iliopsoas muscles) showing a widened, bicornuate uterus. Separate endometrial cavities are seen (arrows), the endometrial echos being thickened because of the premenstrual phase of the cycle.

transverse section. The separate endometrial cavities may be visualized (Fig. 46-19). There is a single cervix, which may also be visualized. With uterus didelphys, two separate uterine horns will be visualized in longitudinal sections. In transverse sections, both uterine horns and also a double cervix are usually seen.

Genital tract obstruction, as from an imperforate hymen, or absence of the vagina will cause primary amenorrhea and perhaps an abdominopelvic mass. Sonography is of great benefit in demonstrating the presence or absence of the uterus and ovaries. In *hematocolpos,* where there is an obstruction to the egress of menstrual blood with distension of the cervix and uterus, ultrasound will readily demonstrate these distended organs (Fig. 46-20).

Keynote

• *Sonography can demonstrate the structure of the uterus and its endometrial cavity. It is useful in the evaluation of uterine congenital anomalies.*

INFERTILITY

Although at this time ultrasound is not being widely applied to the investigation and management of infertility, there are several areas in which it may be of benefit:

1. Establishing presence or absence of the uterus or ovaries in the patient with primary amenorrhea or infertility
2. Determining the size and shape of the uterus and the presence of uterine masses, such as fibroids, that may interfere with implantation
3. Establishing presence of coexistent adnexal masses, for example, from endometriosis or the residua of PID

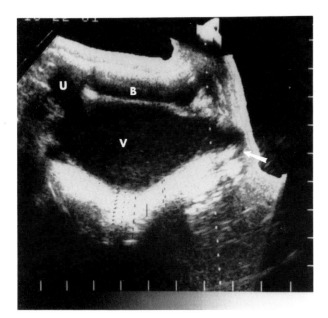

Figure 46-20. Longitudinal section of the pelvis showing the vagina (V) markedly distended with fluid. The presence of low-level internal echos in this fluid is compatible with blood, indicating hematocolpos. The point of occlusion, due to a short-segment vaginal agenesis, is seen (arrow). The uterus (U) and bladder (B) are also demonstrated.

4. Determining certain congenital uterine anomalies
5. Diagnosing ovulation and managing the patient undergoing ovulation induction

With the exception of ovulation induction these areas of application have been covered in other sections. With the resolution available with current generation equipment, it is not uncommon to visualize a developing ovarian follicle, which may be demonstrated from a diameter of 5 mm up to a mean diameter of 20–25 mm immediately before ovulation (Fig. 46-4). Intrafollicular structures representing the cumulus oophorus may occasionally be demonstrated. After ovulation there is a sudden change in the appearance of the follicle with an increase of echos secondary to intrafollicular bleeding. Ultrasound may be used with patients undergoing ovulation induction to determine the response of the patients to gonadotropin. The premature appearance of multiple large follicles is associated with the risk of overstimulation, requiring that the gonadotropin be discontinued immediately.

Keynote

• *Sonography may be used in the management of ovulation induction in determining the number of follicles that are formed and also in timing egg retrieval.*

GYNECOLOGIC ONCOLOGY

In the patient with suspected or proven pelvic malignancy, ultrasound is of value in

1. Diagnosis and characterization of a pelvic mass
2. Assessment of pelvic and abdominal adenopathy
3. Assessment of ascites, omental involvement, or presence of distant metastases
4. Interventional techniques: directed biopsy of masses or enlarged lymph nodes
5. Planning of internal or external radiotherapy
6. Assessment of postoperative complications: fever, hematocrit-level drop, and pelvic masses

Adenopathy

Lymph nodes in the iliac, obturator, and para-aortic chain when enlarged may be visualized by ultrasound. Since such lymph node enlargement may be secondary to causes other than metastatic disease, diagnosis may be confirmed by ultrasound-directed transcutaneous biopsy using a thin aspiration needle.

Ascites

Ascites is detectable by ultrasound before it can be recognized by clinical methods. The distribution of ascites helps to determine whether the ascites is due to a benign or malignant cause. Ascites that shows loculation, contains low-level echos, or does not change appearance with change in the patient's position is more likely to be secondary to malignant disease (Fig. 46-7).

Omental Involvement and Distant Metastases

Omental involvement will be shown by an irregular mass in an anterior peritoneal location, often surrounded by ascitic fluid. Peritoneal metastases as small as 5 mm may be demonstrated.

With an accuracy exceeding that of radionuclide examination, metastatic disease of the liver may be detected as areas of altered echogenicity within the normal liver parenchyma. The sonographic appearance of the metastases is not, however, correlated with the histology of the primary lesion. Pleural effusions secondary to malignancy may be visualized, localized, and aspirated with ultrasound guidance.

Interventional Techniques

Because two-dimensional views are obtained with B-mode ultrasound, directed biopsies of masses or enlarged lymph nodes are possible. Use of an aspiration needle allows sampling of such a lesion with minimal complications. Although the use of aspiration biopsy and diagnosis of enlarged lymph nodes or liver lesions is well established, the use of aspiration biopsy in primary diagnosis of the pelvic mass is considerably more controversial because puncture of a malignant ovarian lesion may lead to peritoneal contamination by malignant cells. Because a persistent adnexal mass requires operative intervention, aspiration biopsy may give no additional useful information. In the patient with treated malignancy who has a recurrent pelvic or abdominal mass, however, biopsy may help differentiate between fibrosis and recurrent disease, greatly influencing the clinical management of the case.

Postoperative Fever or Drop in Hematocrit Level

In cases of unexplained drop in hematocrit level or persistent fever after pelvic surgery, sonography is often of value in demonstrating a hematoma or an abscess collection. Such collections may be related to the pelvic operative site or to the abdominal incision. The transverse (Pfannenstiel's) incision is especially susceptible to postoperative hematoma or abscess formation, characteristically in a subfascial location. Although it may be difficult to distinguish an abscess from a hematoma on sonographic appearance alone, the clinical features combined with sonography should allow an accurate diagnosis. Response of an abscess to therapy may be followed with sonography, or else transabdominal or transvaginal needle aspiration may be accomplished using sonographic guidance.

Keynote

- *Ultrasonic examination may demonstrate pelvic lymphadenopathy and may be used to guide transcutaneous biopsies of these nodes.*
- *Sonography can demonstrate postoperative hematomas and abscesses.*

GYNECOLOGIC UROLOGIC PROBLEMS

Sonography can be used in the evaluation of the bladder and urethra. It allows evaluation of

1. Bladder size and shape, bladder volume, and postvoid residual volume
2. Bladder base and urethrovesical junction (UVJ)
3. Bladder wall thickness and integrity
4. Urethral diverticula.

Bladder Size and Shape

Visualization of the bladder allows assessment of its size and shape and whether the walls are involved by tumor, either primary or by spread from adjacent organs (e.g., from cervical cancer). In cases of neurogenic bladder, for example, the multiple sclerosis patient on drugs to improve bladder function, sonography provides a rapid, noninvasive method of estimating prevoid and postvoid bladder volumes, both before and during therapy. Use of sonography avoids repeated catheterization with its risk of infection.

Bladder Base and Urethrovesical Junction

In the female patient with urinary symptoms of stress incontinence, urgency, and frequency of micturition, two major etiologies are stress incontinence of urine and detru-

sor muscle dyssynergia. In *stress incontinence* the patient involuntarily loses urine when there is a sudden increase of intra-abdominal pressure, for example, from coughing, sneezing, or laughing. In most such patients there is an alteration in the relationship of the bladder and UVJ, this angle becoming wider than normal.

Traditionally, stress incontinence has been investigated radiologically with voiding cystourethrography or static chain cystourethrography. Sonography allows a noninvasive alternative, for it not only will demonstrate the UVJ but will also allow measurement of the descent of the junction when the patient increases abdominal pressure by performing a Valsalva maneuver. In patients with genuine stress incontinence, this UVJ descent is significantly increased. Genuine stress incontinence is often treated surgically, and in the postoperative patient improvement in the UVJ descent should be sonographically demonstrated.

In incontinence secondary to detrusor muscle dyssynergia, there is an alteration in the normal neurogenic control of the bladder, usually resulting in urge incontinence. Such patients will usually demonstrate normal UVJ relationships. Surgery is not helpful and may in fact aggravate the condition.

Bladder Wall Integrity

With sonography the bladder wall is visualized, and any irregularity or mass effect from a primary or secondary tumor may be easily seen. In the patient with pelvic malignancy, involvement of the bladder mucosa will alter the staging and prognosis.

Urethral Diverticula

A urethral diverticulum is relatively uncommon and usually produces recurrent cystitis, incontinence, or both. It is often quite difficult to visualize radiographically at the time of cystography or with endoscopy. When the diverticulum contains urine, however, it is usually readily visualized with sonography.

SUMMARY

Ultrasound has many uses in the field of gynecology. It is used to diagnose and characterize a pelvic mass, found on physical examination, as cystic or solid or complex, uterine or ovarian, or as arising from another pelvic structure. It is of value when PID symptoms respond incompletely to therapy, in the diagnosis and follow-up of endometriosis, in the demonstration of the intrauterine location of an IUD, and in the diagnosis of suspected ectopic pregnancy.

Sonography can be used in the assessment and management of infertility and can be used to monitor ovulation induction. Uterine anomalies can be characterized.

It can be used in the assessment of gynecologic malignancy, both in the evaluation of the primary tumor and in the determination of metastatic disease. It can be used in the assessment of hematomas and abscesses and can be used to guide biopsy and drainage procedures.

Ultrasonography is also used in the evaluation of certain gynecologic urologic problems, such as urinary stress incontinence and urethral diverticula.

REVIEW QUESTIONS

1. Why is pelvic ultrasound performed with the bladder full of urine?

2. What type of information about a pelvic mass can ultrasound provide that can help in its characterization?

3. What is the usual appearance of uterine fibroids?

4. What sonographic findings can be used to differentiate uterine fibroids from uterine carcinoma?

5. Describe the usual appearance of functional ovarian cysts.

6. Describe the usual appearance of corpus luteum cysts.

7. What findings can be used to suggest that an ovarian mass is malignant?

8. What are some of the sonographic findings in a dermoid cyst of the ovary?

9. Under what circumstances should a patient with pelvic inflammatory disease have a sonograpic examination?

10. What is the sonographic appearance of a tubo-ovarian abscess?

11. What is endometriosis? What is its sonographic appearance?

12. What are the methods of determining whether an IUD is in an intrauterine location?

13. What is an ectopic pregnancy? What symptoms are associated with it? What is the role of sonography in the diagnosis of an ectopic pregnancy?

14. What are some of the types of congenital uterine anomalies? What is the role of sonography in their evaluation?

15. What is the role of sonography in infertility?

16. What role does sonography play in gynecologic malignancy?

VOCABULARY

acoustic window
bicornuate uterus
chocolate cysts
corpus luteum cysts
cystic teratoma
decidual cast
dermoid cysts
ectopic pregnancy
endometrial carcinoma
endometrial cavity
endometriosis
fetal pole
functional cysts
gonadotropin
hematocolpos
hydrosalpinx
hysterosalpingogram
intrauterine device
mucinous tumors of the ovary
müllerian ducts
ovarian follicle
pelvic inflammatory disease
powder burns
primary amenorrhea
serous tumors of the ovary
tubo-ovarian abscess
urethral diverticulum
urine stress incontinence
urine urge incontinence
uterine fibroids
uterus didelphys

SUGGESTIONS FOR FURTHER READING FOR CHAPTERS 46 AND 47

Roger C. Sanders, A. Everette James, Jr. *The Principles and Practice of Ultrasonography in Obstetrics and Gynecology,* 3rd Ed. Appleton-Century-Crofts: Norwalk. 1985. (A fine basic and reference text)

B. Felson, Ed. Gynecologic roentgenology. *Seminars in Roentgenology,* **17**(4), 1982.

Hedvig Hricak. MRI of the female pelvis: A review. *American Journal of Roentgenology,* **146**:1115–1122, 1986.

47

ULTRASOUND IN OBSTETRICS

DAVID GRAHAM

KEY CONCEPTS

Radiological

Ultrasound, because of its safety for the fetus, is gaining an ever wider role in obstetric management. Its current main uses are in estimating fetal (gestational) age and detecting intrauterine growth disturbance and fetal malformations. It is also used in the evaluation of third-trimester bleeding, in the detection of fetal death, and in the evaluation of trophoblastic disease.

Estimation of gestational age is based on three main measurements: the crown–rump length (the length of the fetus excluding the limbs), the gestational sac diameter, and the biparietal diameter (of the skull). The first two measurements are used in the first half of gestation, the last in mid-to-late gestation.

Some congenital structural abnormalities of the central nervous system, cardiovascular system, genitourinary system, GI system, and the skeletal system can be detected. In the central nervous system, anencephaly, hydrocephalus, and neural tube defects (mainly meningomyelocele) are the more common detectable lesions. Hydronephrosis, multicystic kidney, and renal agenesis are among the abnormalities sometimes detected in the genitourinary system. In the GI system, duodenal atresia, mesenteric cysts, and diaphragmatic hernias can be detected.

In first-trimester uterine bleeding, ultrasound can determine whether there is a viable fetus in the uterus. In third-trimester bleeding, ultrasound is important in the diagnosis of placenta previa, helping to differentiate the cause of bleeding from placental abruption.

Fetal death in early pregnancy may be detected by seeing either a nonmotile fetus without cardiac activity or by not identifying a fetus or gestational sac at an appropriate gestational age. Fetal death in later pregnancy can be determined by failure to detect cardiac motion. Several secondary signs may also be present: overlapping of the skull bones, scalp edema, abnormal fetal lie, and intravascular gas collections.

Clinical

Neural tube defects including anencephaly and meningomyelocele occur in 1 per 1,000 live births in the United States of America. α-Fetoprotein (AFP) level in the maternal serum is increased in patients with neural tube defects as well as several other conditions. Those with elevated AFP should be screened with sonography.

Intrauterine growth retardation (IUGR) can be detected by sonographic examination. There are two types: early-onset, or low-profile, IUGR, in which the fetus grows at a lower than expected rate from early pregnancy and which is associated with a higher incidence of fetal anomalies; and late-onset, or asymmetric, IUGR, which is often secondary to relative placental insufficiency.

OBJECTIVES

When you complete this chapter you will be able to

1. Identify on selected sonographic studies
   a. A gestational sac
   b. A fetal pole
   c. The fetal skull and abdomen
   d. A twin pregnancy
   e. Placenta previa
   f. A molar pregnancy
2. Describe the two types of IUGR and their significance.
3. List the main causes of first- and third-trimester bleeding.
4. Discuss the concept of placental migration.
5. List the three types of trophoblastic disease, their presumed etiology, and their treatment.

The earliest sonographic evidence of intrauterine pregnancy is a thickening of the normal thin endometrial line as a result of decidual proliferation. This is not, however, infallible evidence of an intrauterine pregnancy, because it may also be seen in some patients in the immediate premenstrual period, in ectopic pregnancy, and in missed abortion. Approximately 5–6 weeks after the last menstrual period, the gestational sac may be seen as a circular collection of echos in the uterus, surrounding a cystic center, the choronic/amniotic sac (Fig. 47-1). At 6–7 weeks of gestation, a small collection of echos, the *fetal pole,* representing the embryo may be seen. The use of real-time equipment allows demonstration of motion and heart motion of the embryo. At approximately 10–11 weeks of gestation, the fetal head may be recognized as a distinct structure, and after this an increasing amount of normal fetal anatomy may be visualized as the pregnancy advances. Although it has been recommended that each pregnant patient have an ultrasound examination during pregnancy, most clinicians perform such an examination only because of certain clinical needs, the most common being:

1. Dating the pregnancy when the last menstrual period is uncertain or when there is a date/examination discrepancy
2. Diagnosing multiple pregnancy
3. Determining certain structural fetal anomalies
4. Diagnosing and characterizing uterine or adnexal masses associated with pregnancy
5. Guiding amniocentesis, reducing the risks of the procedure, and improving the frequency of successful taps
6. Diagnosing fetal IUGR
7. Diagnosing the cause of bleeding during pregnancy
8. Determining fetal death
9. Assessing certain fetal physiological parameters
10. Visualizing a coexistent IUD
11. Investigating postpartum problems, including postpartum fever and hematocrit-level drop.
12. Evaluating trophoblastic disease

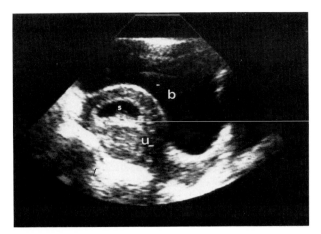

Figure 47-1. Real-time longitudinal scan of the uterus (u) showing a gestational sac (s) representing a 7-week pregnancy, situated in the uterine fundus. b = Bladder.

Keynote

• *Signs of an early intrauterine pregnancy are*

 a. *Thickening of the endometrial line because of decidual proliferation*

 b. *A rounded cystic gestational sac in the uterus at 5–6 weeks*

 c. *A fetal pole within the gestational sac at 6–7 weeks*

 d. *A measurable fetal head at 10–11 weeks (Fetal head can sometimes be seen before this age.)*

GESTATIONAL AGE

One of the most common indications for an ultrasound examination in pregnancy is to date the pregnancy when menstrual dates are uncertain or when there is a discrepancy between dates and uterine size. Several methods are available.

Gestational Sac Diameter

Before the appearance of the fetal pole, the average sac diameter correlates well with gestational age and can be used in dating.

Crown–Rump Length

Up to 12–14 weeks the longest length of the fetus (excluding the limbs) has a linear correlation with gestational age (Fig. 47-2). Measurement of the crown–rump length (CRL) is in fact the single most accurate way of estimating gestational age because there is a rapid increase in size of the CRL over this time, and there is little biologic variation.

Biparietal Diameter

Measurement of the widest diameter of the head, usually taken at the level of the thalami and third ventricle, correlates with gestational age and is the method of choice for dating after 12–14 weeks (Fig. 47-3). The relationship of biparietal diameter (BPD) to gestational age is linear up to 28–30 weeks, and then BPD growth slows and the confidence limits of the measurement widen. At 20 weeks of pregnancy the confidence limits are approximately 7–10 days, but in the last 10 weeks of pregnancy there is a variation of ±21 days. Because of the wide variation in the latter weeks of pregnancy, an estimation of gestational age based on a single BPD obtained after 30 weeks is of limited value.

Keynote

• *Methods of estimating gestational age include*

 a. *Diameter of the gestational sac; useful up to 8–9 weeks.*

 b. *Crown–rump length; useful up to 12–14 weeks of age.*

 c. *Biparietal diameter of the skull; best for dating after 12–14 weeks and up to 30 weeks. After 30 weeks the range of normal variation is greater, limiting accuracy.*

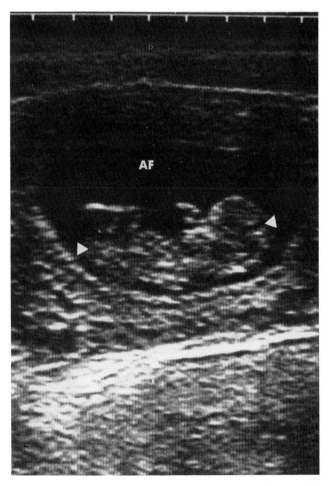

Figure 47-2. Real-time scan of an early pregnancy to show an 11-week embryo. The measurement used for the CRL is shown by arrowheads; the one to the right indicates the fetal head. Fetal limbs are seen anteriorly. AF = amniotic fluid.

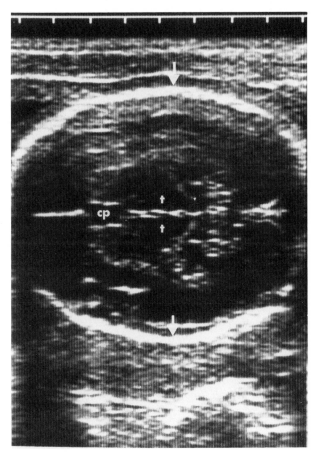

Figure 47-3. Transverse section of the fetal head at the level used to measure the biparietal diameter (arrows). Between the thalami (t) is a thin slit representing the third ventricle. The cavum septum pellucidum (cp) is seen anterior to the thalami.

MULTIPLE PREGNANCY

Multiple pregnancy can be diagnosed as early as can singleton pregnancy by demonstration of two (or more) gestational sacs (Fig. 47–4). There is, however, a discrepancy between the frequency of multiple gestation diagnosed this early in pregnancy and the frequency of multiple pregnancy at term. It has been estimated that only about 30% of multiple pregnancies diagnosed sonographically in the first trimester actually deliver twins, most likely because of a combination of misdiagnosis and a higher than usual early wastage rate. When diagnosed in the second and third trimester most twin pregnancies do progress satisfactorily, although the fetal loss remains higher than in a singleton pregnancy. Ultrasound is of value in multiple pregnancy in

1. Dating the pregnancy.
2. Following fetal growth. In monochorionic twins, twin-to-twin transfusion syndrome may occur, resulting in growth retardation of one infant.

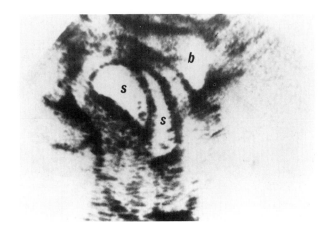

Figure 47-4. Longitudinal section of the uterus showing two gestational sacs (s), each containing a fetal pole, indicating early twin pregnancy. b = Bladder.

3. Diagnosing fetal anomalies, which are more common in twins, especially monochorionic twins.

4. Determining placental anatomy and location and demonstrating a dividing septum, suggesting the most probable type of twin gestation present (Fig. 47-5).

5. Determining fetal position, which will influence the mode of delivery.

Keynote

• *Many multiple pregnancies diagnosed sonographically in the first trimester become singleton pregnancies by term, probably because of early reabsorption of one of the embryos.*

STRUCTURAL ANOMALIES

The use of ultrasound to demonstrate normal and abnormal fetal anatomy is one of the most rapidly expanding applications of the technology. In the subsequent sections normal fetal anatomy and fetal anomalies are discussed by organ system.

Central Nervous System

Use of high-resolution equipment allows visualization of many major intracranial structures including the thalami and third ventricle (Fig. 47-3), cerebellum, cerebral peduncles, lateral ventricles, and some of the major arterial structures. The fetal spine can also be visualized as two parallel lines of echos that widen slightly at the cervical end and, to a lesser extent, in the lumbar area.

Anencephaly. In the anencephalic fetus the normally well-defined cranial outline is replaced by an irregular "nubbin" of tissue representing the base of the skull and the remaining cerebral structures (Fig. 47-6). The diagnosis has been made as early as 13–14 weeks, and although the sonographic findings are characteristic, where there is doubt, an abdominal radiograph should be confirmatory. In approximately 50% of cases there is associated hydramnios.

Hydrocephalus. Because normal lateral ventricles are readily recognized, dilatation may also be seen, usually before an abnormal increase in BPD (Fig. 47-7). Hydrocephalus can be diagnosed from the early second trimester, and its progression can be followed. The spine should also be examined to determine a coexistent spina bifida.

Encephalocele. Encephalocele represents a protrusion of brain, meninges, or both through a defect in a cranial bone, usually in a midline occipital location. Encephalocele is visualized as a cystic, solid, or complex mass adjacent to the head. The cranial bone defect can also be visual-

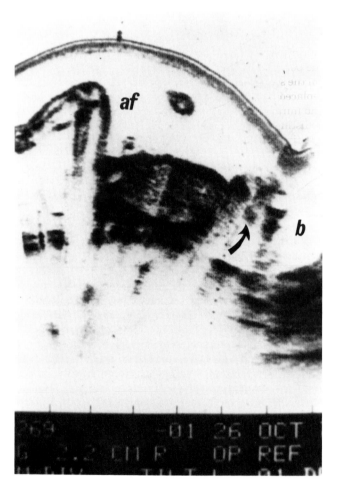

Figure 47-6. Longitudinal scan of the uterus in the third trimester showing an anencephalic fetus lying in a supine position. The remnant of the head is marked (arrow). There is an excess of amniotic fluid present (af). b = Bladder.

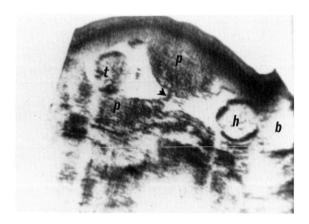

Figure 47-5. Longitudinal section through a uterus in the midtrimester showing a twin pregnancy. There are two placentas (p), anterior and posterior. The head (h) of one infant and trunk (t) of the other are demonstrated. Between the two placentas is an echogenic line representing the sac separation (arrow). b = Bladder.

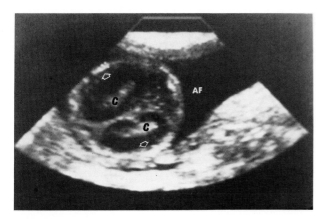

Figure 47-7. Transverse section of a fetal head in midtrimester showing markedly dilated ventricles containing choroid plexus (c). The thin rim of remaining cerebral cortex is seen (arrows). AF = amniotic fluid.

ized. Because there is an associated increased frequency of spina bifida, the spine is also examined.

Hydranencephaly. In hydranencephaly some as yet unknown prenatal insult results in infarction of cerebral tissue perfused by the anterior and middle cerebral arteries. On the sonogram the normal supratentorial structures are replaced by fluid, but structures at the base of the brain and infratentorially are usually spared. Hydranencephaly is distinguished from hydrocephaly by the lack of any remaining cerebral cortex in the former condition. Such distinction is important because of the poorer prognosis of hydranencephaly.

Spina Bifida. Neural tube defects (NTDs), principally spina bifida, occur with an incidence of 1 per 1,000 live births in the United States but are significantly more common in certain areas of the United Kingdom, where the incidence may be as high as 4–7 per 1,000. Once a patient has had an affected infant, there is 5% chance of recurrence of a NTD (not necessarily of the same type) in a subsequent pregnancy. After two affected pregnancies the repeat rate increases to 12%. By measuring the level of the fetal protein AFP in the maternal serum, NTD or certain other fetal anomalies may be detected. Where the AFP level is elevated, increasing the possibility of an open NTD, sonography may be performed. Not only will it correct an erroneous gestational age, diagnose a multiple pregnancy or detect a fetal demise, all of which could also account for an elevated AFP level, but sonography can also allow visualization of the fetal spine and detection of spina bifida. Although closed spina bifida defects may have a normal serum AFP level, these too should be detected by sonography. The normal spine is visualized sonographically as two parallel rows of echos. In spina bifida there is local widening of these parallel echos, often with an adjacent mass representing the meningomyelocele. A small number of spina bifida le-

sions, usually small and in the lower lumbar and upper sacral area may miss sonographic detection.

Cardiovascular System

Fetal cardiac movement may be demonstrated as early as 7 weeks of gestation. The heart, aorta, inferior vena cava, and major tributaries may be visualized (Fig. 47-8). The heart may be investigated by

- Two-dimensional real-time study, allowing demonstration of fetal life, structural cardiac defects, and evaluation of rhythm disorders
- M-mode echocardiography similar to the technique used in the adult, allowing evaluation of chamber size, valve motion, cardiac defects, and arrhythmias

Intrathoracic Lesions

Although normal fetal lungs are seen in little detail, certain intrathoracic anomalies, including pleural effusions,

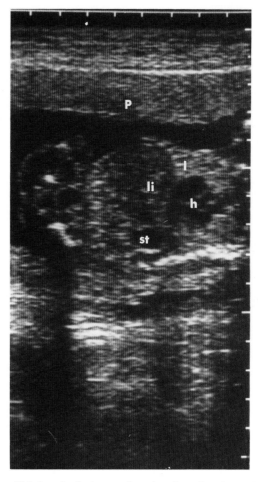

Figure 47-8 Longitudinal coronal section through a fetus showing heart (h), lung (l), Liver (li), and stomach (st). The fetal head (not shown) would be to the right.

diaphragmatic hernias, and pulmonary malformations, may be sonographically visualized.

Genitourinary System

The fetal kidneys and bladder may be visualized from the early second trimester (Fig. 47-9 and 47-10). When the bladder is visualized sequentially over several hours, it can be seen gradually to fill and then empty as the fetus produces urine and voids. External genitalia may be visualized in a small number of instances, the penis and scrotum being more readily recognized than the labia.

Hydronephrosis. Because the renal pelvis can be visualized, hydronephrosis may be recognized prenatally and its progress followed (Fig. 47-11). Prenatally, hydronephrosis is most often caused by a ureteropelvic (UPJ) obstruction. Where there is a complete bilateral urinary tract infection, oligohydramnios is usually present.

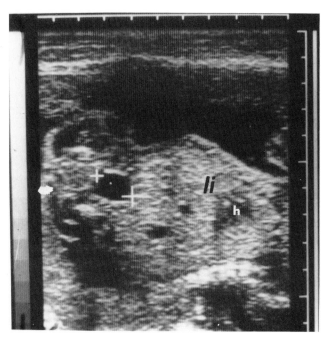

Figure 47-10 Coronal section through a midtrimester fetus showing the bladder (++). The fetal liver (li) and heart (h) are also visualized. AF = amniotic fluid. The fetal head (not shown) would be to the right.

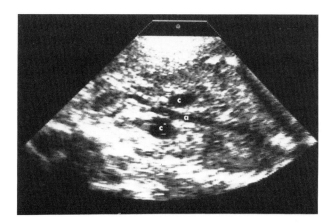

Figure 47-11. Coronal section through a fetus showing cystic masses (c) representing hydronephrotic kidneys on either side of the fetal aorta (a). The fetal outline is poorly visualized because of oligohydramnios, a common accompaniment of bilateral renal obstruction.

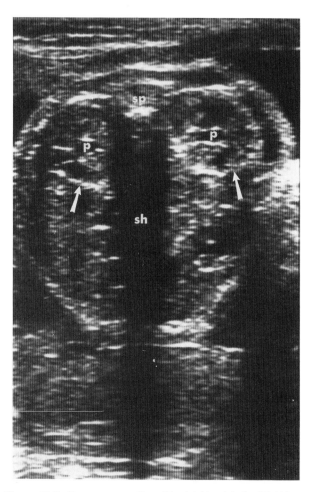

Figure 47-9. Transverse section of the fetal trunk in the third trimester showing fetal kidneys (arrows). In the center of each kidney is a cystic collection of fluid, the renal pelvis (p). The spine (sp) produces shadowing (sh) of a portion of the fetal trunk.

Multicystic Kidney. Multicystic kidney, a renal dysplasia, is recognized by replacement of normal renal structures by numerous cysts of varying size. Occasionally one of the cysts is much larger than the rest, and the appearance of in utero hydronephrosis is simulated.

Polycystic Kidney. In infantile polycystic disease, normal renal parenchyma is replaced by numerous tiny cysts. This condition can be recognized prenatally by enlarged, echogenic kidneys with loss of normal intrarenal anat-

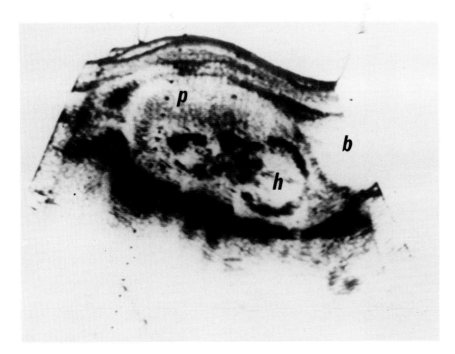

Figure 47-12. Longitudinal section of a uterus at approximately 20 weeks of gestation. There is marked oligohydramnios from renal agenesis, with no visualized amniotic fluid. The fetal head (h) is seen with trunk and small parts to the left of this. The placenta (p) is seen anteriorly; b = bladder.

omy. Theoretically, a fetus affected by the infantile form of adult polycystic disease would be expected to show evidence of cyst formation in the kidneys and the liver.

Renal Agenesis. Renal agenesis is characterized by marked oligohydramnios together with a sonographic inability to demonstrate normal renal structures (Fig. 47-12).

Renal Tumors. Prenatal diagnosis of Wilms's tumor and neuroblastoma can be made from an alteration of normal intrarenal or perirenal anatomy.

Hydrocele. Hydrocele can be seen either as an incidental finding or in association with fetal ascites.

Gastrointestinal System

Normal fetal stomach and bowel can be recognized prenatally, becoming more prominent as pregnancy advances. Real-time examination may show evidence of peristalsis in the visualized bowel. Several GI anomalies can be visualized prenatally.

Duodenal Atresia. Duodenal atresia can be seen as two large cystic masses in the upper abdomen, the sonographic equivalent of the radiological *double-bubble sign.* There is almost invariably maternal polyhydramnios (Fig. 47-13).

Mesenteric Cysts. Mesenteric cysts are recognized as an intra-abdominal cystic mass. There may be polyhydramnios.

Diaphragmatic Hernia. Herniation of bowel into the chest will be recognized by the presence of cystic masses within the fetal thorax. Usually there is associated polyhydramnios.

Skeletal System

Traditionally, skeletal anomalies have been investigated prenatally with radiography; ultrasound now offers an accurate, noninvasive method of visualization of skeletal anatomy. Long bones may be visualized (Fig. 47-14) and measured and compared with available standards.

Dwarfism. By measurement of long bones, various forms of dwarfism, including achondroplastic and thanatophoric, can be diagnosed prenatally.

Osteogenesis Imperfecta. The autosomal recessive type of the condition osteogenesis imperfecta congenita can be recognized prenatally by deformity of long bones and visualization of fractures (Fig. 47-15).

Keynotes

- *Obstetric ultrasound plays an increasing role in the diagnosis of fetal anomalies.*
- *Ultrasound can diagnose anencephaly, hydrocephalus, encephalocele, and hydranencephaly in utero.*
- *Neural tube defects can usually, but not always, be detected by ultrasonic examination.*
- *The normal spine is visualized sonographically as two parallel rows of echos. In spina bifida there is usually local widening of these parallel echos; there may be an associated mass adjacent to the defect.*
- *Both M-mode and two-dimensional real-time studies can evaluate the fetal heart for structural defects and rhythm disorders.*

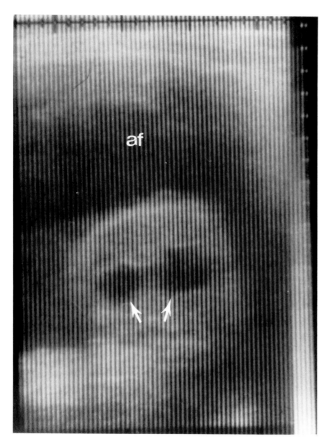

Figure 47-13. Transverse section of the fetal trunk in duodenal atresia. The dilated stomach and proximal duodenum are seen as two cystic collections of fluid (arrows). There is an excess of amniotic fluid (af).

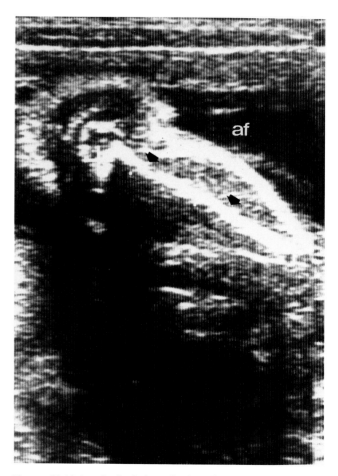

Figure 47-14 Longitudinal view of a fetal femur (arrows) showing the shaft and the femoral neck.

- *Fetal ultrasound can diagnose hydronephrosis, renal cystic disease, renal agenesis, and renal tumors.*
- *Fetal ultrasound can diagnose duodenal atresia, mesenteric cysts, and diaphragmatic hernias.*
- *Fetal ultrasound can diagnose certain types of dwarfism and some cases of osteogenesis imperfecta.*

ADNEXAL AND UTERINE MASSES IN ASSOCIATION WITH PREGNANCY

When, on physical examination, a mass is detected in association with pregnancy, ultrasound is of value in characterizing the lesion as cystic, solid, or complex and also in determining from which organ the mass arises. Most commonly an adnexal mass found in association with pregnancy is a corpus luteum cyst (Fig. 46-6). Sonographically, such cysts appear as simple, well-defined cystic masses. Occasionally they may contain internal echos because of bleeding into their centers. Corpus luteum cysts, being HCG dependent, usually have regressed markedly or disappeared by the early second trimester and, therefore, require no intervention. When an adnexal mass is shown to

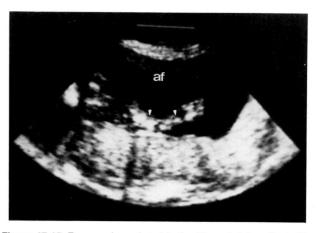

Figure 47-15 Forearm (arrowheads) of a 17-week fetus affected in utero by osteogenesis imperfecta. There is bowing of the limb and irregularity of the visualized bone, secondary to in utero fractures. af = Amniotic fluid.

have a complex internal structure or persists after mid-pregnancy, it is unlikely to be a corpus luteum cyst and will usually require surgical removal.

GUIDED AMNIOCENTESIS

Amniocentesis is the aspiration of a sample of amniotic fluid using a transabdominal approach. Before the widespread application of ultrasound, this procedure was done as a blind procedure, usually through a lower midline approach. Amniocentesis can be performed in the midtrimester for prenatal diagnosis because amniotic fluid contains a number of fetal cells that can be harvested and cultured. Biochemical analysis can be performed on the amniotic fluid or on the cultured cells. In this way, midtrimester amniocentesis is used to

1. Determine fetal chromosomal anomalies, for example, Down's syndrome, by karyotyping cultured cells
2. Determine certain autosomal recessive conditions characterized by biochemical abnormalities determinable in fetal cells or amniotic fluid
3. Diagnose NTD and certain other fetal anomalies by detection of a raised AFP level in amniotic fluid

Ultrasound is an invaluable adjunct in midtrimester amniocentesis, allowing

1. Accurate dating of the pregnancy, allowing choice of an optimal time for the procedure (16–18 weeks), and allowing correct interpretation of AFP levels, which change markedly with gestational age
2. Diagnosis of multiple pregnancy, each amniotic sac may need to be separately tapped
3. Localization of the placenta, given that avoidance of the placenta increases the chances of a successful aspiration and reduces the risk of fetomaternal transfusion
4. Diagnosis of fetal anomalies or fetal demise
5. Fetal localization, reducing the risks of fetal injury

Routine use of ultrasound for guiding amniocentesis will thus reduce the risks of the procedure and increase the chances of a successful procedure.

In late third trimester, amniocentesis may be required to determine

1. Fetal lung maturity, by measurement of the lecithin sphingomyelin (L/S) ratio. A mature L/S ratio is associated with a minimal risk of respiratory distress syndrome after birth.
2. The degree to which a fetus is affected by isoimmunization, by measurement of the amniotic fluid bilirubin level.
3. Presence of amnionitis, by presence of white cells and bacteria.

Again, ultrasound-guided aspiration increases the chance of a successful aspiration and minimizes the risk of fetal injury.

Keynotes

- *Amniocentesis is the aspiration of a sample of amniotic fluid. Ultrasound aids in this procedure.*
- *The amniocentesis specimen is used in the analysis of amniotic fluid chemistry and fetal cells for*
    - a. *The determination of fetal chromosomal abnormalities*
    - b. *Certain fetal biochemical abnormalities*
    - c. *Neural tube defects and certain other fetal anomalies that raise the AFP level*
- *In the late third trimester, amniocentesis can be used to determine*
    - a. *Fetal lung maturity based on the L/S ratio*
    - b. *Isoimmunization*
    - c. *Amnionitis*

INTRAUTERINE GROWTH RETARDATION

An infant who is growth retarded is one who has a birthweight less than the tenth percentile for its gestational age. Two patterns of IUGR are recognized sonographically:

1. Early-onset, or low-profile, IUGR, in which the fetus grows at a lower than expected rate from early in pregnancy. This type of IUGR is associated with a higher incidence of fetal anomalies.
2. Late-onset, or asymmetric, IUGR, in which fetal growth is normal until 28–30 weeks of gestation and then slows. This type of IUGR is most often secondary to relative placental insufficiency as in toxemia or diabetes.

Ultrasound at present offers the only noninvasive method of evaluating fetal growth. There are several screening methods for detecting IUGR:

Total intrauterine volume (TIUV). Measurement of the TIUV represents the volume of the fetus, placenta, and amniotic fluid. Intrauterine growth retardation is usually associated with decreased production of amniotic fluid and thus a decreased TIUV.

Estimated fetal weight. Several techniques have been used to estimate fetal weight. The one most widely used at present involves measuring the abdominal circumference of the fetus (Fig. 47-16) at the level of the umbilical vein, together with the BPD. Intrauterine growth retardation should obviously be associated with a lower than expected fetal weight for gestational age.

Head/abdomen ratio. In asymmetric IUGR there is usually sparing of brain growth unless the process is prolonged and severe. Comparison of the measure-

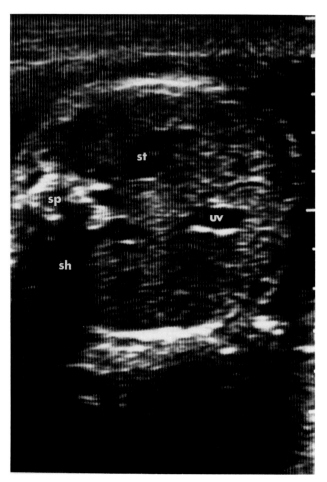

Figure 47-16. Transverse section of the fetal trunk at the level used for measurement of the trunk circumference. The spine (sp) and distal shadowing (sh) are seen, as are the stomach (st) and umbilical vein (uv).

ment of brain growth (the head circumference) with a measure of abdominal size (the trunk circumference) can therefore aid in diagnosing IUGR.

After the initial diagnosis of IUGR, ultrasound can be used in the assessment of fetal well-being by measurement of certain physiological parameters, as in the Fetal Biophysical Profile discussed below.

Keynotes

- *Intrauterine growth retardation (IUGR) is defined as having occurred when an infant has a birthweight less than the 10th percentile for its gestational age.*
- *Early onset IUGR is associated with a higher incidence of fetal anomalies and can be associated with intrauterine viral infections.*
- *Late onset IUGR is most often secondary to placental insufficiency and can be associated with toxemia or diabetes.*

BLEEDING IN PREGNANCY

Approximately 25% of women experience vaginal bleeding at some stage of pregnancy. Most often this bleeding is minor and has no adverse effects on the mother or fetus. Occasionally this bleeding is profuse and associated with considerable maternal and fetal morbidity. The principal causes of vaginal bleeding differ at different stages of the pregnancy.

First-Trimester Bleeding

In the first trimester, vaginal bleeding in a patient thought to be pregnant and who on examination is shown to have a closed cervix is termed a *threatened abortion*. Ultrasound plays a major role in the diagnosis of these patients, for with it the patient can rapidly be categorized as having a viable intrauterine pregnancy or not. A viable intrauterine pregnancy is demonstrated by a gestational sac appropriate to the expected menstrual based fetal age and containing a fetal pole where appropriate, this fetal pole demonstrating evidence of cardiac activity. Patients who have a demonstrated viable intrauterine pregnancy have a significant chance of continuing with the pregnancy, although they may have recurrent bleeding later in pregnancy.

When no viable intrauterine pregancy is demonstrated, the following are possibilities:

1. The patient is not in fact pregnant; an empty uterus and normal endometrial cavity are seen.
2. The patient has a *blighted ovum*. The blighted ovum, or anembryonic pregnancy, is characterized by abnormal development and then resorption of the embryo. The gestational sac that is visualized sonographically may be inappropriately small for the probable dates, have an irregular trophoblastic shell, and contain no fetal pole (Fig. 47-17). Because trophoblast is present and producing HCG, the urinary pregnancy

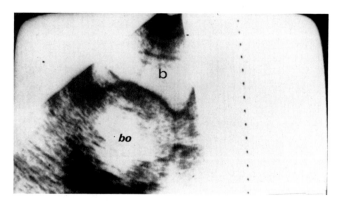

Figure 47-17. Transverse section of the uterus in a patient with first-trimester bleeding. There is a large, irregular fluid-filled structure in the uterus, without a fetal pole and compatible with a blighted ovum (bo). b = Bladder.

test may still suggest pregnancy. Such patients most often will subsequently abort spontaneously. When there is convincing evidence of a blighted ovum, the clinician may intervene and perform a curettage.

3. In the *missed abortion,* where death of the embryo or fetus has occurred several weeks previously, two main sonographic appearances are possible: either a nonmotile fetus without cardiac activity can be recognized, or the uterus, smaller than expected, will contain a nonhomogeneous collection of echos in its center (Fig. 47-18).

4. The patient has an ectopic pregnancy.

Late-Pregnancy Bleeding

Where significant bleeding occurs later in pregnancy, major causes are placenta previa and placental abruption. Bleeding may also occur secondary to local causes in the vagina and cervix. Ultrasound accurately demonstrates placental anatomy and location, making it invaluable for preliminary investigation in late pregnancy bleeding.

Placenta Previa. In placenta previa some portion of the placenta is in contact with the internal cervical os. This situation predisposes the patient to placental separation with resulting vaginal bleeding, especially when the cervix begins to dilate, shearing the placenta. Placenta previa is manifested clinically as recurrent vaginal bleeding usually unassociated with abdominal pain. The vaginal bleeding tends to become more profuse with each episode. Because the lower uterine segment is occupied by placenta, the fetus

is more likely to take an oblique or transverse lie. Where there is total previa at the onset of labor, vaginal delivery cannot be accomplished and a cesarean section should be performed.

Sonography has an important role in the diagnosis of placenta previa because both the placenta and the internal os may be visualized and their relationship evaluated (Fig. 47-19). An important concept established by ultrasound is that of *placental migration.* Serial sonograms during pregnancy show that the position of the placenta relative to the internal os changes as pregnancy advances because of the development of the lower uterine segment. Because of this phenomenon placenta previa is relatively common at 20 weeks but quite uncommon at term. For this reason, when placenta previa is diagnosed sonographically before term, the patient should have a repeat sonogram before any decision is made on the route of delivery.

Placental Abruption. Placental abruption is the separation of a portion of the placenta from the uterine wall before delivery. This results in bleeding in the retroplacental area; the blood may be passed vaginally—a revealed hemorrhage—or remain in a retroplacental location—a concealed hemorrhage. Placental abruption is more common in patients with preeclampsia or vascular diabetes and in older patients, and it is usually associated with abdominal pain and uterine tenderness. Because the bleeding may be mainly in a retroplacental location, the clinical findings may be out of proportion to observed blood loss. Severe placental abruption may be associated with disseminated intravascular coagulation.

While ultrasound has a major role in the diagnosis of placenta previa, the role in placental abruption is more limited because in the majority of cases examined, the sonographic findings are normal even when there has

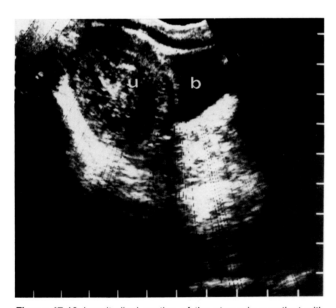

Figure 47-18 Longitudinal section of the uterus in a patient with first-trimester bleeding. The uterus (u), while enlarged, was smaller than expected for the duration of amenorrhea. It contains an inhomogeneous collection of echos compatible with a missed abortion. b = Bladder.

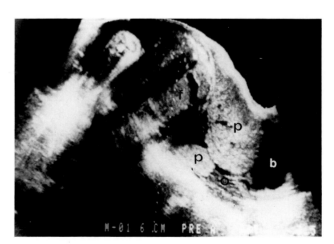

Figure 47-19. Longitudinal section of the uterus in the third trimester. In this case of placenta previa, the lower edge of the placenta (p) overlaps the area of the internal os (o). The lower limbs of the fetus are also shown (f). b = Bladder.

been major placental separation. Less commonly one may visualize a retroplacental collection of blood or separation of the placenta from the wall. In the patient with late-pregnancy bleeding, the major role of ultrasound is, therefore, to diagnose or exclude placenta previa. When placenta previa and local causes of vaginal bleeding have been excluded, the majority of patients will have placental abruption, even though the sonographic appearances are normal.

Keynotes

- *In first trimester uterine bleeding, ultrasound is used to demonstrate whether or not a viable intrauterine pregnancy is present.*
- *When no viable intrauterine pregnancy is present, the patient may*
  a. *Not be pregnant*
  b. *Have a blighted ovum*
  c. *Have a missed abortion*
  d. *Have an ectopic pregnancy*
- *Late-pregnancy bleeding may be due to placenta previa, placental abruption, or local causes in the vagina or cervix.*
- *In placenta previa, some portion of the placenta is in contact with the internal cervical os. The placenta can separate from the placental wall, resulting in vaginal bleeding.*
- *Sonography can demonstrate the relationship of the placenta to the internal cervical os.*
- *During pregnancy, serial sonograms will demonstrate placental migration away from the internal cervical os as the lower uterine segment grows.*
- *The patient with sonographically demonstrated placenta previa earlier in pregnancy should have a repeat sonogram before any decision is made about the route of delivery.*
- *Placental abruption is the separation of a portion of the placenta from the uterine wall before delivery.*
- *In most patients with placental abruption, the sonogram will not demonstrate any placental abnormality; thus the role of sonography in late-pregnancy bleeding is primarily to diagnose or exclude placenta previa.*

FETAL DEATH

The assessment of fetal viability in early pregnancy has already been described. In later pregnancy fetal death in utero (FDIU) may be suspected because of lack of fetal motion reported by the patient or because of inability to hear fetal heart tones. With real-time equipment, the question of possible FDIU may be rapidly and reliably assessed by visualization of the fetal heart and demonstration of cardiac activity. When fetal death has been present for several days, secondary changes may be produced that can be visualized with real-time or static scanners:

1. Overlapping of skull bones (Fig. 47-20), the sonographic equivalent of the radiographic Spalding's sign. Overlapping may occur from skull compression in labor, so this must be ruled out.

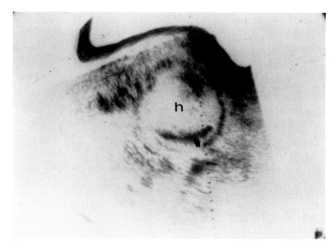

Figure 47-20. Transverse section of a fetal head (h) showing skull bone overlapping (arrow) secondary to fetal death in utero.

2. Scalp edema (similar to the radiographic Duell's sign), shown by a thickening of the normally barely perceptible scalp shadow around the cranial bones.
3. Abnormal fetal lie. After death often bizarre fetal lies are produced.
4. Intravascular gas formation, demonstrated sonographically by foci of shadowing originating within the fetus.

Keynote

- *Fetal ultrasound can be used to confirm suspected fetal death in utero.*

FETAL PHYSIOLOGICAL STATUS

The advent of high-resolution real-time sonographic equipment has opened a new realm of fetal evaluation, the emphasis shifting from visualization of fetal structural anatomy to evaluation of fetal movement and certain physiological functions. It has been shown that fetal well-being is associated with the ability to demonstrate certain functions such as fetal movement, normal fetal tone, and fetal breathing. Conversely, inability to demonstrate such functions is associated with a high incidence of fetal compromise. These functions have been quantitated and combined to form a prenatal planning score, the Fetal Biophysical Profile, which is analogous to the postnatal Apgar score and which has a similar 0–10 point scale, with 0 indicating fetal compromise and 10 fetal well-being. The score measures four sonographically evaluated parameters: fetal movement, fetal tone, fetal breathing, and the amount of amniotic fluid (oligohydramios being associated with fetal compromise). A fifth measurement, fetal cardiac reactivity, is measured with the conventional nonstress test with an external Doppler monitor. The application of real-time ultrasound to fetal physiological assessment is relatively new and undoubtedly will continue to be refined and expanded to include such measurements as fetal cardiac output, end-diastolic volume, quantitation of type of breathing, and visualization of certain neurological reflexes.

Keynote

• *The Fetal Biophysical Profile can be used to assess fetal wellbeing. It is analogous to the postnatal Apgar score and gives a rating from 0 through 10 based on fetal breathing, tone, movement, the amount of amniotic fluid, and the reactivity of the heart.*

COEXISTENT IUD

The IUD continues to be a popular form of contraception because of its minimal side effects. Intrauterine devices are, however, associated with a 2–3% failure rate, depending on type. One of the reasons for inability to visualize an IUD string is retraction of the device into the uterus enlarged by pregnancy. When an IUD and a pregnancy coexist, the spontaneous abortion rate may be as high as 50%; but when an IUD can be safely removed, the spontaneous abortion rate is considerably reduced. Sonographic examination allows visualization of the presence of the device and its relation to the gestational sac (Fig. 46-15). It is not very likely that an IUD situated on the side of the gestational sac adjacent to the fundus can be removed without disrupting the pregnancy, but a device located adjacent to the cervix may usually be retrieved safely. In later pregnancy an IUD, even one known to be intrauterine, may be very difficult or impossible to demonstrate sonographically.

POSTPARTUM PROBLEMS

The postpartum patient, especially after an operative delivery, is subject to two major complications, postpartum fever and postpartum hematocrit-level drop.

Postpartum Fever

After a vaginal delivery or an operative delivery, when postpartum fever occurs, it usually results from endometritis, which usually has the clinical manifestations of fever, uterine tenderness, and foul-smelling lochia and responds promptly to antibiotic therapy. Such patients therefore do not usually require sonographic evaluation. The patient who has had a cesarean section is also prone to develop a hematoma that may become infected and form an abscess. There are several common sites for abscess formation. Abdominal wound abscesses are most commonly subfascial after a Pfannenstiel's (transverse) incision and subcutaneous after a midline longitudinal incision. Abscess formation may also be related to the uterine incision. Clinically, abscess formation is characterized by

a typical spiking fever and suboptimal response to antibiotics. In this clinical situation sonography is indicated to detect an abscess collection, which may then be drained either with a needle under ultrasound guidance or with surgery or else its response to intensive antibiotic therapy may be followed.

Postpartum Drop in Hematocrit Level

After a vaginal delivery, a drop in hematocrit level is usually accounted for by the observed external blood loss. After operative delivery, however, hematoma formation related to an abdominal wound or uterine incision may cause a hematocrit-level drop out of proportion to that measured externally. Sonography again is of value in detecting hematoma formation and in estimating the amount of blood involved.

Keynotes

• *Ultrasonic examination can be useful in evaluating a suspected postpartum abscess, both for diagnosis and for guiding the placement of percutaneous drainage catheters.*

• *Hematoma following operative delivery can be detected by ultrasonic examination.*

TROPHOBLASTIC DISEASE

Trophoblastic disease is a spectrum of disease ranging from the benign hydatidiform mole through the locally invasive chorioadenoma destruens to the malignant choriocarcinoma. Hydatidiform mole is thought to arise from an abnormal gestation and consists of marked trophoblastic proliferation with hydropic distension of chorionic vesicles. The uterus becomes filled with masses of grapelike vesicles of varying size (Fig. 47-21). There is significant production of HCG, resulting in ovarian hyperstimulation and formation of multiple, bilateral theca-lutein cysts. Clinically patients experience bleeding in the second trimester and have a uterus that is usually larger than expected for the duration of amenorrhea. Occasionally the patient may have the signs and symptoms of severe preeclampsia. In approximately 50% of patients with bilateral adnexal masses, the theca-lutein cysts can be palpated. Sonographically the appearances of hydatidiform mole are characteristic, with enlargement of the uterus containing numerous echos and often visible cystic areas. Bilateral theca-lutein cysts are seen in 50% of cases.

Treatment of hydatidiform mole is by uterine evacuation, usually producing a cure. Occasionally there is persistence of the disease and degeneration to form a choriocarcinoma. Choriocarcinoma may also follow a spontaneous abortion or a normal pregnancy. Metastases, most commonly to the lung or brain, are often responsible for the presenting symptoms. Sonographically, the choriocarcinoma, which does not have hydropic vesicles, has a different appearance, usually as a nonhomogen-

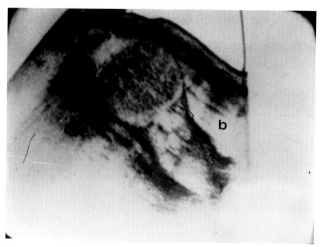

Figure 47-21. Longitudinal section of the pelvis showing a uterus (u) that is enlarged and has a collection of homogeneous echos compatible with a hydatidiform mole. In the cul-de-sac area are seen a number of theca-lutein cysts (arrows). b = Bladder.

eous collection of echos in the endometrial cavity and myometrium.

Keynotes

- *Trophoblastic disease ranges from the benign hydatidiform mole through the locally invasive chorioadenoma destruens to the malignant choriocarcinoma. Ultrasonic examination can detect and differentiate these conditions.*
- *Hydatidiform mole consists of marked trophoblastic proliferation with hydropic distention of chorionic vesicles. It usually appears clinically either with midpregnancy bleeding or with signs of severe preeclampsia.*

SUMMARY

Ultrasonic examination has an important and expanding role in the care of the pregnant patient and fetus. In appropriate clinical settings, it can be used to aid in infertility management, the early diagnosis of pregnancy, and the detection of fetal anomalies; to guide amniocentesis for the detection of fetal biochemical and chromosomal abnormalities; and for the assessment of fetal growth, fetal maturity, and fetal well-being.

The ultrasonic examination can be used in assessing the complications of pregnancy. When first-trimester bleeding is present, an assessment can be made of whether a viable fetus is present in the uterus. When late-trimester bleeding is present, placenta previa may be directly diagnosed and the presence of placental abruption can be inferred. In the patient with oligohydramnios or polyhydramnios, ultrasonic examination can be used to look for fetal anomalies and multiple pregnancies. When there is a discrepancy between fetal size and expected size for duration of pregnancy, ultrasonic examination can be used to better assess the gestational age and fetal viability and to measure possible IUGR.

Postpartum abscesses can be detected by ultrasonic examination and can be drained under ultrasonic guidance. Postpartum hematomas can be detected. Trophoblastic disease can be diagnosed.

REVIEW QUESTIONS

1. What are the ultrasonic signs of an early intrauterine pregnancy?
2. What are the methods for estimating gestational age? At what age is each method of greatest utility?
3. What are the clinical findings suggestive of multiple pregnancy and the sonographic signs confirming it? What is the clinical outcome of multiple pregnancy diagnosed sonographically in the first trimester?
4. Anomalies of which organ systems can be diagnosed sonographically?
5. Which anomalies of the central nervous system can be diagnosed by ultrasonic examination?
6. Which renal anomalies can be detected by ultrasonic examination?
7. What is amniocentesis? What are its applications in the first half of pregnancy? What are its applications late in pregnancy?
8. What is IUGR? What are its two types? What is the clinical significance of each?
9. What is the key finding sought by the ultrasonic examination in the patient with first-trimester bleeding?
10. If no intrauterine pregnancy is found by ultrasonic examination in the patient with first-trimester bleeding, what diagnostic possibilities should be considered?
11. What are the causes of late-pregnancy vaginal bleeding? What diagnoses should be considered if the ultrasonic examination is normal?
12. What is the natural history of placenta previa diagnosed in midpregnancy?
13. What is the clinical management of placenta previa diagnosed in midpregnancy compared with that diagnosed during labor?
14. What are the clinical and sonographic findings in placental abruption?
15. What are the clinical and sonographic findings when fetal death in utero has occurred?
16. What is the Fetal Biophysical Profile and how is it used?
17. What is the application of the ultrasonic examination in the patient with a postpartum abscess or hematoma?
18. What are the types of trophoblastic disease? What is the clinical presentation and sonographic appearance of each form?

VOCABULARY

amniocentesis
amnionitis
anencephaly
Apgar score

hydrocephalus
hydronephrosis
intrauterine growth retardation

biparietal diameter
blighted ovum
chorioadenoma destruens
choriocarcinoma
corpus luteum cyst
crown–rump length
decidual proliferation
disseminated intravascular co-agulation
Down's syndrome
duodenal atresia
encephalocele
Fetal Biophysical Profile

karyotype
lecithin sphingomyelin ratio
meningomyelocele
missed abortion
monochorionic twins
multicystic kidney disease
neural tube defects
neuroblastoma
oligohydramnios
osteogenesis imperfecta
placental abruption
placental migration

fetal pole
α-fetoprotein
gestational sac
HCG
hydatidiform mole
hydranencephaly

placenta previa
polycystic kidney disease
preeclampsia
spina bifida
trophoblastic disease
Wilms's tumor

SUGGESTIONS FOR FURTHER READING

B. Felson, Ed. Obstetrical radiology. *Seminars in Roentgenology,* **17**(3), 1982.

For additional suggested reading see Chapter 46.

PART 4

THE URINARY TRACT

The next six chapters discuss the imaging of the urinary tract. Chapter 48 discusses the methods used for imaging the urinary tract, what they can demonstrate, and their main clinical applications.

Chapter 49 and Chapters 51 through 53 discuss major symptoms of renal disease and their evaluation. Chapter 50 discusses the problem of adverse reactions to contrast media. Chapter 54 discusses radiation hazards.

48

RENAL IMAGING

KEY CONCEPTS

Radiological

There are many imaging methods used in the evaluation of the kidneys. Each demonstrates renal anatomy and physiology to a differing degree. The major anatomic structures that can be evaluated include the perirenal spaces, the renal parenchyma, the papillae, the minor calyces, renal pelvis, ureters, and bladder. The major physiological phases of renal function include the large-vessel, small-vessel, tubular, and collecting-systems phases. The small-vessel phase is often called the *phase of total-body opacification*. The tubular phase is also called the *nephrogram*.

The main imaging methods are:

The intravenous urogram, which uses a radiopaque medicine that is excreted by the kidneys. This method gives excellent anatomic information about the kidney and good physiological information. It does not demonstrate the perirenal spaces well. It is used mainly in the evaluation of renal or ureteral colic, unexplained hematuria, and unexplained flank pain.

The retrograde pyelogram, in which a radiopaque contrast medium is passed through a catheter into the urinary system. This method gives excellent demonstration of the ureteral anatomy and can be used to obtain cultures and cytological material from the collecting system.

The renal sonogram, which gives good information about the anatomy of the retroperitoneal spaces and kidney and is of use in evaluating whether a renal mass is a cyst and in detecting hydronephrosis.

The nuclear medicine ^{99m}Tc 2,3-dimercaptosuccinic acid (DMSA) scan, which demonstrates the location of functioning renal tubules and is of use in evaluating whether an apparent mass of the kidney is a normal variant, hypertrophy of otherwise normal renal parenchyma, or some other kind of mass.

The nuclear medicine excretion study, which is used to measure certain aspects of renal physiological function in evaluating relative function of the right and left kidneys and drainage of the renal collecting systems.

The nuclear medicine renal clearance study, which can estimate the glomerular filtration rate and is used in comparing the function of the right and left kidneys.

The renal angiogram, in which the renal vessels are evaluated. This is used in the evaluation of suspected renal artery stenosis, unexplained hematuria after normal intravenous urography and CT, and in the preoperative evaluation of renal cancer.

The transmission computed tomography study, which gives excellent anatomic information about the perirenal spaces, retroperitoneum, and renal parenchyma, with much less information about the papillary and calyceal anatomy and renal physiology. It is used mainly in the staging of known renal cancer, in evaluating renal masses when the findings of sonography are uncertain, and in defining processes in the retroperitoneal and perirenal spaces.

OBJECTIVES

When you complete this chapter you will be able to

1. Identify the kidneys on selected urograms, sonograms, and nuclear medicine and CT examinations.
2. Use the summary from this chapter to select appropriate imaging examinations for the patient with renal colic, hematuria, a suspected renal mass, acute renal failure, suspected renovascular hypertension, or suspected perinephric abscess and to explain your choice.

3. Describe the differences among the three nuclear medicine techniques and list their different applications.

There are multiple methods of imaging the kidney. Each method differs in the type and proportions of anatomic and physiological information provided. Selection among these techniques requires initially a clinical differential diagnoses, a knowledge of the type of anatomic and physiological abnormality expected, and a knowledge of what each of these methods can demonstrate.

Anatomically, diseases of the kidney and retroperitoneum can be demonstrated by several of these techniques. Some of the types of anatomic abnormalities that can be caused by renal disease are fluid collections around the kidney; masses next to, attached to, or within the kidney; distortion of the shape or location of calyces; abnormalities of the papillae or mucosal surfaces; and filling defects within the kidney.

NORMAL RENAL ANATOMY

The evaluation of renal anatomy consists of nine steps:

1. Is the kidney in a normal place within the body? The normal position is with the hilum centered at the level of the first or second lumbar vertebra. The kidney should be aligned vertically or with its lower pole slightly lateral to the upper pole.

2. Is the kidney of normal size? The normal length of the kidney is equivalant to approximately three and one-half vertebral body heights, or 12–14 cm. Its length decreases with increasing age.

3. Are the perinephric tissues normal? The kidney is normally surrounded by fat.

4. Are the calyces in a normal position within the kidney? The top-to-bottom alignment of the calyces should be similar to the top-to-bottom alignment of the kidney.

5. Is the spacing between the calyces normal? The relationship of one calyx to another is variable; the displacement of calyces is best recognized by finding an area of the kidney that does not appear to be drained by a calyx.

6. Is the parenchyma of the kidney of normal thickness? The thickness of the parenchyma is symmetrical in the right and left kidneys. The poles of the kidney are slightly thicker than the midportion of the kidney.

7. Are the papillae of normal shape? The papillae are normally conical or hemispheric.

8. Are the calyces of normal shape? The calyces normally tightly envelop the papillae.

9. Is there anything other than urine in the collecting system? No filling defects (stones, tumors, blood clots, etc.) should be found within the renal collecting system.

NORMAL RENAL PHYSIOLOGY

The imaging techniques in which medication is given can detect physiological differences in the appearance time of the medicine reaching the kidney, filling the calyces, or draining from the renal pelvis. Differences in volume excreted or in the concentration ability of the kidneys can also be detected.

Radiologists classify the physiology of the excretion of imaging agents into four phases:

1. Major-artery filling
2. Small-vessel and capillary filling (the blood pool phase or the phase of total-body opacification)
3. Tubular localization (the nephrogram)
4. Collecting-system filling (calyceal and pyelographic phase)

Abnormalities seen in the physiological phases can aid in explaining both diffuse and focal abnormalities of the kidneys. As each of the imaging techniques is discussed below, pay attention to the types of anatomic and physiological information that can be obtained.

Keynote

• *All imaging studies provide some anatomic and some physiological information. In many cases, the anatomic changes in several diseases may overlap, and it is only because of their differing physiological changes that they can be differentiated.*

METHODS OF RENAL IMAGING

The methods of renal imaging are

Radiographic methods
  Intravenous urography
  Retrograde pyelography
Sonography
Nuclear medicine imaging
  Using a tubular cell–avid compound [^{99m}Tc 2,3-dimercaptosuccinic acid (DMSA)], chlormerodrin Hg 197)
  Using a glomerular filtration compound [^{99m}Tc diethylene triamine pentaacetic acid (DTPA)]
  Using total clearance agents (iodohippurate sodium I 131)
Angiography
  Arterial
  Venous
  Digital (computer-processed) angiography for anatomy and physiological measurements
Computer-assisted methods
  Transmission computed tomography
    Without contrast
    With contrast agent

Nuclear medicine physiological measurement
Time activity curves (using agents indicated above)
Magnetic resonance imaging

Keynote

- *A time activity curve is a graph demonstrating the change in the radioactivity recorded in a portion of the body over a period of time.*

Radiographic Methods

Intravenous Urogram

Technique

A plain film of the abdomen is taken (Fig. 48-1a). A medicine, a radiographic contrast medium, is then injected. Initially, all portions of the body having blood supply light up; by 2 minutes much of the material is filtered into and concentrated in the renal tubules (Fig. 48-1b); by 4 minutes some is excreted into the calyces (Fig. 48-1c). Peristalsis then fills the renal pelvis, ureters, and bladder (Fig. 48-1d). Films are taken at intervals appropriate for evaluating the patient's symptoms or presumed clinical diagnosis.

Information Provided

Detailed anatomic information about
Thickness of parenchyma
Size of kidneys
Papillary shape (Fig. 48-2)
Calyceal shape (Figs. 48-3 and 48-4)
Renal calcifications (see Chapter 50)
Adequate physiological information about
Parenchymal opacification and appearance time
Very good physiological information about calyceal appearance time (Fig. 48-5) and contrast concentration

Advantages

Demonstrates papillary, calyceal, and renal pelvic anatomic details best of all studies

Disadvantages

Gives little information about perirenal space.
Only major physiological changes can be identified.
Low-frequency hazard of a severe contrast medium reaction

Main Uses

Evaluating
Unexplained hematuria
Urinary calculus disease
Unexplained flank pain

Debatable Uses

Preoperative evaluation in
Prostate surgery
Uterine or ovarian surgery
Rectosigmoid colon surgery
Suspected renovascular hypertension (because computer-assisted angiography is now the probable procedure of choice)
Frequently misused in evaluating
Uncomplicated acute pyelonephritis
Renal failure

Retrograde Pyelogram

Technique

A urologist (or less often a gynecologist) passes a cystoscope through the urethra into the bladder. A plain film of the abdomen is taken. The urologist then places a catheter into one or both ureters. Air or a radiopaque contrast medium is injected via the catheter to fill the region of interest. Films are then taken. Two types of catheter techniques can be used:

1. A catheter with a bulbous tip is placed at the entrance of the ureter into the bladder, occluding it; contrast media is then introduced into the ureter and renal pelvis by retrograde injection.
2. A straight-tipped catheter is passed via the ureter to the site of interest. Air or a contrast medium is then injected, outlining the region of interest.

Cells for cytological evaluation can be collected during this examination.

Information Provided

Air-retrograde method
Whether calcification is within the collecting system or within the parenchyma (Fig. 48-6)
Contrast medium retrograde method
Gives best demonstration of ureteral mucosa
Can demonstrate calyceal and renal pelvis mucosa and lumen when intravenous urography does not solve the problem (Fig. 48-7)

Main Uses

Evaluating
Atypical pericalyceal calcifications
A nonfunctioning kidney
Suspected ureteral stone disease not confirmed or equivocally confirmed on intravenous urography (IVU)
Suspected ureteral abnormality, not adequately delineated by IVU

Main Misuses

Frequently as compensation for improper IVU technique

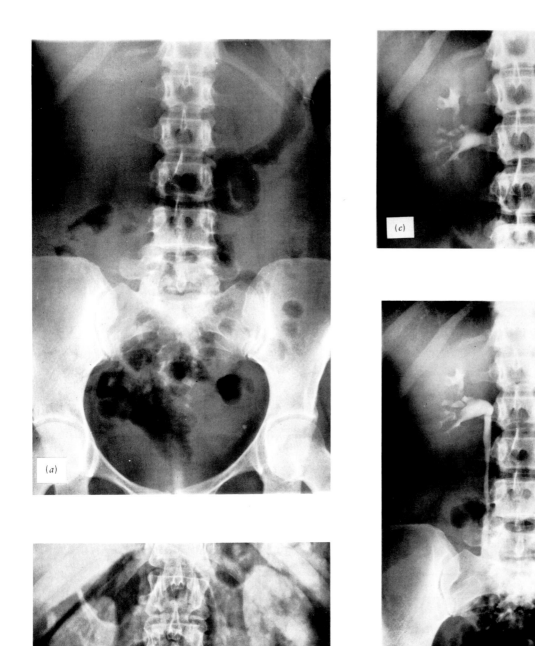

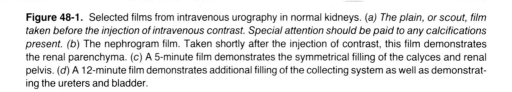

Figure 48-1. Selected films from intravenous urography in normal kidneys. (*a*) *The plain, or scout, film taken before the injection of intravenous contrast. Special attention should be paid to any calcifications present.* (*b*) The nephrogram film. Taken shortly after the injection of contrast, this film demonstrates the renal parenchyma. (*c*) A 5-minute film demonstrates the symmetrical filling of the calyces and renal pelvis. (*d*) A 12-minute film demonstrates additional filling of the collecting system as well as demonstrating the ureters and bladder.

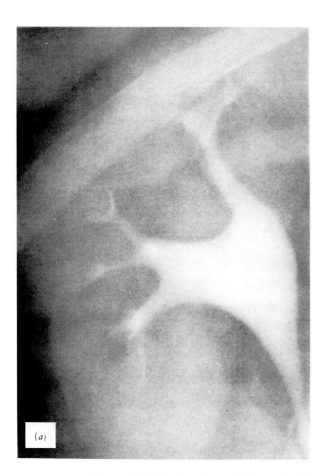
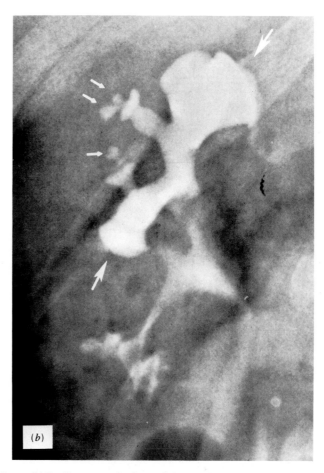

Figure 48-2. Papillary shape. (*a*) Normal papillary shape. (*b*) Papillary necrosis. Several abnormalities of papillary shape are present: There are small pockets of contrast present in the papillae (small arrows). There are two calyces that are clubbed (i.e., rounded with no evidence of papillary impression) (large arrows). These clubbed calyces are the result of the entire papilla becoming necrotic, breaking free of the renal parenchyma, and passing down the ureter. This patient had sickle hemoglobin trait.

Keynotes

- *The delay in calyceal filling caused by either decreased arterial pressure or increased intraparenchymal or collecting-system pressure is the most commonly encountered physiological change resulting from renal diseases shown on imaging studies.*
- *Hematuria is blood in the urine, a common and important sign of renal disease. Commonly seen with urinary stone disease and glomerulonephritis, it can also be an early sign of urinary cancer and tuberculosis.*
- *Renovascular hypertension is high blood pressure resulting from partial obstruction of the renal arteries. This is an uncommon but curable cause of hypertension. The best method for screening for renovascular hypertension is under debate. Of the current proposed methods, those preferred are renal arteriography, computer-assisted arteriography, and the use of an investigational renin-antagonist medicine, which is not yet approved for general use by the Food and Drug Administration.*
- *Pyelonephritis infection of the kidney.*
- *A cystoscope is an instrument that is passed through the urethra to look into the bladder.*

Sonography

Technique

Multiple sonographic images are made in both transverse and longitudinal planes through the kidney (Fig. 48-8).

Information Provided

Size of kidney

Dilation of collecting system (Fig. 48-9)

Sonic texture of renal parenchyma (abnormal in some forms of interstitial nephritis) (Fig. 48-10)

Advantages

Demonstrates perirenal retroperitoneal spaces

Differentiates most renal cysts from renal neoplasms (Fig. 48-11 and 48-12)

Main Uses

Differentiating solid and cystic renal masses

Evaluating acute renal failure to exclude obstruction

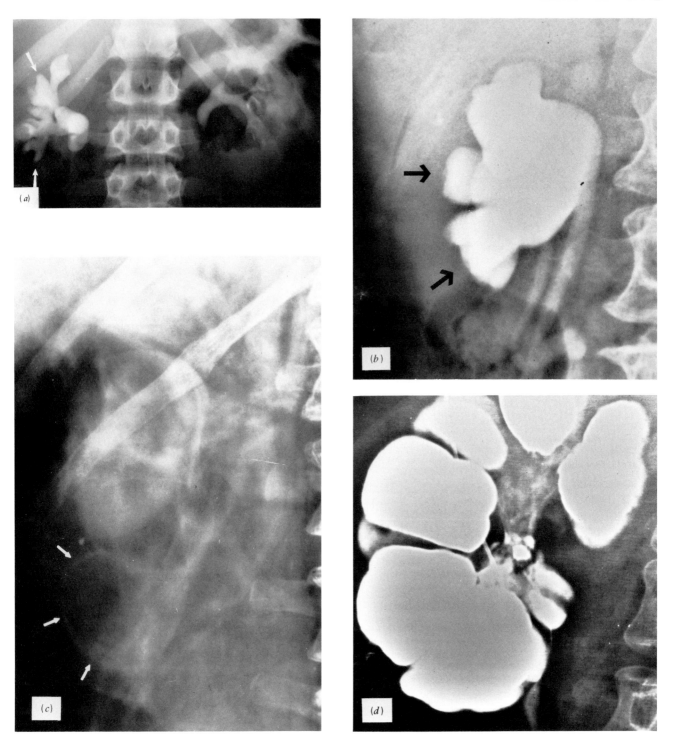

Figure 48-3 The calyceal dilation of hydronephrosis. (*a*) Calyceal dilation from prior pregnancy. The calyces of the right kidney demonstrate mild rounding of their margins (arrows). Mild dilation of the calyces is commonly seen after normal pregnancies. Obstruction of the urinary tract is not present. These films were obtained 5 minutes after the intravenous injection of contrast. If obstruction were present, the excretion into the collecting system would be delayed. (*b*) Moderate hydronephrosis caused by incomplete distal ureteral obstruction from cervical cancer. The margins of the calyces are even more rounded (arrows). This film was obtained 25 minutes after contrast injection. (*c*) Marked hydronephrosis secondary to idiopathic pelvo-ureteric junction obstruction. The calyces are markedly dilated, and only a thin rim of parenchyma (arrows) is visible around them on this intravenous urogram. This is the *rim sign* of hydronephrosis. (*d*) Antegrade pyelogram of the same kidney shown in *c*. A needle has been placed through the skin into the renal pelvis, and contrast medium has been injected, filling some of the markedly dilated calyces.

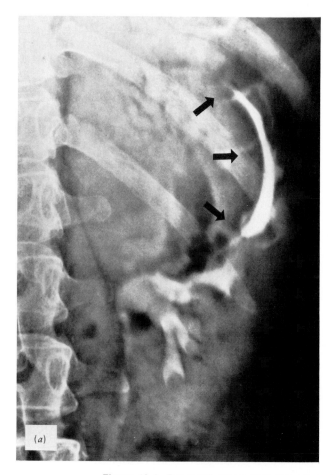 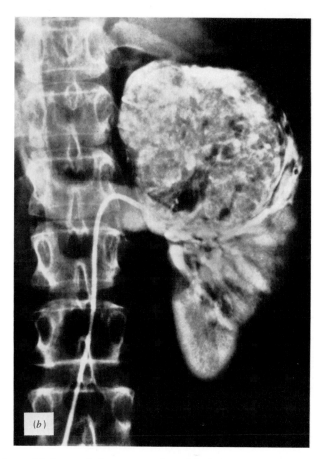

Figure 48-4. Renal cell cancer distorting calyceal shape. (*a*) A mass in the upper portion of the left kidney stretches and displaces the collecting system (arrows). (*b*) An angiogram demonstrates that the mass contains many abnormal vessels indicative of a probable renal cell cancer.

Differenting a cystic renal mass from a neoplastic one
Evaluating for
  Polycystic kidney disease
  Perinephric abscess
  Perinephric hematoma
  Urinoma
  Lymphocele

Main Misuses

As primary evaluation of hematuria
  Will not demonstrate most transitional cell tumors
  Will not show many stones
Dilation of collecting system sometimes misinterpreted
  as being the same as current obstruction; cannot differentiate current obstruction from past obstruction

Debatable Uses

Occasionally a kidney obstructed by retroperitoneal fibrosis will not have a dilated collecting system. An obstructed infected kidney may not have a dilated collecting system.

In these situations, a technique demonstrating the physiology of renal excretion should be used as well.

Keynotes

- *The most common renal mass is a renal cyst. Renal cysts usually require no treatment. The most feared renal mass is a renal cell cancer. Renal sonography can diagnose most renal cysts as being cysts, thus preventing the need for further evaluation or surgery.*

- *Patients with acute renal failure are placed into two groups: with and without urinary tract obstruction. In those with urinary tract obstruction, relief of the obstruction is usually curative. The easiest method of differentiating these two groups is by renal sonography.*

- *Polycystic kidney disease is an uncommon, autosomal, dominant inherited disease in which multiple cysts form in the kidney and liver, eventually resulting in renal failure in the midadult years.*

- *A urinoma is a collection of urine within the soft tissues.*

- *A lymphocele is a collection of lymph within the soft tissues. These are common around transplanted kidneys.*

- *Retroperitoneal fibrosis is fibrosis in the retroperitoneum, an uncommon cause of low back pain. Some cases are associated with methysergide medication.*

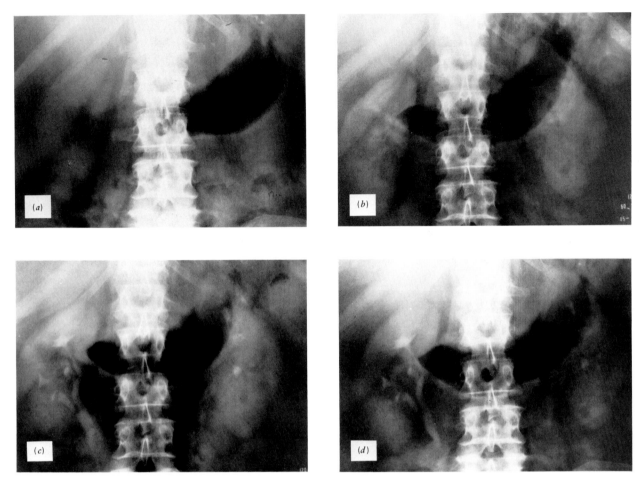

Figure 48-5. Delayed excretion with decreased concentration secondary to renal contusion. Delayed excretion is usually due to a ureteral stone, but any process that increases the pressure within the renal capsule will result in a delay in excretion. Renal injury with swelling is one such cause. (*a*) The scout film demonstrates the renal contours. (*b*) The 90-second film demonstrates the increased opacification caused by contrast in the renal tubules (the *nephrogram phase*). (*c*) The 4-minute film demonstrates early filling of the calyces. More filling is present in the right kidney, indicating a delay on the left side. (*d*) The 7-minute film demonstrates continued delay and incomplete filling of the left kidney and decreased concentration of the contrast on the left. This is the result of the renal contusion.

Nuclear Medicine Imaging

With Tubular Cell–Avid Compound

Technique

Images are obtained after injection of ^{99m}Tc DMSA.

Information Provided

Labeled material attaches to renal tubules, identifying the location of normal renal parenchyma (Fig. 48-13).

Main Uses

The main use for nuclear medicine imaging with ^{99m}Tc DMSA is in differentiating masses caused by excess normal or hypertrophied renal parenchyma from cysts and neoplasms. This problem occurs mainly with a common normal variant: the doubled Bertin's column, which lies

between the upper and middle calyceal groups. Usually, it is possible to differentiate Bertin's columns on the standard IVU, but in some cases, a ^{99m}Tc DMSA scan is needed. Hypertrophy of the renal parenchyma occurs when approximately one-third to one-half of the renal parenchyma is damaged so that it cannot grow normally (in children) or function normally. Sometimes the hypertrophy is mass-like, and ^{99m}Tc DMSA scans can be most helpful.

With a Glomerular Filtration Agent

Technique

A tracer, usually ^{99m}Tc DTPA, is injected intravenously. Serial rapid recordings are made to study the arrival time within the kidney (Fig. 48-14*a*), the rate of tubular passage (Fig. 48-14*b*) and calyceal filling (Fig. 48-14*c*), and the rate of calyceal emptying.

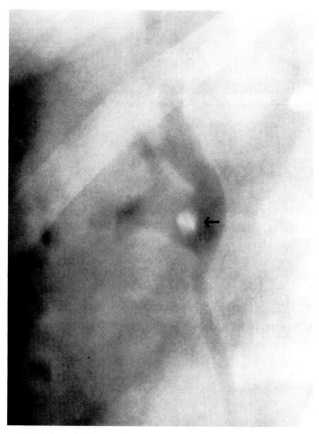

Figure 48-6. An air–retrograde pyelogram of the right kidney demonstrates a calcified stone (arrow) lying in the renal pelvis.

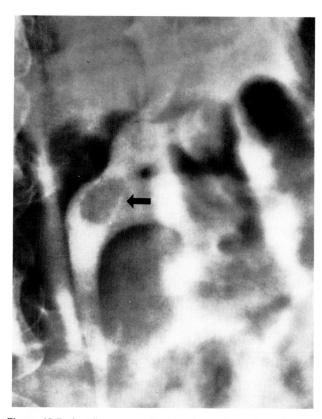

Figure 48-7. A radiopaque contrast medium retrograde pyelogram of the left kidney, obtained in evaluation of a filling defect (arrow) of the renal pelvis. The retrograde method permitted a brush biopsy of this lesion, which on cytological examination proved to be a small transitional cell carcinoma. This lesion had been seen on intravenous urography, but its nature was uncertain.

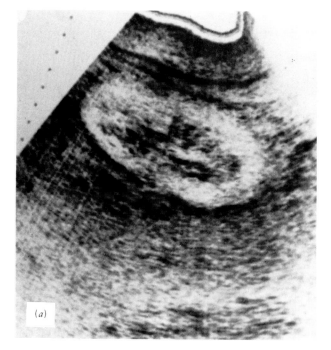

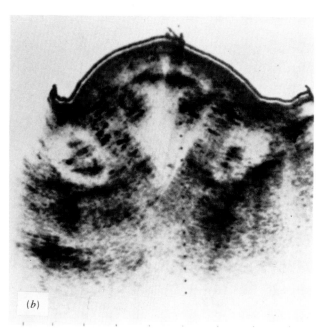

Figure 48-8. Renal sonograms. (*a*) Longitudinal view of a normal kidney. The ovoid, relatively sonolucent structure is the renal parenchyma. Contained within it is the echogenic renal sinus. (*b*) Transverse view of normal kidneys seen in cross section with their sonolucent parenchyma and echogenic sinuses. (Both courtesy R. Sanders, M.D.)

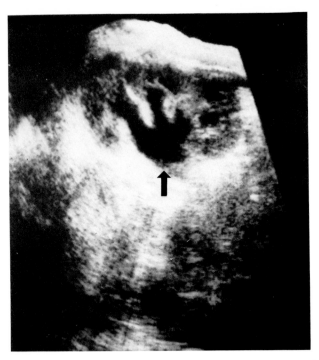

Figure 48-9. Sonogram of a hydronephrotic kidney, longitudinal view. Dilated calyces are seen entering the dilated renal pelvis (arrow). Compare this appearance with Figure 48-3b. Lesser degrees of hydronephrosis may show only a sonolucent structure within the renal sinus, representing the dilated renal pelvis. (Courtesy M. Dunne, M.D.)

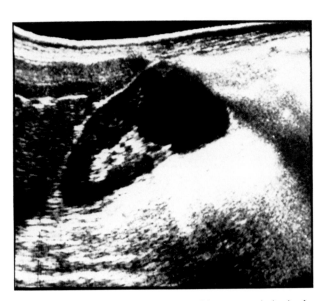

Figure 48-11. Sonogram of a renal cyst. A large, rounded echo-free mass is seen in the lower pole of the right kidney. In addition to the echo-free character of the mass, there is increased through transmission of sound so that posterior to the cyst there are more echos because of the lack of absorption of the sound waves in the homogeneous cyst. (Courtesy M. Dunne, M.D.)

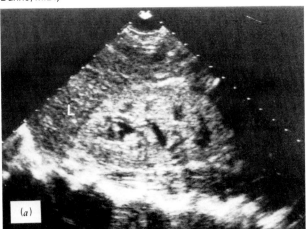

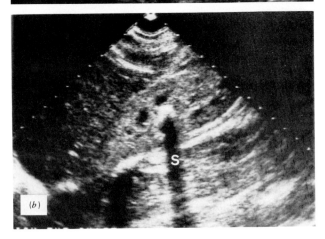

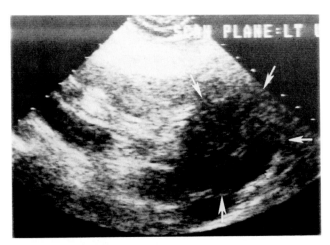

Figure 48-12. Sonogram of a renal cell cancer. There is an echogenic mass (arrows) in the mid and lower portion of the left kidney. The presence of internal echos indicates that this mass is solid and could be a renal cell cancer or abscess.

Figure 48-10. Sonogram of a kidney with arteriolar nephrosclerosis and renal calculus. (a) Longitudinal view demonstrates a very echogenic renal parenchyma, more echogenic than the liver (L). This is a sign of severe interstitial disease. (b) Another section through the same kidney demonstrates the intense echos and sonic shadowing (S) of a renal stone.

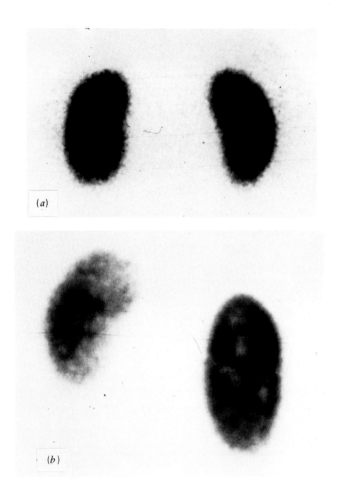

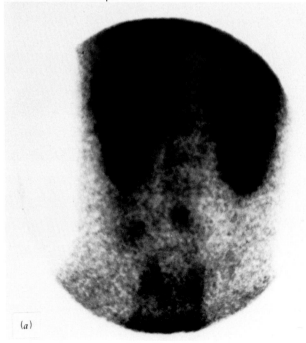

Figure 48-13. ^{99m}Tc DMSA renal scan of normal kidneys. (a) Uniform radioactivity in the renal parenchyma. (b) In this less intense image, differentiation between the renal cortex and medullary tissue is seen. This is an oblique view.

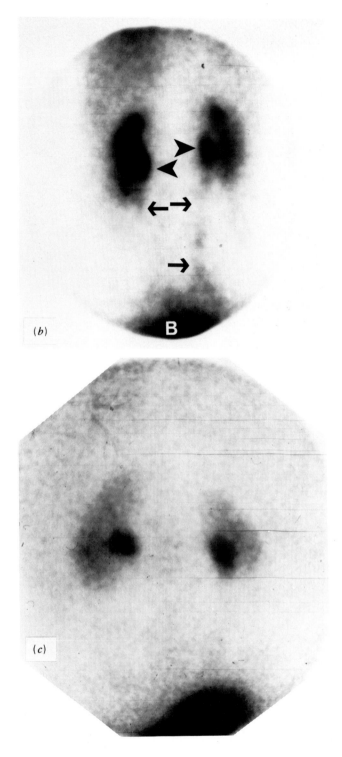

Figure 48-14. Selected views from a ^{99m}Tc DTPA renal scan of normal kidneys. (a) Early renal concentration and blood pool activity. The kidneys demonstrate symmetrical activity and shape. (b) Early excretion phase. Activity can be seen in the renal pelves (arrowheads), ureters (arrows), and bladder (B). (c) Later drainage film demonstrates decreased renal activity persisting in the renal pelves.

Main Uses

Evaluating
   Renal blood flow
      To gauge extent of renal disease
      To exclude renal artery obstruction
   Pyelocalyceal drainage in cases of suspected obstruction of ureter (Fig. 48-15)
   Suspected acute tubular necrosis

With a Totally Cleared Tracer Compound

Technique

A tracer compound, usually iodohippurate sodium I 131, is injected intravenously. Rapid serial image records are made (Fig. 48-16).

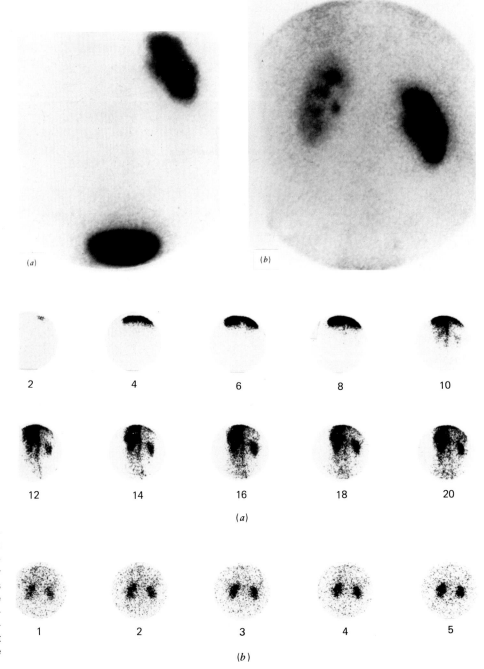

Figure 48-15. Obstruction of the left ureter, in a 99mTc DTPA renal scan, posterior view. (*a*) Intermediate image demonstrates activity in the right kidney and bladder but no activity in the left kidney. (*b*) Later image demonstrates some left kidney parenchymal opacification and partial filling of a dilated renal collecting system.

Figure 48-16. An iodohippurate sodium I-131 serial renal scan of normal kidneys. (*a*) Images obtained at 2-second intervals demonstrate activity in the lungs at the top of the images taken at 4, 6, and 8 seconds. The aorta appears on the 10-second image. The kidneys appear on the 12-second image. (*b*) Images obtained at 1, 2, 3, 4, and 5 minutes demonstrate symmetrical activity in the kidneys.

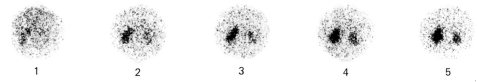

Figure 48-17. Asymmetrical excretion on an iodohippurate sodium I-131 scan, caused by unilateral renal artery stenosis. Images obtained at 1, 2, 3, 4, and 5 minutes demonstrate decreased activity of the left kidney.

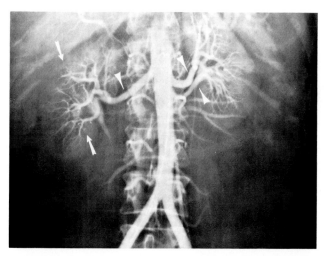

Figure 48-18. Normal aortogram. A catheter has been passed from the right femoral artery to the upper abdominal aorta and contrast injected. The main renal arteries (arrowheads) (there are two to the left kidney) and the intrarenal vessels (arrows) are demonstrated.

Main Uses

Evaluating renal blood flow

Comparing right and left kidneys for renal arterial stenosis (Fig. 48-17)

Evaluating extent of unilateral renal dysfunction

Main Abuse

The main abuse of nuclear medicine imaging with a totally cleared tracer is equating the unilateral renal dysfunction it can demonstrate with the amount of unilateral permanent renal damage. This technique does not evaluate the amount of functional recovery possible.

Keynote

• *Bertin's columns are a normal extension of renal cortical tissue into the more central portions of the kidney, separating the regions of medullary tissue. An unusually thick Bertin's column can be masslike.*

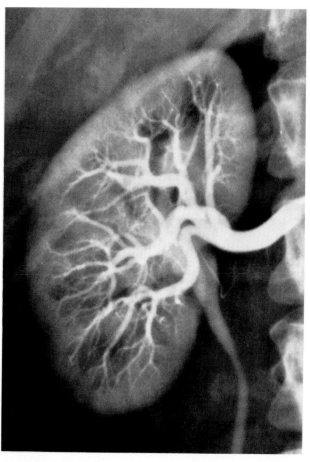

Figure 48-19. Normal selective renal arteriogram. The arborization of the intrarenal vessels is demonstrated. (Courtesy S. Cisternino, M.D.)

Renal Angiography

Arterial Studies

Technique

Two types of studies are done: an aortogram (Fig. 48-18) and a selective renal arteriogram (Fig. 48-19). For each, a catheter is passed percutaneously into the femoral artery and then passed proximally into the midaorta. For the aortogram, the injection of contrast is made into the midaorta above the level of the renal arteries. This will fill the renal arteries of both kidneys. For the selective renal arteriogram, the catheter is positioned so that its tip lies just within the renal artery and contrast medium can be injected directly into the renal artery. After injection of the contrast medium, a series of films is rapidly taken to demonstrate the anatomy of the arteries and some of the larger veins.

Information Provided

The luminal diameter, structure, and distribution of the renal arteries can be studied. Abnormal vessels resulting from disease can be identified (Fig. 48-4 and Fig. 48-20).

Main Uses

Staging of renal cell cancer (CT may be better.)

Investigating unexplained renal-origin hematuria

One method of diagnosing periarteritis nodosa

Investigating suspected renal artery stenosis in patients with high blood pressure

Disadvantages

Slight hazard of injury from angiography and contrast medium

Venous Studies

Although the larger veins can sometimes be adequately studied by arteriography, selective venography can also be performed.

Technique

A catheter is placed percutaneously into the femoral vein and is then directed proximally into either the right or left renal vein. The larger veins are studied by contrast injected into the renal vein. This washes out rapidly because of the large renal blood flow. Investigation of the smaller and intrarenal veins often requires that the flow through the kidney be slowed. The technique used for this is the injection of microquantities of epinephrine into the renal artery, followed by injection of a contrast medium into the renal vein.

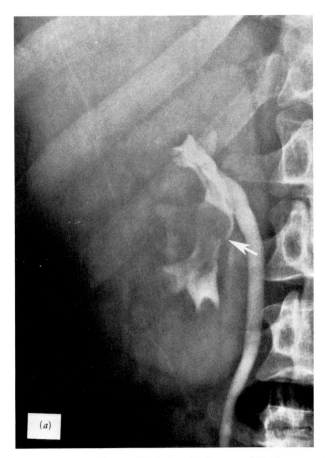
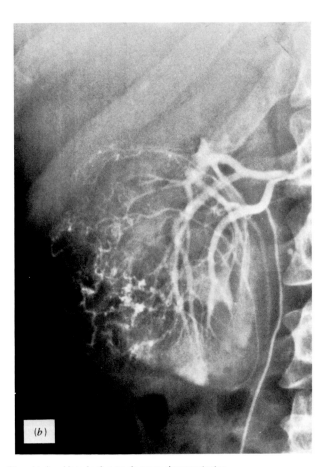

Figure 48-20. Renal cell cancer. (*a*) This urogramlike film obtained late in the angiogram demonstrates a large filling defect (arrow) in the renal collecting system. In patients with renal cell cancer, such filling defects can be caused by blood clot or tumor invasion. This was tumor invasion. (*b*) In the selective renal angiogram, a tangle of abnormal vessels is seen in the lateral portion of the kidney. These new vessels ("neovascularity") have multiple areas of aneurysmal dilation and are of the type seen in renal cell cancer.

Information provided

> Venous anatomy
>
> Venous patency

Main Uses

> Investigating suspected renal vein thrombosis
>
> Investigating unexplained renal hematuria for suspected varices or arteriovenous malformation
>
> Rarely, for localizing an undescended testicle
>
> Investigating and guiding treatment of scrotal varicoceles

Computer-processed (Digital) Angiography

Computer processing of arteriographic images can accentuate differences in radiodensity. For studies of the larger vessels, intravenous injections can be sufficient, but intra-arterial injections of small amounts of contrast produce better images.

Main Uses

> Evaluating renal arteries for stenosis
>
> Physiological measurement of renal parenchymal opacification

---

Keynote

- *Periarteritis nodosa is an uncommon disease with inflammation of multiple small arteries. Symptoms are quite variable depending on the location of the vessels involved.*

Transmission Computed Tomography

Technique

With or without the injection of an intravenous contrast medium, multiple images are made through the kidneys and retroperitoneal structures (Fig. 48-21). Often major vascular structures can be identified.

Information Provided

> Demonstrates
> > Perirenal spaces
> > Renal parenchymal texture and aids in differentiating masses from normal parenchyma (Figs. 48-22 and 48-23)
> > Retroperitoneal lymph nodes

Main Uses

> Staging of known renal cell cancer
>
> Defining process when sonography is uncertain
>
> Differentiating a renal cyst from a renal neoplasm
>
> Defining retroperitoneal spaces and adenopathy

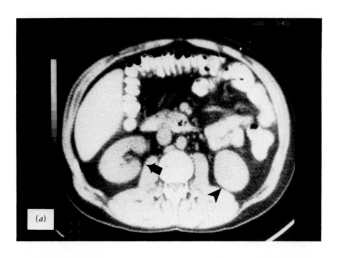

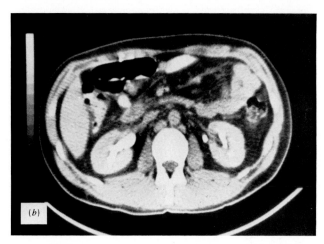

Figure 48-21. CT images of normal kidneys. (*a*) Image obtained without intravenous contrast. The right kidney and its radiolucent sinus (arrow) demonstrate the appearance of the midportion of the kidney. On the left, the lower pole of the kidney (arrowhead) appears as a homogeneous radiodense structure because the section is obtained below the level of the renal sinus. (Courtesy M. Dunne, M.D.) (*b*) Image obtained after the administration of an injected radiographic contrast medium. Within the renal sinus, the collecting system is opacified as an ovoid and branching whiter structure. (Courtesy M. Dunne, M.D.)

Magnetic Resonance Imaging

Magnetic resonance imaging of the kidney can be used to look at internal architecture and differentiate renal sinus fat and medullary and cortical tissue (Fig. 48-24). Currently, MRI it does not appear to offer a clinical advantage over CT, which is cheaper.

SUMMARY

The different methods of imaging the urinary system have been discussed. In practice, the usual approach is to ask yourself the question If I think the patient has———, which study should I use *first?* This summary list will serve as a guide.

Recommended First Choice of Imaging Procedures

1. Unexplained hematuria?
   Cystoscopy and IVU

2. Ureteral colic?
   IVU

3. Suspected renal mass?
   IVU

4. Known renal mass?
   Sonography or CT

5. Calcified renal mass?
   CT

6. Acute renal failure?
   Sonography (for renal size and evidence of hydronephrosis)

7. Transplanted kidney
   Nonfunctioning or suspected rejection?
   Nuclear medicine imaging. Under study: computer-assisted intravenous arteriography

   Suspected urine leak?
   Nuclear medicine imaging
   Perirenal fluid collection?
   Sonography

8. Suspected renal tuberculosis?
   IVU

9. Suspected renovascular hypertension?
   Angiography or computer-assisted angiography

10. Suspected perinephric mass, abscess, or hematoma?
    Sonography or CT

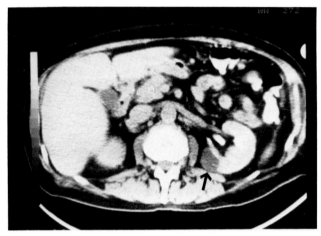

Figure 48-22 A renal cyst demonstrated on CT. In the CT image obtained with contrast enhancement, a small renal cyst is seen in the posterior portion of the left kidney (arrow). This cyst is sharply demarcated from the kidney and is of uniformly decreased radiodensity.

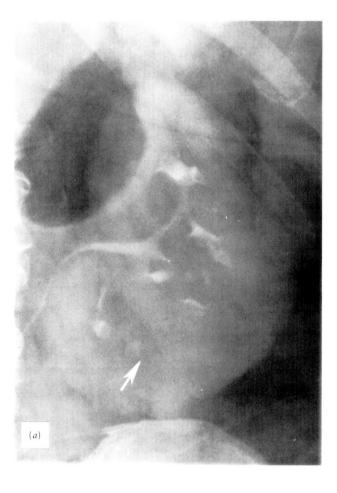

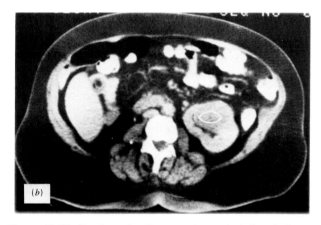

Figure 48-23. Small renal cell cancer demonstrated on both urography and CT. (*a*) View of the left kidney from the IVU demonstrates distortion of the calyces in the lower pole of the kidney (arrow). They are spread apart. (*b*) CT of the kidney demonstrates the left renal mass as an area of decreased radiodensity pressing on the renal sinus. An oval ring shaped marker is placed in the center of the mass.

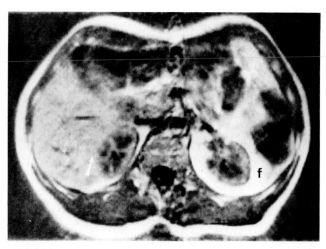

Figure 48-24. MRI of normal kidneys. The kidneys are well seen with their corticomedullary difference well demonstrated. The left kidney is surrounded by fat (f), which appears white with this imaging technique. The right renal cortex blends with the liver (arrow).

REVIEW QUESTIONS

1. Describe the IVU. Which portions of the renal anatomy and physiology are well demonstrated by this technique?
2. Describe the retrograde pyelogram. Which portions of the urinary system does this technique demonstrate?
3. What information does the sonogram yield about the kidney?
4. Describe the three types of nuclear medicine imaging study of the urinary system. What does each demonstrate?
5. What information does renal arteriography yield?
6. What is the preferred method of imaging for each of the following common clinical problems:
    Ureteral colic?
    Hematuria?
    Palpable renal mass?
    Uncontrollable hypertension?
    Acute renal failure?
    Suspected perinephric abscess?

Vocabulary

acute tubular necrosis

Bertin's columns

cystoscope

hematuria

lymphocele

periarteritis

polycystic kidney disease

pyelonephritis

renovascular hypertension

retroperitoneal fibrosis

time activity curve

transitional cell cancer

urinoma

SUGGESTIONS FOR FURTHER READING FOR CHAPTERS 48 TO 53

Charles Ney, Richard M. Fridenberg. *Radiographic Atlas of the Genitourinary System,* 2nd Ed. Lippincott: Philadelphia. 1981. (A fine reference text.)

Alan J. Davidson. *Radiology of the Kidney.* Saunders: Philadelphia. 1985. (A fine reference text)

Anthony F. Lalli. *Tailored Urologic Imaging.* Year Book Medical Publishers: Chicago. 1980.

49

URINARY STONE DISEASE

KEY CONCEPTS

Clinical

The patient with urinary stone disease may have symptoms or signs of ureteral colic, dull or sharp flank pain, blood in the urine, or chronic infection. The patient with a stone in the ureter will often have a progression of symptoms, starting with flank pain, then developing colicy pain that shifts from the flank to the lower abdomen and then to the groin and thigh. Most patients with urinary stone disease will incur no permanent renal damage; a few, however, will have permanent or progressive renal damage.

Staghorn calculi are those that partially conform to the shape of two adjacent calyces. They are often associated with chronic infection.

Medullary sponge kidney is a moderately common idiopathic cause of urinary stone disease in which multiple small calculi form in dilated collecting ducts.

RADIOLOGICAL

About half of all urinary calculi can be identified on plain abdominal films. Those not visible may contain no calcium or may be superimposed on other structures that prevent them from being recognized.

The IVU is the main method used in evaluating a suspected urinary calculus. The main findings sought are visualization of the calculus, demonstration of dilation of the collecting system, and detection of a delay in the filling of the collecting system.

OBJECTIVES

When you complete this chapter you will be able to

1. Identify usual and staghorn calculi and medullary sponge kidney on selected plain abdominal radiographs.

2. Identify on selected IVUs patients with ureteral stone disease.

3. List the three main findings seen on the IVU in the patient with a stone lodged in the ureter.

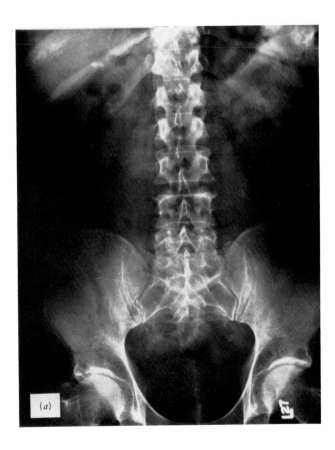

(a)

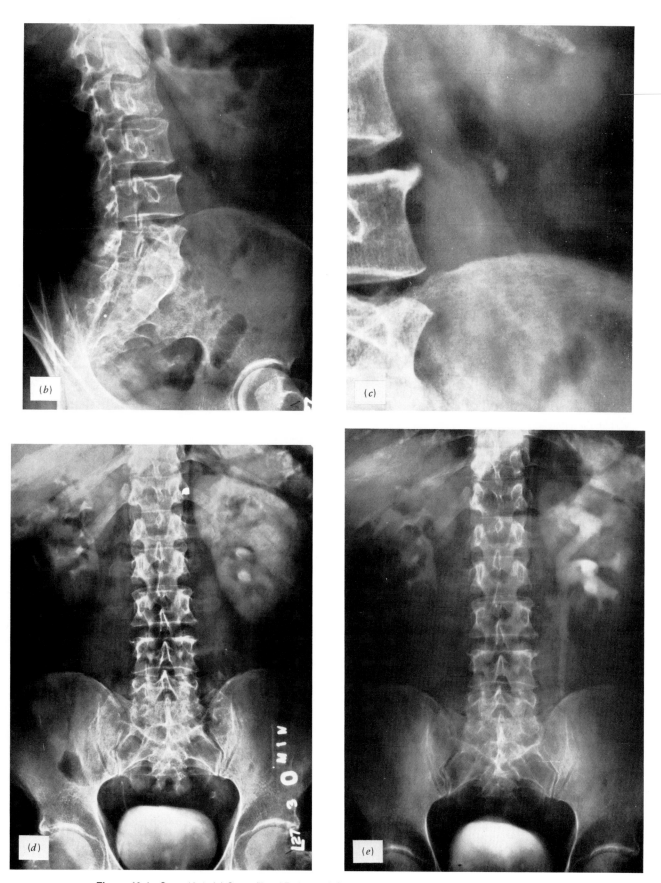

Figure 49-1. Case 49-1. (*a*) Scout film, AP view. (*b*) Scout Film, Oblique view. (*c*) Scout film, Close-up of oblique view. (*d*) 10-minute film. (*e*) 2 1/2-hour film.

4. List the two main symptoms seen in the patient with medullary sponge kidney.

Urinary stone disease usually manifests as flank pain, colic, hematuria, or chronic urinary infection. The IVU is the main method of evaluating these symptoms.

Case 49-1

GK is a 56-year-old farmer who came to our emergency room complaining of severe, agonizing pain. He had initially had a dull pain in his left flank, but this had then changed to sharp, shooting pains down his side into his groin. What do you see on the IVU (Fig. 49-1)?

The films provided are scout films (Fig. 49-1*a, b,* and *c*), a 10-minute film (Fig. 49-1*d*), and a 2½-hour film (Fig. 49-1*e*). What are the findings?

On the scout films, the left kidney outline appears larger than the right. A 7-mm calcification lies lateral to the left transverse process of the second lumbar vertebra (close-up in Fig. 49-1*c*).

On the 10-minute film (FIg. 49-1*d*), the right renal calyces are filled, but the calyces of the left are not yet filled with contrast. The left renal nephrogram is intense.

The 2½-hour film (Fig. 49-*e*), shows filling of the left calyces and ureter.

What is going on? The patient has a stone partially obstructing the left ureter. Because of the increased pressure in the renal collecting system, the pressure on the tubular side of the glomerular membrane is increased, slowing the rate of filtration. The nephrogram is increased both because the kidney is thicker than normal (it's swollen) and because the tubular cells have more time to act to concentrate the contents of the tubules. (There is some research that indicates that the concentration may not be increased, but this is debated.)

Keynotes

- *Scout films are obtained before a radiographic contrast medium is given. This is the best film for detecting calcifications.*
- *Ureteral obstruction increases the pressure in the kidney and slows filtration.*

Case 49-2

Figure 49-2 is from another patient. The 8-minute film (Fig. 49-2*a*) demonstrates a right ureteral calculus (arrow) and no excretion of contrast by the right kidney. No opacification on the right side was seen on this film or on earlier or later films; there was no nephrogram (tubular phase) or calyceal filling. The left kidney functioned normally.

What explains the total lack of function of the right kidney?

Two possibilities: that the pressure in the collecting

system is so high that no filtration can take place (i.e., tubular pressure exceeds arterial pressure less plasma colloid osmotic pressure) or that the tubular cells are so damaged that they cannot resorb salt to concentrate the glomerular filtrate.

Figure 49-2*b* is the same patient 3 weeks later and Figures 49-2*c* and *d*, 4 months later. What do you see?

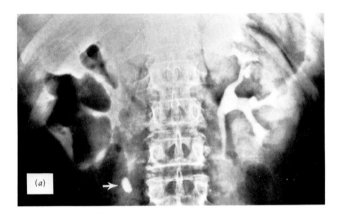

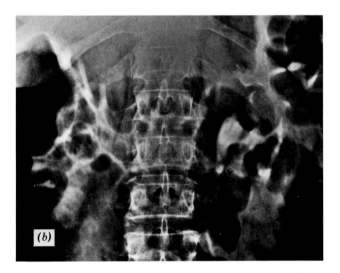

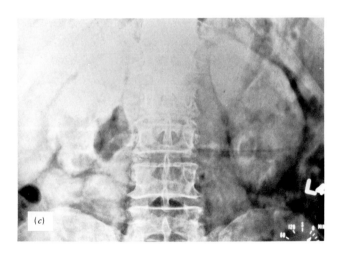

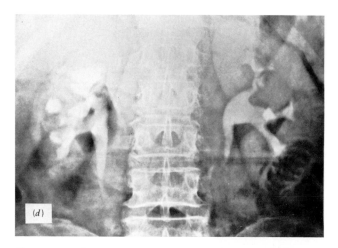

Figure 49-2. Case 49-2. (*a*) 8-minute film, initial study. (*b*) 8-minute film, 3 weeks after initial study. (*c*) 30-second film, 4 months after initial study. (*d*) 8-minute film, 4 months after initial study.

At 3 weeks only a small amount of faint contrast is present in the collecting system. At 4 months the kidney is much smaller than on the other side but the concentration is almost back to normal.

What does this mean? That obstruction with pressure high enough to prevent a visible nephrogram can result in permanent damage to the kidney; but also that even a severely damaged kidney can repair itself, and the full history of why the kidney is poorly functioning is necessary before function can be assumed to be permanently lost.

___

Keynote

- *Uncommonly, ureteral obstruction can increase the intrarenal pressure to a level that prevents blood flow and can cause ischemic damage.*

___

STAGHORN, OR DENDRITIC, CALCULI

Certain renal calculi conform to the shape of part or all of the renal collecting system. Those that fill at least two adjacent calyceal groups are called *staghorn,* or *dendritic, calculi* (Fig. 49-3). They are most often seen in patients with chronic renal infection.

MEDULLARY SPONGE KIDNEY

Medullary sponge kidney is a moderately common idiopathic renal process in which the collecting ducts are dilated. About half the patients will have symptoms either from hematuria or from small stones that form in the dilated collecting ducts and then pass down the ureter. In about half the patients, multiple small calculi can be seen

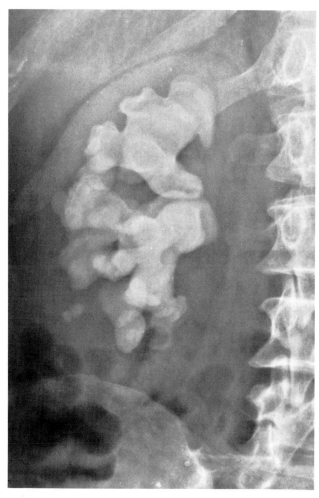

Figure 49-3. Staghorn, or dendritic, calculus. This patient has a proteus infection.

in the medullary portion of the kidney (Fig. 49-4). Dilated collecting ducts can often be identified on urography.

___

Keynotes

- *Staghorn calculi are those that correspond in shape to the renal collecting system.*
- *Medullary sponge kidney is an occasional cause of urinary stone disease.*

___

SUMMARY

The patient with a stone obstructing the ureter demonstrates several changes on IVU. The stone itself may be calcified and detected on the scout films. A delay in the nephrogram and in calyceal filling can be present. The nephrogram can be more intense. The collecting system can be dilated. The stone can be seen to pass down the ureter.

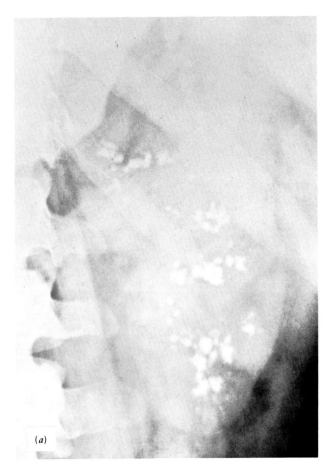
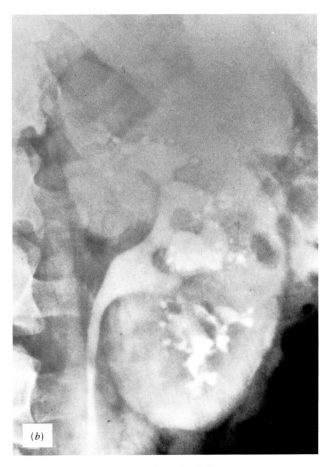

Figure 49-4. Medullary sponge kidney. (a) The plain film demonstrates multiple small renal calcifications. (b) The film from the urogram demonstrates that many of these renal calicifications lie in the medullary portion of the kidney, some of them in dilated collecting ducts.

Seeing the calcified stone and seeing the dilated calyces can establish the diagnosis, but about half the stones are not seen or only poorly seen. Detecting the physiological change of delayed excretion may be the only sign of ureteral obstruction by a stone.

Conversely, not all ureteral stones cause obstruction, so a lack of dilation and a lack of delay in the excretion do not mean that no ureteral stone is present. You must, therefore, look carefully for delayed excretion, calcified stones (seen best on the scout film) and noncalcified stones (seen best as areas of radiolucency on the filled films).

REVIEW QUESTIONS

1. What are the anatomic changes indicative of ureteral stone disease?
2. What are the physiological changes of ureteral stone disease?
3. Why is the nephrogram of increased radiodensity in ureteral stone disease with obstruction?
4. How can the nephrogram indicate which patients are at especially high risk for permanent renal damage from ureteral stone disease?

VOCABULARY

dendritic calculus   staghorn calculus
medullary sponge kidney

SUGGESTIONS FOR FURTHER READING

Errol O. Singh, Reza Malek. Calculus disease in the upper urinary tract. *Seminars in Roentgenology,* **17**:113–132, 1982.
John R. Thornbury, Timothy W. Parker. Ureteral calculi. *Seminars in Roentgenology,* **17**:133–139, 1982.

For additional suggested reading see Chapter 48.

50

CONTRAST MEDIA REACTIONS

KEY CONCEPTS

Clinical

Reactions to iodinated radiographic contrast media vary from mild to severe, with the mild reactions occurring in up to 10% of patients, the severe ones being much less frequent. The clinician, in deciding whether or not to select a study that involves the administration of radiographic contrast, should decide whether the benefit to be gained exceeds the risk. Once the physician has decided, he or she should explain and counsel the patient on the desirability of the study and the risk.

There are several patient conditions that increase the risk of radiographic contrast media. The clinician should be aware of these and discuss the problems with the radiologist and the patient. Conditions that increase the risk of reaction include previous reactions, asthma, severe dehydration, multiple myeloma with dehydration, current treatment with the hyposoluble sulfa drugs, marked hyperuricemia, renal insufficiency, and renal insufficiency associated with diabetes. Diabetic patients without renal insufficiency may be at slightly increased risk of developing renal impairment compared with the normal population.

OBJECTIVES

When you complete this chapter you will be able to

1. List the minor reactions to the iodinated radiographic contrast media.
2. List the conditions that predispose the patient to develop a reaction to iodinated contrast media.
3. List the severe reactions to iodinated radiographic contrast media, and give an estimate of their frequency.

Contrast media reactions vary in their frequency and severity. The physician referring a patient for a study involving the admin-

istration of radiographic contrast should be aware of the level of risk involved and discuss the risk and the reason for the study with the patient. The radiologist should carefully follow the patient and be alert and ready to treat any developing complication.

Case 50-1

What Is Wrong with This Patient?

This 62-year-old lawyer complained that he had had increasing difficulty urinating and often had to wake up at night to "pee." He had had a sigmoid colectomy for cancer 4 years before and had no symptoms related to that. On examination, his prostate was moderately enlarged. An IVU (Fig. 50-1) was obtained. What does it show?

The scout film (Fig. 50-1a) demonstrates metallic-radiodensity sutures from the sigmoid colectomy. The left kidney is larger than the right.

The 2-minute nephrogram film (Fig. 50-1b) demonstrates equal nephrograms. The kidneys have smooth margins.

The 7-minute film (Fig. 50-1c) shows again the nephrogram. No contrast is seen in the collecting system.

By 20 minutes (Fig. 50-1d), minimal contrast is present in the collecting systems, which are thin and incompletely filled.

What Does This Mean?

By 7 minutes, excretion into the collecting system should be at its maximum. If the time labels are correct, something must be limiting the clearance of contrast from the kidneys. What might do this?

What affects flow across the glomerular membrane?

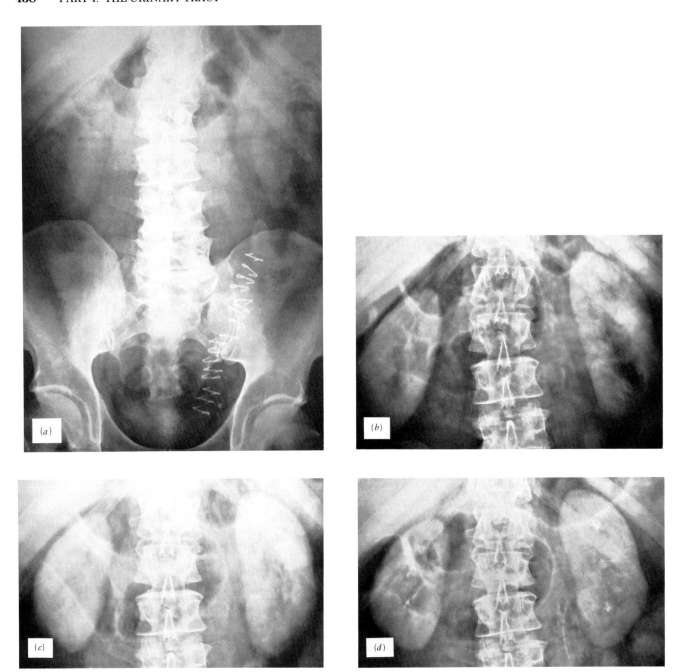

Figure 50-1. Case 50-1. (*a*) Scout film. (*b*) 2-minute film. (*c*) 7-minute film. (*d*) 20-minute film.

According to Starling's law of fluid transport, the factors that affect filtration should be the net difference in hydrostatic pressure, the net difference in oncotic pressure, and the membrane permeability. Within the physiological states detectable by IVU, only differences in the hydrostatic pressure have sufficient effect to be visualized. Changes in permeability and oncotic pressure do not result in enough difference to be seen.

What would affect the net difference in hydrostatic pressure?

A fall in blood pressure or an increase in the pres-

sure on the tubular side of the membrane would slow filtration. The following list includes some of the things that would decrease the rate of filtration:

Decreased blood pressure
    Heart failure
    Hypotension
    Shock
    Coarctation of the aorta

Increased tubular pressure
  Obstruction of
    Tubule
      Necrosis
      Urates
      Sulfa drugs
      Tamm-Horsfall protein in
        Myeloma
        Dehydration
    Ureter
      Stone
      Tumor
  Acute swelling of kidney within capsule
    Acute pyelonephritis
    Acute glomerulonephritis
    Renal contusion
    Renal vein thrombosis

The Whole (or Intact) Nephron Hypothesis

Often students suggest that diseases like chronic pyelonephritis or chronic glomerulonephritis will result in a delay in the appearance time of contrast within the kidney. With rare exceptions, these conditions do not. The reasons for this are two: the first is the whole, or intact, nephron hypothesis; and the second is that as nephrons are lost, the renal collecting system usually shrinks so that there is less collecting system to fill.

The intact nephron hypothesis states that the nephron either functions or fails to function as a unit: that most of the physiological changes seen in patients with renal failure can be explained if one considers that there are a group of nephrons that are diseased and not working at all and another group that are normal. While this hypothesis is not strictly true, is it applicable in this case: In the kidney with chronic disease, those nephrons that are functioning function at a normal rate of speed. Thus renal calyceal filling occurs at a normal time. The diseased kidney will excrete less urine, but the effect on the filling of the calyces and pelvis is minimal because, most of the time, as the kidney loses nephrons, its collecting system becomes smaller. There may be less urine excreted, but there is less collecting system to fill.

Back to Our Patient

When the resident sees that there was no excretion into the collecting system at 7 minutes, he checks the patient and finds his blood pressure is 80/60 with a pulse of 48! What is happening?

Yes, the patient is in shock, but why is the pulse 48 rather than 148?

Vagal overactivity. The patient has had a vasovagal attack.

This case was treated by placing the patient in Trendelenburg's position and infusing fluids, but it could also have been treated with atrophine.

The patient had a reaction to the contrast medium.

Keynotes

- *The nephron is a glomerulus and its tubule.*
- *A vasovagal attack is a brief episode of vagal hyperactivity that results in bradycardia, hypotension, sweating, pallor, and syncope. It is one of the reactions to contrast media injection.*
- *Trendelenburg's position is a position in which the patient is placed inclined 30–40°, head down, usually supine. It is used as a method of increasing the return of blood to the heart to compensate for blood loss or blood pooling in vasodilated patients.*

All of the above is to introduce the problem of contrast media reactions. These reactions vary from minor annoyances to predictable dangers to unpredictable catastrophies. Contrast media reactions can be divided into three groups:

Minimal
Severe predictable
Severe unpredictable

The minimal reactions are annoyances for the patient. The predictable severe reactions, *because* they are predictable, should be preventable. The unpredictable reactions can occur in any patient, young or old, sick or healthy, and are of major concern.

Keynote

- *If you can predict a complication, you can usually prevent it.*

MINIMAL REACTION

Hot feeling
Metallic taste in mouth
Hives
Nausea
Vomiting
Bronchospasm in asthmatics
Angina in patients with cardiac angina

Most patients having an IVU find the experience uncomfortable. Because some patients may vomit, it is important that patients not eat so that their stomachs will be empty. Asthmatics should take their asthma medicine before the study; patients with angina, their angina medicine.

Keynote

- *Patients to receive an intravenous contrast medium should not be given anything to eat, to protect them should they vomit.*

SEVERE PREDICTABLE REACTIONS

While not every patient with these conditions will develop the complication, these patients are at increased risk:

> Patients with
> > Severe dehydration
> > Dehydration associated with
> > > Myeloma
> > > > Renal shutdown can occur if patient is dehydrated. Normal hydration is usually protective.
> > > Hyposoluble sulfa drug administration
> > > > Renal shutdown can occur if patient is dehydrated. Normal hydration is usually protective.
> > > Renal failure
> > > > Renal failure will worsen with dehydration. Effect of contrast agent without dehydration debated.
> > > Marked hyperuricemia (greater than 12 mg%)
> > > > Renal shutdown can occur. Hydration is *not* protective.
> Diabetic patients with
> > Creatinine greater than 5 mg%
> > > Moderate risk of increased renal failure. Normal hydration is *not* protective.
> > Creatinine less than 5 mg%
> > > Increasing risk with increasing creatinine levels. Some risk of renal shutdown at all levels. Effect of hydration in decreasing level of risk debated.

The severe predicatable reactions are separated from the others because if you can predict that a patient is at much increased risk of having a reaction, you can prevent it by not doing the study or by modifying the technique of the study.

Some of the predictable reactions occur in the patient who has been dehydrated for the IVU. These reactions can be usually prevented if the patient is normally hydrated with a urine specific gravity of about 1.010. The renal shutdown occurring in patients with myeloma or nondiabetic renal failure or who are on hyposoluble sulfa drugs will usually not occur if the patient is normally hydrated. The clinical need for the study and the risks should be carefully compared.

Those patients with marked hyperuricemia (over 12 mg%) and diabetic patients with creatinine level over 5 mg% are at serious risk of developing permanent renal damage from IVU. Hydration does not seem to protect them, and in these patients IVU should not be done except for the strongest of clinical reasons.

The diabetic patient without renal insufficiency has a slightly increased risk of developing renal shutdown from IVU. The incidence is approximately 1:1,000, and the renal shutdown is usually, but not always, transient. The diabetic patient with mild renal insufficiency is at increased risk of renal shutdown compared to the nondiabetic.

Keynotes

- *The patient with multiple myeloma, renal failure, or who is on hyposoluble sulfa drugs is at increased risk if dehydrated. Hydration is largely, but not completely, protective.*
- *Patients with marked hyperuricemia (over 12 mg%) and diabetic patients with creatinine level over 5 mg% are at increased risk. Hydration is not protective.*

SEVERE UNPREDICTABLE REACTIONS

The most feared reactions to IVU are the severe unpredictable reactions:

> Renal shutdown
> Hypotension
> > Vasovagal
> > Nonvasovagal
> Laryngeal edema
> Cardiac arrest
> Anaphylactoid reaction
> Death

The vasovagal reactions occur in approximately 1 in every 500 urograms and are easily controlled, if recognized. Clinically significant renal shutdown occurs in approximately 1 in every 1,500 patients and is usually mild and transient. The other more serious reactions occur with a frequency of about 1 in 2000 with death occurring in most studies in 1 in 30,000 to 1 in 60,000. While anyone can develop a reaction, people with an allergic history or cardiac disease are at increased risk. It is important that urography be performed only where facilities for emergency resuscitation are available.

WHAT DO YOU TELL THE PATIENT ABOUT UROGRAPHY?

Because urography is important in the evaluation of the urinary tract, but possibly of some danger to the patient, the patient is entitled to a clear explanation of the procedure and its hazards. If I were the patient, I would want to be told

> Why I need the study
> What the hazard is
> What the hazard of not having the study is
> Whether there is another, safer way to acquire the same information

and, since you will be telling me that I might die from the procedure, I would like some time to think it over.

Fortunately, medical ethics and the law correspond in this case, and this is the information you are required (in Maryland and in many other states) to provide to the patient long enough before the procedure is done to allow the patient to think it over and change his or her mind.

It is usually best for the clinician rather than the radiologist to obtain the consent. It is hard for the radiologist to know the hazard to the patient of not having the study because that depends on the clinical index of suspicion that something might indeed be found to be abnormal on the test.

CONTRAST MEDIA AND CT

The same types of contrast media are often used in CT examinations, and the same reactions can occur.

THE PATIENT WITH A PREVIOUS SEVERE REACTION

The patient with a previous life-threatening reaction to a contrast medium can be studied, but the reason for the study should be definite. If another, safer study could give the same information, the urogram should not be done.

Currently, a multicenter study is evaluating the best method for handling patients with a prior severe reaction. Until those results are available, it is best to discuss the problem with your own radiologist. One technique is to premedicate the patient with 100 mg of hydrocortisone the evening before the study. The morning of the study, the patient is given an additional 100 mg of hydrocortisone and 0.6 mg of atropine. Two physicians and a nurse should be present so that resuscitation can begin immediately if necessary. Unfortunately there is little scientific information to support the effectiveness of this form of premedication, and the results of the multicenter controlled study are eagerly awaited.

SUMMARY

Many patients find the IVU an unpleasant, uncomfortable study.

The minor reactions to intravenous contrast media include: a hot feeling, a metallic taste in the mouth, hives, nausea, vomiting, bronchospasm in asthmatics, and angina in patients with cardiac angina.

The severe predictable reactions occur in patients who are severely dehydrated and in those with dehydration along with myeloma, nondiabetic renal failure, or taking hyposoluble sulfa drugs. In these patients, a normal state of hydration markedly decreases the risk. Patients with marked hyperuricemia (12 mg% or greater) and diabetic patients with renal failure (creatinine level 5 mg% or greater) are at great risk, and hydration is not protective.

The severe unpredictable reactions include renal shutdown, hypotension, laryngeal edema, cardiac arrest, anaphylaxis, and death.

A proper informed consent should be obtained before the administration of a contrast medium and should include telling the patient why she or he needs the study and what if any alternative methods might be as useful but less risky. The consent should be obtained long enough before the procedure so that the patient can think over the information and change her or his mind.

REVIEW QUESTIONS

1. Describe the application of Starling's law of fluid transport to the interpretation of the IVU.
2. Describe the whole (or intact) nephron hypothesis. Describe how it affects what you see on IVU in chronic pyelonephritis.
3. What are the minor reactions to contrast media?
4. What are the severe predictable reactions to intravenous contrast media?
5. What are the severe unpredictable reactions to intravenous contrast?
6. Write out what you think you should tell a patient with ureteral colic and a suspected ureteral calculus about the IVU in order to obtain a proper informed consent.

VOCABULARY

anaphylactoid reaction

hyperuricemia

multiple myeloma

nephron

Trendelenburg's position

vasovagal attack

whole, or intact, nephron
    hypothesis

SUGGESTIONS FOR FURTHER READING

M. Amiel, Ed. *Contrast Media in Radiology, Appraisal and Prospects: First European Workshop.* Proceedings, Lyon, 1981. Springer-Verlag: Berlin, 1982.

G. Ansell. An epidemiologic report on adverse reactions in urography: ionic and nonionic media. *Diagnostic Imaging* 9, #4, part 2. P. 6–10. 1987.

For additional suggested reading see Chapter 48.

51

HEMATURIA

KEY CONCEPTS

Clinical

The patient with red urine needs careful evaluation. The urine may be red from foods, medicines, hemoglobin not in red cells, red blood cells, or red blood cell casts. Each of these requires a different type of evaluation. In general, the patient with red blood cells may require an imaging work-up; the others do not.

Red blood cells in the urine with no red cell casts can be caused by urinary stones, bladder infection, renal cell cancer, transitional cell cancer, tuberculosis, an injury, or an idiopathic vascular bleed.

Radiological

The patient with unexplained hematuria, with red cells in the urine, should have an evaluation of the entire urinary tract: the kidneys, ureters, bladder, and urethra. Cystoscopy is usually the preferred method for evaluating the bladder; the IVU is usually the preferred initial imaging procedure for the kidneys and ureters. The ureters may be adequately demonstrated on the intravenous urogram; if not, then retrograde ureterograms may be necessary.

OBJECTIVES

When you complete this chapter you will be able to

1. List the steps in the evaluation of a patient with red urine.
2. List three etiologies for each potential type of red urine: food dyes and medicine, hemoglobin with no red cells, red cell casts, and red cells with no casts.
3. List the steps in the evaluation of the patient with red blood cells in the urine.

51-1, A True Story

BA is a 59-year-old woman who has always received her care from the Obstetrics and Gynecology Clinics at our hospital. Her records, starting at age 17, document five normal pregnancies and deliveries, colds, physicals, Pap smears, and the like, and thus it is not surprising that when she started "peeing blood" at age 59 she returned to the gynecology clinic for care.

Seen by a gynecology resident, she had a pelvic examination (normal for age and parity) and cystoscopy (so much blood that nothing could be seen). Intravenous urography was scheduled for several days later, and the patient was told to return in 2 weeks to learn the results of the tests. No urinalysis and no blood count were done.

Two weeks later, urinating less blood, she was seen again, recystoscoped (normal), told the results of her IVU (normal), and told to return in 1 month for further evaluation. She was asked to bring in two urine specimens for cytology (eventually reported as "atypia," which implies inflammation, but with cancer still possible). Again no urinalysis and no blood count were done.

She returned 1 month later, was seen by a different gynecology resident, was recystoscoped (normal), and was asked to bring in several more urines for cytology (marked atypia). The patient was told to return in 1 month.

This pattern continued: always seen by a new resident, always recystoscoped. In the eighth month, two urine cytology results were reported positive for transitional cell carcinoma. This was noted by a new gynecology resident, who recystoscoped the patient and, find-

442

ing nothing, told the patient to return in 1 month and to submit two more urine specimens for cytology.

For the next 2½ years the pattern continued: cystoscopy and urine cytology. There was still no urinalysis recorded on the chart, and even with all the bleeding, no blood count was recorded.

Clearly the residents were making mistakes. If you had a patient who complained of urinating blood, what diagnosis would you think of? How would you evaluate the patient?

Finally, after 2½ years, a new resident saw the patient, noted the history, recystoscoped the patient, reviewed the chart, and wrote a full-page note. He ended it by saying, "I don't know where she is bleeding from," and referred the patient to the Urology Clinic.

Arriving in the Urology Clinic several weeks later, a 2½ year history of "peeing blood" is noted, the patient is recystoscoped (normal), urines are sent for cytology (marked atypia), and a new IVU is ordered. There is no record of a urinalysis or blood count.

Films from the IVU are in Figure 51-1. What do you see?

There is at least one filling defect in the right upper pole calyx, and the mucosa near it appears nodular. The scout tomogram (Fig. 51-1b) shows faint calcification at the site of the filling defect.

What could the patient have?

The urology resident, noting the abnormal urine cytologies, tells the patient that she probably has cancer and has to have her right kidney, ureter, and part of her bladder removed (this is the standard operation for transitional cell cancer of the kidney). The resident has not read the x-ray report. B.A. said that she wanted some time to get her affairs in order.

Two months later, admitted and prepared for surgery, but still without a recorded urinalysis or blood count, the patient signs the consent form.

The resident, reviewing the chart, finds the radiologist's report: "1 cm calcified stone in the right upper pole calyx with reactive mucosal changes."

Why is this a stone and not transitional cell cancer

of the kidney? Because transitional cell cancer of the kidney does not calcify (it does in the bladder, but not in the kidney).

The next day the resident removes the portion of the kidney containing the stone. There is no cancer pres-

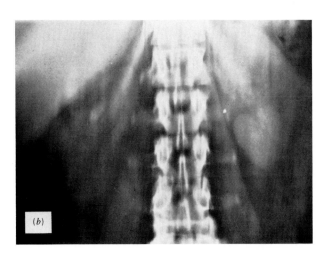

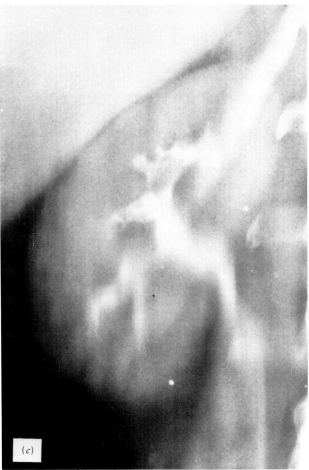

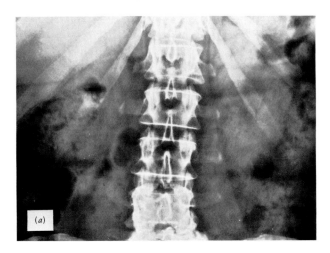

Figure 51-1. Case 51-1. (a) Scout film of the kidneys. (b) Tomographic scout film. (c) Tomographic 8-minute film selected to best demonstrate the upper pole collecting system of the right kidney.

ent; the cytology results return to normal, and the patient is cured.

In the record of the hospitalization, there is no recorded urinalysis or blood count.

This is a true story, but bad medical care. If you had a patient who complained of bloody urine, what diagnosis would you think of? How would you evaluate the patient? If you were one of the physicians in the Gynecology Clinic, how would you prevent this failure to reach a diagnosis? How would you prevent the repeated nonproductive evaluation of the patient?

THE DIFFERENTIAL DIAGNOSIS OF RED URINE

The differential diagnosis of red urine is based on a careful urine analysis and the medical history. Possible findings on urinalysis include

1. Red urine, no hemoglobin
    A. Phenazopyridine HCl (a drug taken as a urinary analgesic)
    B. Rifampin (a drug taken for tuberculosis)
    C. Ingestion of red licorice
    D. Ingestion of beets
2. Myoglobin
    A. Skeletal muscle injury or infection
    B. Idiopathic
3. Hemoglobin, no red cells
    A. Urine left standing too long, lysis of red cells
    B. Hemolysis
        (1) Immunologic
        (2) Enzymatic, such as glucose-6-phosphate dehydrogenase (G-6-PD) deficiency
        (3) Structural
            a. Hypersplenism
            b. Sickle cell disease
            c. Hereditary spherocytosis
4. Red cell casts
    A. Glomerulonephritis
5. Red cells, no casts
    A. Urinary stones
    B. Renal cell cancer
    C. Transitional cell cancer
        (1) Kidney
        (2) Ureter
        (3) Bladder
    D. Glomerulonephritis
    E. Tuberculosis
    F. Papillary necrosis (necrosis of the papillae usually associated with sickle cell disease or trait, diabetes with infection, or excessive use of phenacetin)
    G. Vascular malformations
    H. Bladder infection
    I. Trauma

Of these, the most common renal causes of hematuria are

1. Acute glomerulonephritis
2. Urinary stone disease

WORK-UP OF THE PATIENT WITH RED URINE

1. History and physical examination.
2. Urinalysis.
3. Blood count and looking at a blood smear.
4. Sickle preparation.
5. If red cell casts are seen, imaging techniques are of limited value.
6. If red cells are seen without red cell casts:
    A. Visibly red urine.
        (1) *Immediate* cystoscopy and IVU. These should be performed immediately because it helps in identifying the site of bleeding if the studies are done while the patient is actively bleeding.
    B. Microscopic hematuria.
        (1) Cystoscopy and intravenous urography at a convenient time.

PREVENTION OF THE CLINIC SYNDROME

In many clinics, patients receive less than ideal care because the clinic situation does not permit time to review the patient's chart and because often the patient will be seen by a different physician on each visit. How do you prevent these problems?

If the clinic setting does not permit a preview of the charts, then you should feel responsible to hold the charts on your patients so that you can review them later at a slack time. This may result in disagreements with the clerks or medical records librarians, but if you are firm and explain why this will result in better care, you will usually be able to hold the charts for a while. When you review the chart later, you can, if you find something that needs further attention, call the patient back.

It is helpful to keep a list of each patient's name and unit number so that the chart can be repulled for you to review if it is removed or if you remember something important after you've returned the chart.

How do you prevent repetitive nonproductive work-ups?

By indicating in your notes what action you intend to take should a test's results be abnormal and what action you would take if they were normal. Thus, even if you don't see the patient yourself, the next physician who does will know what you were planning to do and is more likely to move the work-up to the next stage.

Obviously, the best method for preventing both problems would be restructuring the clinic format to prevent these problems, but this type of reorganization is usually not possible for the student, intern, or resident to accomplish.

Keynote

• *Before you order a test, decide what you would do for the patient if the results were either positive or negative. Record your plan in the chart to remind yourself or to aid the next physician who sees the patient. This is a simple method of improving care and lowering its cost.*

SUMMARY

The patient with red urine needs a history, physical examination, and most important, a careful urinalysis. A red urine without blood cells in it can be due to food dyes, drugs, intravascular hemolysis, myoglobinopathy, or poor techniques of urinalysis. The patient with red cell casts has some form of glomerulonephritis, needs a serum titer of streptococcus antibody, and may need a renal biopsy. The patient with red blood cells not explained as being due to acute bladder infection or traumatic injury needs cystoscopy to evaluate the bladder and an IVU to evaluate the kidneys and ureters.

The most common causes of hematuria are cystitis, rupture of a periprostatic vein, glomerulonephritis, and urinary stone disease. The most feared causes of hematuria are tumors of the bladder, ureter, or kidney. A complete work-up is required in every case of unexplained hematuria in someone in the cancer age group.

It is not uncommon for patients being cared for in a clinic situation to receive suboptimal care. This is often because the physician caring for the patient does not really know a lot about the patient and cannot review the chart in the time available in a busy clinic. It is the responsibility of anyone who cares for a patient to review the chart for missed information and to write directive notes to explain what should be done if the results of any test that is ordered are positive.

REVIEW QUESTIONS

1. Explain the work-up of the patient with red urine.
2. What is the role of the urinalysis in this work-up?
3. Which patient with red urine should have immediate cystoscopy and urography?
4. How would you evaluate the patient with red cell casts in his or her urine?
5. Have you had problems adequately caring for patients in the clinics you have rotated through? Based on the problems you have seen, how would you try to improve the patient's care?

VOCABULARY

cellular atypia	myoglobin
cystoscopy	papillary necrosis
G-6-PD deficiency	phenazopyridine HCl
glomerulonephritis	rifampin
hereditary spherocytosis	transitional cell cancer
hypersplenism	

SUGGESTIONS FOR FURTHER READING

For suggested reading see Chapter 48.

52

RENAL CYSTS, TUMORS, AND PSEUDOTUMORS

KEY CONCEPTS

Radiological

There are two types of renal pseudotumor, the congenital type that occurs in approximately 5% of normal people, and the acquired type that occurs in the scarred kidney. The congenital type can usually be recognized as a pseudotumor because it will usually have one or more short calyces. In the scarred kidney, a pseudotumor may have to be confirmed as hypertrophied renal parenchyma with a ^{99m}Tc DMSA scan.

The renal cyst is best differentiated from a renal cancer by sonography or CT. Because sonography is less expensive, it is preferred.

The presence of a renal mass should be suspected on IVU when the margin of the kidney cannot be seen, when there is an unexplained bulge in the renal margin, when there is displacement of calyces, or when a focal lack of nephrogram is present.

OBJECTIVES

When you complete this chapter you will be able to

1. Identify renal tumors and pseudotumors on selected IVUs.
2. List the four findings that suggest the presence of a mass on IVU.
3. Indicate the method of further evaluation of a mass seen on IVU that
   a. Is suggestive of a renal pseudotumor.
   b. Shows vessels on the vascular phase of the IVU.
   c. Has calcium in it.
   d. Has no specific diagnostic features.

Renal cell cancer represents 1% of all cancers. Renal cysts are common in patients over the age of 50. Renal pseudotumors occur in about 5% of people. The identification of renal masses and their differentiation from renal pseudotumors forms are an important aspect of kidney imaging procedures.

RENAL PSEUDOTUMORS

Congenital Renal Pseudotumors

There are two types of renal pseudotumors: congenital and acquired. Though the congenital ones can be defined in different ways, about 5% of people have at least one kidney with a congenital renal pseudotumor. Fortunately, most of these can be immediately identified on the IVU (Figs. 52-1 and 52-2) and need no further work-up. These congenital renal pseudotumors almost always occur between the upper and middle calyceal groups of the kidney. They result from the way the kidney forms from multiple renal lobes.

The *renal lobe* is the basic unit from which the embryologic kidney forms. It consists of a cup-shaped boundary of cortex within which is a pyramid of medulla draining through a papilla into a minor calyx. These early lobes fuse in the embryo and are usually symmetrically arrayed around the renal pelvis. In about 5% of kidneys, the fusion of the lobes is less orderly, and between the upper and middle calyceal groups, a lobe is displaced medially so that it lies deeper within the kidney, separating the upper and middle calyceal groups.

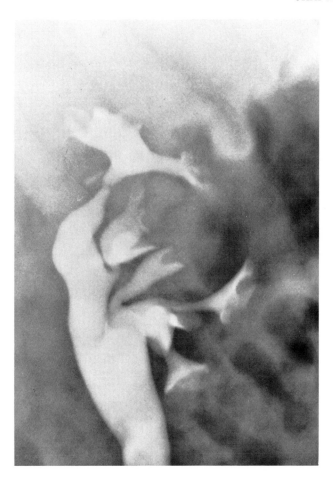

Figure 52-1. Congenital renal pseudotumor. A rounded pseudo-mass lies between the upper and middle portions of this left kidney. There are several short calyces draining it. This is a typical appearance of a congenital renal pseudotumor.

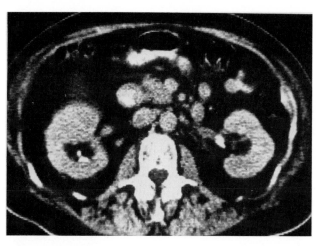

Figure 52-2. A congenital renal pseudotumor seen on CT. The asymmetric thickness of the renal parenchyma of the right kidney is due to a renal pseudotumor. These can be differentiated from a true renal tumor because the radiodensity and appearance of the pseudo-tumor are identical to the normal parenchyma, by their small size, and by their location between the mid and upper portions of the kidney. Contrast this to the mass shown in Figure 48-23b. Although the appearance of that renal cell cancer is similar, it is of lesser radiodensity on the enhanced CT scan. (Courtesy N. Whitley, M.D., University of Maryland Hospital.)

Acquired Renal Pseudotumors

Acquired renal pseudotumors are moderately uncommon. Renal hypertrophy can result in a pseudotumor appearance in the kidney. When moderate unilateral renal damage is present, generalized hypertrophy of the undamaged kidney can occur, resulting in a unilaterally large kidney. When both kidneys have regions of moderate disease, the areas of more normal renal tissue can hypertrophy in a masslike way (Fig. 52-6), displacing calyces as any new growth would. The clue to suspecting them is to see evidence of bilateral renal damage with focally small or scarred portions of the kidney in addition to the larger masslike regions. If the diagnosis is uncertain, a renal scan with ⁹⁹ᵐTc DMSA or glucoheptonate will resolve the problem. Sonography can be used, but it is less sensitive and certain.

The main method of correctly identifying this renal pseudotumor is to note that because a renal lobe must drain into a calyx, a calyx must also drain the renal pseudotumor. Often these pseudotumor calyces are shorter than normal (because the lobe is displaced within the medullary space).

True masses should not have short calyces. Because they are new growths, they should push calyces away from the mass (Fig. 52-3) rather than drain it. To be certain, however, it is helpful to reconstruct mentally the calyceal positions in three dimensions, using oblique views, because, occasionally, a mass will push a calyx directly backward, projecting it in a foreshortened shape.

In the uncommon case where the diagnosis of renal pseudotumor is uncertain based on its anatomic structure, a ⁹⁹ᵐTc DMSA or glucoheptonate nuclear scan can be performed to confirm the diagnosis by showing normal activity at the site of the mass (Figs. 52-4 and 52-5).

Keynotes

- *The congenital renal pseudotumor is a normal variant of kidney structure that resembles a mass. It usually lies between the upper and middle calyceal groups and usually has short calyces draining it.*
- *Congenital renal pseudotumors drain into calyces; masses displace calyces.*
- *Acquired renal pseudotumors are masslike growths of hypertrophied renal tissue that occur in scarred kidneys. They displace calyces. Because they are normal renal parenchyma, they will take up renal tissue–avid scanning agents such as ⁹⁹ᵐTc DMSA or glucoheptonate.*

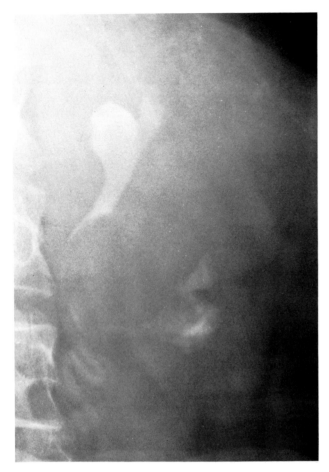

Figure 52-3. A renal cell cancer occurring in the mid left kidney. The mass displaces and distorts the shape of the calyces. No short calyces drain it. Note also that portions of the upper lateral margin of the kidney cannot be seen.

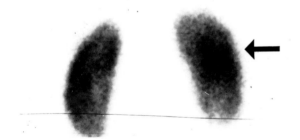

Figure 52-4. 99mTc DMSA scan. Normal posterior view with a moderately uniform appearance of radioactivity. Slight increase in activity (arrow) between mid and upper poles of the right kidney is the location of the congenital renal pseudotumor.

TRUE RENAL MASSES

Renal cysts and renal neoplasms are the more common of the true renal masses. Abscesses and other complications of infection (discussed in Chapter 53) can be masslike but are less common.

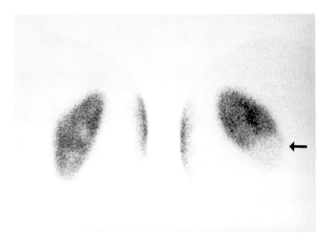

Figure 52-5. 99mTc glucoheptonate scan. Oblique views of kidneys in a patient with a renal cell cancer of the lower pole of the left kidney. The focal area of decreased radioactivity (arrow) is the location of the renal cell cancer.

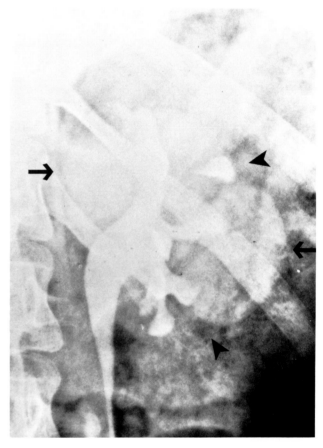

Figure 52-6. Acquired renal pseudotumors in a patient with severe bilateral chronic pyelonephritis. Arrows indicate the sites of two focal areas of renal hypertrophy, each displacing calyces. Arrowheads indicate the locations of several focal renal scars caused by the pyelonephritis. (Courtesy R. Sanders, M.D.)

Identification

Renal masses are usually identified by one of four signs:

1. Inability to see a normally located margin of a portion of the kidney
2. A bulge in the renal margin
3. Displacement of calyces
4. Focal lack of nephrogram

Inability to See a Normally Located Margin of the Kidney. The normal kidney is surrounded by fat, which is of different radiodensity than the water radiodensity or contrast radiodensity of the kidney. Thus it should be possible to see the margin of the kidney all the way around (Fig. 52-7a). It may be necessary to combine the portions of the margin from several films, but inability to see any portion (except that near the renal pelvis) should be interpreted as suspicious for a renal mass (Fig. 52-7b). This is the most frequent sign seen on the IVU not done with tomography.

Bulge in the Renal Margin. The margin of the normal kidney is smooth, but two types of normal bulges occur. The most common is a bulge near the lateral margin of the left kidney near the spleen (the splenic hump).

This can be differentiated from a true mass because a true splenic hump will usually have a long, narrow calyx draining it.

The second kind of bulge that can occur is due to a lack of complete fusion of the renal lobes (renal lobation or lobulation). When the renal lobes come together, a small indentation can be left between the lobes, making each lobe simulate a focal bulge. This can be identified because the calyx at the site of the bulge is not displaced.

Other bulges are likely to be true renal masses (Fig. 52-8).

Displacement of Calyces. Many masses displace calyces, but calyces can appear displaced by renal pseudotumors as well. How can you tell that a calyx is displaced? By finding a portion of renal parenchyma that does not seem to be drained by a calyx. It would appear easy to measure the distance between calyces and note two that were too far apart, or to look for asymmetry in spacing; but these simplistic methods do not work because the natural variation in calyceal shape and spacing is too great. Marked asymmetry is not unusual between the two kidneys or even between the upper and lower poles of the same kidney.

The only rule that seems to work is that given above: calyceal displacement is identified by finding a portion of renal parenchyma that does not seem to be drained by a calyx (Fig. 52-3). This rule is based on the embryology of the kidney. Each renal lobe has a draining calyx. When more lobes fuse, the calyces are larger or more complex in shape, but they still drain the parenchyma. New masses will not have draining calyces.

Focal Lack of Nephrogram. When tomography is done as part of the IVU, rounded regions of lack of nephrogram

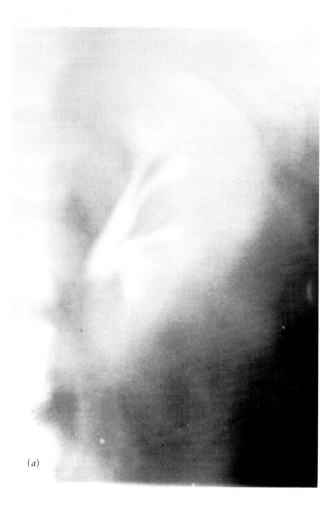

(a)

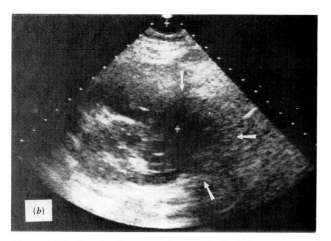

(b)

Figure 52-7. Renal cell cancer, detected by inability to see renal margin. (a) Tomographic section through the left kidney. The inferior lateral margin of the left kidney cannot be seen on this or on the other tomographic sections obtained. The orientation of the calyces is abnormal, with the inferior calyces pushed toward the midline. (b) This sonogram demonstrates a large echogenic mass (arrows) at the lower pole of the left kidney. Note the poor through transmission of the sound, a sign that the mass is solid.

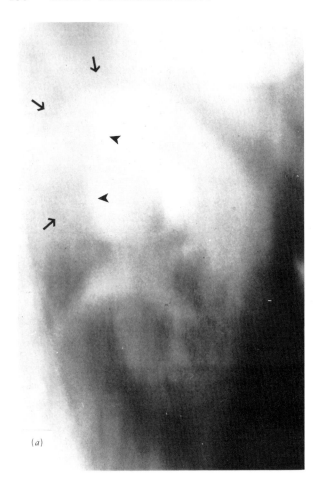

(a)

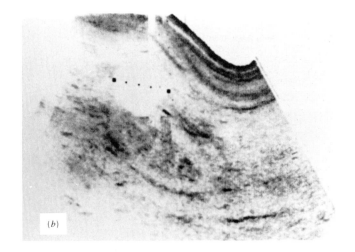

(b)

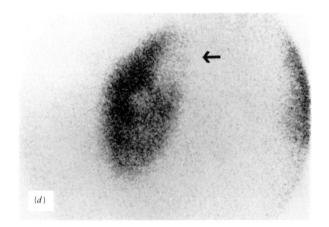

(d)

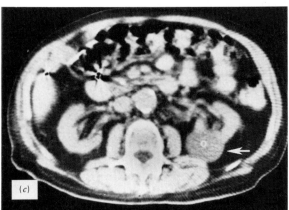

(c)

Figure 52-8. Renal cyst demonstrated as an extra contour and bulge of the kidney. (*a*) Tomographic section demonstrates two margins of the upper pole of the left kidney. Arrows indicate the margin of a renal cyst. Arrowheads indicate the slightly indistinct margin of the upper pole of the kidney. (*b*) A sonogram confirms the presence of a well-demarcated, sonolucent mass fulfilling the criteria for a benign cyst. The clinical work-up should have stopped at this point. Note the increased through transmission of the sound with increased echoes on the far side, a sign of its cystic nature. (*c*) A CT also demonstrates the presence of the renal cyst (arrow). (*d*) A ^{99m}Tc glucoheptonate scan (posterior oblique view) demonstrates the focal lack of activity in the renal cyst (arrow). These last two studies were unnecessary confirmation and only added to the cost and length of the patient's work-up.

indicative of renal masses can sometimes be seen (Fig. 52-9). If the tomogram is taken very early in the vascular phase (the phase of total-body opacification), those masses with vessels in them may show evidence of their vascularity (Fig. 52-10). If taken in the nephrogram phase, both cysts and cancers will appear as regions of lack of nephrogram. Bowel gas overlying the kidney may simulate a focal lack of nephrogram.

Evaluation

Once you have found a true renal mass, how should you evaluate it? The evaluation of a known renal mass depends on what has been learned about it from the IVU. Four possibilities exist:

1. The mass may have an appearance suggestive of a renal pseudotumor.

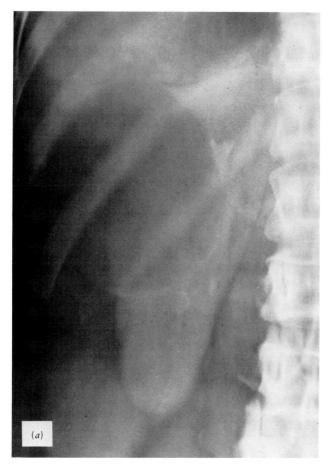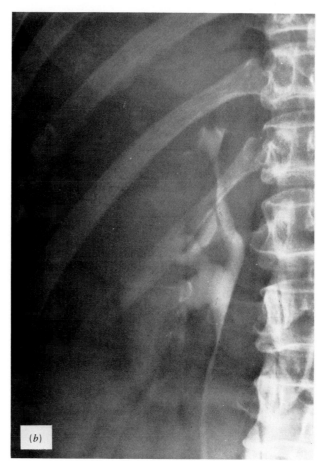

Figure 52-9. Renal cyst showing a focal lack of nephrogram. (*a*) Tomographic section obtained during the nephrogram (tubular) phase. A large renal cyst is demonstrated in the mid right kidney as a focal lack of nephrogram. (*b*) Later in the study, the nephrogram has faded and the mass is much harder to detect. At this time, the inability to see the renal margin at the site of the cyst is probably the most obvious sign of its presence.

2. The mass may be clearly vascular on the vascular phase film.
3. The mass may contain calcium.
4. The mass may have no specific determining feature.

Each of these possibilities demands a different method of imaging evaluation.

Mass Suggestive of a Renal Pseudotumor. The mass that is definitely a renal pseudotumor as previously described with short calyces and in a classical location between the upper and middle calyceal groups needs no further evaluation. The mass thought to be a pseudotumor, but without sufficient confirming evidence, is probably best evaluated with a 99mTc DMSA or glucoheptonate scan because this will provide a positive diagnosis. Sonography and CT can also be used to evaluate a suspected renal pseudotumor, but these techniques base this diagnosis on the exclusion of renal cysts and renal cancers rather than on direct identification.

Vascular Mass on the Vascular Phase of the IVU. The vascular mass on an IVU cannot be a renal cyst; either a CT scan or an arteriorgram can be used to stage the mass for surgery.

Calcified Mass. Calcification in a mass usually prevents its complete sonographic characterization because the calcium prevents the transmission of sound. If the calcium is more than minimal, the mass will usually be avascular or may have only a few small vessels, thus making angiographic evaluation difficult. Computed tomography is probably the procedure of choice in evaluating calcified masses.

Masses with No Diagnostic Features. Masses without calcium and without evidence of vascularity on the IVU can be evaluated either with sonography or CT; because sonography is cheaper, it is usually preferable except in very obese patients.

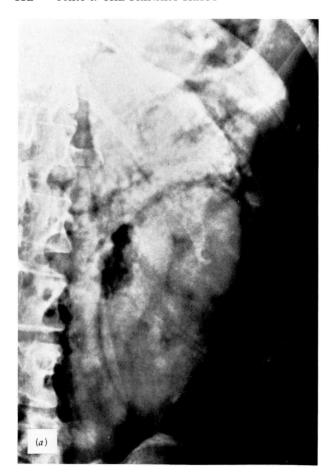
(a)

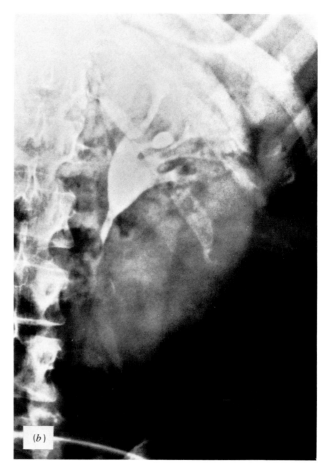
(b)

Figure 52-10. Renal cell cancer. Vascularity demonstrated on a film obtained during the vascular phase (the phase of total-body opacification) of the IVU. (*a*) Film obtained during the vascular phase of an IVU. (*b*) When the calyces are filled, the vascular channels seen in *a* have disappeared. The calyces are displaced upward by the lower pole renal mass. (*c*) A selective left renal arteriogram demonstrates the marked vascular supply of this renal cell cancer. (*d*) A late film from the left renal arteriogram demonstrates filling of the vascular structures (arrows) demonstrated on the vascular phase film of the IVU. Compare with *a*.

Keynotes

- *If you cannot see the margin of the kidney, you cannot exclude a renal mass. This is true for all imaging modalities: sonography, CT, and radiography. Because there is not an identifiable tissue limit on tracer images, tracer images cannot be used to exclude a mass growing from the margin of the kidney.*

- *The differentiation of a normal renal bulge from a true mass is possible because a normal renal bulge will have a calyx extending into it. The bulge due to a mass will displace the calyx.*

- *True renal masses will not be drained by the calyceal system.*

- *On the earliest film of the IVU, it is sometimes possible to see vessels or a tumor blush within a mass. This excludes the diagnosis of renal cyst.*

MAGNETIC RESONANCE IMAGING

At the present time, although MRI images of renal masses can be produced, the technique does not appear to offer any clinical advantage over CT. Further investigation may, in the future, define a role for this new technique in the evaluation of the kidney.

SUMMARY

The most common types of renal mass are the renal pseudotumor, the renal cyst, and the renal cell cancer. These masses are usually detected on IVU or as unexpected findings on other imaging modalities. There are two types of renal pseudotumors, congenital and acquired. In most cases, the congenital pseudotumor can be diagnosed by noting its location (usually between the upper and middle calyceal group) and by identifying the congenitally short calyces that drain it. Should the diagnosis be uncertain, it can be confirmed by a renal scan with ^{99m}Tc DMSA. The acquired renal pseudotumor is a focal area of renal hypertrophy. These occur only in severely scarred kidneys, so the presence of scarring is a major indicator of the diagno-

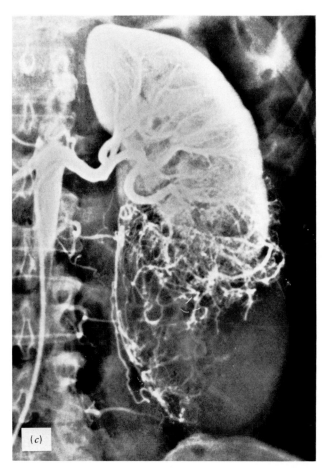

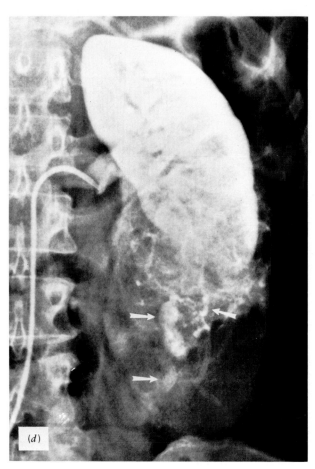

Figure 52-10. (Continued).

sis. The diagnosis can be confirmed with a renal scan with
^{99m}Tc DMSA.

Renal cysts and renal cell cancers can be identified on
urographic studies because the margin of the kidney cannot be seen, because a bulge is seen in the renal margin,
because of the displacement of calyces, or because there is
a focal lack of nephrogram.

Once a renal mass is found and the diagnosis of renal
pseudotumor discarded, the work-up depends on the specific findings seen on urography. If the mass is clearly
vascular on the early films from the IVU, computed tomography or angiography should be used to stage the lesion. If
the mass is calcified, CT is the preferred imaging method.
If the mass has no specific identifying features, the mass
can be evaluated with either sonography or CT.

REVIEW QUESTIONS

1. What is a renal pseudotumor? What types are there? How can
   you differentiate these types from a true renal mass?

2. What are the imaging signs of renal masses?

3. What are the common diagnoses for renal masses?

4. Once the mass is identified, how should one kind of mass be
   distinguished from another?

VOCABULARY

calyx ^{99m}Tc DMSA
renal cell cancer ^{99m}Tc glucoheptonate
renal lobe

SUGGESTIONS FOR FURTHER READING

Beverly G. Coleman, Peter H. Arger. Sonography of renal adenocarcinoma. *CRC Critical Reviews in Diagnostic Imaging*,
19:203–255, 1983.

For additional suggested reading see Chapter 48.

53

INFECTION AND THE KIDNEY

KEY CONCEPTS

Clinical

Pyelonephritis is divided into acute and chronic conditions. Simple acute pyelonephritis in the adult is a brief, limited disease that usually does not need imaging evaluation, unless it is recurrent or fails to respond to therapy. The two main indicators that the acute infection is other than simple acute pyelonephritis are that there are an absence of pyuria and failure to respond to appropriate therapy within 72 hours. Diabetic patients seem to have an increased incidence of complications from renal infection and should be monitored closely.

Renal infection is more severe in the presence of ureteral obstruction. Other complications include renal and perirenal abscesses. Some of these abscesses contain gas. When the gas spreads along tissue planes, the condition is called "emphysematous pyelonephritis."

Chronic pyelonephritis can occur with and without vesicoureteral reflux. The patients with reflux, especially children, can develop severe renal damage. Those infections unassociated with reflux usually produce little or no permanent renal damage.

Radiological

Imaging studies performed during an episode of acute pyelonephritis may demonstrate slight renal enlargement, a slightly inhomogeneous nephrogram (on CT), and ^{67}Ga- avid kidneys.

The child with renal infection should have an imaging work-up. The male child with either cystitis or pyelonephritis should have a voiding cystourethrogram and an evaluation of the kidneys, either with an IVU or a renal sonogram. The girl with pyelonephritis should have a voiding cystourethrogram or a nuclear medicine voiding cystogram and well as evaluation of the kidneys with urography or sonography. The girl with her second episode of cystitis should have a similar evaluation. Many clinicians do not evaluate the first episode of cystitis in girls.

OBJECTIVES

When you complete this chapter you will be able to

1. List the three situations in which you should suspect complicated acute pyelonephritis.
2. Describe the difference between chronic pyelonephritis with and without vesicoureteral reflux.
3. List and explain the differences in the work-up of the child, male or female, with bladder or renal infection.

Renal infection is usually classified into acute and chronic forms. In general, the acute form is more common, rapidly responds to therapy, and does not require radiological investigation. The chronic form is less common, more difficult to manage, and often does require radiological investigation. This chapter discusses renal infection in the following categories:

1. Acute pyelonephritis
2. Complications of acute pyelonephritis
3. Chronic or recurrent pyelonephritis in a patient with reflux of urine from the bladder to the kidney
4. Recurrent acute pyelonephritis in a patient with no reflux of urine from the bladder

454

ACUTE PYELONEPHRITIS

Acute pyelonephritis is an acute self-limited infection of the kidney associated with a high fever, chills, and flank pain. The usual organism is *E. coli,* and the usual treatment is antibiotics and hydration. Response to the antibiotics can be seen within 48–72 hours. Imaging studies are in general not indicated during the acute phase because they do not affect the initial therapy. If performed, a urogram will demonstrate slightly enlarged and poorly functioning kidneys. The kidneys will be ^{67}Ga avid (Fig. 53-1), and CT scanning may show an inhomogeneous nephrogram.

Complications

Some patients with acute pyelonephritis do not follow a typical course. When the course is atypical, imaging studies may be useful. The major complications of acute pyelonephritis are

1. Ureteral obstruction from
   a. Stone
   b. Sloughed papillae
2. Focal abscess formation in or around the kidney
3. Emphysematous pyelonephritis

When to Suspect Complications

1. Pyuria is minimal or absent in a patient with clinically suspected pyelonephritis.
2. Ureteral colic is frequent or more than minimally painful.
3. Ureteral colic preceded the onset of fever.
4. The fever does not lyse within 48–72 hours.
5. The patient has diabetic vascular disease or is in a state of ketoacidosis.

Ureteral Obstruction. Two groups of patients can have a combination of acute pyelonephritis and ureteral obstruction: those with urinary stone disease and those with diabetic vascular disease. In the patients with urinary stone disease, illness often starts with symptoms of ureteral colic and then fever develops. Ureteral colic is usually severe in these patients; the fever is prolonged and unresponsive to therapy. Renal damage from the infection can be extensive. Depending on the degree of ureteral obstruction present, pyuria may be less than expected, minimal, or absent. Intravenous urography is the imaging method of choice when you suspect this disease.

In diabetic patients with acute pyelonephritis renal papillae can slough, and these sloughed papillae can obstruct the ureter. In these patients, the symptoms of infection usually precede the onset of ureteral colic. In some patients the function of the kidney may be so compromised that urine output is minimal and ureteral colic may not occur. In some of these patients, the kidney will infarct and develop emphysematous pyelonephritis requiring emergency surgical drainage and nephrectomy.

Because the symptoms vary widely in the diabetic with complicated acute pyelonephritis, and because it may be difficult to distinguish uncomplicated from complicated acute pyelonephritis in these patients, the clinician's index of suspicion should be high, and imaging studies should be obtained on even minimal suspicion of a developing complication.

The imaging procedure to use can be debated. Intravenous urography, followed by retrograde pyelography if the kidney does not function, is almost always definitive; the diabetic patient is, however, at increased risk of contrast media reactions, especially if renal function is already limited. Sonography can often show the abnormality, but in some patients the kidney is functioning so poorly that ureteral obstruction will not result in dilation of the collecting system. [99m]Tc DTPA studies may be abnormal from the acute pyelonephritis and may not definitely show that the abnormality is obstruction. Sonography is a good first choice, followed by retrograde pyelography if dilation of

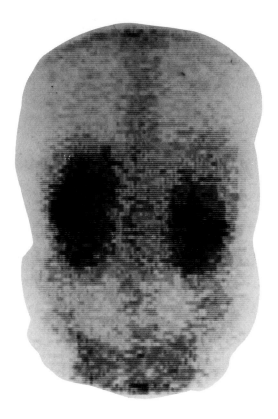

Figure 53-1. Gallium 67 scan of the kidneys demonstrating bilateral uptake in a patient with bilateral acute pyelonephritis.

the collecting system is shown. If sonography is normal, a
^{99m}Tc DTPA study should be performed.

Focal Renal or Perirenal Abscess. A focal renal abscess
may be suspected because fever fails to lyse on appropriate
antibiotics in 48–72 hours or because pyuria is minimal or
absent. These abscesses are best looked for by sonography
or CT (Figs. 53-2 and 52-3), sonography being preferable
because it is less expensive. Each of these techniques permits evaluation of the perirenal tissues, a common site of
abscess formation. Urography is usually not sufficiently
helpful to be required initially in the work-up; if, however,
the sonography is normal and complicated acute
pyelonephritis is still suspected, urography may disclose

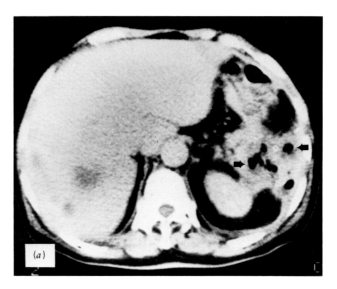

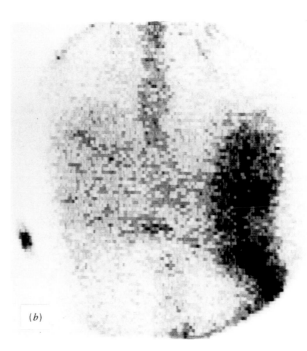

Figure 53-3. (a) CT section of a left perirenal abscess demonstrating multiple small pockets of air (arrows). The small focal radiolucencies in the liver are metastases from colon cancer. (b) This ^{67} Ga
scan demonstrates the extent of the inflammatory process.

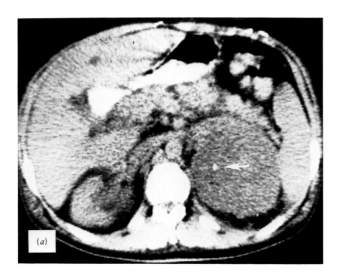

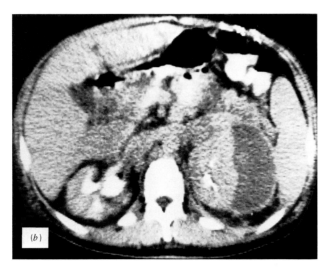

Figure 53-2. CT scan of the abdomen in a patient with a perirenal
abscess on the left side. (a) Section obtained before the injection of
intravenous contrast demonstrates a flank mass on the left containing a small focal calcification (arrow). (b) Section obtained after the
injection of intravenous contrast demonstrates the left kidney compressed by the perirenal abscess. (Courtesy N. Whitley, M.D., University of Maryland Hospital.)

an obstruction of the collecting system that sonography
has missed. In some patients with acute pyelonephritis,
the kidney parenchyma may be so swollen that collecting-
system distention cannot occur; in others, urine output
may be so low that there is insufficient urine to distend
the obstructed collecting system.

Emphysematous Pyelonephritis. Emphysematous pyelonephritis is an uncommon complication of acute pyelonephritis; it occurs in diabetic patients. In these patients, the

renal parenchyma is destroyed by the infection. Gas is present at the site of the destroyed kidney. The patients are usually moribund and most will die, though occasionally, thorough drainage of the renal bed may save the patient. Diagnosis can be made on a plain abdominal film by seeing gas within and around the kidney (Fig. 53-4). Sonography can also establish the diagnosis by showing multiple echogenic foci at the site of the kidney.

Keynotes

- *Imaging studies of the kidney are not needed in most patients with acute pyelonephritis.*
- *The acute complications of acute pyelonephritis are associated with ureteral obstruction or abscess formation.*
- *Suspect complicated acute pyelonephritis when*
  - *a. Pyuria is minimal or absent.*
  - *b. Ureteral colic preceded the onset of fever.*
  - *c. The fever does not lyse within 72 hours.*
  - *d. The patient has diabetic renal or vascular disease.*
- *Obstruction with urinary infection results in the formation of a large abscess. Fever is prolonged and renal damage may be extensive.*
- *Sloughing of a papilla is one of the forms of papillary necrosis. Papillary necrosis is associated with diabetes, infection, sickle cell disease, phenacetin, and renal infarction.*
- *Sonography is usually the safest and most sensitive method of detecting hydronephrosis. In the presence of severe renal infection, the collecting system may not dilate in response to ureteral obstruction, either because the kidney is too swollen or because urine output is too low to distend the calyces.*
- *The urogram does not adequately demonstrate the structures surrounding the kidney. Because the abscesses may be intrarenal or perirenal, sonography or CT imaging is preferred.*
- *In emphysematous pyelonephritis, gas produced by the infection spreads within and around the renal parenchyma. The kidney is severely damaged by this type of infection.*

CHRONIC PYELONEPHRITIS WITH VESICOURETERAL REFLUX

Chronic or recurrent pyelonephritis in a patient with reflux of urine from the bladder to the kidney has two different patterns depending on whether the patient is a child or an adult. The childhood form is more important.

Childhood Form

In the child, acute pyelonephritis can occur with or without reflux of urine from the bladder to the kidney. Those children who do not have reflux will almost always have a normal looking kidney following the resolution of the acute infection. Those children with reflux, however, will develop scarred kidneys and can develop renal failure if the condition is not recognized and treated.

The kidney affected both by acute infection and reflux will often have a decreased rate of growth in the regions affected, and some retractile scars may also form (Fig. 53-5). These scars can be differentiated from other renal indentations in several ways. Most of the time, the scar of reflux pyelonephritis lies directly over the calyx. Retrac-

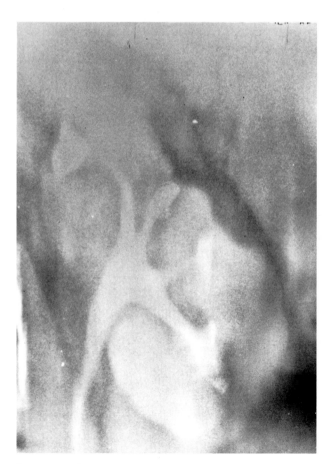

Figure 53-5. Focal scars of chronic pyelonephritis in a patient who had vesicoureteral reflux and pyelonephritis in childhood. The parenchymal scars overlie calyces that are blunted.

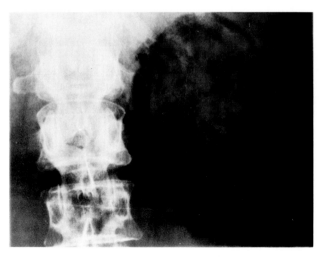

Figure 53-4. Emphysematous pyelonephritis. This focused view of the left flank demonstrates focal and streaklike collections of gas in and around the kidney.

tion and scarring of the parenchyma will deform the papillae, resulting in blunted or clubbed calyces.

The indentations of the renal margins that lie between the calyces are developmental variants. They occur because the kidney is a result of the fusion of a group of renal lobes. In the center of each lobe is the draining calyx. The indentations at the lines of fusion of the lobes, therefore, lie between calyces rather than opposite them. These indentations are called *fetal lobation* or *fetal lobulation*. *Renal infarcts* are usually broader scars that extend from one lobe to the one adjacent to it. They are thus wider than the indentations of fetal lobation.

In the child with recurrent episodes of reflux associated pyelonephritis, each episode scars the kidney more. When the scarring is sufficient to cause renal failure, focal hypertrophy of the kidney can occur. Those regions of the kidney that are not scarred overgrow and can displace calyces as though neoplastic masses were growing in the kidney (see Fig. 52-6). If there is any clinical suspicion of neoplasm, a ^{99m}Tc DMSA scan can be done to show that the mass has functioning renal tubular cells, indicating that it is benign.

This clinical entity of reflux associated pyelonephritis is important because it is a preventable cause of renal failure. In order for the scarring and eventual renal failure to occur, both infection and reflux must recur. If you prevent the reflux or prevent the infections, the renal scarring will not progress. For this reason, any child with a single episode of acute pyelonephritis should be investigated to discover whether the child also has vesicoureteral reflux. Usually this study is delayed until at least 6 weeks after the acute infection because some children will reflux during an episode of cystitis but not at other times. The time selected for obtaining the voiding cystourethrogram varies among institutions. In most, the voiding cystourethrogram is obtained 6–8 weeks after the acute infection has been treated. In others, the study is obtained at the time of the acute infection. Both techniques have good justification, and you should determine what the standard is in your institution.

Evaluation of the Child with Cystitis. The child with pyelonephritis should be evaluated after the first infection with both urography and voiding cystography. The evaluation of the child with cystitis is different. Because bladder infections in boys are unusual, evaluation is indicated after the first episode of infection. In girls, bladder infections are much more common; the usual opinion is that the evaluation should be made only after the second infection. There is, however, some disagreement on this last point, and some physicians will evaluate girls after the first episode of bladder infection.

For both boys and girls, the voiding cystogram is usually performed first. If no reflux is demonstrated, some radiologists will evaluate renal size and shape with sonography instead of IVU.

Demonstration of Vesicoureteral Reflux. There are two methods used for demonstrating the presence of vesicouret-

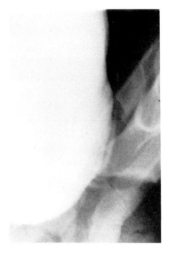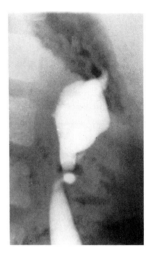

Figure 53-6. Two views of a voiding cystourethrogram obtained during fluoroscopy. The contrast was placed in the bladder via a catheter and is seen to reflux into the left kidney.

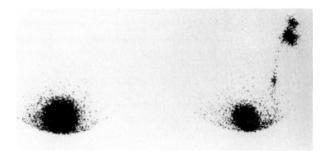

Figure 53-7. Views from a nuclear medicine–voiding cystogram. In the right-hand image, activity is seen in the left kidney, ureter, and bladder. (Courtesy D. Moses, M.D.)

eral reflux: voiding cystourethrography using a radiographic contrast medium (Fig. 53-6) and isotope-voiding bladder imaging (Fig. 53-7). In both tests, the urethra is catheterized and the agent is placed in the bladder. Serial images are made as the child voids. The major advantage of the isotope cystogram is that the radiation dose is much lower than with the radiographic cystogram. The major advantage of the radiographic cystogram is the demonstration of urethral anatomy. In girls, significant urethral abnormalities are unusual, and isotope cystography is thus preferred by some clinicians. In boys, urethral abnormalities are more common and are often discovered through urinary infections. For this reason, radiographic-voiding cystourethrography is preferable for boys for the initial evaluation and isotope cystography for follow-up evaluation if necessary.

Should a child have reflux and a history of acute urinary infection, several methods of treatment can be used: long-term antibiotic suppression of urinary infection or simple reimplantation of the refluxing ureter to prevent further reflux. In some children, reflux will stop as the child grows. This will usually occur by age 5, so, most of the time, children under age 5 are treated with suppressive antibiotics and those past 5 by surgery. There is much disagreement over what the correct management is, and different policies may be followed in your institution.

Adult Form

The adult with recurrent episodes of acute pyelonephritis who also has vesicoureteral reflux usually does not develop the scarring of the kidney seen in children with this disease. An occasional adult, however, will show the development of very similar scars, though usually not as deep or numerous as in children.

Keynotes

- *Recurrent renal infection can result in a severely scarred kidney when urine reflux from the bladder to the kidney is present and in little scarring when it is absent.*
- *The indentations in the margin of the kidney from chronic pyelonephritis are directly over the damaged calyx. Those from fetal lobation lie between the calyces. Those from renal infarcts are broad, deep scars.*
- *Focal areas of hypertrophy have occasionally been mistakenly removed on the suspicion of cancer. In a scarred kidney with a focal mass, the possibility of focal renal hypertrophy should be considered.*
- *Children with urinary infection should always be evaluated for the possibility of urine reflux. All children with pyelonephritis and boys with cystitis should be investigated after the first episode of infection. Girls with cystitis are usually investigated only after a second episode of infection.*

REPEATED PYELONEPHRITIS WITHOUT REFLUX

Most patients with acute pyelonephritis do not have urine reflux from the bladder to the kidney. In these patients, the scars that occur from infection are microscopic and cannot be identified on imaging studies. With each episode of infection, the kidney swells and then comes back to normal size. Repeated acute pyelonephritis usually does not result in the scarred kidneys seen in chronic pyelonephritis with reflux.

Keynote

- *To avoid confusion in terminology, you may call repeated episodes of pyelonephritis without reflux "recurrent acute pyelonephritis" and those with pyelonephritis with reflux and renal scarring "chronic pyelonephritis with reflux."*

SUMMARY

The evaluation of urinary infection is based on the site of infection (kidney or bladder), the age of the patient (child or adult), and preexisting disease (diabetes). Acute pyelonephritis usually requires no imaging in the adult. Only when a complication of acute pyelonephritis is suspected are imaging studies indicated. The child with acute urinary infection should have imaging studies to look for the possible presence of vesicoureteral reflux and renal anomalies and scars.

Complications of acute pyelonephritis should be suspected in the patient whose renal colic preceded the onset of fever, in the patient whose fever fails to lyse within 48–72 hours, and in the patient with diabetic renal or vascular disease.

The child with urinary infection and urine reflux from the bladder can develop a scarred kidney and eventually may develop renal failure. Each child should be evaluated with both urography and voiding cystourethrography after an episode of pyelonephritis. Boys should be evaluated after a single episode of cystitis, girls after two episodes.

Recurrent acute pyelonephritis unassociated with reflux usually does not result in a scarred kidney.

REVIEW QUESTIONS

1. Describe the role of imaging procedures in acute uncomplicated pyelonephritis.
2. What clinical features should indicate the possible presence of a complicated pyelonephritis?
3. What are the complications of acute pyelonephritis?
4. What is the difference between recurrent acute pyelonephritis and chronic pyelonephritis associated with vesicoureteral urine reflux?
5. How should the child with urinary infection be evaluated? What are the differences for bladder infection and renal infection? What are the differences in the evaluation of boys and girls?

VOCABULARY

emphysematous pyelonephritis	sloughed papillae
	ureteral colic
pyelonephritis	vesicoureteral reflux
pyuria	voiding cystourethrography

SUGGESTIONS FOR FURTHER READING

For suggested reading see Chapter 48.

54

RADIATION HAZARDS

KEY CONCEPTS

Radiological

There is insufficient data about the doses used in diagnostic imaging to judge the risk involved in radiation exposure accurately. Extrapolation from higher dose levels and other species suggests that there is a low degree of risk for the development of genetic damage and fetal damage at doses that are used in diagnostic imaging. The data relating low levels of radiation to the development of neoplasia are very limited.

Diagnostic imaging uses gamma and x-radiation for most examinations. Sound waves are used in sonography. Electromagnetic waves are used in MRI.

Radiation damage is caused both by direct hits inducing ionization and by producing free radicals that can react with other atoms.

Clinical

Counseling of a pregnant woman exposed to radiation is usually based on the Swedish rule, where the recommendation is based on the dose of radiation received by the fetus. This requires a calculated estimate of the dose received.

The best way for the clinician to limit the hazard of radiation is to eliminate unnecessary studies. The best way for the radiologist to limit radiation is by using the lowest amount that can yield the information required.

OBJECTIVES

When you complete this chapter you will be able to

1. List the types of radiation used in diagnostic imaging.

2. List the three potential types of radiation damage that might occur from the dose levels used in diagnostic imaging.

3. Discuss the Swedish rule and how it should be applied to patients whose fetuses received 0.5, 5, and 11 rads of radiation.

Large doses of radiation are harmful. Small doses, such as those used in diagnostic imaging, may or may not have a small risk to them. While experts debate whether there is a threshold dose below which radiation is safe, it is best to consider it potentially harmful but at a very low level of risk. In general, if a study using radiation is indicated on a clinical basis, the potential risk is so low that the study should be obtained. The only time special care is necessary is in the pregnant woman because, based on information from animal experimentation, the fetus is thought to be more likely to be damaged by a small amount of radiation than is the adult.

In general, it is abdominal irradiation that results in a significant exposure to the fetus. With nuclear medicine procedures, it is a combination of radiation from the mother's bladder with the possible transplacental passage of the radioactive isotope that can result in significant fetal exposure.

Keynotes

- *Though appropriate and complete data are not available, the radiation used in diagnostic imaging should be considered dangerous but with a low level of risk.*

- *The fetus is probably at increased risk of radiation damage compared with the adult.*

TYPES OF HAZARDS

There are three types of hazard that must be considered: the induction of neoplasia, genetic damage that will become manifest in future generations, and fetal damage.

There is no good evidence linking small amounts of radiation with neoplasia.

There is, based on extrapolation from higher doses, suggestive evidence that the radiation doses used in diagnostic radiology could induce genetic damage that would become detectable in future generations.

In experimental animals, fetal damage can be demonstrated at low doses, possibly at 10 rads, and definitely at 25 rads. These are close enough to the doses used in diagnostic radiology to arouse concern and caution.

Keynote

• *The three possible hazards of low doses of radiation are the induction of neoplasia, genetic damage, and fetal damage.*

DATA EXTRAPOLATION

Experimental data derived at the radiation doses used in diagnostic imaging is not available either in humans or animals. For this reason, risk estimates are based on extrapolation from animal experiments at moderately higher doses and from human exposures at much higher doses. There has been extensive discussion about which method of extrapolation should be used because the different methods proposed for extrapolation of the data would result in different risk levels.

Keynote

• *Risk estimates at the low doses used in diagnostic imaging are estimated by extrapolating from documented risks at higher doses and from other animal species.*

TYPES OF RADIATION

There are four types of radiation that can be encountered: gamma or x-radiation, beta radiation, alpha radiation, and neutron radiation. Of these only gamma and x-radiation are used in diagnostic imaging. Gamma and x-radiation have the longest path in and through the body and the lowest energy deposition.

Keynote

• *Gamma and x-radiation are the types of radiation used in diagnostic imaging.*

BASIS OF THE RADIATION EFFECT

Radiation induces detectable changes in tissues by injuring DNA. In some cases genes are damaged. In others chromosomal damage can prevent DNA replication and thus cell division or result in cell death. Cancer and genetic damage most likely are the result of gene damage. Fetal damage can be the result of gene damage or the failure of division of key progenitor cells. The basis of both types of change is radiation-induced ionization, in which the radiation displaces an electron from an atom or molecule. These ions then result in damage either because the ionization has occurred directly in the DNA or by the production of ions of non-DNA atoms (called free radicals) that then interact with DNA.

In some cases, it appears that more than one ionization may be necessary to have an effect. Some theorists propose that the induction of neoplasia may require DNA changes in several adjacent cells. DNA damage does not always result in genetic abnormalities. Many sites of DNA damage are in noncritical regions of chromosomes. In some cases intracellular DNA repair mechanisms repair the damage.

In the developing fetus, radiation can cause a malformation either by inducing a genetic change or by interfering with the division of a few progenitor cells, cells that are critical to the development of an organ or part of an organ.

Keynote

• *Radiation induces its damage by ionization of DNA and by the production of free radicals that can react with other DNA.*

TYPICAL DOSE LEVELS

Most imaging studies uses doses of less than 1 rad. There are several that use up to 3 rads. Computed tomography examinations are usually less than 5 rads. Multiple studies in a short period of time are probably addititive.

LEVEL OF RISK

The level of risk is debated. The best attitude to have is that the risk is low, but real, and thus to avoid unnecessary exposures. With the fetus, because data is lacking, the Swedish rule is often followed. This approach uses critical decision doses of 1 and 10 rads and requires an accurate estimate of the radiation, the patient receives. The patient whose IVP is shown in Figure 54-1 can serve as an example.

What do you see in Figure 54-1? An IVU, and the woman is pregnant.

What should you do? Advise her to have an abortion? Ignore the risk? What?

What should be done is to estimate the dose the fetus

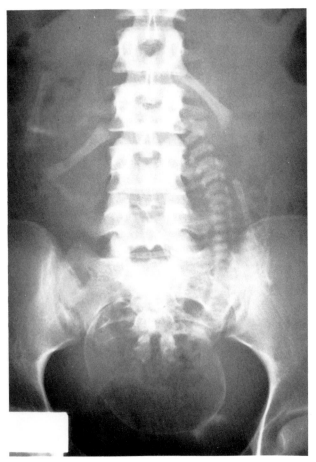

Figure 54-1. This one-film IVU was performed because this pregnant woman developed ureteral colic. The urinary system is visualized and is mildly dilated as a result of the pregnancy. The fetal bones are easily seen within the abdomen.

received. To do this, a radiation physicist or radiation safety officer calculates the dose based on the number of films, the size of the films, the part of the body irradiated, the settings or probable settings on the machine, the type of machine, and the approximate energy distribution of the x-ray beam.

In this case, the radiologist knew the patient was pregnant and obtained only the one film. The dose was calculated at 0.68 rads.

Is this a critical dose?

If you follow the Swedish rule:

A dose of less than 1 rad calls for reassuring the patient.

A dose of 1–10 rads calls for careful genetic counseling.

A dose greater than 10 rads calls for working with a genetic counselor and usually recommending a theraputic abortion.

Thus, with a dose calculated at 0.68 rads, this patient should be reassured that the risk is very low.

Keynotes

- An evaluation of the radiation hazard to an individual should be based on a calculated estimate of the dose received.
- The Swedish rule is used to decide what to tell a pregnant woman about the risk from the radiation her fetus has received.

RECOMMENDATIONS

With the many uncertainties concerning whether there is a risk and, if there is, how much, the recommended policy is:

1. Don't do unnecessary studies.
2. Limit the radiation used in each study to the minimum that will yield valid information.
3. If the patient is pregnant, use sonography if possible; limit the number of films taken, if possible.

Keynote

- The best way to limit radiation exposure is to eliminate unnecessary studies and to limit the amount of radiation used with each study.

SUMMARY

The data to indicate whether or not the low doses used in diagnostic imaging are harmful are not available. Decisions must therefore be made based on extrapolations from exposures at higher doses and in different animal species. Based on what is known, the extrapolations suggest that there is probably a delayed genetic effect that will be manifest in future generations and that there is a potential for fetal damage. It is therefore advisable to limit patients' radiation by following the recommendations in this chapter.

REVIEW QUESTIONS

1. What are the three potential hazards of low doses of radiation?
2. What is the usual range of doses of diagnostic imaging examinations?
3. What would you tell a pregnant patient who needed an x-ray study?
4. What types of radiation are used in diagnostic imaging.
5. What are free radicals?
6. What is the Swedish rule? How is it applied?
7. How can you avoid having your patient exposed to excess doses of radiation?

VOCABULARY

alpha radiation	ionization
beta radiation	neutron radiation
extrapolation	rad
free radicals	x-radiation
gamma radiation	

SUGGESTIONS FOR FURTHER READING

Merle K. Loken. Low level radiation: Biological effects. *CRC Critical Reviews in Diagnostic Imaging,* **19:**175–202, 1983.

Committe on the Biological Effects of Ionizing Radiations. *The Effects on Populations of Exposure to Low Levels of Ionizing Radiation: 1980.* National Academy Press: Washington, D.C. 1980.

PART 5

THE SKELETAL SYSTEM

In many radiology departments, examinations of the skeletal system constitute 20–30% of the examinations. The skeleton can be evaluated with conventional radiography, nuclear medicine bone scans, and CT. Bone stops the sound waves of ultrasound, preventing its use. Bone produces only a minimal response of signal in MRI; the bone marrow, however, produces a strong MRI signal, so magnetic resonance may come to have an important clinical role in evaluating the bone marrow.

The next five chapters discuss the imaging of the skeletal system. Chapter 55 is an introduction to skeletal anatomy and physiology. Chapter 56 gives an approach to the evaluation of fractures. Chapter 57 surveys processes that result in the destruction and production of bone. Chapters 58 and 59 discuss the applications of imaging to arthritis, first from the viewpoint of the clinician and then from the vantage of the radiologist.

55

THE SKELETAL SYSTEM: INTRODUCTION

KEY CONCEPTS

Radiological

An accurate interpretation of bone images often requires that you evaluate both the physiology and anatomy reflected in the image. In the child, bone growth is more rapid that in the adult, with growth occurring at the growth plate and under the periosteum. In the adult, bone continues to be active; there is a slow turnover of bone and a slow expansion of the diameter of the bone. Changes occur slowly unless incited to activity by an injury.

The child's bone consists of four parts: the epiphysis (at the end of the bone), the growth plate, the metaphysis (the flare), and the diaphysis (the shaft). Adult bone is similar but lacks the growth plate. Structurally, bone consists of an outer cortex of compact bone and an inner medulla consisting of plates of bone called *trabeculae*. Disease can affect any of these structures.

Surrounding the cortex of the diaphysis and metaphysis is a layer of tissue that can form bone, the periosteum. The periosteum normally produces bone slowly, but when activated by disease, it can produce bone rapidly. The pattern of periosteal-produced new bone reflects the rate at which the bone is formed.

OBJECTIVES

When you complete this chapter you will be able to

1. Identify on selected radiographs and bone scans the epiphysis, growth plate, metaphysis, and diaphysis.
2. Identify patterns of active periosteal bone formation.
3. List three patterns of abnormality in the epiphysis, three patterns of disease in the growth plate, and three patterns of disease in the metaphysis.
4. List three causes of transverse white lines in the metaphysis.

The diseases of the skeletal system can be divided into those of bone, joints, muscles, nerves, and vessels. In this book only the diseases of bone and joints are discussed. Conventional radiographic techniques can provide information about bone and joint anatomy and physiology. Nuclear medicine scans with ^{99m}Tc phosphate complexes show regions of new bone deposition and help in finding regions of abnormally increased bone turnover. Nuclear medicine imaging with sodium pertechnetate Tc 99m phosphate complexes can show regions of hyperemia and can image the synovial inflammation in the inflammatory arthritides. Nuclear medicine imaging with gallium citrate Ga 67 can demonstrate regions of soft tissue, bone, or joint infection. The transmission computed tomogram can be used to image the muscles, soft tissues, and bones of the pelvis and extremities. It is most useful in evaluating the bones of the pelvis, scapula, and the sternoclavicular joints.

Because the structure of bone changes slowly, it is all too easy to think of bone as a static tissue, unchanging and fixed. Bone, however, responds to the stresses placed upon it by normal activity and by diseases in predictable and repetitive patterns. It is the challenge of the bone radiologist to decipher the pattern, deduce the physiological response that the bone is making, and then diagnose the process that is inciting this pathophysiological change. The evaluation of the bone image requires a knowledge of both normal bone physiology and normal bone anatomy.

Keynote

• *The evaluation of bone disease on imaging studies is based on the analysis of bone physiology and anatomy.*

NORMAL BONE PHYSIOLOGY

In the Child

In the child, active growth is present. This growth occurs at two places, along the growth plate and adjacent to the periosteum. During periods of rapid growth, changes in the length of the bone can be seen on films taken at monthly intervals. The bone deposition at the periosteal surface progresses more slowly, and changes can be seen only at intervals of many months. Studied by ^{99m}Tc phosphate complex bone scans, active deposition of bone is shown as focal increased activity at the sites of the growth plates (Fig. 55-1).

In the Adult

In the adult there is a continuous turnover of bone: bone is slowly and continuously removed and replaced. The trabecular bone tends to be replaced more slowly than it is formed, so that the trabeculae become more widely separated with increasing age. (Fig. 55-2a and b). The cortical bone tends to be resorbed slowly on its internal (endosteal) side and to be slowly replaced on its periosteal side so that the diameter of the bone increases with increasing age. If studied by radiographic technique, little change is seen from film to film from year to year; changes are only seen when films are viewed over several years. Images made with ^{99m}Tc phosphate complexes show minimal uptake and activity in all bones (Fig. 55-2c).

Keynotes

- *In the child, bone growth takes place both at the growth plate and under the periosteum. These sites of growth can be seen on radiographs and bone scans.*
- *There is a continuous, normal, slow replacement of bone resulting in a slow change in the appearance of bones throughout life.*
- *The slow replacement of bone results in minimal bone activity on ^{99m}Tc phosphate complex bone scans.*

NORMAL BONE ANATOMY

In the Child

The child's bone can be divided into four parts (Fig. 55-3):

1. Epiphysis
2. Growth plate
3. Metaphysis
4. Shaft

Each of these has its characteristic appearance on the radiograph. In addition, each of these sections of the bone (except for the growth plate) is divided into

1. Cortex
2. Medulla

The *cortex* is the outer portion of the bone; the *medulla*, the inner portion. These are the portions of the bone that can be evaluated in all normal children.

In addition, outside the *cortex* but lining its surface in both the metaphysis and shaft is a thin layer of fibrous tissue, the periosteum. The periosteum is normally invisible because it is of water radiodensity and blends with the overlying layer of muscle, which is also of water radiodensity. Periosteum lifted from the surface of the bone will, however, promptly form a layer of new bone, and this new periosteal-formed bone will be visible. Periosteal new bone is normal in the child 3–12 months of age (Fig. 55-4), when it can be seen because of rapid growth. At other ages, visible periosteal-formed bone that is separated from the cortex is always abnormal.

In the Adult

The bone in the adult differs from that in the child in that growth has ceased and the water-radiodensity portion of

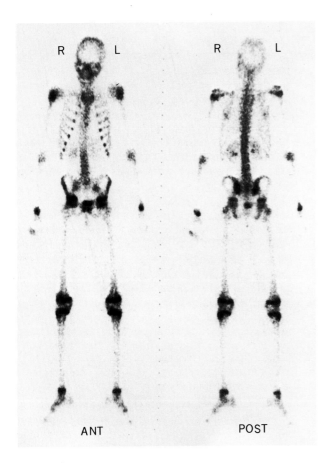

Figure 55-1. A ^{99m}Tc phosphate complex nuclear medicine bone scan in a normal 9-year-old child. Increased activity is seen in the growth centers.

the growth plate is no longer there (Fig. 55-1*a*). In most patients, the calcified portion of the growth plate also disappears, but in a few it remains as a 1-mm-thick line of radiodensity (Fig. 55-5). The adult bone is divided into

1. Epiphysis
2. Metaphysis
3. Shaft

Keynotes

- *The child's bone consists of four parts: the epiphysis, the growth plate, the metaphysis, and the shaft. Each has a characteristic normal appearance that can be changed by disease.*
- *The cortex is the outer shell of bone in which bone is densely formed. The medulla is the inner portion of the bone and consists of more widely spaced plates of bone separated by bone marrow.*
- *A single lamella (or line) of periosteal-formed bone running almost parallel to the cortical surface is normal in the young child (aged 3–12 months). At other ages, visible lines of periosteal-formed bone are indicative of disease.*
- *The adult's bone consists of three parts: the epiphysis, the metaphysis, and the shaft.*

EPIPHYSIS

The *epiphysis* is an articulating end of a bone where growth occurs or has occurred.

Defining Characteristics

1. Presence of an appropriate amount of ossification for the age of the patient
2. Number of ossification centers
3. Regular margin
4. Aligned with shaft of bone
5. Thickness of surrounding rim of ossification and calcification

Basis of Abnormalities

1. Delayed or accelerated appearance of ossification centers in metabolic disturbances. Bone age of patient can be calculated using reference books.
2. Increased number of ossification centers in certain congenital diseases. Fragmentation of ossification centers in Legg-Perthes disease.
3. Irregular margin in injuries, in Legg-Perthes disease, and as a normal variation.
4. Displacement of an epiphysis in a fracture. An eccentric epiphysis can be a normal variation.
5. Increased thickness of the surrounding rim of ossification in scurvy and lead poisoning; decreased thickness in rickets.

The child's epiphysis is formed of cartilage in the fetus. Most of the epiphyses are still cartilaginous at birth. Because cartilage is of water radiodensity, its structure usually cannot be identified and separated from the surrounding muscles. As the child grows, the epiphyses develop regions of ossification within them (Fig. 55-6*a*, *b* and *c*).

Most epiphyses develop only one center of ossification, but occasionally an epiphysis may develop several. Multiple small foci of ossification may appear during the earliest stage of epiphyseal ossification. Each epiphysis has its own expected age of development. Standard references give the ages for the development of epiphyses. Marked delay in the development of the epiphyses may be due to malnutrition, rickets, or hypothyroidism. Delay of the ossification of the proximal femoral epiphysis beyond the age of 1 year may be due to congenital subluxation or dislocation of the hip.

An injury may displace an epiphysis. If the epiphysis is still cartilaginous, the displacement may be very difficult to recognize.

The ossification center of the epiphysis is usually smooth and regular in its margin; however, the lateral portion of the acetabular roof and the medial and lateral femoral condyles are usually irregular in margin in late childhood (Fig. 55-7).

Keynotes

- *The epiphysis is the end of the bone where it articulates with another bone and where growth occurs or has occurred.*
- *The main patterns of epiphyseal abnormality are (1) delayed or accelerated formation of the centers, (2) fragmentation of the centers, (3) irregularity, (4) fractures and displacements, and (5) surrounding ring(s) of increased radiodensity.*
- *Some epiphyses are ossified at birth; others develop ossification as the child grows.*

GROWTH PLATE

The *growth plate*, also known as *epiphyseal plate* and *physis*, is the site of growth that adds to the length of bone; growth occurs by enchondral bone formation (cartilage maturing and being replaced by bone).

Defining Characteristics

1. Two portions (Fig. 55-8).
   a. Water radiodensity (radiolucent) band adjacent to the epiphysis.
   b. Thin layer of radiodense calcified cartilage adjacent to the metaphysis. This merges on radiographs with a thin metaphyseal white line of cartilage-cored trabeculae (called *primary trabeculae*).

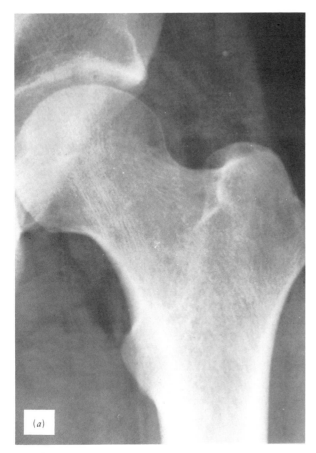
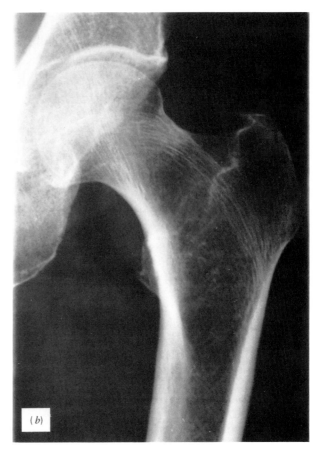

Figure 55-2

2. Width of the water-radiodensity cartilage: thickness varies with age of patient and the bone radiographed (Fig. 55-6a, b, and c and 55-8).

3. Presence of the line of radiodense calcified cartilage.

4. Width of the radiodense line of calcified cartilage.

Basis of Abnormalities

1. Narrowing of the zone of water-radiodensity (from injury, infection, or normal aging)

2. Widening of the zone of water-radiodensity cartilage (from rickets or renal failure)

3. Absence of the line of calcified cartilage (from rickets or renal failure)

4. Widening of the line of calcified cartilage and the adjacent metaphyseal white line of cartilage-cored trabeculae (from scurvy or lead poisoning)

5. Fragmentation of the line of calcified cartilage (from scurvy or injury)

The growth plate is composed of cartilage and calcified cartilage (Fig. 55-8). The cartilaginous portion (the portion closest to the epiphysis) is of water radiodensity and blends in radiodensity with the adjacent muscle. The calcified portion of cartilage appears as a white line along the metaphyseal side of the growth plate. Its thickness is greater in children exposed to much sunlight than in those who are not. Thus, the pictures shown are appropriate for a temperate climate such as Baltimore. In northern climates, the zone of calcification may be thinner; in tropical climates it will usually be a little thicker.

Several important diseases affect the appearance of the growth plate. Rickets, scurvy, poisoning with lead or phosphorus, and fractures can all affect the growth plate. Thus it is important that its structure be understood.

Width

The growth plate is widest in young children and decreases in width throughout childhood and into the teenage years (Fig. 55-6a, b, and c and 55-8). The plate is thickest in areas that grow more—thus at the knee, shoulder, and wrist. Infection or fractures may cause the plate to close too early, and with growth stopped, deformity will occur. Comparison with the other side of the body is always quite helpful.

In rickets, the water-radiodensity portion of the growth plate is thickened, the metaphysis is often cupped, and the white line is absent (Fig. 55-9). The calcified portion of the growth plate is thickened in scurvy (Fig. 55-10) and in lead poisoning (Fig. 55-11).

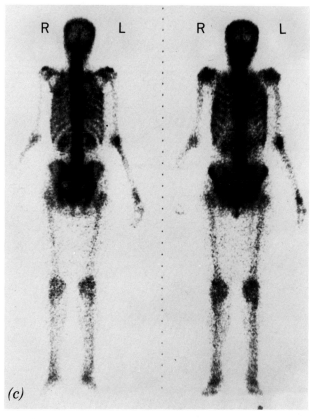

(c)

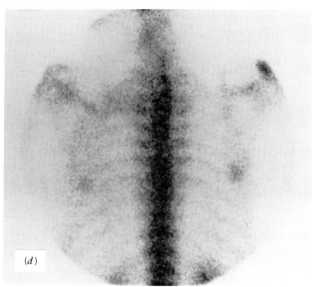

(d)

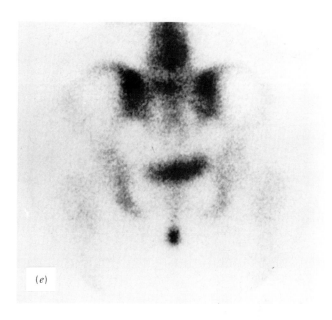

(e)

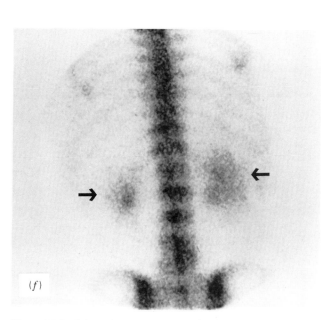

(f)

Figure 55-2. Selected views of normal bones. (*a*) The normal proximal femur at age 27. (*b*) The same bone at age 73. In the younger bone, the trabeculae (the white lines within the bone) are closely spaced and extend into the shaft of the bone. In the older bone, many of the trabeculae have been resorbed, and those that remain are preserved along the lines of major stress within the bone and may be slightly thickened. (*c*) 99mTc phosphate complex nuclear medicine bone scan, normal posterior view. Activity is seen in all the bones. (*d*) Posterior view of the upper rib cage and thoracic spine. (*e*) Posterior view of the pelvis. Activity is also seen in the bladder. (*f*) Posterior view of the thoracolumbar spine, with tracer activity in the kidneys (arrows) reflecting tracer excretion by the kidneys. Views *d*, *e*, and *f* are gamma camera images. This machine records images of smaller portions of the body.

Keynotes

- *The growth plate is a site of bone growth and lies between the epiphysis and metaphysis. At this site, bone growth develops by enchondral bone formation (by the growth of cartilage and then the replacement of that cartilage by bone).*

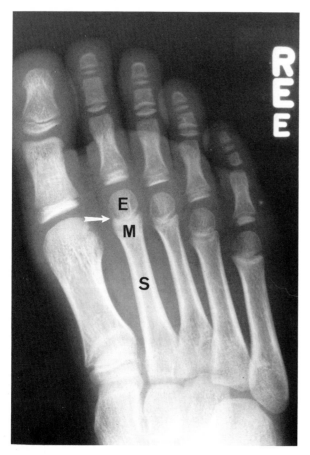

Figure 55-3. A normal forefoot of a child. E = epiphysis, arrow = growth plate, M = metaphysis, S = shaft.

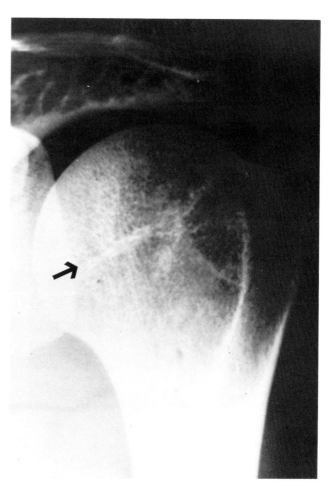

Figure 55-5. View of the proximal left humerus showing a residual white line (arrow) of the child's growth plate persisting into adulthood.

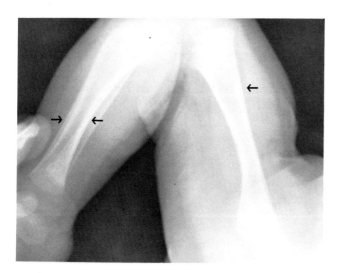

Figure 55-4. Physiological (normal) periosteal reaction of the young child. This 4-month-old has a thin line of periosteal new bone (arrows) along the shafts of the tibia and femur. Linear periosteal new bone is a normal finding between the ages of 3 and 12 months.

- *The patterns of abnormality of the growth plate include (1) narrowing or widening of the cartilage space, (2) absence of the white line of calcified cartilage, (3) widening of the white line of calcified cartilage and the adjacent metaphyseal white line of cartilage-cored trabeculae, and (4) fragmentation of the white line of calcified cartilage.*
- *Longitudinal bone growth may be limited if an infection or a fracture results in early closure of the growth plate.*
- *In rickets, the growth plate will be widened, the white line will be thinned or absent, and often the metaphyseal bone will have a cup shape.*
- *In lead poisoning in children, the white line of the growth plate and of the cartilage-cored trabeculae of the metaphysis will be thickened. Often flecks of lead (from lead paint) can be seen in the colonic feces on abdominal films.*

METAPHYSIS

The *metaphysis*, also known as the *zone of remodeling, zone of flare,* and *cutback zone,* is the portion of the bone

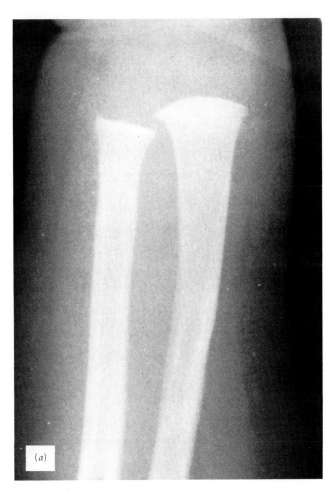 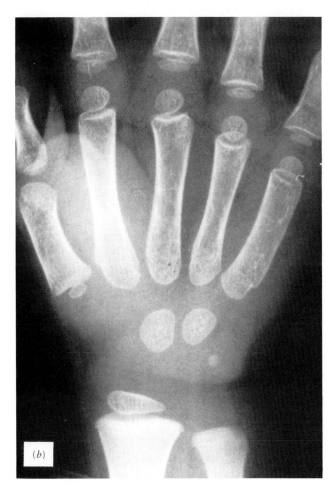

Figure 55-6. AP view of a normal child's wrist. (*a*) At 4 months of age. (*b*) At 2 years of age. (*c*) At 8 years of age. Note the progressive ossification of the carpal bones and the progressive narrowing of the growth plate.

between the growth plate or the epiphysis and the shaft of the bone, in other words, the flared portion of the bone.

Defining Characteristics

1. Angle of the flare
2. Pattern of the trabecular bone

Basis of Abnormalities

1. Decreased flare; triangular metaphysis (from thalassemia, Gaucher's disease, or prolonged lack of use)
2. Increased flare (from osteogenesis imperfecta or healed rickets)
3. Decreased trabecular bone (from osteopenia)
4. Focal absence of trabecular bone (from variation, osteomyelitis, or tumor)
5. Irregular trabecular bone (from Paget's disease)
6. Lines crossing the metaphysis (from leukemia, neuroblastoma, or after an illness)
7. Increased trabecular bone (from osteopetrosis)

The metaphysis, or zone of remodeling, is the portion of the bone that flares outward. The amount of flaring (trumpeting) is decreased (i.e., the margins of the metaphysis are triangular rather than trumpet shaped) in thalassemia, Gaucher's disease, and Pyle's disease (Figs. 55-12 and 55-13). The trumpeting is increased in some patients with osteogenesis imperfecta, in some patients with hemophilia, and in some with juvenile polyarthritis.

The cortex of the metaphysis varies in thickness. It is thinnest near the growth plate and wider as it merges into the cortex of the shaft (Fig. 55-12). The cortex is thinnest where the diameter of the bone is greatest, thickest where the bone diameter is least.

The bone in the medulla is composed of plates of bone called *trabeculae* that on radiographs appear to be lines. In most bones, the lines originate along the entire width of the calcified portion of the growth plate and then run gently toward the periphery of the metaphysis. In normal bone, the trabeculae decrease in number from the growth plate to the diaphysis, and in adults few trabeculae are seen in the medullary canal of the diaphysis.

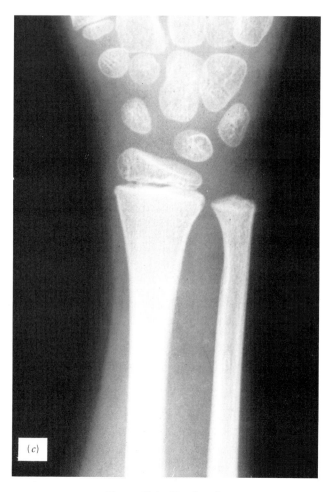

Figure 55-6. (Continued).

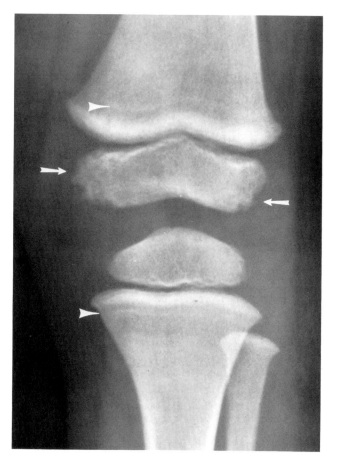

Figure 55-7. AP view of a normal knee at age 5. The irregularity of the distal femoral epiphysis (arrows) is normal. The faint white lines (arrowheads) parallel to the growth plate are a variant called "post–growth-arrest lines." The growth arrest occurs during childhood illnesses. The lines become visible as growth resumes, moving the white line into the metaphysis.

Keynotes

- *The metaphysis is the flared portion of the bone, where the diameter of the bone changes from the wider diameter of the epiphysis to the narrower diameter of the shaft. In the child, the narrowing takes places through active bone removal and replacement.*
- *The degree of flaring of the metaphysis can be increased or decreased in disease.*
- *The width of the cortical bone in the metaphysis is thickest where the diameter of bone is least, thinnest where the diameter of the bone is greatest.*

SHAFT

The *shaft,* also known as the *diaphysis,* is the central portion of the bone, where the walls are roughly parallel. There is little trabecular bone in the medullary portion of the shaft.

CORTEX

Thickness

The thickness of the cortex varies with the diameter of the bone. It is thin when the diameter of the bone is wide and thick when it is narrow. The cortex of the shaft, like the metaphysis, can be affected both by age and by disease. The thickness of the cortex is greatest in the teenager and progressively decreases with increasing age. When the cortex is thinner than usual for any age, osteopenia (decreased bone) is present. The usual cause of osteopenia that thins the cortex is osteoporosis. The cortex is thicker than normal when it is continuously stressed. It is thicker in the laborer than in the office worker.

Margin

The margin of the cortex is usually smooth. Rough, irregular margins can be seen, however, along the attachments

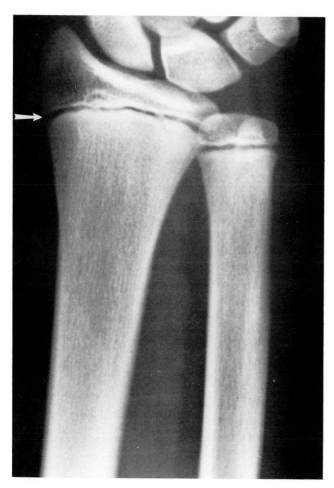

Figure 55-8. AP view of distal radius at 12 years of age. The blacker line (arrow) crossing the bone is the epiphyseal plate.

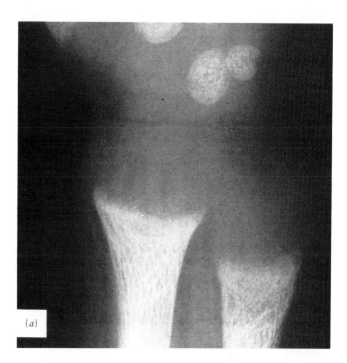

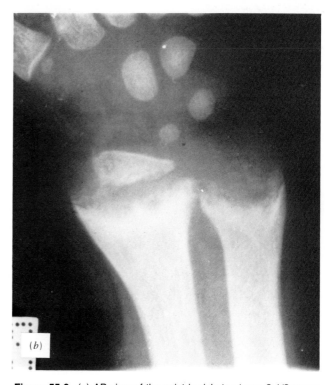

Figure 55-9. (a) AP view of the wrist in rickets at age 2 1/2 years. The cuplike shape of the metaphysis and the absence of its white line are seen. (Courtesy, Pediatric Radiology Teaching File, Johns Hopkins.) (b) AP view of the wrist in a 4-year-old child with rickets. The growth plate is widened (compare with Fig. 55-6b and c), and there is absence of the white line in the metaphysis.

of ligaments and tendons. These irregularities of surface are greatest along the posterior margin of the femur, along the lateral margin of the tibia, and along a portion of the lateral margin of the upper humerus at the insertion of the deltoid muscle (Fig. 55-14).

In other locations, an irregular thick cortex usually means that infection is or was present (Fig. 55-15) or that the patient has Paget's disease (Fig. 55-16).

Corticomedullary Junction

The cortex should be distinct from the medulla. When the cortex of the bone is of almost the same radiodensity as the medullary portion of bone, disease is usually present. When the radiodensity is the same in cortex and medulla, but overall normal or of increased radiodensity, myelofibrosis with myelosclerosis is probably present (Fig. 55-17). When the density of cortex and medulla is about the same but the overall density is decreased, osteomalacia or rickets is probably present. The renal osteodystrophy associated with renal failure can result in equal density of both

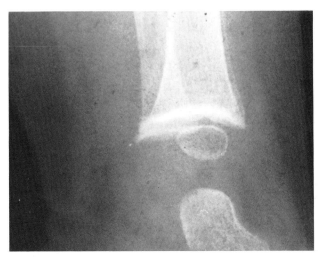

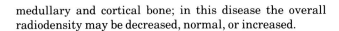

medullary and cortical bone; in this disease the overall radiodensity may be decreased, normal, or increased.

MEDULLARY BONE

The lines of the trabeculae of the medullary bone in general run from the epiphysis in the adult or from the physis of the child and gently spread outward to merge with the cortex of the metaphysis. There are very few trabeculae in the medullary portion of the diaphysis. A few thinner trabeculae run transversely from trabeculum to trabeculum. With increasing age, the number of these transverse trabeculae decreases and the thickness of the trabeculae running in the long axis of the bone increases (Fig. 55-1a and b). Trabeculae that lie in the direction of the stress applied to the bone are thick. Trabeculae perpendicular to the direction of stress are usually thin.

Disoriented trabeculae that are both thin and thick, but positioned in random directions, are usually from Paget's disease (Fig. 55-16). The trabeculae in the epiphysis and metaphysis can be absent when they are destroyed by disease. Usually the disease that destroys them is ei-

Figure 55-10. Lateral view of the ankle in a young child with scurvy. The white line of the distal tibial metaphysis is thickened, and the bone is osteoporotic. The white line around the epiphysis is also thickened. (Courtesy Pediatric Radiology Teaching File, Johns Hopkins.)

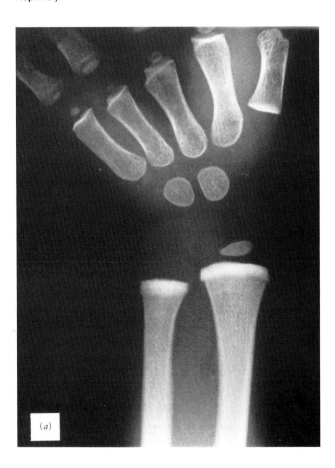

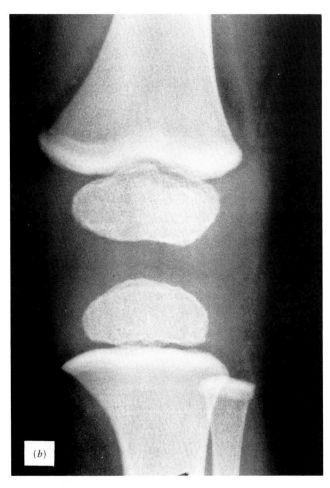

Figure 55-11. Lead poisoning. The white line of the metaphysis is thickened. Several flecks of radiopaque lead paint are seen in the colon (arrows) of this 2 1/2-year-old child. (a) An AP view of the wrist. (b) An AP view of the knee. (c) An AP view of the abdomen.

ther infection or cancer. Because they are so thin, the loss of calcium that occurs may be quite difficult to detect until much bone is lost. In general, a loss of bone 2 cm in diameter must be present before the bone loss can be seen.

Nuclear medicine imaging techniques will detect a cold region at sites of trabecular loss, but this usually must be 2 cm in diameter to be seen. Most of the time, however, processes destroying trabecular bone will also result in the deposition of new bone. Tracer imaging is a most sensitive method of detecting this new bone deposition, and these sites of new bone deposition will show as a hot region on the bone scan (Fig. 55-18).

Lines in the Metaphysis or Shaft

Transverse white lines in the medullary portion of the metaphysis or shaft of the bone are normal only when they do not involve the cortex. Transverse lines limited to the medullary portion of bone (see Fig. 55-7) are due to previous illness that occurred many months or years before. These are common and occur in most people. Transverse white or dark lines crossing both the medullary and cortical bone are always a sign of disease. They can represent

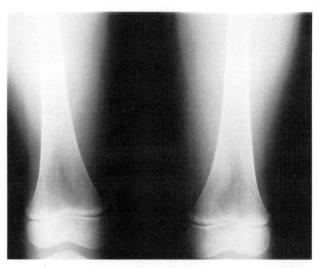

Figure 55-12. AP view of both distal femurs, normal appearance.

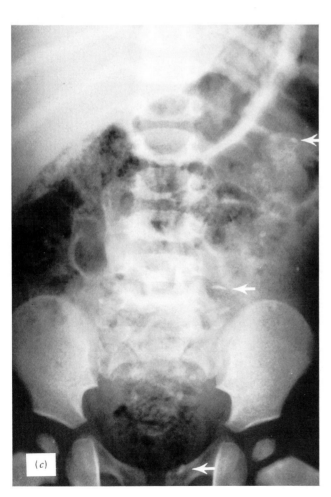

Figure 55-11. (Continued).

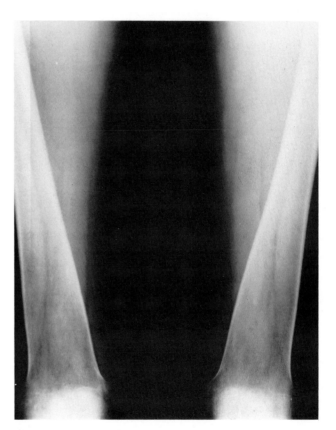

Figure 55-13. AP view of both distal femurs in a patient with Gaucher's disease. The metaphyses are wider and less trumpet shaped.

impacted fractures, healed or healing fractures, or stress fractures (see Chapter 56).

Radiolucent oblique lines through the cortex in the metaphysis or shaft can be due to the channels through

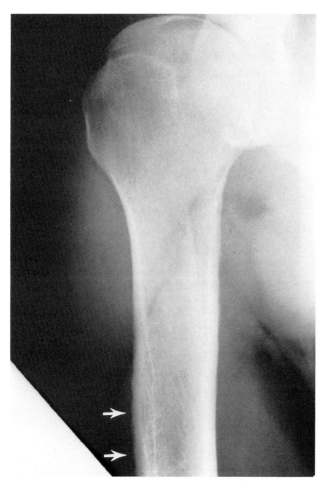

Figure 55-14. The normal irregularity (arrows) of the cortex at the insertion of the deltoid muscle into the shaft of the humerus.

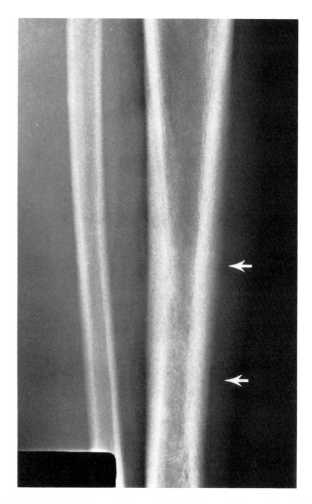

Figure 55-15. The irregularity and indistinctness of the anterior tibial cortex (arrows) is indicative of osteomyelitis.

which blood enters the medulla (Fig. 55-19). They can usually be identified because they are directed away from the faster growing epiphysis (away from wrist, shoulder, and knee) and on close observation have smooth margins with a very slight increase in radiodensity along those margins. This slightly radiodense margin often extends into the medullary canal.

Keynotes

- *The shaft of the bone is its midportion where the cortical walls are roughly parallel.*
- *Osteopenia means decreased bone mass. It implies bone loss caused by osteoporosis, osteomalacia, or hyperparathyroidism. Because it can be difficult to distinguish these three causes of bone loss on radiographs, the term osteopenia is used to describe all three processes.*
- *Most of the outer margin of the cortex is smooth; the cortex can, however, have irregularities at the sites of tendon and ligament insertions. Although these irregularities are usually small ones,*

- *larger areas of tendon insertion irregularity are seen in the lateral humeral cortex and the posterior aspect of the femur.*
- *The corticomedullary junction is usually distinct on radiographs because of the different amounts of bone in the cortex and medulla. Indistinctness of this junction occurs in diseases in which the amounts of bone are more similar. Diseases that decrease the bone in the cortex (such as rickets and osteomalacia) as well as diseases that increase the amount of medullary bone (such as renal osteodystrophy, myelosclerosis, and extensive bone infarction) can result in an indistinct corticomedullary junction.*
- *As bone becomes osteopenic, those trabeculae in major areas of stress will persist longer than those subject to less stress.*
- *Processes that destroy bone trabeculae will usually be detected earlier by nuclear medicine bone scanning than by radiography.*
- *White lines crossing only the medullary portion of the metaphysis are common and of no current clinical significance. They are due to previous disease that briefly interrupted bone growth; they are therefore called post–growth-arrest lines, or more simply, Park's lines, after an early describer.*
- *Vascular grooves are normal oblique lines running through the cortex; care should be taken not to confuse them with fractures.*

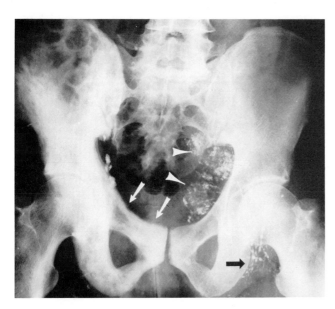

Figure 55-16. Paget's disease is present in the right hemipelvis. The cortex is thickened and irregular (white arrows), and the trabecular pattern is irregular. The patient has had a lymphangiogram, and several lymph nodes (white arrowheads) are partially filled with contrast. Several lymphatic channels are also demonstrated (black arrow).

PERIOSTEAL BONE

The periosteum covers most of the outer margin of the cortex and is absent only within joints and at site of tendon and ligament insertion. The periosteum is of water radiodensity and cannot be separated from the shadow of the surrounding muscle. The bone that is formed by the periosteum *can* be seen; it is this bone that is searched for on the radiograph.

The cortical bone of the diaphysis in a child and of the diaphysis and metaphysis in an adult is largely the result of periosteal bone formation. The periosteum continuously forms a small amount of bone throughout life. This normal periosteal new bone is continuous with the cortical bone, and no space of separation can be identified.

Periosteal Bone in Disease

Periosteal bone resulting from disease is separated from the margin of the cortex by a zone of water radiolucency. It results when the periosteum is lifted off the cortex by disease. The pattern of this periosteal new bone (periosteal reactive bone) is determined by the speed at which the periosteum is lifted from the bone and the time that the periosteum has remained at each potential position. It takes approximately 14 days for the periosteal bone to be abundant enough to be seen on a radiograph; it can be seen on bone scanning in 2–3 days. Bone scanning is thus more sensitive for the detection of early periosteal new bone.

The radiograph, however, permits the differentiation of

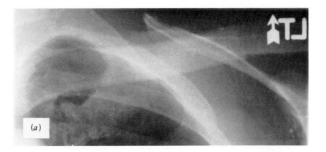

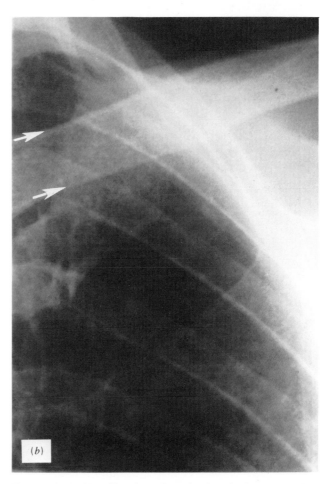

Figure 55-17. Myelofibrosis and myelosclerosis demonstrated in the clavicle. (*a*) The clavicle in this patient with myelofibrosis demonstrates an almost uniform radiodensity with the cortical margin almost merging into the medullary shadow. (*b*) A normal clavicle is shown for comparison. The clavicle in this older patient demonstrates the changes of osteoporosis with thin cortices; however, the corticomedullary junction (arrows) is detectable.

the pattern of periosteal new bone. A single thin layer of periosteal new bone (Fig. 55-20) is the earliest detectable periosteal new bone. It results from a single displacement of the periosteum. Once present, two things can happen to it. If the process that has elevated the periosteum has been

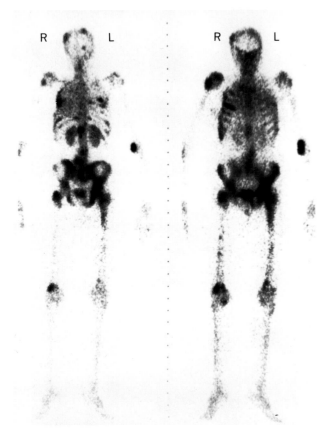

Figure 55-18. A bone scan obtained in a patient with metastatic breast cancer demonstrates many areas of increased and asymmetric activity. These areas demonstrate the active formation of bone made in response to the metastases.

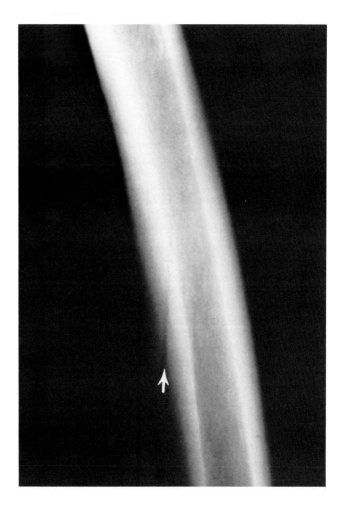

Figure 55-19. The normal vascular groove (arrow) of the femur is seen running obliquely through the cortex. It should not be confused with a fracture.

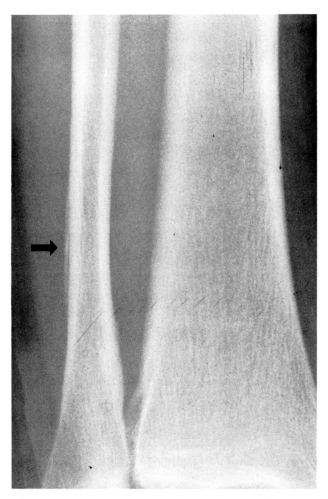

Figure 55-20. A single lamella of periosteal new bone (arrow) lies adjacent to the fibula. This was formed in response to cellulitis in the overlying soft tissues.

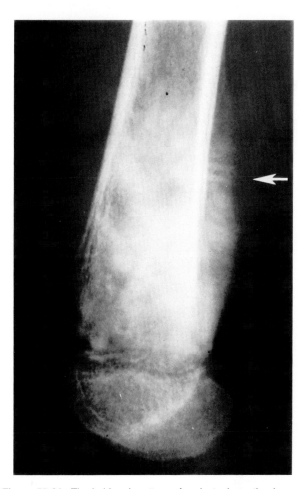

Figure 55-21. The hairbrush pattern of periosteal reaction in a patient with an osteogenic sarcoma of the distal femur. Multiple bands (arrow) of periosteal bone are directed perpendicular to the distal femur.

controlled, the thin band of periosteal new bone will slowly and progressively thicken until it blends with the outer margin of the cortex. If the process that elevated the periosteum continues, a second and then multiple lines of periosteal new bone will form. These multiple layers are called *onionskinning.*

If the periosteum is expanding at a steady rate of speed, too fast for lamellae of periosteal new bone to form, the periosteal bone will appear as streaks perpendicular to the cortical surface (Fig. 55-21). This hairbrush or sunburst appearance indicates rapid lifting of the periosteum.

Where there is rapid lifting of the periosteum, the portions of periosteum at the margin of the process move more slowly, and the triangular lamellae (Fig. 55-22) of bone layed down are called Codman's triangles, so this pattern, too, indicates a rapid lifting of the periosteum. The radiograph thus tells much about the speed of expansion of the process causing periosteal new bone.

Keynote

- *The periosteum normally forms bone throughout life. Bone formation is more rapid at periods of rapid growth. Growth can be accelerated at foci of disease that lift the periosteum or result in hyperemia near the periosteum.*

SUMMARY

This chapter has discussed the normal appearance of bone in the child and adult as seen on radiographs and ^{99m}Tc phosphate complex bone scans. The child's normal bone is divided into four parts: the epiphysis, growth plate (physis), metaphysis, and shaft (diaphysis). The adult bone is divided into three parts: the epiphysis, metaphysis, and shaft. Each bone also consists of a cortex and medulla. The normal appearance of each of these structures has been

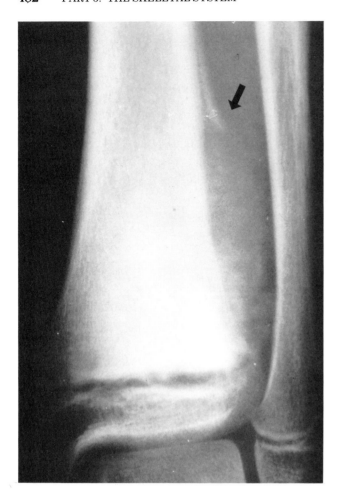

Figure 55-22. The Codman's triangle (arrow) pattern of periosteal reaction seen in a patient with an osteogenic sarcoma of the distal tibia.

discussed and contrasted with some of the diseases that can affect them.

REVIEW QUESTIONS

1. How do imaging studies document the slow physiological turnover of bone?
2. Where does bone growth occur in the child?
3. What are the four parts of a child's bone?
4. What are the three parts of an adult's bone?
5. What are the differences between the cortex and medulla of a bone?
6. What forms of periosteal-formed bone are normal? What forms are abnormal?
7. What are the main patterns of abnormality seen in the epiphysis? In the growth plate? In the metaphysis? In the diaphysis?
8. When does epiphyseal ossification occur?
9. What processes can limit the longitudinal growth of a bone?
10. What is rickets? What is its appearance on radiographs?
11. What are the forms of osteopenia?
12. Where do irregularities of the cortical margin occur?
13. What processes decrease the distinctness of the corticomedullary junction?
14. What happens to the cortex and the trabeculae in osteoporotic bone?
15. What is the appearance of vascular grooves?

VOCABULARY

cortex	osteoporosis
diaphysis	Paget's disease of bone
epiphysis	periosteum
Gaucher's disease	physis
Legg-Perthes disease	post–growth-arrest lines
medulla	rickets
metaphysis	scurvy
osteomalacia	thalassemia
osteopenia	trabeculae

SUGGESTIONS FOR FURTHER READING FOR CHAPTERS 55 TO 59

Theodore E. Keats, Thomas H. Smith. *An Atlas of Normal Developmental Roentgen Anatomy.* Year Book Medical Publishers: Chicago. 1977.

Theodore E. Keats. *An Atlas of Normal Roentgen Variants That May Simulate Disease.* Year Book Medical Publishers: Chicago. 1984.

George B. Greenfield. *Radiology of Bone Diseases,* 4th Ed. J.B. Lippincott: Philadelphia. 1986.

Jack Edeiken, Philip J. Hodes. *Roentgen Diagnosis of Disease of Bone.* Williams & Wilkins: Baltimore. 1984.

56

INTRODUCTION TO FRACTURES

KEY CONCEPTS

Radiological

Displaced fractures are easy to recognize, but there are many fractures that are difficult to recognize. For these, the three main findings suggesting fracture are soft tissue swelling, joint effusions, and minimal changes in bony contour.

Joint effusions can often be recognized because the joint capsules are usually surrounded by fat and this fat is displaced outward by the fluid within the joint. The presence of fat within the joint fluid usually indicates that a fracture is present. Films taken with a horizontal x-ray beam may demonstrate a fat-fluid level within the joint. Bone can respond to sudden stress in three ways: it can bend and spring back, bend and stay bent, or fracture.

When evaluating a radiograph for the possible presence of fracture, five questions should be posed:

1. Is there a fracture or is the radiolucent line seen a vascular groove or a growth place?
2. Is the fracture open to the outside?
3. Are there any coexistent injuries or fractures?
4. Does the fracture involve the adjacent joint or growth plate?
5. Is there an injury to adjacent organs?

Clinical

The presence of a joint effusion may indicate a fracture. In the elbow, where fractures can be very difficult to see, many clinicians will treat the patient with an elbow effusion for fracture even when no fracture can be seen.

OBJECTIVES

When you complete this chapter you will be able to

1. Identify displaced fractures of the extremities on selected radiographs.
2. Identify fractures of the elbow and wrist on selected radiographs.
3. List five pairs of fractures that can occur together.
4. List and explain the three types of response that bone can have to sudden stress.

The lesions of the skeleton you are most likely to see are the fractures, so it is fitting to begin with a discussion of them. If you know that a normal knee looks like the one in Figure 56-1a, you should have no difficulty identifying the fragmented tibial plateau in Figure 56-1b. Or, if you know that the normal alignment of the ankle is that shown in Figure 56-2a, then the fractures shown in Figure 56-2b should present no difficulty. The key is knowing what the normal bone should look like.

But while most fractures do show the amount of displacement shown in Figures 56-1b and 56-2b, these fractures are so easy to recognize from an examination of the patient, that the radiograph adds little diagnostic information. Far more important is learning how to recognize the subtle fractures and how to use the configuration of one fracture to predict the presence of another unsuspected injury. The hard-to-see fractures are the ones that are emphasized here. To find them, careful observation is often necessary. The clues to subtle fractures are:

1. Soft tissue swelling
2. Joint effusions
3. Minimal changes in bony contour

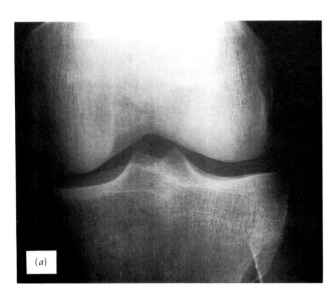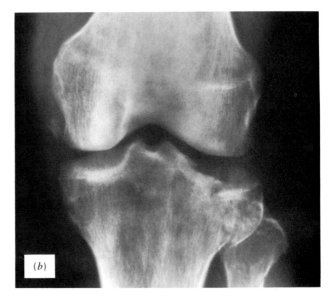

Figure 56-1. (a) AP view of the normal knee. (b) Fracture of the lateral tibial plateau with depression of the fragments. There is a smaller fragment of fractured bone near the medial femoral condyle.

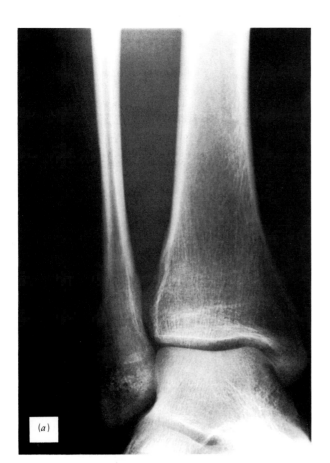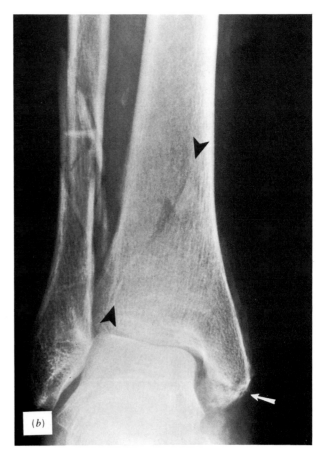

Figure 56-2. (a) Normal ankle. (b) Fractures of the tibia and fibula. There are multiple fragments of bone at the fibular fracture site. The tibial fractures are more difficult to see. The fractures of the medial malleolus (arrow) and posterior portion of the tibia (arrowheads) could be more easily seen on other views.

PRINCIPLES OF FRACTURE RECOGNITION

Soft Tissue Swelling

Most radiographs include far more bone than is actually injured. A radiograph of the hand (Figure 56-3a) includes many bones, but only one may be injured. Though every bone contour must be checked, swelling is a guide to the

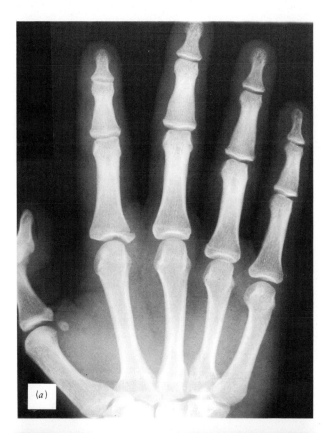

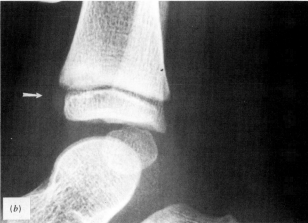

Figure 56-3. (a) Swelling as a guide to a fracture of the base of the index finger. There is an area of bone contour irregularity on the ulnar side of the base of the proximal phalanx of the index finger. (b) Swelling (arrow) as a sign of an undisplaced fracture through the growth plate of the distal tibia in a child. This fracture would be classified as an undisplaced Salter-Harris type I fracture (see Fig. 56-21).

regions most likely injured. Sometimes swelling may be the only sign of an undisplaced fracture. In Figure 56-3b, there is focal swelling (arrow) adjacent to the distal tibial growth plate; it indicates an undisplaced fracture through the growth plate.

The normal soft tissues of the extremities include muscle, fat, vessels, and nerves. Muscle and fat show a sharp demarcation (Fig. 56-4a), which is disrupted by swelling (Fig. 56-4b). When injured, the fat becomes edematous and appears trabeculated (Fig. 56-4b). When looking at radiographs, look for evidence of swelling, then check the nearby bones carefully.

Joint Effusions

Each joint capsule in the extremities is surrounded by fat. Joint effusions displace this fat outward from the joint, and this outward displacement can be recognized on the radiograph.

In the elbow (Fig. 56-5), the fat anterior to the distal humerus can be seen (Fig. 56-5a) lying directly in front of the distal humerus shaft when no effusion is present. When fluid distends the capsule, the fat is displaced away from the anterior portion of the humerus (Fig. 56-5b). Posterior to the humerus, fat can be seen only in the presence of an effusion (Fig. 56-5b and c).

In the knee (Fig. 56-6), the suprapatellar fat normally contains the thin water-radiodensity suprapatellar bursa (Fig. 56-a). This fat is displaced when the suprapatellar bursa is distended by fluid (Fig. 56-6b).

Fat-Fluid Level. Sometimes the effusion contains fat (Fig. 56-7). Figure 56-7b is a lateral view of the knee taken with a horizontal x-ray beam to show layering. In the fluid in the suprapatellar bursa, a fat-fluid layer can be recognized because of the difference in radiodensity of the two types of fluid. The presence of fat within the joint fluid almost always indicates that a fracture has occurred. If no fracture is seen, treatment should nonetheless be that for an undisplaced fracture.

Changes in Bone Contour

The cortex responds to a sudden stress in a sequential pattern:

Elasticity   The bone bends and springs back.
Plasticity   The bone bends and stays bent.
Fracture   The bone bends and then breaks.

Because bone has these three responses, elastic, plastic, and fracture, a bone subjected to injury can have components of each response. A fracture can be *complete*, that is, through all of the cortical tissue at one level, or *incomplete*. Incomplete fractures can show just bending (Fig. 56-8a) or breakage of bone on one cortical margin and plastic bending on the other (the *green-stick fracture*) (Fig. 56-8b). The plastic component of the green-stick fracture is important because the bent cortex will spring back to its bent

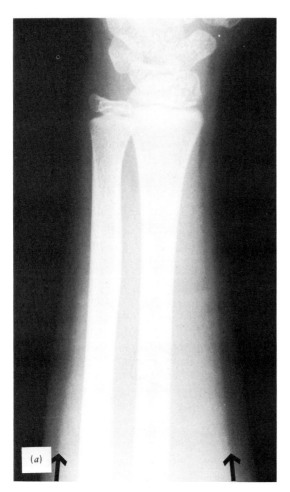

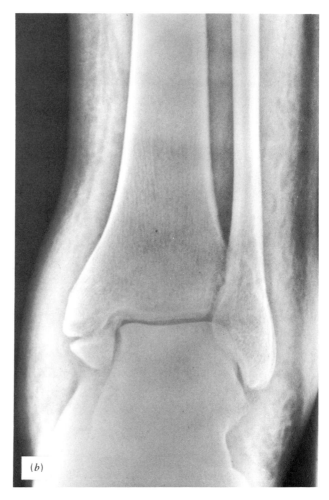

Figure 56-4. Soft tissue appearance. (*a*) Normal distinct fat-muscle deliniation (arrows). (*b*) Swelling around the ankle caused by injury and fracture. The fat near the medial malleolar fracture is uniformly white from extensive edema. That near the fibula and more proximal tibia is reticulated from moderate edema.

position, resulting in recurrent deformity after fracture reduction.

You must learn the normal contours of bones in order to be able to identify these subtle fractures. Two important regions of skeletal injury illustrate the fracture abnormalities that can be seen in those regions: the elbow and the distal radius.

Keynotes

- *Swelling makes the muscle-fat plane indistinct and gives fat a reticulated appearance.*
- *Joint effusions displace the pericapsular fat outward.*
- *In the normal elbow, fat is seen along the anterior portion of the distal humerus. None is seen posterior when the elbow is flexed. An elbow effusion displaces the fat anteriorly away from the bone and posteriorly so that it can be seen.*
- *Knee effusions push the anterior fat pad away from the bone and enlarge the suprapatellar bursa.*
- *A fat-fluid level in a joint almost always indicates a fracture.*

- *Injured bone can spring back (be elastic), bend (be plastic), or break (fracture).*
- *A complete fracture is one that goes through the entire cortex of bone. An incomplete fracture is one that only passes through part of the cortex.*
- *The green-stick fracture is an incomplete fracture in which one cortex is bent and the other is broken.*

FRACTURES OF THE ELBOW

Fractures of the radial head and of the distal humerus can illustrate the principles of fracture recognition.

Fractures of the Radial Head

Criteria of Normal

No joint effusion

Smooth contours, except for minimal irregularity at the remnant of the growth plate

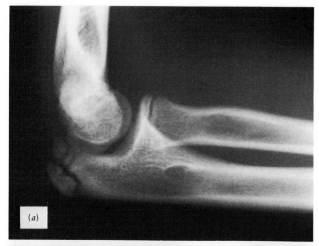

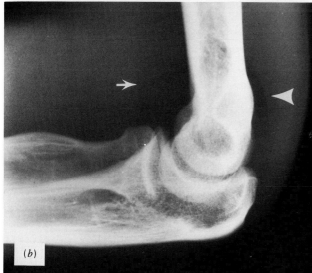

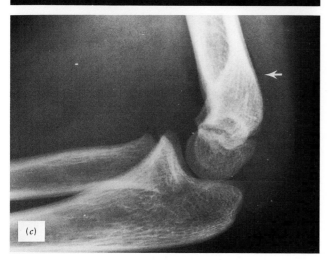

Figure 56-5. (*a*) A normal child's elbow demonstrating the normal anterior fat pad of the elbow. The multiple separate bony portions are the growth centers. (*b*) An elbow effusion in a patient with a radial-head fracture not seen on this film. The anterior fat pad (arrow) is visible (see also Fig. 56-17*b*). (*c*) Minimal effusion in the elbow. Only a sliver of the posterior fat pad (arrow) is visible.

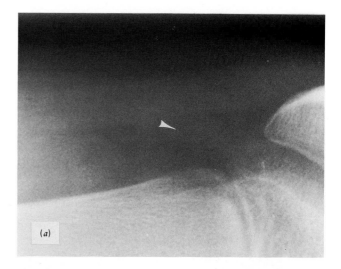

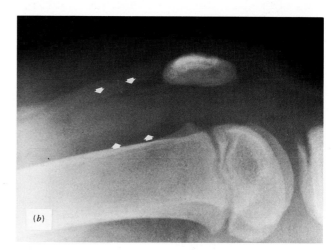

Figure 56-6. Lateral views of the knee. (*a*) Normal appearance of the suprapatellar space (arrowhead). (*b*) An effusion distends the suprapatellar bursa (arrows).

Smooth Contours. Figure 56-9 demonstrate the normal shape of the radial head and neck. The margins are smooth. The density of the bone is uniform with some trabecular bone identifiable as thin lines within the margins of the bone. In Figure 56-9*b*, there is a thin white line crossing the midportion of the radial head; this is a remnant of the growth plate.

Subtle Fractures. Figure 56-10 demonstrates several types of fractures of the radial head and neck. Look for the contour and density abnormalities. The legends discuss the locations of the fractures. Each of these fractures is difficult to see, and in the book, each is magnified many times. It may be necessary to use a magnifying lens to see the radial head fractures on actual radiographs.

If you missed one of these fractures, what might happen to the patient? Every fracture damages the bone bordering the fracture line, and this damaged bone undergoes resorp-

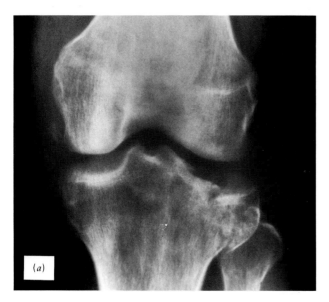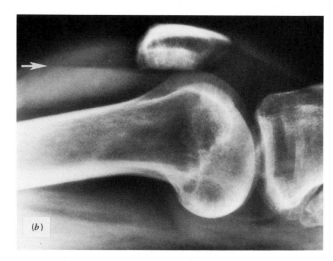

Figure 56-7. A lateral tibial plateau fracture with a fat-fluid level in the suprapatellar bursa. The presence of fat in a joint effusion usually indicates the presence of a fracture. (*a*) AP view demonstrating the lateral tibial plateau fracture. (*b*) Horizontal-beam lateral view demonstrating the fat-fluid level (arrow) in the suprapatellar bursa.

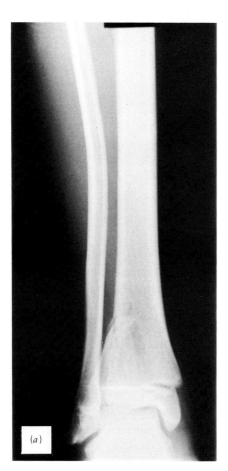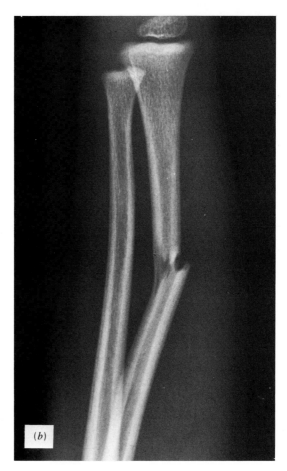

Figure 56-8. Fractures with plastic deformity of bone. (*a*) Plastic bowing of the fibula associated with a distal tibia fracture through the growth plate and metaphysis (Salter-Harris type II). (Courtesy J. Brown, M.D.) (*b*) Green-stick fracture of the radius with a slight ulna plastic bow.

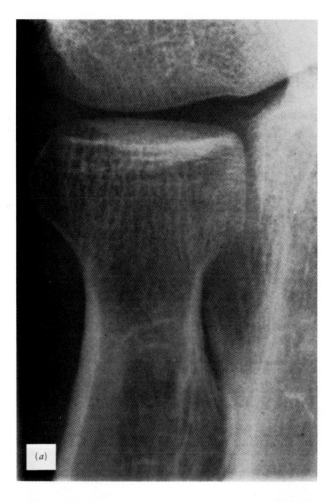

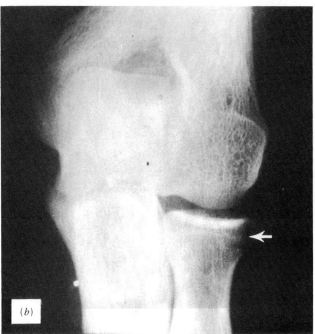

Figure 56-9. (a) Normal radial head. (b) Normal radial head with a calcified remnant of the growth plate (arrow).

tion. If the elbow is not immobilized, the fragments can displace, and this can result in arthritis within the joint.

Because many fractures of the radial head are almost impossible to see, most orthopedic surgeons will treat a patient for fracture if a joint effusion is seen. In some of these patients, a follow-up radiograph 2 weeks later may demonstrate the fracture, now easier to see because of the resorption of injured bone around the fracture line.

Figure 56-11 demonstrates the right and left elbows of a 6-year-old child. What do you see?

Several lines cross the bone ends. These represent the growth plates. At the proximal end of the radius, there is asymmetry. On the right side, the radial head epiphysis (or ossification center) can be seen; on the left, it is absent. Usually, the ossification centers are bilaterally symmetrical. What do you think has happened to this child?

He has fractured off the left growth center, and it is hidden within the joint.

Fractures of the Distal Humerus

Fractures of the distal humerus are common in children but can be difficult to recognize. In general, these fractures occur from a fall on the outstretched hand, and the distal humerus is driven back. Figure 56-12 demonstrates lateral views of the right and left elbows of a 6-year-old child. How do they differ?

The soft tissues of the right side are much increased. There is an effusion within the joint demonstrated by displacement of the fat pad, and the distal right humeral alignment is straighter than that of the left: it has been displaced backward.

Recognition of these distal humeral supracondylar fractures depends on the recognition of the joint effusion and the displacement of the distal humeral condyles. The latter can be recognized most easily by drawing the two lines along the distal humeral shaft in the lateral view as shown in Figure 56-13. The first line runs along the anterior margin of the humeral shaft and should (in normal elbows) bisect the capitellum. The second line runs along the midhumeral shaft and should lie just posterior to the capitellum. The distal humeral condyles can be displaced anteriorly or posteriorly by fracture, but posterior displacement is more common.

Danger of Missing a Distal Humeral Fracture. Posterior displacement of the humeral condyles limits elbow flexion, but the hidden danger of this fracture is the effect that the marked swelling common in these fractures can have on the blood supply to the forearm. Ischemia of these muscles can occur after these fractures and, if not recognized, the muscles of the forearm can infarct and hand and wrist function can be lost. This complication is called *Volkmann's ischemic contracture.*

Keynotes

- *The white-line remnants of the growth plate can persist into adult life and simulate fractures.*

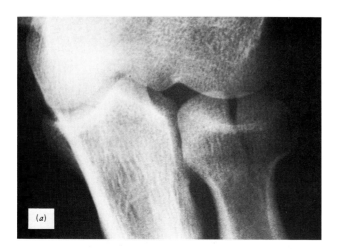

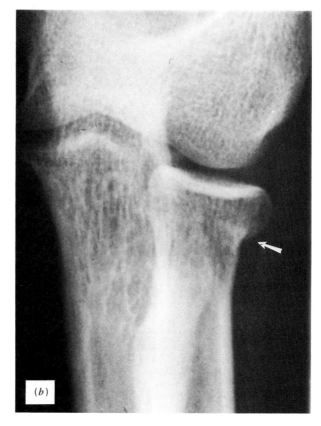

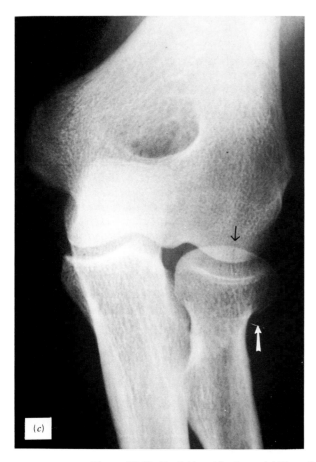

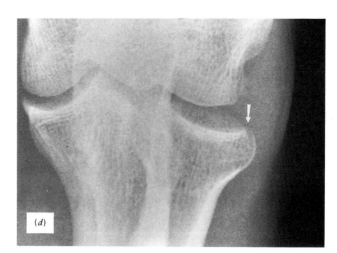

Figure 56-10. Radial-head fractures. (*a*) Linear fracture through the radial head. (*b*) Impacted fracture of the radial neck. The white line at the head-neck junction (arrow) is the fracture. (*c*) Marginal fracture of the radial head. A subtle contour irregularity (white arrow) is present. The line of the fracture (black arrow) is just visible crossing the radial head. Its limited visualization is due to its not being in the plane of the x-ray beam. (*d*) A fracture of the margin of the radial head (arrow) is demonstrated as a slight interruption of the white line of the bony margin.

490

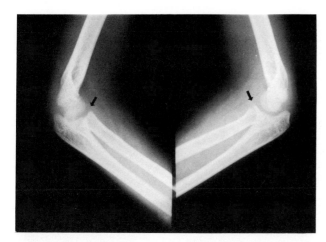

Figure 56-11. Missing radial-head epiphysis. The radial-head epiphysis (arrow) can be seen on the right but not (arrow) on the left. It has been displaced by a fracture and is hidden in the joint space.

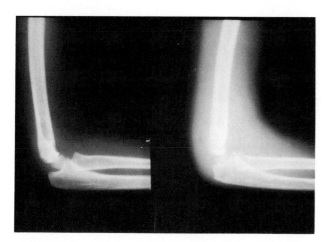

Figure 56-12. Supracondylar fracture of the humerus. The elbow on the right side of the figure is swollen, and the alignment of the distal radius is distorted compared with the elbow on the left.

- *In the injured elbow, a joint effusion usually indicates the presence of fracture. Even if the fracture cannot be seen on the radiograph, the patient is treated.*
- *On the lateral view, a line drawn along the anterior cortex of the distal humerus should bisect the capitellum. A line drawn along the midhumeral shaft should lie just posterior to the capitellum.*
- *Volkmann's ischemic contracture is due to infarction of the muscles of the forearm. It can follow a fracture of the distal humerus.*

FRACTURES OF THE WRIST

Fractures of the Distal Radius

Fractures of the distal radius are also common fractures. Some are easy to recognize by comparing the normal (Fig. 56-14) with the fractured forearm (Fig. 56-15), but diffi-

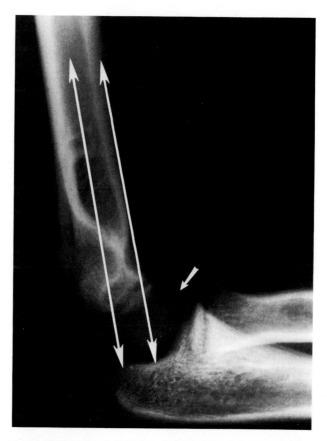

Figure 56-13. Lateral elbow view with lines drawn. The anterior humeral line and the midhumeral line demonstrate the normal relationship of these lines with the capitellum (arrow). Compare these with the elbows shown in Figure 56-12.

cult-to-see fractures also occur in this location. Usually the lateral view is the most helpful in evaluating the distal radius

Alignment of the Distal Radius on the Lateral View: Normal Criteria

1. Smooth contour
2. Anterior angulation of the distal radial articular surface
3. Uniform radiodensity, except for a white line representing the remnant of the growth plate

Smooth Contour: Figure 55-14 represents the contour of the normal distal radius in an adult. Figure 56-15 demonstrates the angular disruption of the dorsal surface of the radius in a patient with a *Colles's fracture.* Figure 56-16*a* demonstrates the normal contour of the distal radius in a 7-year-old child. Figure 56-16*b* and *c* demonstrates two types of fractures in children. In Figure 56-16*b*, the epiphyseal growth center is displaced dorsally along with a small portion of the distal metaphysis of the radius. This type of fracture is described as a *Salter-Harris* type II *fracture.*

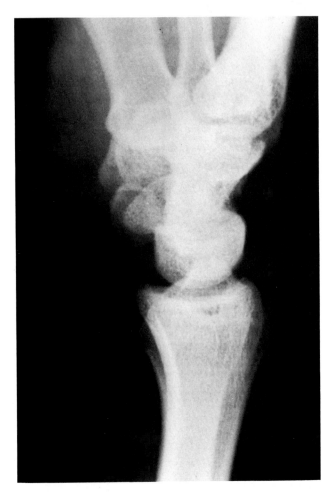

Figure 56-14. Normal distal radius in the adult. Note the alignment of the distal radial articular surface to the shaft of the radius.

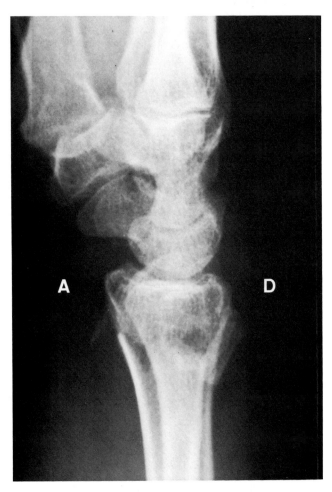

Figure 56-15. Lateral view of the wrist in a patient with a Colles's fracture. The distal articular surface is inclined dorsally. Compare this to the normal in Figure 56-14. A = anterior, D = dorsal.

Figure 56-16c and *d* demonstrates a bulge in the dorsal and medial part of the cortex of the distal radius with a normal anterior cortex. This type of fracture is called a *buckle,* or *torus, fracture.*

Anterior Inclination of the Distal Radial Articular Surface.

Most fractures of the distal radius occur from a fall on the pronated outstretched hand. This directs more force along the dorsal surface of the radius, impacting and compressing this margin more than the anterior margin. This results in decreased anterior angulation or actual posterior angulation of the distal articular surface. Figure 56-14 demonstrates the normal anterior inclination. Figure 56-15 demonstrates the alignment after a Colles's fracture.

Keynotes

- *Colles's fracture is a fracture through the distal radius with dorsal displacement of the distal fragment; it is often associated with fracture of the ulnar styloid.*
- *Buckle, or torus, fracture is a fracture of childhood in which the cortex bulges outward at the fracture site.*

GENERAL APPROACH TO THE EVALUATION OF FRACTURES

Using the elbow and distal radius as examples, certain principles in fracture identification have been stressed. In a book of this length, it is not possible to discuss all possible fractures, but there are certain queries that aid in the evaluation of all fractures:

1. Is there a fracture?
   a. Normal lines that can be confused with fractures must be eliminated:
      Vascular grooves
      Growth plates
2. Is the fracture open to the outside?
   a. Air or foreign material in soft tissue or adjacent joint
3. Are there any coexistent injuries or fractures?
4. Does the fracture involve the adjacent joint or growth plate?

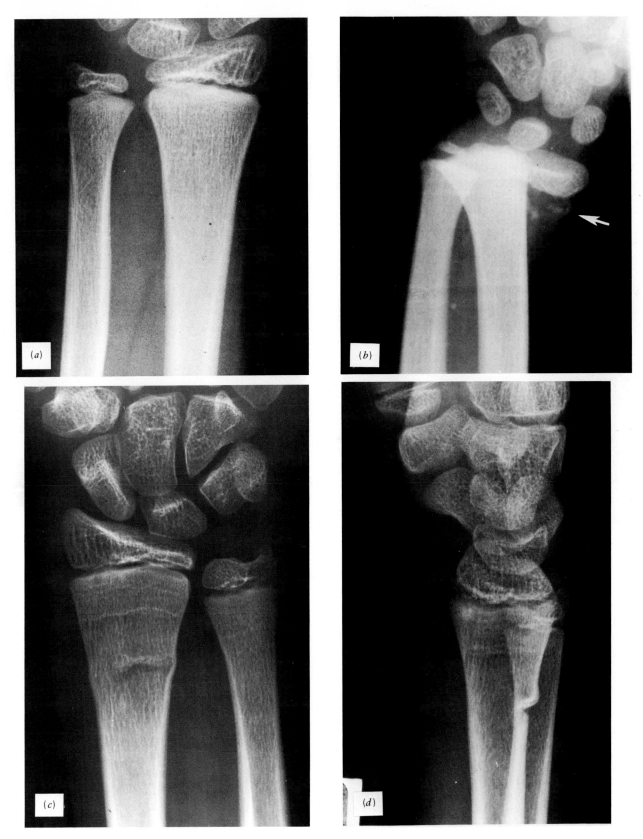

Figure 56-16. (*a*) Normal child's wrist. Compare the position of the distal radial epiphysis with that in *b*. (*b*) Salter-Harris type II fracture of the distal radial growth plate and metaphysis. An arrow indicates the metaphyseal fragments. (*c*) PA view of a distal radial torus, or buckle, fracture. The buckling of the cortex is easily seen. The white lines crossing the metaphysis are post–growth-arrest lines and are a sign of previous illnesses. (*d*) Lateral view of the same fracture.

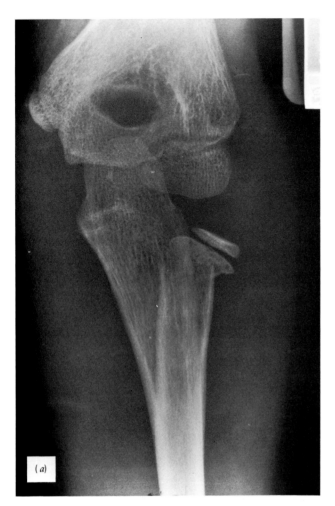
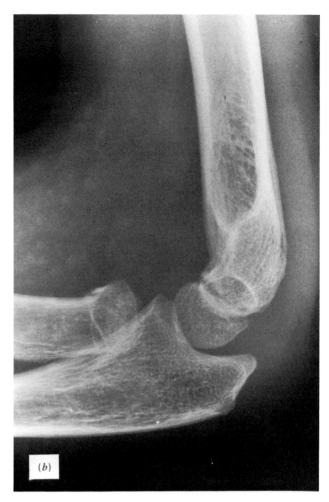

Figure 56-17. Fracture of the radial neck in an 8-year-old child. There is angulation, interruption and overlap of the cortex, and interruption of some of the trabecular lines in the medulla. (*a*) AP view. (*b*) Lateral view. A joint effusion elevates the anterior fat pad.

5. Is there any injury to adjacent organs?
   a. Vessels?
   b. Nerves?
   c. Muscles?
   d. Visci?

Is There a Fracture?

Fractures can be recognized as radiolucent lines crossing the cortex of the bone (Fig. 56-17), as interruptions of the trabecular bone, and as regions of increased bone density (Fig. 56-18) when the bone is impacted (pushed together so that more bone is compressed into a smaller volume). Vascular grooves and growth plates can be confused with fracture lines.

Vascular Grooves. Vascular grooves run obliquely through the cortex of a bone. The direction of obliquity is predictable, which aids in diagnosing them. Each tubular

bone has two ends, and these ends almost always grow at different rates. The outer portion of the groove is always closer to the center of rapid growth than is the inner portion. This is because the bone on the inner cortex is always formed before the outer cortical bone. With growth, this inner and older cortex is displaced further from the side of bone growth than is the outer and newer cortex.

Figure 56-19*a* demonstrates the vascular groove of the proximal phalanx of the index finger. Almost all longitudinal growth of this phalanx occurs at the proximal end. The vascular groove runs from the outer proximal portion of the phalanx to the inner distal portion.

Figure 56-19*b* demonstrates the vascular groove of the femur. The distal end of the femur grows more than the proximal end of the femur. The vascular groove runs from outer distal to inner proximal, reflecting the differential growth.

Figure 56-20*a* demonstrates the vascular groove of the humerus seen en face. Contrast this to Figure 56-20*b*, which demonstrates a subtle fracture of the femur seen en

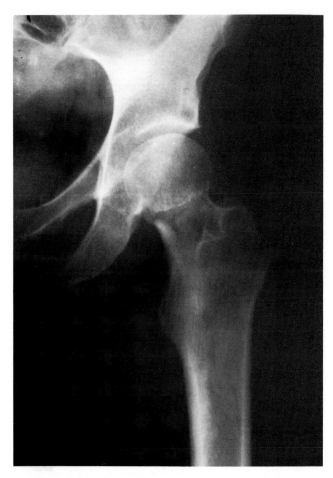

Figure 56-18. An impacted fracture of the femoral neck. The white line and the adjacent radiolucent lines crossing the midfemoral neck are components of the fracture. (From Freedman, M.: *Radiology of the Postoperative Hip.* Copyright 1979, John Wiley & Sons, Inc. Reprinted with permission.)

face. The vascular groove has slightly sclerotic (whiter) margins, whereas the fracture does not.

Growth Plates. Growth plates are radiolucent lines crossing bones near their ends that can be confused with fractures. Growth plates can be recognized because they always have a denser white line along their metaphyseal portion. This white line is due to the growth plate's replacement by bone.

In some people this white line of growth plate may persist many years into adulthood (Fig. 56-9*b*). This can be differentiated from an impacted fracture by knowledge of the normal location of growth plates. Figure 56-9*b* represents the typical location of the radial-head growth plate in the midradial head. Figure 56-10*b* shows the white line of an impacted fracture at the radial-head—radial-neck junction. Recognizing the difference in location is the key to differentiating the fracture from the normal growth plate remnant. Fractures can occur *through* the growth

plate, resulting in widening of the plate or displacement of the epiphysis.

Is the Fracture Open to the Outside?

A fracture open to the outside provides a site of entry for microorganisms that could lead to infection. Skin wounds can be seen on physical examination. In some patients, air or foreign matter within the soft tissues or an adjacent joint can indicate that the wound is open to the outside. These fractures require careful cleaning and debridement.

Are There Coexistent Injuries?

Ligamentous Injuries. Certain types of fractures involving joints can occur only if a ligament at another part of the joint is torn. The radiological analysis for the coexistent ligamentous injury is complex and beyond the scope of this book. But physical examination will always show tenderness and often swelling at the site of ligamentous injury, and ligamentous injury should be suspected when there is focal tenderness and no fracture is identified on the radiograph.

Fractures. Certain fractures occur in pairs or triplets. When one fracture is found on a radiograph, look for others. Because adjacent joints can be injured, physical examination of the entire extremity should be done whenever a fracture of one part is suspected.

Common Coexistent Fractures

Distal radius and styloid process of the ulna

Distal radius and scaphoid bone

Distal radius and radial head (at elbow)

Supracondylar fracture of the distal humerus and surgical neck fracture of the proximal humerus

Adjacent ribs

Fractures of the pelvis (often in pairs)

Tibia and fibula at the ankle

Medial malleolus and any part of the fibula

Calcaneus, tibial plateau, and lumbar spine

Does the Fracture Involve the Adjacent Joint or Growth Plate?

Joint. Fractures can enter joints along an articular or nonarticular surface. Extension into a joint can be identified by seeing an extension of the fracture into the joint or by identifying a joint effusion in the adjacent joint.

When a fracture enters a joint, free fragments called *loose bodies* can be scattered in the joint. Sometimes these will get caught between the bone ends, causing pain or limited motion (called *locking*) or resulting in a sudden reflex relaxation of the adjacent muscles (called *giving way*).

When a fracture enters a joint at an articular surface, the resulting irregularity and cartilage damage can result

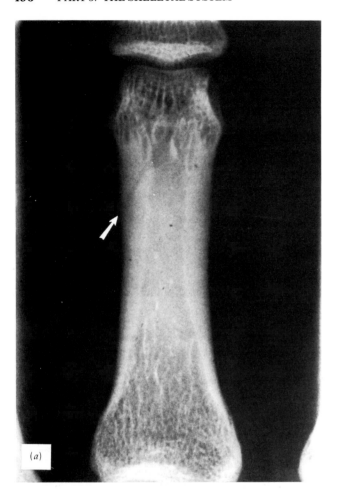
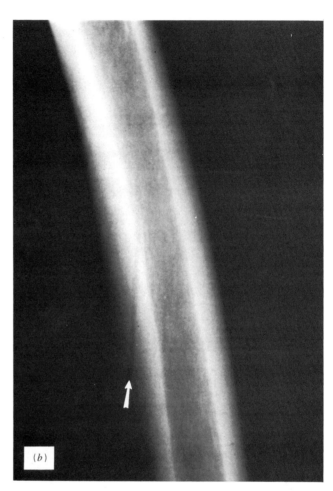

Figure 56-19. Vascular grooves. (*a*) Index finger (arrow). (*b*) Femur (arrow). Because the distal femur grows faster than the proximal femur, the inner portion of the groove grows to lie proximal to the outer portion of the groove.

in degenerative arthritis. Fractures that enter the articular margin must be reduced accurately to decrease the chance of late arthritis.

Growth Plate. The weakest area of bone in a child's limb is usually the cartilaginous growth plate. This growth plate can be at either one or both ends of a bone; it can be at an articular end or at the site of tendon insertion. Growth occurs from a proliferation of cartilage starting at the epiphyseal end of the bone with maturation occurring as the portion moves closer to the metaphysis. The metaphyseal edge of the growth plate is bordered by a white line representing initial calcification of mature cartilage. Fractures that occur through the epiphyseal side of the cartilage can damage the proliferating cartilage cells, often limiting future growth. Fractures through the metaphyseal side of the growth plate affect growth much less commonly.

Salter and Harris divided growth plate fractures into five types (Fig. 56-21). Types one and two involve only the metaphyseal side of the growth plate and carry a good prognosis for future growth. Types three and four involve the epiphyseal side and future growth potential may be limited. The type five injury is a crush injury of the plate. In this injury the growth potential is usually lost.

Are There Injuries to Adjacent Organs?

In some fractures, the fracture itself is of little consequence, but a coexistent injury to a nerve or artery may result in a much poorer prognosis. These associated injuries may be of greater importance than the fracture. When you see a fracture, always consider what organ lies adjacent to it that might be injured. Remember also always to evaluate the blood supply and innervation distal to the fracture. Fractures of the left lower ribs can be associated with splenic rupture.

Keynotes

• *An impacted fracture is a fracture in which bone is pushed closer together by the injury.*

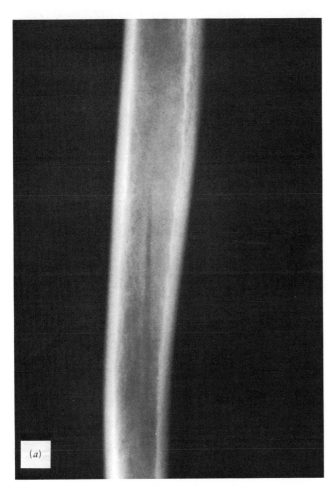 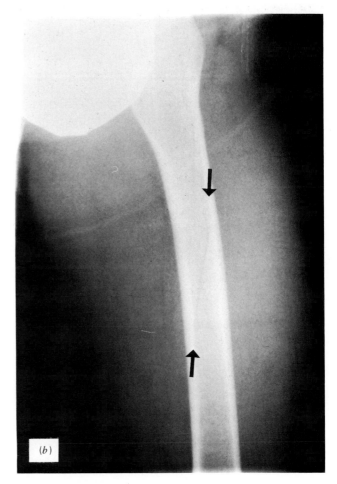

Figure 56-20. A vascular groove versus a fracture. (*a*) Vascular groove seen en face in the humerus. Both margins of the groove are lined by a border of increased radiodensity. (*b*) Subtle linear fracture of the femur (arrows). Note the different appearance and the lack of sclerotic margins.

- *Air in the soft tissues or within the joint in association with an acute fracture usually means that the fracture is open and potentially contaminated.*
- *Debridement is the removal of dead and injured tissue.*
- *A fracture that enters a joint can result in irregularity of the articular surface, predisposing to arthritis. It can produce free fragments within the joint that can cause locking and giving way.*

SUMMARY

In this chapter the radiological diagnosis of fractures has been discussed. In evaluating the radiograph for a possible fracture, the identification of soft tissue swelling and joint effusions may point to the presence of fracture. Swelling often shows as enlargement of the soft tissues or as a disruption of the normally distinct margin between the fat and muscle in the extremities. Joint effusions can be recognized by the displacement of the fat that normally surrounds all joint capsules.

Vascular grooves and growth plates and their rem-

nants can be confused with fractures. Vascular grooves are oblique radiolucent lines that pass through only one cortex of a bone. Often there is a fine band of radiodensity that extends from them into the medullary canal. Growth plates in the child show a band of water radiodensity marginated on the metaphyseal side of the bone by a thin band of calcified cartilage and denser bone. In the adult the thin band of denser bone and cartilage may persist for many years.

If you know the normal structure of bone, most fractures will be obvious because they result in major deformity. The undisplaced fractures and impacted fractures may be much more difficult to detect, and they require careful inspection for identification. Areas of difficulty covered in this chapter include the difficulty in diagnosing some fractures of the distal radius, of the radial head and neck, and of the distal humerus.

Fractures through the growth plate have been classified by Salter and Harris into five groups: Type I fractures involve only the growth plate. Type II fractures involve the growth plate and metaphysis. Type III involve the

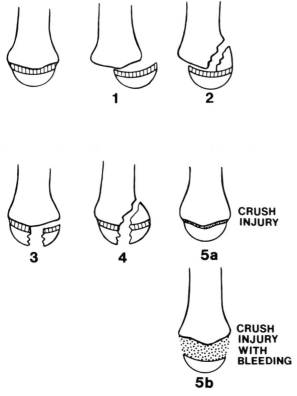

Figure 56-21. Salter-Harris fractures through the growth plate. The first drawing represents the normal appearance. Type I is a fracture through the growth plate. Type II is a fracture of the growth plate and adjacent metaphyseal bone. Type III is a fracture of the growth plate and epiphysis. Type IV is a fracture of the growth plate, epiphysis and metaphysis. Type V is a crush injury of the growth plate that at the time of the acute injury may appear with the growth plate wide, narrow, or of normal width. (Illustrative Services, Art Department, University of Maryland, School of Medicine.)

growth plate and epiphysis. Type IV involve the growth plate and both the epiphysis and metaphysis. Type V are crush injuries to the growth plate. The frequency of interference with growth increases with the higher numbers.

REVIEW QUESTIONS

1. What is the appearance of soft tissue swelling on the radiograph?
2. What is the appearance of joint effusions?
3. What is the significance of a joint effusion in the patient with an acute injury?
4. What does it mean to say that a bone has three responses to injury: elastic, plastic, and fracture?
5. What is an incomplete fracture? A complete fracture?
6. What should be done with a patient who has an elbow injury, a joint effusion, but no evidence of fracture on the radiographs? Why?
7. What two lines can help in detecting subtle fractures of the distal humerus in children?
8. What is the normal alignment of the distal radial articular surface? What type of fracture changes it?
9. What are the lines in a normal bone that might be confused with fracture? How would you distinguish them from a fracture?
10. What might you see on a radiograph that might tell you that a fracture was open? What should be done with an open fracture?
11. What problems can result from a fracture that enters a joint?
12. What are several of the potential pairs of fractures that can occur from the same injury?
13. How do you tell whether a ligamentous injury is present?
14. Describe the Salter-Harris classification of fractures and its significance.

VOCABULARY

buckle fracture	locking
Colles's fracture	loose bodies
complete fracture	open fracture
debridement	plastic
elastic	Salter-Harris fractures
fat-fluid level	suprapatellar bursa
giving way	torus fracture
green-stick fracture	Volkmann's ischemic contracture
impacted fracture	
incomplete fracture	

SUGGESTIONS FOR FURTHER READING

B. Felson, Ed. Fractures I and II. *Seminars in Roentgenology,* **8** (1, 2), 1978.

Lee F. Rogers. *Radiology of Skeletal Trauma.* Churchill Livingstone: New York. 1982. (A fine reference text)

For additional suggested reading see Chapter 55.

57

DISEASES WITH INCREASED DESTRUCTION AND FORMATION OF BONE

KEY CONCEPTS

Radiological

Most processes that result in the destruction of bone also result in the formation of new bone. With minimal or early processes, it is the formation of bone that can be detected with the bone scan. With larger areas of involvement, changes can be seen on radiographs and CT. When the destructive process does not result in the formation of new bone, the bone scan may be normal. This occurs primarily with multiple myeloma.

Focal destructive disease processes are usually called *lytic processes*. Processes resulting in more bone being produced than destroyed are called *osteoblastic processes*. Diffuse destructive disease results in osteopenia.

Lytic and osteoblastic disease are usually evaluated by their patterns. A lesion may be focal or diffuse, single or multiple, or have a well-defined or poorly defined margin. It may have periosteal new bone or a soft tissue mass associated with it. In addition the age of the patient and the location of the lesion aid in establishing a diagnosis.

Osteopenia can be recognized on radiographs when it is moderate to severe. It can be quantitated with a nuclear medicine technique, photon absorptiometry, or by CT bone mineral analysis.

Osteomyelitis will demonstrate its first imaging abnormality on bone scans obtained 2–3 days after the onset of symptoms. Radiographs usually become abnormal at 10–14 days and initially demonstrate periosteal reaction. After 3–4 weeks, focal areas of bone destruction can be seen.

Paget's disease of bone can be lytic, osteoblastic, or mixed lytic and osteoblastic. Its identifying radiographic characteristics are the presence of thickened and irregularly oriented trabeculae and thickened cortices.

OBJECTIVES

When you complete this chapter you will be able to

1. Identify osteolytic and osteoblastic lesions on selected radiographs.
2. Identify hot lesions on selected bone scans.
3. List the sequence of imaging abnormalities seen in osteomyelitis.
4. List the diagnostic features of Paget's disease of bone.
5. List three methods of evaluating osteopenia.

Most processes in the body that damage or destroy bone also result in the formation of new bone. Those lesions in which more bone is destroyed than is formed are considered lytic bone lesions; those diseases in which more bone is formed than is destroyed are osteoblastic or sclerotic lesions. Whether a lesion is lytic or osteoblastic relates to the balance of the two forces of bone destruction and bone deposition. Four different groups of processes are seen:

1. Diseases in which bone lysis predominates
   A. Myeloma
   B. Most metastases, especially
      (1) Lung
      (2) Kidney
      (3) Metastases from most cases of
         a. GI cancer
         b. Bladder cancer
         c. Squamous cell cancer

2. Diseases in which lysis is followed by increased bone formation
   A. Paget's disease of bone
   B. Infection
   C. Bone infarction
3. Diseases in which osteoblastic processes predominate
   A. Fracture healing
   B. Most metastases from
      (1) Prostate cancer
      (2) Medullary carcinoma of the thyroid
4. Diseases that may have or can have lytic and osteoblastic foci at the same time
   A. Metastases from
      (1) Breast cancer
      (2) GI cancer
      (3) Prostate cancer
      (4) Bladder cancer

Keynote

• Whether a lesion in bone appears lytic or osteoblastic depends on the balance between bone destruction and bone production.

PATTERNS OF LYTIC DISEASE

Lytic disease is evaluated using the following criteria:

1. Is the lesion solitary, one of many lesions, or is the bone loss diffuse?
2. Is the process limited within the bone, or does it permeate widely throughout the bone?
3. Is the margin of the lesion sclerotic?
4. In what bone and in what part of that bone is it?
5. How old is the patient?
6. Is there periosteal reaction or a soft tissue mass associated with it?

Is the Lesion Solitary, One of Many, or Diffuse?

Solitary Lesions. Solitary lesions can represent solitary metastases, a single focus of a nonneoplastic process such as osteomyelitis, or uncommonly a primary bone tumor.

Multiple Lesions. Multiple lytic lesions are usually due to metastatic disease, and thus when many are seen, that is the usual first diagnosis. Sometimes the multiple lesions are identified because symptoms direct you to them, and you take radiographs (Fig. 57-1). When this is not the case, a bone scan is the most useful secondary screening method for determining whether the first lesion found is solitary or one of many (Fig. 57-2).

Before 1970 the preferred method of looking for multi-

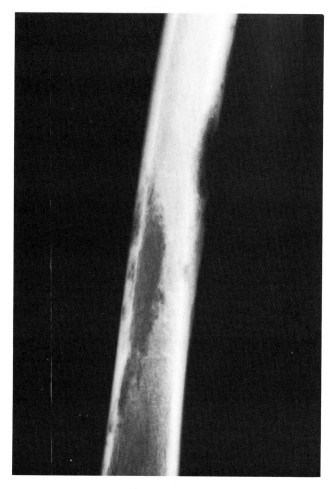

Figure 57-1. Metastatic lung cancer. Two adjacent destructive lesions of the midfemur result from lung cancer metastases.

ple metastases was with a radiographic skeletal survey. This is no longer so because the survey is less sensitive than the bone scan. Currently, the preferred method is to begin with a bone scan, then, if that is normal, take a single view of the pelvis and a lateral view of the skull. The two radiographs are obtained because occasionally the bone is so saturated with metastases that it is diffusely hot; the change being diffuse rather than focal, it could be missed.

In a patient with extensive metastases, the bone may absorb most of the bone-scanning tracer, leaving none available for renal excretion. (Compare the normal in Fig. 55-2f with Fig. 57-2b). The absence of renal excretion on the bone scan can indicate the extent of bone uptake and can be a clue that diffuse saturation metastases are present.

The only disease that commonly can affect bone and not result in a positive bone scan is multiple myeloma. In this disease a skeletal survey should be done in the search for metastases. Sometimes the lytic lesions in myeloma are unusually diffuse and destructive (Fig. 57-3). Despite the severity of the disease, the bone scan may still be normal.

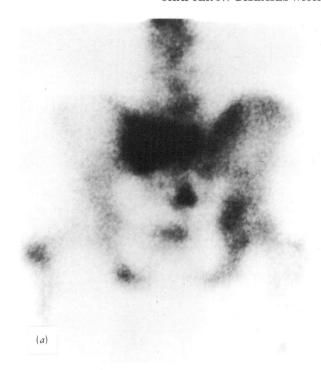

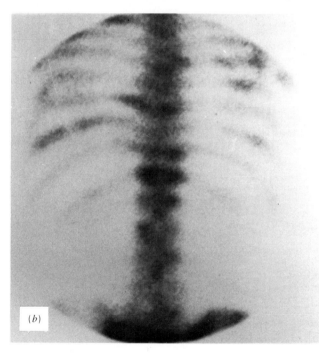

Figure 57-2. ⁹⁹ᵐTc phosphate complex bone scan demonstrating multiple sites of metastases to bone from metastatic breast cancer. (*a*) View of the pelvis. Areas of increased activity are seen in the sacrum, left ilium, and left acetabulum. (*b*) View of the lower thoracic spine and lumbar spine. Multiple focal areas of increased activity are seen in the vertebrae and ribs. There is lack of activity in the kidneys, indicating that there are enough focal hot spots of activity in bone to leave little or no tracer to be excreted by the kidneys.

Diffuse Bone Loss. Diffuse bone loss is called *osteopenia.* The most common form of osteopenia is osteoporosis, and two types seen: acute and chronic. In acute osteoporosis, such as that occurring when a patient has a fracture and is placed in a cast, multiple small regions of bone loss can occur (Fig. 57-4). The same pattern can be seen after acute paralysis, as from a stroke. This pattern is seen in a minority of immobilized patients, but when it occurs, it is specific. More often osteoporosis affects the trabecular bone and cortex. Subacute osteoporosis can also cause more focal resorption adjacent to the growth plate, either before or after it has closed (Fig. 57-5), and can result in more focal resorption just under the articular cartilage, leaving a remnant white line of calcified cartilage (Fig. 57-6).

Chronic generalized osteoporosis results from an imbalance in the slow turnover of bone with bone resorption exceeding bone formation. Either bone resorption is increased or bone formation is less than the normal bone resorption or both are increased.

In osteoporosis, there is loss of trabecular bone quantity. The interconnecting trabeculae are lost first, making the trabeculation lying in the line of stress more distinct (Fig. 57-7). When the loss of bone is due to lack of use (and in some patients in whom the loss of bone is due to steroid use) the stressed trabeculae become more distinct but do not thicken. In osteoporosis of aging, the stress trabeculae become thicker than normal (see Fig. 55-2*b*). In patients who had disuse osteoporosis and then resumed activity, those trabeculae remaining will hypertrophy.

Chronic osteoporosis also affects the thickness of the cortex, which also varies, however, with the age and sex of the patient, with the amount of activity the patient is involved in, and with the diameter of the bone. These multiple variables make it difficult for the novice to use cortical thickness for the identification of osteoporosis. It is easier to use the previously described changes in the trabecular bone pattern to establish this diagnosis.

In addition to the evaluation of osteopenia by radiographs, a nuclear medicine technique, bone absorptiometry, can be used. In this technique, a special machine is used to transmit gamma rays of one or two energies through selected bones. The amount of transmission correlates with the amount of calcium in the path of the gamma-ray beam and can be used to quantitate the amount of bone present.

An alternate quantitative method, CT bone mineral analysis, uses a CT scanner to scan the patient's spine while the patient lies on a special bone-density phantom. Comparisons can be made between the amount of absorption of the CT's x-ray photons in the patient's spine and in the calcium standards in the bone-density phantom.

Is the Process Limited within the Bone, or Does It Permeate Widely throughout the Bone?

Certain types of processes spread rapidly through bone, causing the resorption of many small focal areas of bone. This pattern is called the *permeative pattern* (Fig. 57-8). It is seen mainly in the most aggressive tumors and infections

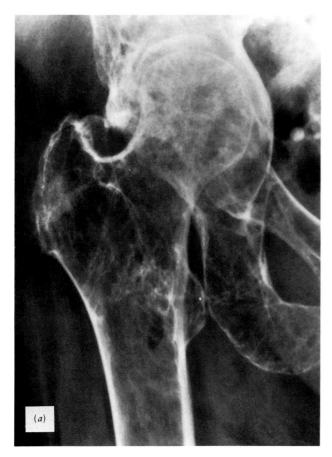

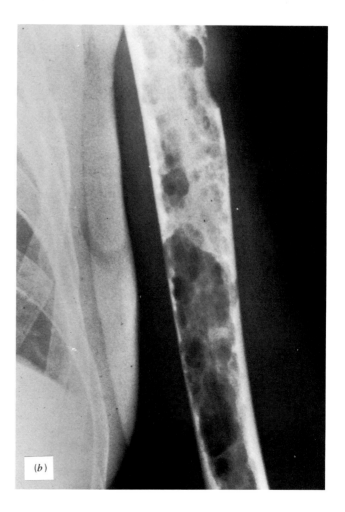

Figure 57-3. Multiple myeloma with extensive areas of bone destruction. (*a*) Proximal femur and hip. (*b*) Humerus.

including fibrosarcoma, Ewing's sarcoma, and some osteosarcomas; in some cases of metastatic lung and breast cancer; and in aggressive infections caused by *Salmonella* and *Staphylococcus aureus*.

Most lytic processes within bone are much more localized. The margin of the lesion can be identified, and because the shape appears similar to a country on a map, the pattern is called *geographic* (Fig. 57-9).

Is the Margin of the Lesion Sclerotic?

Sclerosis in the margin of a lesion indicate that it is expanding slowly enough so that the body has had a chance to lay down a visible layer of bone in response to it. In almost all lytic processes, bone is being laid down in response (as shown on the bone scan), but then this reactive bone is destroyed so that it is never of sufficient quantity to be seen on radiographs. Only when the lesion expands slowly or when it has stopped expanding, will sclerosis form around it (Fig. 57-9).

In What Bone and in What Part of the Bone Is It?

Certain types of processes occur in certain bones. For example, it is unusual to see metastatic disease in the

peripheral skeleton of the adult. Metastases are usually in the skull, spine, pelvis, upper humerus, or upper femur. Conversely, the hand-and-foot syndrome of infarction in young children with sickle cell disease occurs only in the hands and feet.

Most lytic processes in bone favor a particular portion of bone. Chondroblastoma of bone occurs only in the epiphysis. Osteomyelitis in children is usually metaphyseal; if the child has sickle cell disease, however, osteomyelitis in the diaphysis can also occur.

How Old Is the Patient?

The age of the patient affects the diseases likely to be present. In an infant who is under 1 year of age, osteomyelitis frequently spreads to the adjacent joint, resulting in a pyarthrosis. In a child who is older than 1 year of age, osteomyelitis is usually limited to the metaphysis. Certain tumors occur in children, others in young adults, and others in older adults. One should usually limit diagnoses given to those appropriate to the patient's age.

Is There Periosteal Reaction or a Soft Tissue Mass Associated with the Lesion?

Periosteal reaction (new bone formation) and the presence of a soft tissue mass indicate that a lesion has ex-

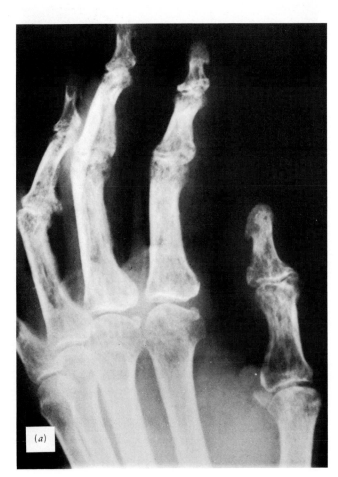
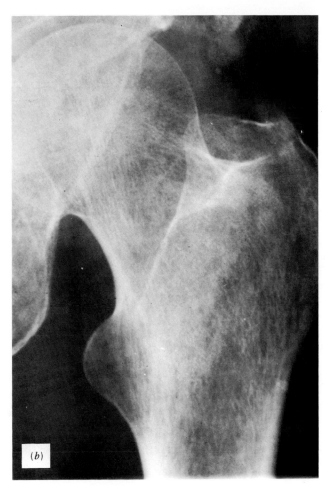

Figure 57-4. Lacunar osteoporosis. This acute form can result from immobilization, hyperemia, or a stroke. (*a*) In the hand after a distal radial fracture. Multiple focal areas of bone loss can be identified. (*b*) In the proximal femur after a stroke. Multiple focal areas of bone loss can be identified. Compare with Figure 55-2*a*.

tended beyond the normal limits of bone. This is a sign of aggressiveness in the lesion. The actual pattern of periosteal new bone formed is indicative of how rapidly the lesion is expanding (as discussed in more detail in Chapter 55). An example of how periosteal new bone formation is used in the evaluation of disease is in the diagnosis of osteomyelitis.

Osteomyelitis. The initial image findings of osteomyelitis result from the elevation of the periosteum and the deposition of periosteal new bone. This new bone deposition is first seen on tracer studies with ^{99m}Tc phosphate complexes. It is often visible within 2–3 days (Fig. 57-10*a* and *b*). Gallium 67 scanning will also be positive for infection. Radiographic changes lag 10–14 days behind the disease process because it takes that long for the bone deposited by the periosteum to be abundant enough to be seen.

In most cases, the clinical diagnosis of osteomyelitis has been made in 10 days, and treatment has usually been started. Radiographs can be used to evaluate the effectiveness of treatment. If the treatment has been effective, the radiograph may show normal bone or a thin layer of periosteal new bone (Fig. 57-11). If the process is controlled, follow-up radiographs should show progressive thickening of this periosteal bone until it merges with the margin of the cortex. Areas of bone destruction should heal (Fig. 57-12). When treatment is delayed, additional bands of periosteal new bone may develop, but 10–14 days after effective therapy, no new bands should develop. If treatment is ineffective, new periosteal bone will continue to form, and focal areas of cortical or trabecular bone loss may develop. Sometimes the osteomyelitis may progress to a subacute state with the area of bone lysis becoming well defined (Fig. 57-13). Less often the infection will incite a sclerotic reaction in the bone, representing a more chronic pattern (Fig. 57-14).

Keynotes

• *Major criteria for the evaluation of lytic bone lesions:*

  a. One or many?

  b. Limited or diffuse?

  c. Sclerotic margin?

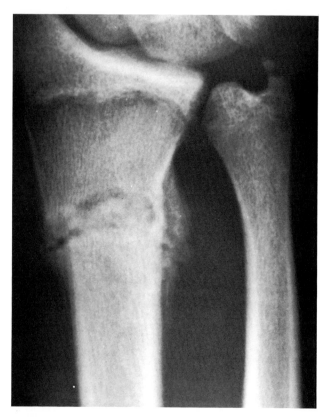

Figure 57-5. Acute osteoporosis of the distal radius and ulna associated with a healing distal radial fracture. In this teenager, the maximal resorption is present in the metaphysis adjacent to the growth plate. This is a common site of bone resorption in children whose growth plates are still open. Callus is present adjacent to the radial fracture and is a sign of partial healing. There is also a small chip fracture of the ulnar styloid process.

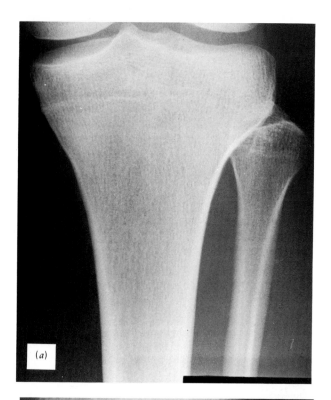

(a)

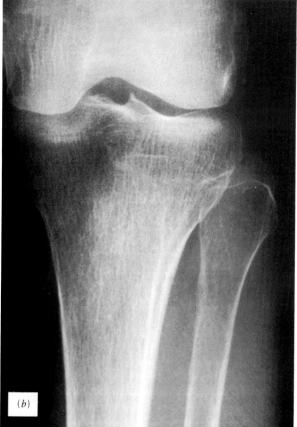

(b)

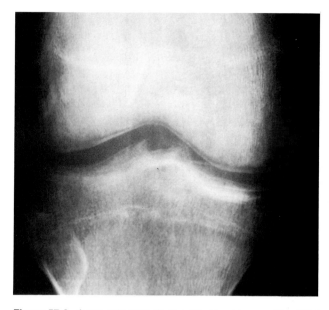

Figure 57-6. Acute osteoporosis in a 38-year-old man with a tibial fracture. Maximal resorption is taking place just under the articular cartilage and is best seen in the distal femur. This is a common pattern of osteoporosis.

Figure 57-7. (a) Normal tibia and fibula. (b) Moderately osteopenic tibia and fibula, chronic. In the chronically osteopenic bones, the trabeculae are fewer, are mainly aligned with the longitudinal axis of the bone, and appear thicker. The cortex of the tibia and fibula are thinner. This is a typical appearance of chronically osteopenic bone.

504

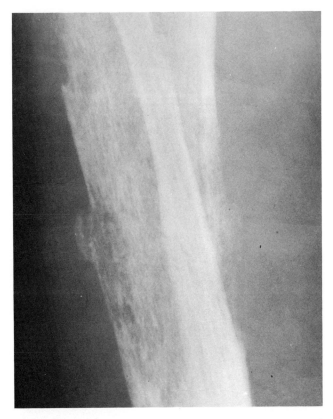

Figure 57-8. Permeative pattern of bone destruction demonstrated in the proximal tibia. This patient had breast cancer metastatic to bone.

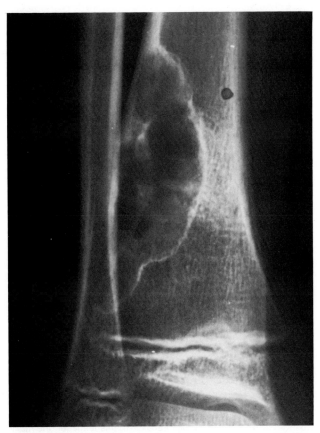

Figure 57-9. Geographic destructive lesion of the distal tibia. This nonossifying fibroma (fibroxanthoma) of bone has resulted in a well-defined, sharply marginated area of bone loss. The bone adjacent to the lesion is denser (whiter) than normal, indicating that it has hypertrophied to buttress the tibia, making it stronger.

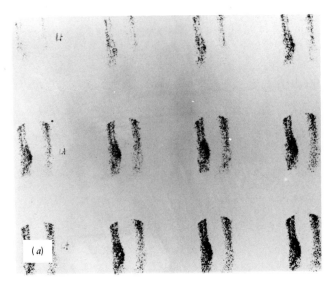

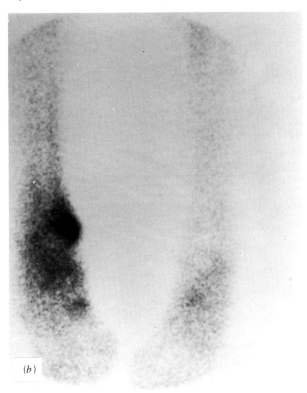

Figure 57-10. Osteomyelitis of the medial malleolus of the tibia. (*a*) Serial images from the vascular phase of the ⁹⁹ᵐTc phosphate complex bone scan demonstrate increased flow to the medial portion of the right distal tibia. (*b*) An equilibrium view from the same bone scan demonstrates increased activity of the medial malleolus. The overall increase in activity on the right side is caused by the hyperemia demonstrated on the vascular phase. (*c*) A radiograph of the ankle demonstrates a slight spotty osteopenia of the medial malleolus.

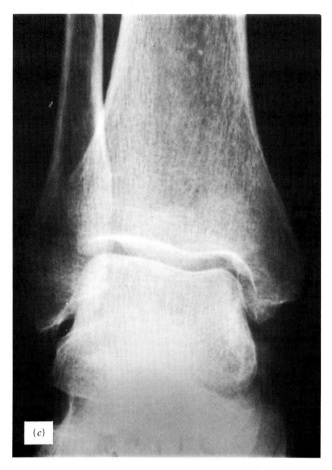

Figure 57-10. (Continued).

d. *Which bone or part of bone?*

e. *Patient's age?*

f. *Periosteal reaction? Soft tissue mass?*

- *Preferred evaluation for possible bone metastases: bone scan with radiographs of abnormal areas. If scan is normal: AP view of pelvis and lateral skull. In multiple myeloma: radiographic skeletal survey.*

- *Osteopenia is a decreased amount of bone. It can be due to osteoporosis, osteomalacia, rickets, hyperparathyroidism, and congenital decreased bone formation (osteogenesis imperfecta).*

- *Patterns of osteoporosis:*

  a. *Acute:*

     Lacunar

     Trabecular bone loss

  b. *Chronic:*

     Trabecular bone loss

     Cortical thinning

- *Those tumors and infections expanding most rapidly in bone have a permeative pattern. Those tumors and infections expanding less rapidly have a geographic pattern.*

- *A nonexpanding or slowly expanding lesion will develop a band of sclerotic bone around it.*

- *Always consider the age of the patient before you suggest possible diagnoses.*

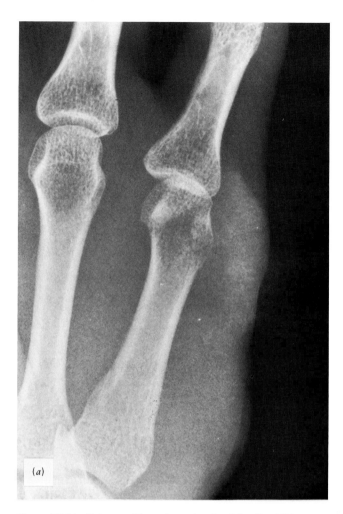

Figure 57-11. Osteomyelitis and pyarthrosis of the distal fifth metacarpal caused by *Pseudomonas* infection. (*a*) The initial film at presentation demonstrates a narrowed fifth metacarpophalangeal joint indicative of joint infection, periarticular osteoporosis indicative of hyperemia, and moderate focal soft tissue swelling. (*b*) The radiograph obtained 35 days later demonstrates destruction of the lateral portion of the distal metaphysis and moderate periosteal new bone (arrow) along the medial portion of the shaft.

- *The diagnosis of osteomyelitis is best made by using the clinical symptoms confirmed by a bone scan or combined bone and gallium scan. Radiographic changes are delayed for 10–14 days.*

PATTERNS OF OSTEOBLASTIC DISEASE

Bone density can be increased by several types of processes. In part, these processes can be predicted from the pattern seen on the radiograph. Increased bone can form as a buttress to help support a portion of bone weakened by another process. This type of buttressing occurs at the margin of a process in which bone has been lost, for example, from a slow-growing tumor or from injury (Fig. 57-9).

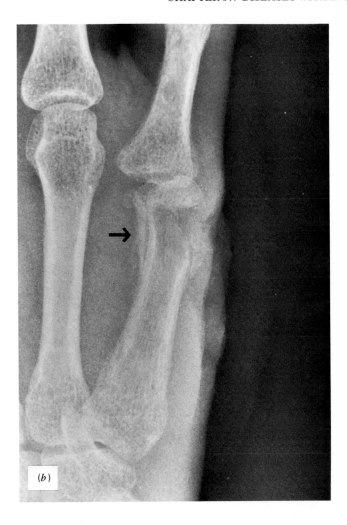

(b)

mogeneity; but when it is diffuse and homogeneous, diffuse increased bone radiodensity is best detected by observing the absence of margination at the corticomedullary junction (see Fig. 55-17). This distinct margin, normal in Figure 55-17b, cannot be identified in Figure 55-17a because the medullary portion of bone has become filled with bone. Diffuse increased bone radiodensity occurs in myelosclerosis, in diffuse bone infarction (especially in patients with sickle cell disease), in some patients with renal failure, and in some patients with metastatic carcinoma of the prostate.

Paget's Disease

Paget's disease of bone is a common process in which bone density can be increased. In Paget's disease, accelerated osteolysis is followed by accelerated bone deposition. Because of the speed of the process, it is possible to see osteolytic areas, osteoblastic areas, or areas of mixed lytic and osteoblastic change (Figs. 57-20 and 57-21). The main aid in identifying a process as Paget's disease is that the bone formed in Paget's disease is usually thicker than normal bone. The cortices are thicker, the bones are enlarged, and the trabeculae are often disorganized and may not lie in the lines of stress (Fig. 57–20). Paget's disease can result in bone pain and narrow nerve channels causing neuropathy and, rarely, can undergo malignant change. But most patients with Paget's disease have no symptoms of the disease. Because Paget's disease is common, it frequently must be distinguished from osteoblastic metastases. The main method of differentiation is recognition of the expansion of bone that is seen essentially only in Paget's disease. Only rarely will metastatic cancer expand the bone.

Focal Disease

The increased bone can form as a direct response to the tumor or infection. Usually in these processes, because the process permeates into the surrounding bone, the edge will be ill-defined, and the sclerosis will seem to radiate into the surrounding bone (Fig. 57-15).

Sclerosis can develop in a nonexpanding bone process. Because the process is not expanding, the margins of the sclerosis are moderately well defined. The most common processes to have this appearance are the bone island (Fig. 57-16) and bone infarct (Fig. 57-17). Unfortunately, some metastases (particularly breast cancer and prostate cancer metastases to bone) will sometimes have well-defined margins as well (Fig. 57-18). Sometimes this well-defined margin indicates that the process is in remission, having responded to effective therapy.

Diffuse Disease

Diffuse increased bone density is harder to detect than focal increase. When the process is diffuse, but inhomogeneous (Fig. 57-19), it can be recognized because of its inho-

Keynotes

- *A buttress of bone will often form around a chronic area of bone loss, helping to support the bone and helping to prevent fracture.*
- *An osteoblastic lesion that permeates into the surrounding bone is usually an active process. One that is well defined is more often (but not always) inactive.*
- *Diffuse increase in bone density can be detected because the corticomedullary junction becomes indistinct.*
- *Paget's disease of bone is a process of unknown etiology in which there is rapid resorption of bone, usually followed by the rapid deposition of new bone. The new bone laid down is more haphazard in its orientation. Cortices are usually thickened, and the trabeculae are often oriented in many different directions.*

SUMMARY

Most processes that injure bone result in a combination of bone lysis and bone deposition. The processes in which bone lysis predominates are called *lytic processes;* those in which bone deposition predominates are called *osteoblastic.* The

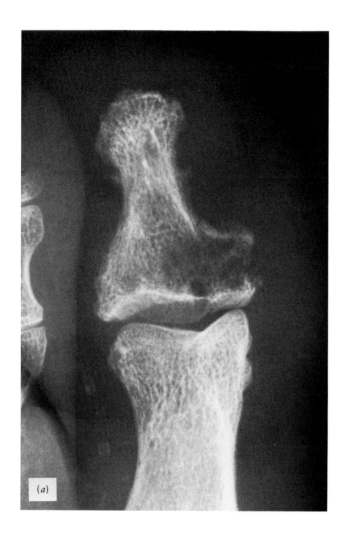

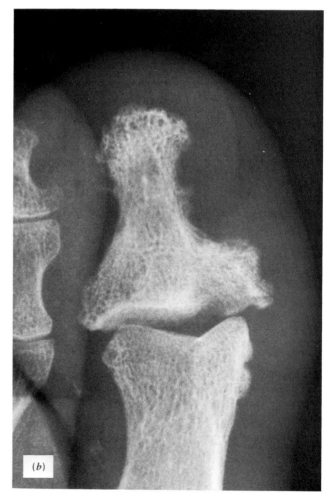

Figure 57-12. Osteomyelitis of the great toe. (*a*) During the acute infection, bone destruction is present. The soft tissues are markedly swollen. (*b*) Four months later, the infection cured, the bone has reformed in a near-normal pattern.

508

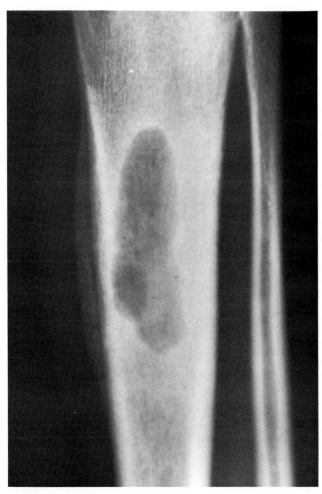

Figure 57-13. Cystic osteomyelitis. This large, lytic, well-defined lesion of the proximal tibial shaft is surrounded by a thin rim of denser bone. Periosteal reaction is seen anteriorly. Cystic osteomyelitis in this pattern can be seen when antibiotics are given in insufficient quantity or duration to cure the infection.

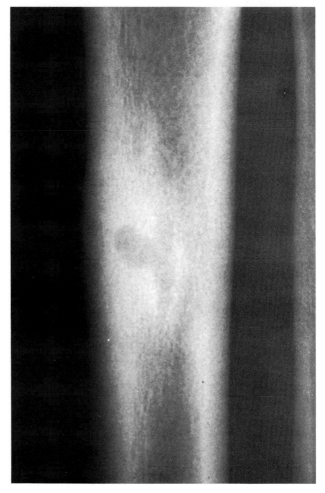

Figure 57-14. Surrounding a focal lytic area of infection is a sclerotic reaction to infection. In addition to the rounded lytic area, there is also a linear tractlike extension of the lytic area. Tracts like this are common in sclerotic osteomyelitis. This particular form of osteomyelitis is called a *Brodie's abscess.*

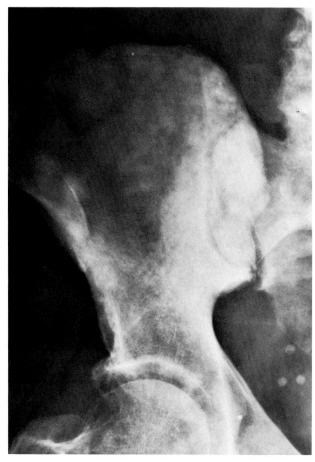

Figure 57-15. Osteoblastic metastases from metastatic prostate cancer. Multiple areas of increased bone are seen in this section of the pelvis. This is one of the typical patterns of metastatic prostate cancer. (Courtesy M. Vaccaro, M.D.)

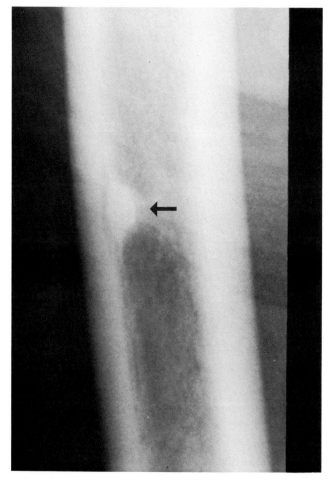

Figure 57-16. This bone island (arrow) in the midshaft of the femur is sclerotic and well defined. Bone islands are a common asymptomatic variant of skeletal ossification.

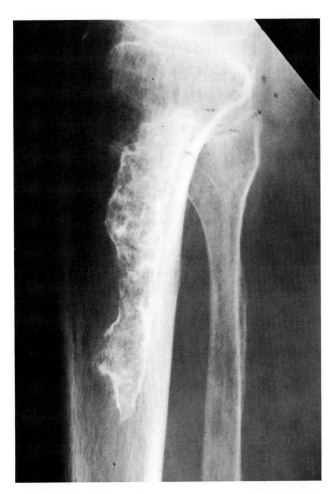

Figure 57-17. This bone infarct occurred in a chronic alcoholic. Bone infarcts occurring in medullary bone are symptomatic when the infarct occurs but then become asymptomatic. During the early phase when the patient is symptomatic, the bone radiograph usually appears normal, but a bone scan may show decreased or increased activity. The typical calcification pattern of a late bone infarct is that of a serpentine, densely calcified rim, with lesser degrees of calcification within it.

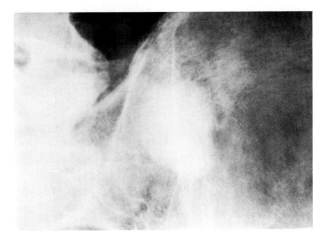

Figure 57-18. This well-defined osteoblastic metastasis in the ilium occurred in a patient with metastatic prostate cancer.

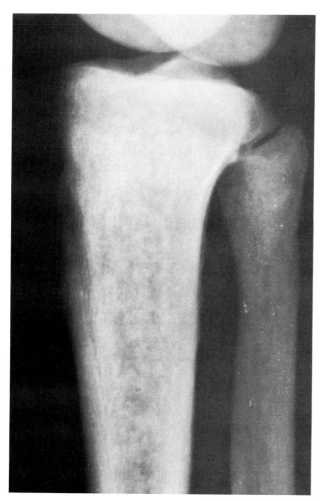

Figure 57-19. Extensive bone infarction in a patient with sickle cell anemia. The marked sclerotic reaction is inhomogeneous, aiding in its detection.

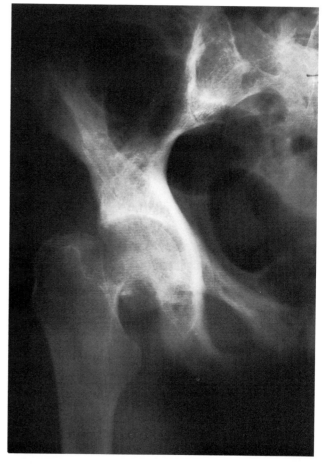

Figure 57-20. Paget's disease of the right hemipelvis and a femoral neck fracture. There is cortical thickening best seen in the acetabulum and a disordered trabecular pattern best seen in the supra-acetabular portion of the ilium and in the ischium. (Reprinted from Freedman, M., *The Radiology of the Postoperative Hip* with permission of John Wiley & Sons, Inc. Copyright 1979.)

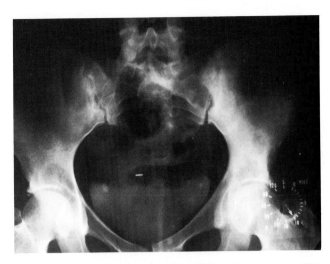

Figure 57-21. Paget's disease of the left ilium, biopsy proven. This patient demonstrates a pattern of increased bone radiodensity in the left hemipelvis without cortical thickening or apparent disorder of the trabeculae. This pattern can occur in Paget's disease but is more often seen in metastatic disease. For this reason, a biopsy was performed.

bone scan is the most sensitive imaging method for detecting new bone formation, even if it is only the minimal response seen in areas of predominant bone lysis.

Criteria for evaluating a lytic process in bone include: Is the lysis solitary, multiple, or diffuse? How widely does it spread through the bone? Does the lytic area have a sclerotic margin? In what bone and in what part of that bone does the lysis occur? How old is the patient? Is there periosteal reaction or a soft tissue mass associated with it? Based on these criteria, a limited differential diagnosis is usually possible.

The current preferred method for evaluating whether a lesion is solitary or multiple is the bone scan. If the bone scan is normal, it is sometimes helpful to obtain a pelvis film and a lateral skull film to exclude diffuse disease. Some patients with multiple myeloma have lytic bone disease with no new bone formation. For this reason, the bone scan in multiple myeloma may not detect areas of bone destruction. In the patient with multiple myeloma, a radiographic skeletal survey should be performed.

Osteoporosis is identified by studying the trabecular pattern and evaluating the cortical thickness. Osteoporosis results in a loss of trabeculae outside the lines of stress and, in its common form, thickening of the trabeculae lying along the lines of stress. Cortical thinning also occurs. Osteoporosis can be quantified by photon absorptiometry or CT bone mineral analysis.

The earliest response of bone to infection that can be imaged is a nonspecific hyperemia. Within several days, the bone scan can reveal reactive bone formation, and gallium scanning can detect the infection. Radiographs become abnormal at 10–14 days, showing early periosteal new bone. If the disease is not treated, new bands of periosteal new bone form, and areas of lysis within the original bone can develop.

Osteoblastic disease can result from the buttressing support surrounding a destructive lesion, in direct response to the bone process as with osteoblastic metastases, or as a reactive process as in Paget's disease of bone.

REVIEW QUESTIONS

1. Why is the bone scan usually abnormal in the patient with a lytic destructive bony lesion?
2. In which bone processes does bone lysis predominate? In which does bone production predominate?
3. Why is the criterion of single, multiple, or diffuse lesions useful in differential diagnosis?
4. What is the importance of the criterion of geographic versus permeative pattern?
5. What does a sclerotic margin of a lytic lesion mean?
6. Give examples of the importance the location of a lesion has for its differential diagnosis.
7. How does the age of the patient help in differential diagnosis?
8. What is the importance of periosteal reaction or a soft tissue mass in association with a lytic lesion of bone?
9. Of what importance is the distinctness seen in the margin of an osteoblastic bone lesion?
10. What is a bone island?
11. What is Paget's disease of bone? What are its radiographic findings?
12. What are the imaging patterns seen in osteomyelitis?

VOCABULARY

osteoblastic processes

geographic pattern

hand-and-foot syndrome of sickle cell disease

lytic processes

multiple myeloma

osteopenia

osteoporosis

Paget's disease of bone

permeative pattern

skeletal survey

SUGGESTIONS FOR FURTHER READING

For suggested reading see Chapter 55.

58

CLINICAL EVALUATION
OF THE PATIENT WITH ARTHRITIS

J. WOLFE BLOTZER

KEY CONCEPTS

Clinical

Most rheumatic diseases share the presence of arthritis with a variety of cutaneous and visceral features. The diagnosis is clinical and based on such host factors as age and sex, the patterns of joint involvement, and the associated extra-articular features. Only in certain cases are radiological features essential to diagnosis. This chapter discusses the clinical evaluation of the patient with arthritis. Chapter 59 discusses the radiology of arthritis.

Arthritis is classified by its clinical presentation into four groups: acute monarticular, acute polyarticular, chronic monarticular and chronic polyarticular arthritides. The most important causes of acute monarticular arthritis are infection and crystal-induced arthritis (gout and pseudogout).

Osteoarthrosis is a common disease of the elderly. The pain of osteoarthrosis is deep and aching and worsens as the day progresses. Because osteoarthrosis is so commonly present in the elderly, care must be taken not to ascribe the patient's pain to osteoarthrosis when some other process may be superimposed on it, causing the pain.

Not all pain felt in the joint is caused by joint disease. Referred pain from cervical spondylosis, neoplasms of the lung, diaphragmatic irritation, and cardiac disease can simulate the symptoms of arthritis.

Radiological

Radiographs are of greatest use in the diagnosis of a chronic monarthritis. Radiographs can be used to assess the degree of joint damage and the effect of therapy in the patient with a chronic polyarthritis but have a limited role in diagnosis. While radiographs in the patient with acute arthritis may be abnormal, the findings are often nonspecific and often not useful.

OBJECTIVES

When you complete this chapter you will be able to

1. List 4 causes each of
   a. Acute monarthritis
   b. Acute polyarthritis
   d. Chronic monarthritis
   d. Chronic polyarthritis
2. List four symptoms you should specifically ask for in evaluating a patient with each of the four types of arthritis.
3. Describe the appropriate evaluation of a patient with an acute monarthritis.
4. Discuss the symptoms and radiographic findings in pulmonary osteopathy.

Most systemic rheumatic diseases are of unknown cause. Thus, etiologic diagnosis is not feasible. Rheumatic diseases share the presence of arthritis with a variety of cutaneous and visceral features. They are discriminated from each other on the basis of host factors (age, sex, etc.), the patterns of joint involvement, and, most important, the associated extra-articular features. Because these entities are defined clinically, not radiologically, their diagnosis depends on the analysis of a carefully performed and thorough history and physical examination. Only in certain instances are radiographic features essential to diagnosis.

Radiographic studies may suggest a diagnosis, but they cannot substitute for the history and physical examination. Laboratory tests are helpful, but their correct selection and interpretation depend on a complete understanding of the patient's clinical problem. For example, *Reiter's syndrome* is defined clinically by the triad of arthritis, urethritis, and conjunctivitis plus associated mucocutaneous features (painless mouth ulcers, circinate balanitis, and keratoderma blennorrhagica). Although radiographs may demonstrate a fluffy calcaneal spur, joint effusions, or sacroiliitis, these same radiographic findings can also be seen in both psoriatic arthritis and ankylosing spondylitis. Diagnosis, treatment, and prognosis all depend on a correct diagnosis, a clinical diagnosis. Table 8-1 lists some of the extra-articular features of the seronegative arthritidies.

In the cases that follow, emphasis is on the clinical history and physical examination that are essential to accurate diagnosis. While radiographs might have been requested in any of these cases, in only some were they necessary, and in others they are never requested. As you read the histories, try to solve the diagnostic problem, and before you see what was done, try to decide if a radiograph would help in diagnosis or treatment.

The cases are arranged according to the classification of arthritis, based on its clinical presentation, into four groups:

Acute monarticular arthritis
Acute polyarticular arthritis
Chronic monarticular arthritis
Chronic polyarticular arthritis

Combinations of the groups can occur. When a patient with a chronic polyarticular arthritis has an acute flare in symptoms, it may indicate just a flare of the chronic polyarthritis, or it could indicate superimposed acute monarticular arthritis.

Keynotes

- *A thorough history and physical examination is the basis of rheumatic diagnosis.*
- *The radiograph plays only a limited role in the diagnosis of rheumatic conditions.*
- *Don't be a passive reader: ask questions of the text, the same way you would ask them of a teacher. Each positive and negative finding in the cases is there for a reason. Can you figure out what it is?*
- *The four general clinical categories of arthritis are:*
  Acute monarticular
  Acute polyarticular
  Chronic monarticular
  Chronic polyarticular

ACUTE ARTHRITIS

Acute Monarthritis

Case 58-1

A 68-year-old woman presents a 5-day history of heat, redness, and swelling of the right shoulder. Any movement of the shoulder is extremely painful. The patient is unaware of any fever, chills, recent weight loss, or other health complaints and has recently been in good health, apart from her shoulder.

The physical examination reveals an elderly woman, not in distress apart from her shoulder. Any motion of the shoulder in any direction is painful. An effusion can be seen and palpated. The shoulder is warm and tender.

This patient's shoulder radiograph is shown in Figure 58-1. What does this mean?

The patient has an acute monarticular arthritis and

TABLE 58-1. EXTRA-ARTICULAR FEATURES OF THE SERONEGATIVE ARTHRITIDES

Disorder	Definition	Skin, Muscosal Lesions	Genital	Ocular	Other
Reiter's disease	Arthritis + urethritis ± conjunctivitis	Keratodermia blennorrhagicum, ungual lesions, painless mouth ulcers	Circinate balanitis	Conjunctivitis, acute iridocyclitis	Aortic insufficiency
Psoriatic arthritis	Arthritis + psoriasis	Psoriasis and/or psoriatic ungual lesions	—	—	—
Behçet's disease	Triad of uveitis + mouth & genital ulcers	Erythema nodosum, skin reactivity to pinprick, painful mouth ulcers	Painful genital ulcers	Uveitis	Thrombophlebitis, CNS Involvement
Crohn's disease	Arthritis + Crohn's disease	Erythema nodosum	—	Uveitis	Radiological or pathological diagnosis
Ulcerative Colitis	Arthritis + colitis	Pyoderma gangrenosum, stomatitis, gingivitis, erythema nodosum	—		Bloody diarrhea; requires X-ray or endoscopic confirmation
Whipple's disease	Arthritis + Whipple's disease	—	—		Malabsorption, CNS Involvement; requires a tissue diagnosis
Relapsing polychondritis	Arthritis with chondritis	—	—		Chondritis of ears, nose, trachea

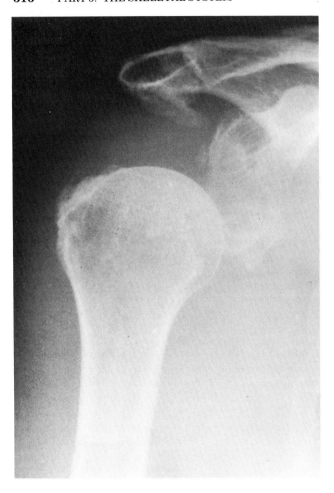

Figure 58-1. Case 58-1. Right shoulder with the humeral head displaced inferiorly in relation to the glenoid fossa and acromion. This can be a sign of muscle weakness or of joint effusion. New bone formation is present adjacent to the greater tuberosity, representing a degenerative change seen in the older patient.

no other symptoms or findings. Consult the following list of possible causes.

Acute Inflammatory Monarthritides

Nongonococcal suppurative (bacterial) arthritis
Gonococcal arthritis
Gout
Pseudogout
Reiter's disease
Psoriatic arthritis
Arthritis of Crohn's disease
Arthritis of ulcerative colitis
Whipple's disease
Behçet's syndrome
Relapsing polychrondritis

All these causes may also apply to oligoarticular or even polyarticular arthritis.

Which seem to you to be appropriate for this patient's clinical history? How would you determine the correct diagnosis?

Acute monarthritis is a common rheumatic problem. In general, acute arthritis of whatever entity (bacterial, viral, psoriatic, colitic, etc.) initially has a nonspecific appearance on radiographs. The usual finding is, as in Figure 58-1, a joint effusion, without specific findings to aid in the differential diagnosis. Often, the presence of the effusion can be ascertained by physical examination.

The critical entity to consider and exclude in any new-onset monarthritis is a bacterial infection, for it is a rapidly destructive but curable form of arthritis. Essential for diagnosis and appropriate therapy is the isolation of the etiologic agent from the joint fluid. Aspiration, Gram stain, and culture of the joint fluid is the key diagnostic test.

In sexually active patients, the gonococcus is the most common offender, but it is also the most difficult to confirm. Isolation of the gonococcus from synovial fluid is difficult; if gonococcal arthritis is suspected, urethral or cervical cultures should be obtained.

A synovial fluid white cell count greater than 50,000 per cubic millimeter or a glucose level less than half the serum value suggests bacterial arthritis. A white cell count greater than 100,000 per cubic millimeter is almost always due to infection.

Gout and pseudogout are common causes of acute severe monarthritis. While they are not rapidly destructive and will not (unlike infection) produce irrevocable damage if the diagnosis is missed on the first attack, they are quite painful and respond rapidly to therapy. The diagnosis of gout and pseudogout—crystal-induced arthritis—is based on the demonstration of the appropriate crystals on polarized-light microscopy.

In this case, you have a shoulder radiograph that demonstrates an effusion but is otherwise nonrevealing. The synovial fluid white cell count is 63,000 cubic millimeters. The Gram stain result is negative. Polarized-light microscopy discloses no crystals. What is your diagnosis?

The next day, cultures demonstrate growth of *Salmonella choleraesuis* and appropriate antibiotic therapy is instituted. As in most cases of acute monarthritis, the radiograph was abnormal but not helpful because a joint effusion is not specific enough to guide therapy.

Acute Polyarthritis

Case 58-2

This 32-year-old nurse complains of pain and swelling of 18 hours' duration in her wrists, metacarpal phalangeal joints, and proximal interphalangeal joints. She denies having a rash, fever, chills, hair loss, dry eyes or mouth, Raynaud's phenomenon, chest or abdominal pain, mouth or nasal ulcerations, numbness, or weakness. For 2 weeks, she has felt ill and anorexic. On physical examination, mild swelling and tenderness of the symptomatic joints are noted. Within an hour of the evaluation, the patient reports the development of a number of large urticarial lesions.

How do you go about this diagnosis?

The basis for deciding how to evaluate the patient further is a knowledge of the clinical possibilities:

Acute Inflammatory Polyarthritides

Gonococcal Polyarthritis/Dermatitis

Reiter's Disease

Viral arthritis¨

   Hepatitis B

   Rubella and others

Systemic lupus erythematosus

Rheumatoid arthritis

Acute rheumatic fever

Lofgren's syndrome (Erythema nodosum syndrome presentation of acute sarcoidosis.)

Serum sickness

Arthritis of inflammatory bowel disease

Lyme disease

Erythema nodosum

Other considerations include adult Still's disease, arthropathy of hemoglobinopathies such as sickle cell disease, vasculitis syndrome (anyphylactoid purpura, Wegener's granulomatosis, etc.), polyarticular gout, and palindromic rheumatism.

Your clinical description depends heavily on the patient's replies to questions about the list of symptoms that might indicate a possible disease to explain the polyarthritis this patient has. Can you match up the symptoms list with the list of possible acute polyarthritides? For example, which diseases might a rash indicate? Rubella or systemic lupus erythematosus. What about the others?

Is there also a role for imaging studies in the evaluation of acute polyarthritis? Yes, but not for joints. You need to know for each item on the list of polyarthritides whether an imaging study would support a diagnosis. It certainly might be useful in the arthritis of chronic bowel disease. For patients with ankle arthritis or periarthritis and with erythema nodosum lesions on the pretibial areas, you should consider the acute syndrome of sarcoidosis, Lofgren's syndrome, and a chest radiograph showing the hilar adenopathy or interstitial disease of sarcoid would certainly support this diagnosis.

So what is this patient's diagnosis? The clinical history gives you clues.

The patient's antecedent history of malaise together with her nursing history suggest hepatitis B arthritis.

Liver enzyme levels prove to be elevated, the patient proves positive for hepatitis B surface antigen, and 3 days later she becomes jaundiced.

Joint radiographs and other imaging studies were not necessary. The diagnosis was based on the history and the results of carefully selected laboratory tests.

Keynotes

- *In the patient with an acute monarticular arthritis, the first tests should be the examination of the joint fluid for evidence of infection or crystal-induced arthritis (gout or pseudogout).*
- *Raynaud's phenomenon is a vasospastic response, usually in the fingers, leading to decreased perfusion, color change, and pain. It is seen in several of the rheumatic diseases.*
- *"What one knows, one sees" applies to all medicine. The more you know in any field of endeavor, the more you recognize and the more interesting the field becomes.*

CHRONIC ARTHRITIS

With subacute arthritis (2–6 weeks of symptoms) and chronic arthritis (more than 6 weeks of symptoms), imaging studies are useful, sometimes to help establish the diagnosis, other times to assess the amount of joint damage that has occurred.

Chronic Monarthritis

Case 58-3

This 64-year-old woman is referred for evaluation of osteoarthritis of the left hip. A retired housekeeper, she has a 3-year history of bilateral hip pain. The pain is constant, deep, and aching and is exacerbated by walking and getting out of chairs and gets worse as the day proceeds. Many of her joints are stiff in the morning but loosen up after about 10 minutes. Her joint pains had been slowly worsening over many years, but in the last 8 months, the left hip has become extremely painful. The patient does not remember whether the left hip pain became worse gradually or suddenly. The pain is now so severe that she can only walk a few steps.

The patient denies weight loss, night sweats, fever, rash, and malaise. She had a cerebral thrombosis on the left side several years ago and has had bilateral iliofemoral bypass grafts for peripheral arterial insufficiency.

Physical examination demonstrates bilateral loss of the range of motion in both hips, the left worse than the right. The left hip range of motion is extremely painful. Arterial pulses are very weak in both feet.

What do you think is going on? What are the clinical possibilities?

Subacute and Chronic Monarthritides

Osteoarthrosis (degenerative joint disease, osteoarthritis)

Mechanical internal derangement

Chronic infection with bacteria, mycobacteria, or fungi

Chronic idiopathic monarthritis (i.e., inflammatory arthritis, all other causes excluded)

Avascular necrosis of bone

Osteochondritis dissecans

Neoplasms of synovium or bone

Fractures (usually of the hip or pelvis in patients with underlying metabolic bone disease)

Paget's disease of bone

Synovial chondromatosis/osteochondromatosis

Osteomyelitis

Pigmented villonodular synovitis

*See also list of acute monarthritis in case 58-1.

Of course most of the diseases listed as causes of acute inflammatory monarthritis can continue into a subacute or chronic stage and should also be included in your differential considerations.

Which of these conditions should you consider now that you know this patient's history of a chronic, slowly progressive oligoarthritis that rapidly worsened in just one joint?

Her history of previous iliofemoral artery bypass surgery and the weak arterial pulses should certainly suggest the claudication of arterial insufficiency. But the pain of intermittent claudication should be intermittent and effort related. It also should not produce painful limitation of hip motion. Arterial insufficiency can be excluded as a cause of this patient's symptoms.

Is the diagnosis osteoarthrosis (degenerative joint disease)? Osteoarthrosis can be diagnosed clinically in the hands by the presence of the pathognomonic Heberden's and Bouchard's nodes usually in association with first carpometacarpal joint involvement. In other joints, confirmation of a clinical diagnosis of osteoarthrosis requires compatible radiographs. The pain of osteoarthrosis is a deep, aching pain that is use related. The pain worsens as the day goes on, with peak pain between 4 PM and 10 PM. Morning stiffness is less than 30 minutes. Does osteoarthrosis explain this patient's symptoms? Certainly her long history of slowly progressive, constant, deep, and aching pain, worsening as the day proceeds, is characteristic of this entity. But the rapid worsening is unexpected; some other process may be superimposed on her osteoarthrosis.

Avascular necrosis, neoplasms, chronic hip infection, a pathological fracture, or a rapid asymmetric unilateral worsening of her osteoarthrosis are all considerations. In this patient, as in all patients with chronic joint pain, radiographic studies are indicated (Fig. 58-2). What do you see?

There are changes of very minimal osteoarthrosis of both hips with small osteophytes on the margins of the acetabulum. But the major finding is a displaced fracture of the femoral neck. The borders of this fracture are sclerotic, indicating the fracture has been present for many months. Even in retrospect, the patient is unable to recall any injury or any acute onset of symptoms.

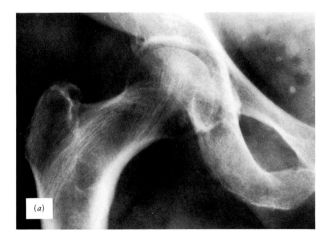

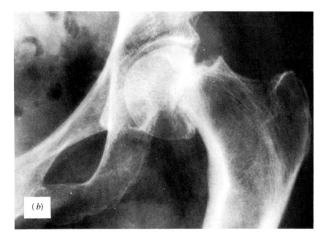

Figure 58-2. Case Example 58-3. (*a*) Right hip. (*b*) Left hip.

Case 58-4

A 62-year-old retired steelworker is referred by his family physician for treatment of "osteoarthritis of the shoulder unresponsive to therapy." The patient has had 6 months of progressive left shoulder pain. The pain is not exacerbated by movement of the shoulder, nor is it relieved by rest. The patient notes no swelling, morning stiffness, history of trauma, or complaints in other joints. He admits to a 15-lb weight loss over the last 6 months.

Physical examination of the joints reveals a full range of motion without pain.

What do you think is going on? Does this patient have arthritis?

One of the hallmarks of arthritis is pain on movement of the joint. Because this patient does not have pain on movement of the symptomatic shoulder, he cannot have an arthritis, tendonitis, or bursitis. He therefore must have referred pain. Most pain referred to the shoulder comes from cervical spondylosis, neoplasms of the lung, diaphragmatic irritation, or cardiac disease.

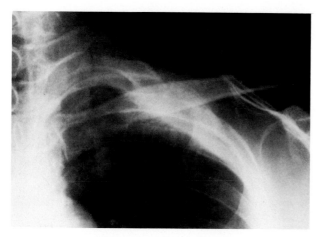

Figure 58-3. Case 58-4. Left lung apex. There is thickening of the apical pleura and a moth-eaten appearance of the bone of the left second rib.

In this case, radiographs (Fig. 58-3) reveal the diagnosis. What is it? A mass in the apex of the lung with destruction of adjacent bone: a form of lung cancer, a Pancoast tumor, that often invades the brachial plexus and causes referred pain. Because the physical examination indicated that this patient did not have arthritis, a more complete evaluation leads to the discovery of the true cause of the pain.

Case 58-5

A 22-year-old senior in college has a 4-year history of arthritis of the right hip. The right hip pain has been continuous. It is exacerbated by walking and somewhat relieved by rest. The hip feels stiff for 3 hours in the morning. The patient states that numerous right hip radiographs have been normal. He denies urethritis, abdominal complaints, mouth or genital lesions, and ocular complaints. He has had severe cystic acne since age 16.

Physical examination reveals an obese male with acne-scarred face and back. There is some atrophy of the right quadriceps muscle. There is slight limitation of motion of the right hip. The hip is painful only on extreme flexion (which would also stress the sacroiliac joint). The right sacroiliac joint is extremely tender on all maneuvers involving the joint.

Is this inflammatory disease? Yes, because of the morning stiffness. Is it hip joint disease? No, because hip arthritis should result in pain on motion of the hip. Is this sacroiliac joint disease? Yes, because stress applied to the right sacroiliac produces pain, indicating presumed sacroiliac joint involvement. Radiographs (Fig. 58-4) are indicated for confirmation.

What form of arthritis might this patient have?

This patient's symptoms clearly implicate the right sacroiliac joint as the site of his arthritis. The numerous normal hip radiographs had not included the sacro-

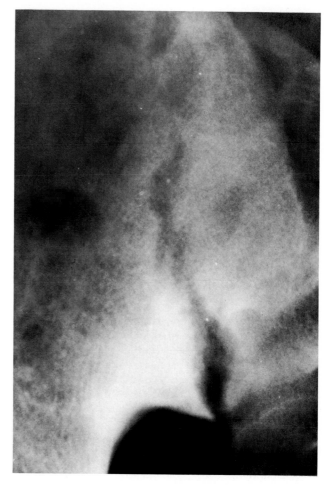

Figure 58-4. Case 58-5. The right sacroiliac joint. There is irregularity of the margins of the joint with sclerosis along the iliac side.

iliac joint. The sacroiliac joint views (Fig. 58-4) demonstrate an erosive sacroiliitis of the right sacroiliac joint. In the absence of extra-articular features, the patient probably has a spondylitic variant or atypical ankylosing spondylitis.

Treatment with indomethacin brings marked symptomatic relief.

Imaging studies are an integral part of the diagnostic evaluation of chronic arthritis. In this case, incomplete physical examinations failed to reveal the site of this patient's arthritis. Radiographs were obtained of the wrong region, and the diagnosis was not established.

Chronic Polyarthritis

Imaging studies are important in the evaluation of chronic polyarthritis. They are used both to help establish the diagnosis and to evaluate the degree of joint damage. A combination of clinical follow-up with radiological follow-up is used to evaluate the rate of progression of the disease and the effect of drug therapy in stabilizing the arthritic process.

Case 58-6

This 26-year-old woman was referred with a 3-month history of a symmetrical additive polyarthritis involving the shoulders, elbows, wrists, metacarpophalangeal (MCP) joints, proximal interphalangeal (PIP) joints, knees, ankles, and metatarsophalangeal (MTP) joints. She complains of 5 hours of morning stiffness, swelling, malaise, easy fatiguability, and a 5-kg weight loss. She denied hair loss, nasopharyngeal ulcers, photosensitivity, psoriasis, other skin lesions, chest or abdominal pain, seizures or psychosis, dry eyes or dry mouth, and Raynaud's phenomenon.

Physical examination reveals a chronically ill appearing young woman with limitation of motion of the shoulders, wrists, PIP joints, and MCP joints. Tenderness and swelling are present in the elbows, wrists, MCP and PIP joints, knees, ankles, and MTP joints. Bilateral epitrochlear adenopathy is noted. Grip strength is 20% of normal. Radiographs at this time demonstrated periarticular osteoporosis, a nonspecific finding of inflammatory arthritis.

What do you think this patient has? Why are the radiographs almost normal and nonspecific? When do you think the radiographs might become abnormal?

First, what are the clinical possibilities? As you look at this list of diagnostic possibilities, consider each of the symptoms listed in the history, those that are positive and those that are negative, and which symptoms are associated with which diseases:

Chronic Polyarthritides

Noninflammatory synovial fluid
   Osteoarthrosis (degenerative joint disease, osteoarthritis)
   Hypertrophic osteoarthropathy
   Reflex sympathetic dystrophy
   Sarcoid arthritis
   Synovial Amyloidosis
Inflammatory joint fluid
   Rheumatoid arthritis
   Systemic lupus erythematosus
   Psoriatic arthritis
   Reiter's disease
   Chronic gouty arthritis
   "Rheumatoid" form of calcium pyrophosphate deposition disease
   Arthritis of Crohn's disease
   Arthritis of malignancy
   Systemic sclerosis
   Primary Sjögren's syndrome

Is this a systemic inflammatory arthritis?

Yes. There are systemic symptoms of malaise, easy fatiguability, and weight loss; there is morning stiffness.

Looking at the listing of the inflammatory diseases, the symptoms the patient does not have help you to eliminate diseases. For example, abdominal pain would probably be a symptom if the patient had the arthritis of Crohn's disease. Dry eyes or dry mouth should have been mentioned for the diagnosis to be Sjögren's syndrome. Psoriasis should usually accompany psoriatic arthritis.

Why are the radiographs almost normal?

Because the patient has had symptoms for 3 months. In general, 6 months has to pass before radiographs start demonstrating joint changes in the chronic polyarthritides. At 3 months, radiographs will sometimes demonstrate swelling, joint effusions, or periarticular osteoporosis, but not specific findings that help in classifying the arthritis.

Should radiographs be obtained this early?

Yes, because several of the diseases do demonstrate early radiographic changes. These include hypertrophic pulmonary osteopathy and, in some cases, the "rheumatoid" form of calcium pyrophosphate deposition disease.

The next stage in the work-up of this patient is an analysis of the clinical possibilities and a selection of any radiological and laboratory tests that might contribute to the diagnosis.

The most likely diagnosis in this patient, based on the history and physical examination, is rheumatoid arthritis because this is the most common inflammatory polyarthritis in the United States and occurs in 0.5% of the population. Systemic lupus erythematosus (SLE) is the next most common.

To establish the diagnosis of rheumatoid arthritis, use the criteria of the American Rheumatism Association (ARA):

Diagnostic Criteria for Rheumatoid Arthritis

1. Morning stiffness
2. Pain on motion or tenderness in at least one joint
3. Joint swelling in at least one joint
4. Swelling in one other joint
5. Symmetrical joint swelling
6. Skin nodules
7. Typical radiographic changes
8. Positive rheumatoid factor
9. Poor mucin precipitate from synovial fluid
10. Characteristic synovial histologic changes
11. Characteristic histologic changes in nodules

*Numbers 1–6 must be present for at least 6 weeks.

Rheumatoid Arthritis Diagnostic Criteria Exclusions

1. Malar rash of SLE
2. LE cells/clearcut SLE
3. Periarteritis nodosa

4. Muscle weakness/dermatomyositis
5. Systemic Sclerosis
6. Rheumatic fever
7. Clinical picture of gout
8. Tophi
9. Infectious arthritis

10. Articular tuberculosis
11. Reiter's disease
12. Reflex sympathetic dystrophy
13. Hypertrophic osteoarthropathy
14. Neuroarthropathy
15. Ochronosis
16. Sarcoidosis
17. Multiple myeloma
18. Erythema Nodosum
19. Leukemia/lymphoma
20. Agammaglobulinemia[†]

[†]The two ARA lists are reprinted from *Arthritis and Rheumatism Journal,* copyright 1982. Used by permission of the American Rheumatism Association.

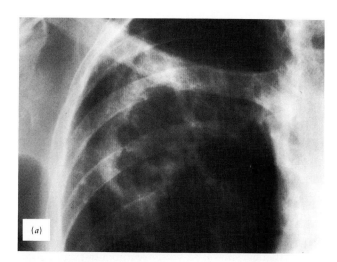

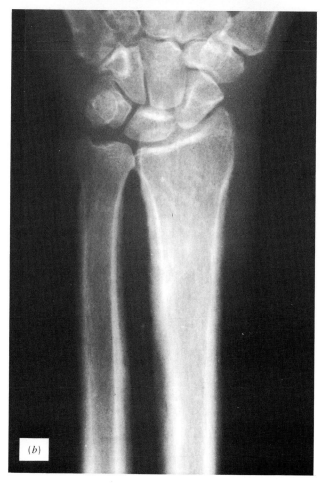

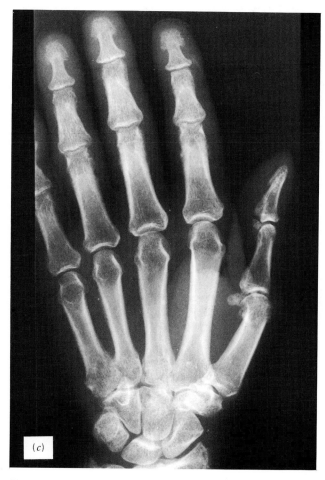

Figure 58-5. Case 58-7. (*a*) Radiograph of the right upper lung. There is a thick-walled, somewhat irregular cavity. (*b*) Distal right forearm. There is a fluffy, thick periosteal new bone formed along the margins of the distal radius and ulna. (*c*) Left hand. There is a small amount of irregular periosteal new bone along the proximal and middle phalanges and very minimal linear periosteal new bone along the shafts of each of the metacarpals.

For a diagnosis of rheumatoid arthritis, at least 5 positive ARA criteria must be present, and all 20 ARA exclusion criteria must be absent. These lists include clinical, laboratory, and radiological criteria. The typical radiological changes are discussed in Chapter 59.

In this patient, the clinical evaluation reveals no evidence of SLE. The laboratory evaluation demonstrates seronegativity for rheumatoid factor, fluorescent antinuclear antibody, and syphilis. Hemolytic anemia, leukopenia, lymphopenia, and thrombocytopenia are absent, and the urinalysis results are normal. At this point, the clinical diagnosis is probable rheumatoid arthritis. Later clinical follow-up supports this diagnosis.

Case 58-7

This 48-year-old man on the thoracic surgery service was seen for evaluation and therapy for a 3-year history of rheumatoid arthritis. He gave a history of a slowly progressive, symmetrical, additive polyarthritis with 3 hours of morning stiffness and profound gel phenomenon. There were no complaints of dry eyes or mouth, skin eruptions, or other associated symptoms. In the past 6 months the patient had developed a nonproductive cough and lost 10 lbs., which caused him to seek medical attention. A chest radiograph (Fig. 58-5a) revealed a cavitary right-upper-lobe mass, which led to his admission on the thoracic surgery service. Physical examination revealed clubbing of fingers and toes, which the patient said had come about over the past few years. Tenderness and swelling of the wrists, MCP and PIP joints, knees, ankles, and toes were noted. Tenderness was also present over the phalanges between the joints, and on the long bones of the extremities. Radiographs of the long bones and hands were requested (Fig. 58-5b and c). Extensive periosteal elevation was noted without evidence of erosions.

What do you make of this clinical picture? What do the radiographs tell you?

In this case, the clinical impression of hypertrophic pulmonary osteopathy is confirmed by the radiological demonstration of periosteal elevation. This radiological investigation had been suggested by the physical examination finding of tenderness of the bones between the joints. At surgery the pulmonary mass proved to be a pulmonary carcinoma. The presence of malignancy and arthritis should always raise the issue of hypertrophic pulmonary osteopathy. Recognition of this connection 3 years earlier by the treating physician might have led to early diagnosis of the patient's neoplasm. Chest radiography is essential to this diagnosis.

Keynotes

- In people over the age of 40, osteoarthrosis is so common that you should look for other diseases that might coexist with it. In people under the age of 40, osteoarthrosis is usually secondary to some other form of arthritis or process.

- Avascular necrosis is also called aseptic necrosis, osteonecrosis, and ischemic necrosis. It is due to a loss of blood supply to the epiphyseal end of a bone.

- Hypertrophic pulmonary osteopathy is a process in which patients with a limited variety of lung processes, chronic infections, malignancies, and cirrhosis develop painful distal extremities associated with periosteal new bone formation. In the United States, the most common cause is lung cancer.

- Even with complete and repeated evaluations, the clinical findings in a patient with arthritis may succeed only in supporting, but not confirming, the diagnosis. Even with the most careful evaluation, a definite diagnosis may not be reached in the rheumatic diseases.

SUMMARY

Diseases of joints are divided into four groups: acute monarticular, acute polyarticular, chronic monarticular, and chronic polyarticular. Most rheumatic diseases are clinical entities. For most, radiography is an adjunct to the clinical evaluation, not the basis of diagnosis.

Joint radiography is useful in the diagnostic evaluation of acute traumatic lesions, chronic monarthritis and polyarthritis, and chronic joint pain without signs of inflammation. Radionuclide scanning is useful when evaluating for tumor, infection, osteonecrosis, and reflex sympathetic dystrophy. Radiographs are usually required to establish the diagnosis of Paget's disease, spondylitis, fractures, avascular necrosis, and, in large joints, osteoarthrosis.

Because osteoarthrosis and Paget's disease are common in older patients, their presence does not necessarily indicate that they are the cause of the patient's pain.

The key to accurate diagnosis of the rheumatic diseases is a careful history and physical examination and analysis of the data derived from them. To interpret the data, a knowledge of the possibilities and parameters is essential.

REVIEW QUESTIONS

1. Can radiographs be used to establish the nature of a rheumatic disease? Under what circumstances?
2. What are the four basic categories of arthritis?
3. Which rheumatic diagnoses can be confirmed by radiographs?
4. What are the common processes that result in an acute monarticular arthritis?
5. What are the common processes that result in an acute polyarticular arthritis?
6. What are the common processes that result in a chronic monarticular arthritis?
7. What are the common processes that result in a chronic polyarticular arthritis?
8. Describe the symptoms and findings in patients with crystal-induced arthritis.
9. What are the symptoms and signs of Reiter's syndrome?
10. Describe Raynaud's phenomenon.
11. What symptoms and signs indicate that joint pain is due to joint disease and is not referred pain?

VOCABULARY

calcium pyrophosphate deposition disease (pseudogout)
crystal-induced arthritis
distal interphalangeal
  joint
gout
Lofgren's syndrome
metacarpophalangeal joint

polyarthritis
proximal interphalangeal joint
psoriasis
pulmonary hypertrophic
  osteopathy
Raynaud's phenomenon
Reiter's syndrome
rheumatic diseases

monarthritis
osteoarthrosis (osteoarthritis/
  degenerative joint disease)
osteonecrosis

rheumatoid arthritis
suppurative arthritis
systemic lupus erythematosus

SUGGESTIONS FOR FURTHER READING

For suggested reading see Chapter 55.

59

THE RADIOLOGY OF ARTHRITIS

KEY CONCEPTS

Radiological

The first step in evaluating diseases of the ends of bones is the classification of these diseases into disease that is primarily a disease of bone and disease that is primarily disease of a joint. This chapter focuses on diseases of synovial joints. There are two types of synovial-lined joints: those in which the bone ends articulate directly and those in which the articulation occurs via a meniscus. When a meniscus is present, it can be damaged by trauma and can degenerate.

There are several patterns seen in diseases of the synovial joints. Periarticular osteoporosis can result from lack of use or from hyperemia. A joint effusion can result from injury or inflammatory diseases. Joint narrowing indicates destruction of cartilage. The loss of cartilage can lead to a loss of the bone under the cartilage, resulting in skip areas and erosions. Bone (osteophytes) can form at the margins of joints. Cartilage can calcify.

Joint injury can result in traumatic effusions, fractures into the joint, and meniscal damage. A meniscus can be evaluated by arthrography with a contrast medium injected into the joint to outline the meniscus.

Joint infection initially results in a joint effusion and often in periarticular osteoporosis. Later, joint narrowing can occur.

Rheumatoid arthritis can result in periarticular osteoporosis, joint effusions, loss of articular bone (in a pattern called an *erosion*), and joint narrowing.

Gout usually demonstrates no osteoporosis because the attacks are intermittent. The joints often appear normal or demonstrate changes of degenerative joint disease. Less commonly, erosions are seen but have a different pattern from those of rheumatoid arthritis.

Degenerative joint disease demonstrates asymmetric joint narrowing and osteophyte formation at the margin of joints.

Clinical

Joints with meniscal damage may present recurrent effusions, joint locking, or joint giving way.

Infected joints produce joint pain and swelling. Aspiration and culture is the prime diagnostic method. Radiographic changes occur late and reflect the damage caused by the infection.

The diagnosis of gout and pseudogout often depends on the analysis of the joint fluid under polarized light.

OBJECTIVES

When you complete this chapter you will be able to

1. Differentiate joint and bone disease on selected radiographs.
2. Correctly classify arthritis as rheumatoid arthritis or degenerative joint disease on selected radiographs.
3. List six types of changes in joints that can occur with joint disease.
4. Describe a typical clinical history of a patient with rheumatoid arthritis. Of a patient with an infected joint. Of a patient with degenerative joint disease.

Diseases of the skeletal system may affect primarily the bones or the joints. This chapter concerns primarily diseases that affect the *joints*, which are the connections between two adjacent bones. There are three types:

Joints of the extremities, which have a synovial lining
Vertebral bodies which are separated by a flexible disc
Joints of the skull, which are separated only by cartilage with little or no movement possible

Different types of disease processes affect each kind of joint. The more common types of arthritis affecting synovial joints are degenerative, septic, and rheumatoid. Joints with an interposed disc can be afflicted by degenerative disc disease with or without disc herniation. The spondyloarthropathies (ankylosing spondylitis, Reiter's syndrome, psoriatic arthritis, and juvenile polyarthritis) affect both disc joints and synovial joints along with their surrounding connective tissue. The cartilage-jointed joints of the skull can be affected by traumatic separation. Only the diseases of synovial joints are discussed in this chapter.

The synovial-lined joints include all of the joints of the extremities, the joint between the odontoid process and the first cervical vertebra, the facet joints of the spine, the temporomandibular joints, the acromioclavicular joints, the sacroiliac joints, and the vertebral-rib joints. The structure of these joints takes two forms: *direct articulating* and *indirect articulating via a meniscus.*

In the more common direct articulating form, the articulating ends of bones are covered with hyaline cartilage. Synovial fluid which coats and nourishes the cartilage, is contained in a joint space lined by synovium. The joint space has the potential to accommodate a wide range of motion.

In the less common form, the bone ends do not directly articulate, but rather articulate via a fibrocartilaginous disc. This type of joint occurs in the knee, the wrist, the acromioclavicular joint, the sternoclavicular joint, and the temporomandibular joint. The cartilaginous disc can degenerate or tear and cause symptoms, and this adds to the types of disease that can affect these joints.

Keynotes

- *The three types of joints:*
  Cartilage-joined joints
  Disc-articulated joints
  Synovial-lined joints
- *There are two kinds of synovial-lined joints: direct articulating and articulating via a fibrocartilaginous meniscus. The joints with a meniscus are subject to the same diseases as those joints that directly articulate plus meniscal tears and degeneration.*

THE PATTERNS OF CHANGE IN DISEASES OF SYNOVIAL JOINTS

Six patterns are commonly seen in patients with disease of synovial joints:

1. Periarticular osteoporosis can result from decreased activity in response to pain or from increased vascularity from inflammation or injury.

2. A joint effusion can result from injury or inflammatory disease. In many joints, the effusion can be recognized because the fat that normally lies around the joint capsule is displaced by the expansion of the intracapsular space. In some patients with fractures entering the joint, fat can be recognized as a layer of lesser radiodensity lying on top of the denser blood. (See Figs. 56-5, 6, and 7.)

3. Joint narrowing is an important sign of joint disease. It is easy to recognize if the narrowing is asymmetric, but it can be difficult to diagnose when the narrowing is concentric. A mental image of the normal range of joint thickness is most helpful.

Most joints need to be stressed to demonstrate the extent of joint narrowing (Fig. 59-1). Weight bearing films of the knees and ankles may be needed. The shoulder (glenohumeral joint) is best stressed by having the arm abducted 45°, the wrist by having the patient make a tight fist. Only the hip joint will usually have enough muscle tone at rest to demonstrate the true amount of joint narrowing.

4. Skip areas and erosions represent loss of the articulating bone from the effect of adjacent synovial pressure or interference with cartilage nutrition. The earliest lesion is called a *skip area*. The skip area is an interruption in the

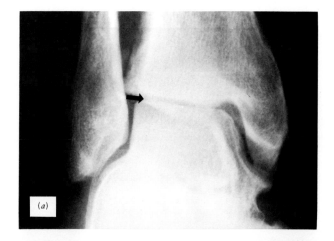

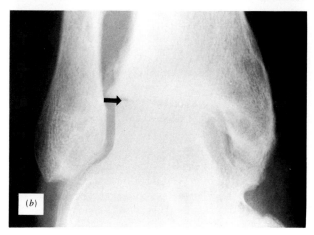

Figure 59-1. Posttraumatic degenerative arthritis of the ankle. (*a*) Non-weight-bearing view. There is moderate narrowing of the joint space (arrow) superiorly. (*b*) Weight-bearing view. The joint space (arrow) between the top of the talus and the adjacent tibia essentially disappears.

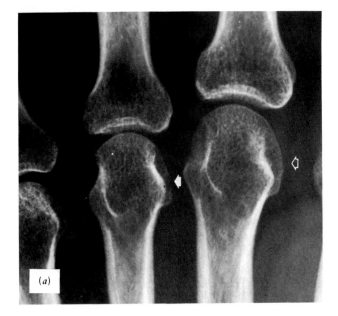

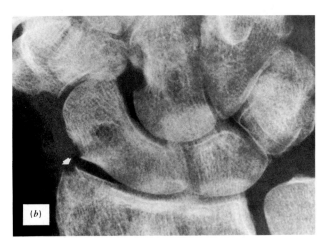

Figure 59-2. Skip areas and erosions in rheumatoid arthritis. (a) The white line forming the margin of the third metacarpal head (open arrow) is complete. That of the fourth metacarpal head is interrupted (solid white arrow). This interruption is called a *skip area*. (b) There is a prominent erosion of the radial styloid process (arrow).

thin line of bone and calcified cartilage that lines the bone end. (Fig. 59-2a).

Erosions represent the progression of this process with the destruction of the trabecular bone underlying the subarticular plate. Erosions can have inner margins that are sclerotic or can have no defined inner margin (Fig. 59-2b). A well-defined or sclerotic inner margin indicates that the process is inactive or had a recent period of inactivity permitting partial healing.

5. *Osteophytes* (Fig. 59-3) are focal regions of bone formation at the margins of joints. They usually result from abnormal motion at the joint. They may not form in the presence of an inflamed synovium.

6. Calcification of the articular cartilage (Fig. 59-4) oc-

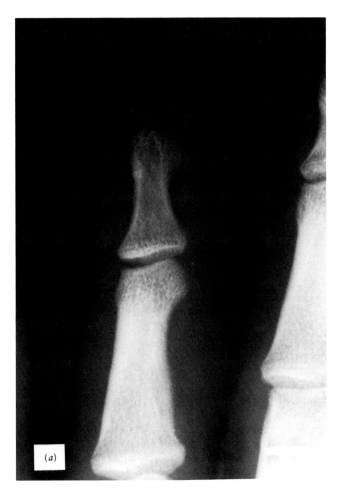

Figure 59-3. Normal appearance and degenerative arthritis of the distal interphalangeal joint of the index finger. (a) Normal appearance of joint, oblique view. There is a normal width of the joint space and smooth contours of the bones. (b) Degenerative arthritis, oblique view, and (c) PA view. The joint is markedly narrowed, and large, bony projections called osteophytes are present.

curs with calcium pyrophosphate deposition disease, called pseudogout because of its similarity in symptoms to gout. Calcified articular cartilage can also be seen associated with degenerative arthritis, hyperparathyroidism, Wilson's disease, and ochronosis.

Other less common manifestations of disease in synovial joints include focal calcifications within joints, enlargement of the ends of bone, and cyst formation with the ends of bones, none of which are discussed in this book.

Keynotes

- *Periarticular osteoporosis is diminished bone around a joint caused by hyperemia and decreased use to avoid pain.*
- *True joint width can be determined only when the joint is stressed.*
- *Skip areas and erosions are due to focal loss of the cartilage, calcified cartilage, and the subarticular plate of bone.*

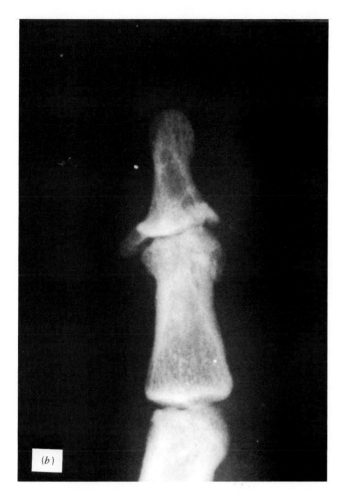
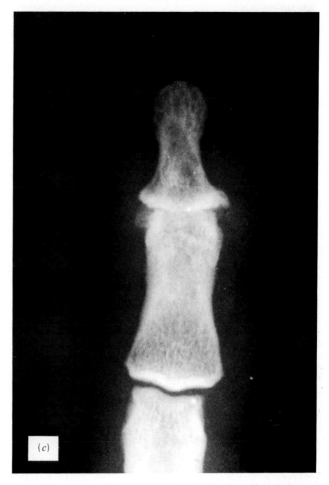

Figure 59-3. (Continued).

- *The inner margin in an active erosion is usually nonsclerotic. If the disease is intermittently and briefly active, as in gout, the margin is sclerotic. If the inflammatory arthritis becomes inactive, the erosion's inner margin becomes sclerotic.*
- *Calcified articular cartilage is also called chondrocalcinosis. Most often it indicates a propensity for the development of pseudogout.*

THE COMMON DISEASES OF SYNOVIAL JOINTS

Traumatic Diseases

There are three types of traumatic diseases:
Traumatic effusion
Fracture into a joint
Meniscal damage

Traumatic Effusion. Injury to the synovial lining of a joint can result in hemorrhage into the joint. No fracture has to be present, but in certain joints, a fracture may be so hard to find that a traumatic effusion is considered to indicate a hidden fracture. This is of greatest importance in the elbow, where distal humeral and radial-head fractures are easy to miss.

In the larger joints, the effusion can be tapped and studied. If no fat is found in the fluid, it is likely that no fracture is present. Fat in the fluid implies that the joint cavity communicates with the bone marrow, indicating probable fracture.

Fracture into a Joint. Fractures into joints (osteochondral fractures) result in joint effusions. Often a disruption of the margins of a bone can be recognized, indicating the site of fracture. Fractures into joints can result in three complications:

1. Loose bodies free in the joint
2. Joint surface irregularity eventually resulting in degenerative joint disease
3. Abnormal healing from either
    a. Interruption of the vascular supply to the fractured bone (often called *osteochondritis dissecans*) (Fig. 59-5)
    b. Interference with callus formation from the
        Absence of periosteum
        Anticallus effect of synovial fluid

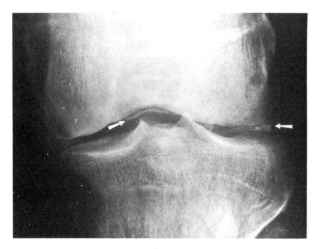

Figure 59-4. Chondrocalcinosis in the knee. Calcification (arrows) is present in the joint cartilage and menisci.

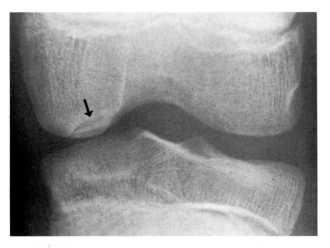

Figure 59-5. Osteochondral fracture of the medial femoral condyle (arrow). These fractures heal poorly, and the fragment may become loose within the joint.

Meniscal Damage. In those joints with a meniscus (such as the knee, the ulnocarpal joint of the wrists, the acromioclavicular joint, and the temporomandibular joint), the meniscus can be damaged by trauma. A damaged meniscus can result in several symptoms:

1. Recurrent joint effusions.
2. *Locking,* an inability to move the joint through a full range of motion. This is often intermittent.
3. *Giving way,* the sudden reflex relaxation of muscles when the meniscus is trapped within the joint. This usually occurs in the knee.
4. Weakness. This usually occurs in the wrist and is often limited to the motions used for turning a water faucet or twisting off a lid of a jar.

The damaged meniscus cannot be directly seen on radiographs. The usual diagnostic method is the physical exami-

nation. In those patients in whom the examination is equivocal, arthroscopy or an arthrogram can be done. The arthrogram consists of a series of radiographs obtained after a contrast medium has been injected into the joint. The contrast medium can be air, the contrast used for urography, or a combination of air and urographic contrast media. In Figure 59-6a, the normal meniscus of the knee can be seen as a triangular structure. Figure 59-6b shows the tracking of contrast medium within the meniscal tear.

Infectious Diseases

Infection in a joint results in joint pain. An effusion is almost always present and can be identified on physical examination in some joints and by radiographic techniques in others. The hyperemia caused by the infection usually results in osteoporosis, and the lysosomes released from dam-

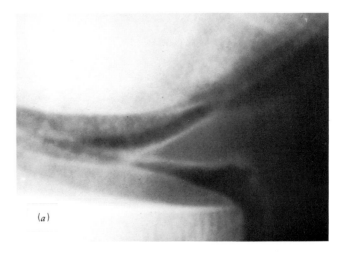

(a)

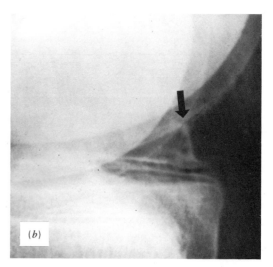

(b)

Figure 59-6. Knee arthrograms from two patients. (a) The normal triangular shape of the medial meniscus is demonstrated. The meniscus is coated by contrast medium and surrounded by air. (b) A tear (arrow) through the base of the medial meniscus.

aged leukocytes destroy cartilage, resulting in symmetrical narrowing of the joint space and, in some cases, in fusion across the joint.

When there is clinical suspicion of infection, joint aspiration, with microscopic examination and culture of the joint fluid, is the best method of evaluation.. Most joint infections show no radiographic change beyond the presence of the effusion for 2–3 weeks from the onset of the disease. It takes at least 2–3 weeks to see the radiographic changes of cartilage narrowing and bone destruction (Fig. 59-7).

Nuclear medicine imaging studies with ^{67}Ga can demonstrate the presence of joint infection. On a normal joint scan with ^{67}Ga, the joint space can be seen. When joint infection is present, the gallium in the synovium will surround and therefore hide the joint space.

Inflammatory Diseases

The common inflammatory diseases are

Rheumatoid arthritis
Gout
Pseudogout

Rheumatoid Arthritis. Radiographs play an important role in the diagnosis and follow-up of rheumatoid arthritis. Joint effusion is an early but nonspecific sign. Other changes usually take a minimum of 6 months of disease activity before they can be seen. Periarticular osteoporosis, followed by erosion, followed by symmetrical joint narrowing, followed by subluxation is the pattern of joint disease. The diagnosis depends on a combination of findings, not on a single finding.

Radiographs are also useful in following the progress of rheumatoid arthritis. Each joint is individually compared to look for stabilization or progression of bone erosions and cartilage narrowing. The inner margin of erosions is stud-

ied. Active disease erosions show trabeculae with no limiting margin of bone at the inner limit of the erosion. A margin of bone in the inner margin of the erosion indicates lack of activity.

Gout and Pseudogout. The acute inflammatory arthritides gout and pseudogout are best diagnosed by their history of sudden onset and by the examination of the joint fluid under polarized light. Radiographs play a limited and secondary role in most patients.

Gout. The radiographs in gout usually show normal bone density (the bone is not osteoporotic) because the attacks of gout are intermittent, acute, and brief. The joint usually looks normal except for swelling; changes of typical degenerative joint diseases are common. Less commonly, erosions or tophi are present. *Tophi,* which are focal deposits of urate in periarticular locations, often are of increased radiodensity (Fig. 59-8a and b). Erosions in gout usually have well-marginated inner margins with a thin layer of bony demarcation (Fig. 59-8c).

Pseudogout. Calcium pyrophosphate deposition arthropathy is best diagnosed by joint fluid polarized-light microscopy. Often radiographs will demonstrate calcification of the articular cartilage or menisci in this disease, but the demonstration of this chondrocalcinosis only indicates the propensity for developing this disease and does not indicate that the disease is active.

Degenerative Joint Disease: Osteoarthrosis

Degenerative joint disease is the most common joint affliction. Often a history of very slowly progressive, intermittent joint pain in an aging patient is sufficient to make the diagnosis. Radiographs when obtained may demonstrate joint narrowing and the formation of osteophytes at the margins of the bone ends. The appearance on the radiograph may not correlate with the severity of the symptoms.

Keynotes

- *Fractures into joints (osteochondral fractures) have a propensity to heal poorly. Sometimes fragments become avascular and break free into a joint.*
- *Symptoms of meniscal tear include locking, giving way, and weakness.*
- *Infection in a joint is best confirmed by aspiration of fluid from the joint, microscopic examination, and culture. A small amount of radiographic contrast should be injected into the joint when no fluid is found to confirm that the needle was actually within the joint rather than next to it.*
- *The early diagnosis of rheumatoid arthritis is based on clinical criteria. Radiographs are usually not supportive until 6–12 months after the onset of the disease.*
- *The most frequent radiographic finding in the patient with an acute attack of gout is either a swollen joint with normal bony contours or a swollen joint with the changes of degenerative arthritis. More specific changes of gout are uncommon.*

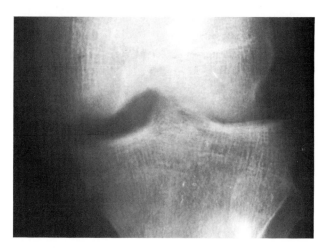

Figure 59-7. Knee joint infection. The bones are osteopenic, the medial ends of the bones are partially eroded, and the joint space laterally is narrowed. These are all findings suggestive of infection.

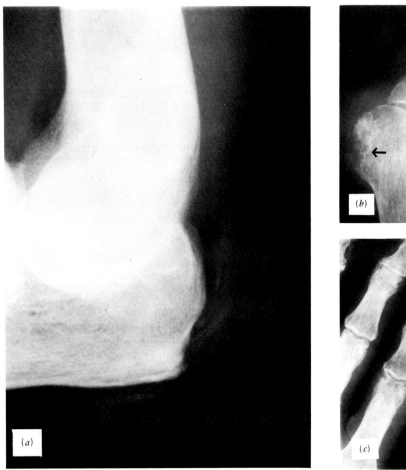

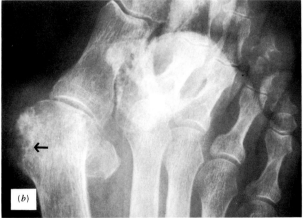

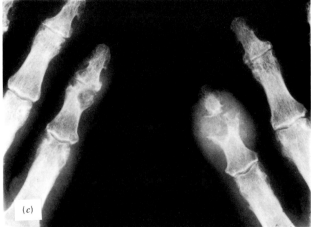

Figure 59-8. Three different patients demonstrating some of the radiological findings of gout. (*a*) Calcified tophaceous material adjacent to the olecranon of the elbow in a patient with gouty olecranon bursitis. (*b*) Podagra. Faintly radiodense tophaceous material is seen adjacent to the first metatarsal head, which is eroded along its medial margin (arrow). (*c*) Classic, well-defined erosions of gout, in this case demonstrated in the fingers.

- *Pseudogout is a disease resembling gout in its severe painful attacks but caused by the deposition of calcium pyrophosphate crystals rather than urate crystals.*
- *In degenerative joint disease, asymmetric joint narrowing and osteophytes are the most frequent findings.*

CLINICAL CASES

Case 59-1

RM is a 46–year–old man who came to the emergency room after stepping on a nail. The wound was cleaned, the tetanus vaccination history was reviewed, and the patient was started on gentamicin. A radiograph (Fig. 59-9*a*) demonstrated no radiopaque foreign matter in the wound.

Mr. RM returned 10 days later with increasing pain and complaints that the pain was so severe that he could not put any weight on the ball of this foot. His follow-up radiograph is shown in Figure 59-9*b*. What do you see?

The fourth MTP joint is slightly narrowed. The bone around the joint is less radiodense than that of the other metatarsals. Your diagnosis?

Joint space infection. The likely organism?

Pseudomonas is the organism most likely involved after puncture wounds of the foot. The treatment?

Open drainage and debridement of tissues. This was unsuccessful, and the bone had to be resected. Joint infections often do not respond to antibiotic treatment alone. In many cases, open debridement and drainage is necessary.

Case 59-2

This 48-year-old man has had intermittent pain in the back of his thigh for 5 years; often he forgets its presence until a sudden move reminds him of it. Finally, he comes in concerned about what it is and what can be

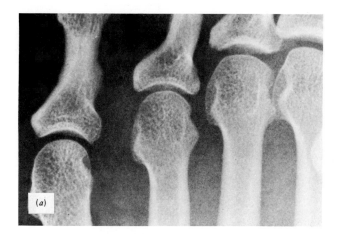
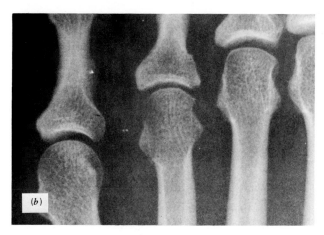

Figure 59-9. Case 59-1.

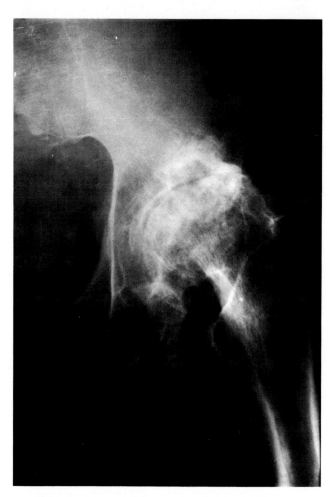

Figure 59-10. Case 59-2. (Reprinted from Freedman, M.: *Radiology of the Postoperative Hip* with permission of John Wiley & Sons, Inc. Copyright 1979.)

done for it. The examination reveals limited abduction and external rotation of the hip. Radiographs are in Figure 59-10. What do you see?

The joint is moderately narrow. Large osteophytes

have formed at the margin of the joint. The joint margins are irregular. These are the typical findings of degenerative arthritis.

Case 59-3

This 42-year-old woman started developing stiffness in her hands when she was 30. Her fingers seemed to "gel" overnight and in cold weather but loosened up during the day. Her knuckles seemed swollen to her.

On examination, the MCP joints were swollen and warm. Joint motion was normal. At that time the disease was limited to both hands and wrists, with symmetrical swelling over the joints and adjacent to the ulna styloid processes. Radiographs were normal except for the swelling. A close-up view of the MCP joints is shown in Figure 59-11a.

The disease remained active and spread to involve multiple joints. Films were obtained every 12–24 months to document the progression of the disease. Figure 59-11b demonstrates the appearance of the MCP joints 22 months after clinical presentation, and Figure 59-11c, after 43 months of disease.

Figure 59-11d and e demonstrates the knee at the time of clinical presentation and at 13 months. Figure 59-11f demonstrates the ankle at 13 months. Figure 59-11g and h demonstrate the wrist at 22 and 43 months.

What is your diagnosis?

The radiographs demonstrate osteopenia and erosions around many joints. The symptoms, course of the disease, and radiographs all indicate that the patient should have rheumatoid arthritis. The patient tested seropositive for rheumatoid factor.

Over many years, treatment with aspirin, gold, physiotherapy, and night-time splinting was used. The close-ups of the most recent films (Fig. 59-11c and h) demonstrate that the inner margin of some of the erosions is now lined with bone. This corresponds to a relative lack of clinical findings of active synovitis in this patient.

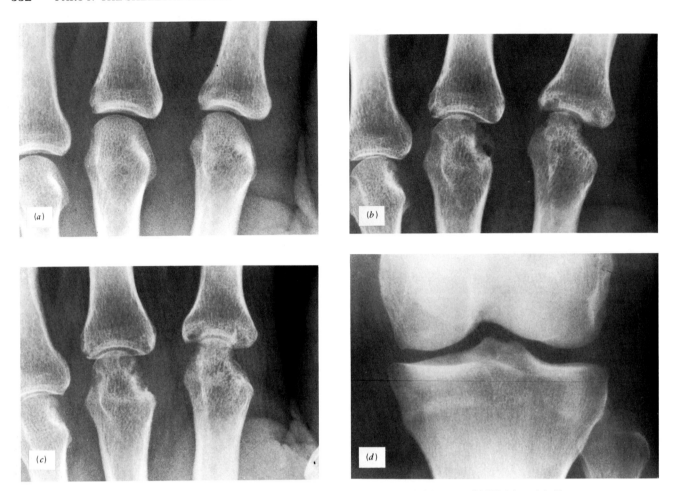

Figure 59-11. Case 59-3. (*a*) Initial view of MCP joints. (*b*) 22-month follow-up of MCP joints. (*c*) 43-month follow-up of MCP joints. (*d*) Initial view of the knee. (*e*) 13-month follow-up of the knee. There is focal bone loss (arrow). (*f*) View of the ankle at 13 months. There is focal bone loss (arrow). (*g*) View of wrist at 22 months. (*h*) 43-month follow-up of the wrist. At this time the erosions are well defined, and some have bone in the margin of the erosions, a sign of relative inactivity of the inflammatory disease.

ADDITIONAL EFFECTS OF JOINT DISEASE IN CHILDHOOD

In children, diseases affecting the synovial joints may have two consequences that do not occur in the adult. Infectious arthritis, rheumatoid arthritis, and hemophilic arthritis each cause hyperemia, which in turn can cause overgrowth of the epiphyseal end of the bone (Fig. 57-12). In many cases this overgrowth may limit motion at the joint. The hyperemia can also result in excessive longitudinal growth or in an early fusion of the epiphyseal plate growth center. Thus in the child, arthritis may result in a deformity both from enlarged, misshaped bone ends and from a long or short overall bone length.

Summary

The common forms of disease affecting synovial joints are due to injury, inflammation, and infection. The traumatic forms include traumatic effusions, osteochondral fractures, and meniscal tears. Fractures into joints may heal poorly and may leave loose fragments of bone or cartilage within the joint space. Fragments that become avascular and may detach are called areas of *osteochondritis dissecans*. Loose bodies and meniscal tears may result in a sudden giving way of the joint or in locking of the joint, preventing full extension.

Joint infection early in its course manifests only an effusion. Gallium scans are positive early, but are usually not needed because aspiration of the suspect joint will be diagnostic. Late changes in infective arthritis include joint narrowing and joint fusion.

Inflammatory diseases of joints include rheumatoid arthritis, gout, and pseudogout. In rheumatoid arthritis, early changes include soft tissue swelling, joint effusions, skip areas, and erosions. Later changes include symmetrical joint narrowing, subluxations, and ulnar deviation of the phalanges. The most frequent finding in gout is soft tissue swelling. The changes of degenerative arthritis are

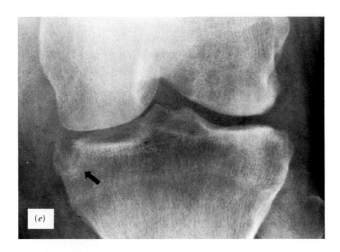

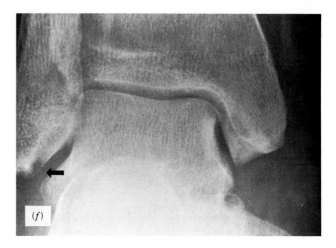

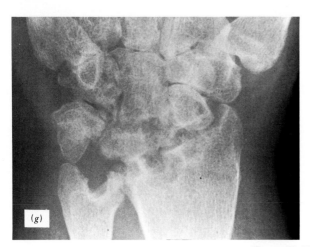

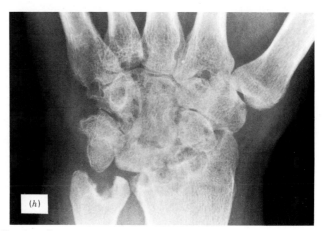

Figure 59-11. (Continued).

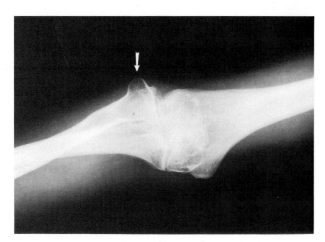

Figure 59-12. Overgrowth of the radial head (arrow) associated with hemophilia. Compare this radial head with those in Figure 56-9.

often present. Less frequently, well-defined erosions and radiodense tophi may be seen. In pseudogout, calcium pyrophosphate crystals are present within the joint fluid. Calcification of the articular cartilage is frequently present.

Degenerative arthritis shows asymmetric joint narrowing and the formation of osteophytes, bony growths at the edges of joints. There is often a discrepancy between the degree of severity of the radiographic changes and of the severity of clinical symptoms.

REVIEW QUESTIONS

1. What are the three types of joints? What types of diseases commonly affect them?
2. What are the two types of synovial-lined joints? How do they differ?
3. What is periarticular osteoporosis? What can cause it?
4. What types of processes can cause a joint effusion?
5. What is the difference in significance of symmetrical and asymmetric joint narrowing?
6. How should joint narrowing best be demonstrated? Give examples in different joints.
7. What is the significance of skip areas and erosions? In what diseases do they occur?
8. What are osteophytes? In what diseases do they occur?
9. What is the significance of calcified articular cartilage? What are some of the diseases in which it occurs?

10. What are the problems that can result from fractures into joints?
11. What are the symptoms of a meniscal injury?
12. How is an arthrogram performed?
13. What are the radiographic findings in joint infection?
14. What are the early and late radiographic findings in rheumatoid arthritis?
15. What are the potential radiographic findings in gout? In pseudogout?
16. What are the radiographic findings in degenerative joint disease?

VOCABULARY

arthrogram
calcium pyrophosphate deposition arthropathy
loose bodies
meniscus
osteochondral fracture
degenerative joint disease
erosions
fibrocartilage
giving way
gout
hyaline cartilage
joint
locking
osteochondritis dissecans
osteophytes
pseudogout
rheumatoid arthritis
skip areas
synovial joint
tophus

SUGGESTIONS FOR FURTHER READING

B. Felson, Ed. The "other" arthritides. *Seminars in Roentgenology,* **17,** 1982.

For additional suggested reading see Chapter 55.

PART 6

THE BRAIN AND SKULL

Starting in the early 1970s, rapid advances in neurodiagnostic testing have greatly changed and improved the clinical practice of neurology and neurosurgery, making these fields more accurate and safer. Computed tomography and digital angiography have had the major impact so far. In the future, MRI and positron emission tomography will futher expand the capabilities of the neuroradiologist.

The following three chapters discuss the evaluation of the plain skull film for evidence of skull and brain disease, cranial CT and neuroangiography.

60

PLAIN-FILM RADIOGRAPHY OF THE SKULL AND BRAIN

HARRY C. KNIPP

KEY CONCEPTS

Radiological

The ability to recognize abnormalities of the skull on radiographs requires a knowledge of the normal pattern and its variants. Linear radiolucencies may be normal vessels or fractures; focal radiolucencies may be normal areas of venous confluence or metastases.

Skull fractures may be linear or depressed. The linear fractures have sharp margins and tend not to branch. Depressed skull fractures may be seen in tangent as focal areas of depression or en face as areas of bony overlap with increased radiodensity. Basilar skull fractures may be quite difficult to detect.

Cranial CT is currently the preferred method for the identification of brain neoplastic disease, though MRI may replaced it in the future. Abnormalities can, however, be seen on skull radiographs including the signs of increased intracranial pressure, focal areas of calcification, and areas of bone destruction or bone formation in the skull. Increased intracranial pressure may, in a child, result in spreading of the sutures. In the adult, the main effect is erosion of the dorsum sellae. Shift of the pineal gland can be caused by a mass or brain edema and can be seen if the pineal gland is calcified.

Infectious disease of the sinuses may demonstrate mucosal thickening, fluid collection with air-fluid level, or opacification of the paranasal sinuses.

Sellar enlargement can result from endocrine or nonendocrine tumors. Endocrine tumors that secrete active hormones may be quite small and difficult to detect.

OBJECTIVES

When you complete this chapter you will be able to

1. Identify correctly on radiographs
   a. Normal vessels
   b. Linear and depressed skull fractures
   c. Venous lakes
   d. Lytic and blastic metastases
   e. Sellar erosions
   f. Sutural spreading
   g. Blow-out fractures of the orbit
   h. Sinusitis
2. List three causes of sutural widening.

If you question an average group of physicians on their ability to evaluate routine PA and lateral radiographs of the chest, most will reply that they feel reasonably competent and confident in the majority of cases. But question them on their skills at interpreting skull and facial films and their confidence rapidly fades. Perhaps they are intimidated by the complex bony structures of the base of the skull and face, but there may also be some innate trepidation relative to the important, sensitive, and still somewhat mysterious organs that lie within. This need not be the case, however. As with any of the many initially intimidating aspects of the practice of medicine, knowledge of basic anatomy, common sense, and a lot of practice will make the job of evaluating these radiographs much easier and more comfortable.

THE NORMAL SKULL

Lateral, PA, and Towne Views

Figure 60-1*a, b,* and *c* illustrates the basic radiographic projections used to evaluate the skull. Concentrate first

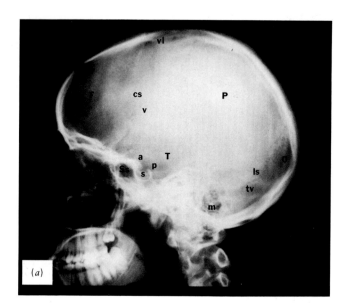

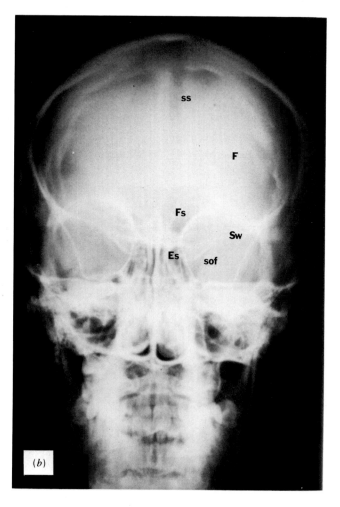

Figure 60-1. The four basic radiographic projections of the skull: (a) lateral view; (b) PA, or Caldwell, view; (c) Towne view; and (d) base view. On the four images, major anatomic landmarks are labeled: F = frontal bone, O = occipital bone, P = parietal bone, Pt = petrous portion of temporal bone, Sw = sphenoid wing, T = temporal bone, Es = ethmoidal sinus, Ms = maxillary sinus, Fs = frontal sinus, Ss = Sphenoid sinus, cs = coronal sutures, ls = lambdoidal sutures, ss = sagittal suture, fl = foramen lacerum, fm = foramen magnum, fo = foramen ovale, fs = foramen spinosum, s = sella turcica, a = anterior clinoid process, p = posterior clinoid process, m = mastoid air cells, od = odontoid process, c1 = C1 vertebra, v = vascular grooves, vl = venous lakes, tv = transverse venous sinus groove, sof = superior orbital fissure.

on the calvaria, the largest and perhaps easiest area to evaluate. Note the various suture lines (cs, ls, ss) joining the many bones that make up the cranial vault. These interdigitated lines are obviously more prominent in children and eventually fuse when brain growth ceases later in life, becoming slightly less sharply defined. Some of the conditions discussed below are manifested by sutural changes.

Observe the structure of the various cranial bones: flat bones comprised of the dense inner and outer skull tables with the *spongiosa* sandwiched in between. The radiographic density of the calvaria will vary with the thickness of these structures in different areas; hence the somewhat more radiolucent appearance of the thinner temporal regions, for example. These areas can be distinguished from the more abrupt density changes of destructive lesions discussed later in this chapter. In addition to the radiolucencies seen in the temporal region, there are other, more focal areas of radiolucency.

Vascular Radiolucencies

Arterial Markings. The blood vessels (v) adjacent to the inner table of the skull produce shallow grooves in the cra-

nial bones. The branching pattern is the sign that these are vessels (usually arteries), rather that fractures.

Venous Markings. Venous structures are often more irregular in pattern and can appear as radiolucencies within the calvaria. Some of these are linear branching radiolucencies; others are focal radiolucencies called *venous lakes* (vl). These may be confused with focal destructive lesions but can often be differentiated by identifying the venous linear channels that course into them. The grooves of the normal cerebral venous sinuses (tv) should also be noted.

Normal Intracranial Calcifications

Often normal intracranial calcifications are visible. The most noteworthy and useful of these is calcification of the pineal gland, a consistent midline stucture. This calcification occurs normally and, when present, should measure within 1–2 mm of the centerline when viewed in the Towne (AP) projection (Fig. 60-1c). A significant deviation of this calcification, when present, suggests a midline shift such as might be caused by an enlarging intracranial mass.

Other normally occurring calcifications include those of the falx, usually seen in older people as linear vertical cal-

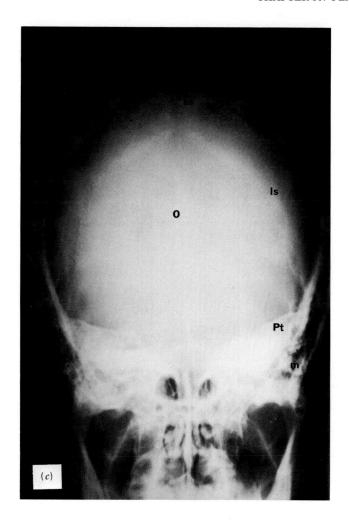

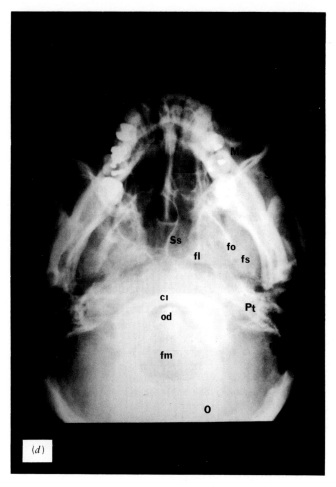

cific densities in the midline. Calcification of the glomus of the choroid plexus may be seen as mottled calcific radiodensities bilaterally, 2–3 cm lateral to the pineal region in the areas of the posterior aspects of the lateral ventricles.

Several types of abnormal intracranial calcifications may be visible and are discussed later in the chapter. The following list summarizes the various normal and abnormal types of intracranial calcifications.

NORMAL CALCIFICATIONS

Pineal gland	Midline marker
Habenular commissure	C-shaped, anterior to pineal
Dural	Plaque like, in falx or on convexities
Choroid plexus	Bilateral at atria of lateral ventricles

PATHOLOGICAL CALCIFICATIONS

Neoplastic	10–15% calcify overall
Craniopharyngioma	60–70% calcify in various shapes
Oligodendroglioma	50–60% calcify, usually punctate
Ependymoma	20–30% calcify
Meningioma	15–20% calcify, often densely
Astrocytoma	10–15% calcify, often lower grade lesions
Infectious	
Tuberculoma	2–3 cm, dense, coarse
Toxoplasmosis	Small flecks or dense collections
Cytomegalovirus	Multiple, small, often periventricular
Cysticercosis	Small, less than 1 cm
Abscess	Uncommon, usually an old lesion
Vascular	
Arteriovenous malformation	30% calcify, punctate or in vessel wall
Aneurysm	Ringlike, in wall
Atherosclerosis	Usually in carotid siphon
Miscellaneous	
Sturge-Weber syndrome	Serpentine cortical calcification

Tuberous sclerosis	Multiple irregular calcifications in ventricular region
Basal ganglia	Usually bilateral, may be related to congenital metabolic disorders
Subdural hematoma	Unusual, curvilinear calcifications in older lesions

The Base View

The base view of the skull (Fig. 60-1*d*) is included in many examinations. Although at first glance it may seem threateningly complex, if you focus on a specific area of interest, valuable information can often be gained. For example, notice how well the bony margins of the maxillary (Ms) and sphenoid sinuses (Ss) are seen. The zygomatic arches are often well demonstrated, too. The bony margins of the middle cranial fossae formed by the sphenoid bones are readily visible, as are the mastoid air cells of the petrosa (Pt). Several important foramina can also be seen, as labeled on Figure 60-1*d*.

As you can see, the base view can be a big help in the radiographic evaluation of a number of areas that may be of clinical interest. If you are interested in unraveling the many overlapping structures in greater detail, compare the base and other views with an actual skull specimen in the company of your trusty anatomy books. You will be surprised how fascinating this can be.

Specialized Views

Several auxillary views of the skull and facial bones have been devised over the years in an attempt to clarify particularly complex areas, such as the paranasal sinuses and the delicate structures of the temporal bone.

The Waters View of the Face. Figure 60-2*a* demonstrates the Waters projection of the face. Notice how clearly the maxillary sinuses (Ms) are seen. This view is used to evaluate suspected sinusitis or trauma to the facial region. Other specialized views are used to demonstrate the nasal bones, orbits, and mandible and temporomandibular joints.

The Stenvers View. Figure 60-2*b* is a Stenvers view of the temporal bone. This is one of several projections used to demonstrate the structures of the middle and inner ears and mastoid region. When you are involved in evaluating the skull and face radiographically, as with any other area of the body, don't hesitate to consult with the radiologist or technologist. With a little clinical information, they may be able to tailor the examination in such a way as to clarify a complex area or eliminate needless studies.

Keynotes

• *The sutural lines demarcate the bones of the calvaria. Disease may be manifest in widening or premature fusion of the sutures.*

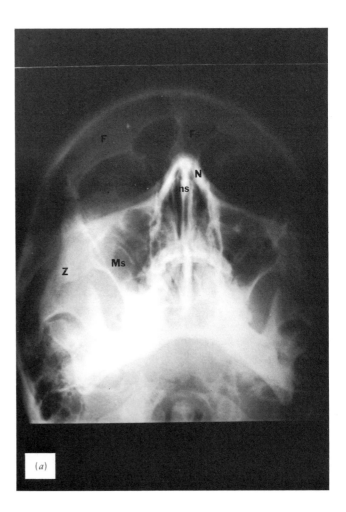

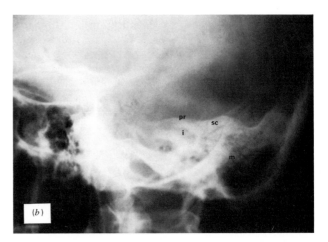

Figure 60-2. (*a*) Waters projection of the face, a view primarily used to evaluate the maxillary sinuses and the bones of the face and orbits. Several important landmarks are labeled: F = frontal bone, N = nasal bone, Z = zygomatic bone, Fs = frontal sinus, Ns = nasal septum, Ms = maxillary sinus. (*b*) Stenvers view of the temporal bone. This is used primarily to evaluate the petrous ridge, the inner ear, and the mastoid air cells. Several important structures are labeled: pr = petrous ridge, m = mastoid air cells, i = internal auditory canal, sc = semicircular canals.

- *The calvaria varies in thickness, resulting in relative radiolucency in the temporal bone and basal portion of occipital bone. These areas of radiolucency can be confused with destructive metastatic lesions.*
- *Branching radiolucencies are due to arterial grooves on the inner surface of the skull. Wider linear radiolucencies represent venous channels in the central diploic layer of the skull. The venous channels can converge on 1–2 cm radiolucencies representing venous structures called venous lakes.*
- *The calcified pineal gland is a useful midline marker. its shift from midline is a sign of focal brain swelling, mass, or focal brain atrophy.*
- *The best way to learn the detailed anatomy of the skull is to compare radiographs with a dried skull specimen using an anatomy text to supply the names of structures.*

DISEASES AFFECTING THE SKULL

The rest of this chapter is a basic discussion of several of the major pathologies of the skull and face and how plain-film radiographs can assist you in diagnosing and treating your patients.

Trauma

The radiographic evaluation of head trauma often includes skull and facial roentgenograms. Although there is a low diagnostic yield for skull films in the absence of otherwise clinically obvious abnormalities, these examinations continue to be used in many emergency rooms. Skull films are of great use in the evaluation of facial trauma but are, in general, of limited use in the evaluation of brain trauma. if a brain injury is suspected, brain CT is recommended.

Figure 60-3 is the skull series of a patient seen the Emergency Department after falling down a flight of steps. He appeared neurologically intact on examination but gave a history of a brief loss of consciousness. Even in the absence of any clinical abnormality, the history of the loss of consciousness is a reasonable indication for obtaining skull films. What do you see on the skull radiographs?

The radiographs revealed an easily seen fracture of the right parietal bone. The PA view is normal, but note the long linear radiolucency crossing the right parietal bone horizontally in the lateral view. The radiolucent line does not branch and is quite straight. This readily distinguishes the fracture from the many branching vascular grooves. Note also that the radiodensity change from the cortex to the fracture line is slightly more abrupt than at the vascular markings.

Linear Skull Fracture. Linear skull fractures, sometimes obvious, are often subtle. They must be differentiated from the sutures and vascular grooves of the normal skull. The interdigitation of the sutural lines usually make this differentiation obvious, but in the pediatric skull, the more prominent sutures and developmental fissures may send you to the nearest anatomy reference book. The vascular grooves of the skull branch in a treelike fashion (as in Fig.

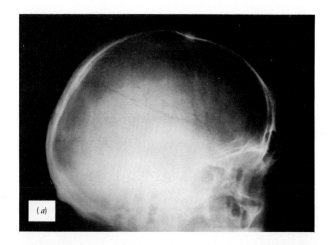

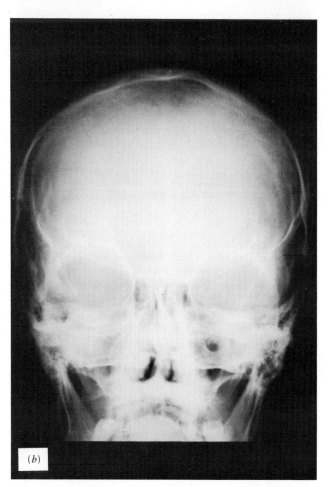

Figure 60-3. Lateral (*a*) and PA (*b*) views from the skull series of an elderly man who injured his head during a fall.

60-1) with a gradual change in bony radiodensity at their margins. Linear fractures are usually more sharply contoured and lack the gentle, branching vascular pattern. Their diminished radiodensity is an abrupt change from the adjacent cortical bone, as is evident in Figure 60-3.

Depressed Skull Fracture. Depressed fracture fragments may be seen in views tangential to the fracture site. When viewed en face, a double bony radiodensity may be seen when the edge of the fragment overlaps the adjacent calvaria. Figure 60-4 is the initial pair of radiographs of a patient assaulted with a hammer. What do you see?

Note that the overlapping radiodensities in the frontal view (Fig. 60-4*a*) create a double density; the depressed fragments are visible because this view is relatively tangential to the area of the fracture. Now examine the lateral view (Figure 60-4*b*). In this case, the severe right frontal fracture is barely visible because none of the fragments overlap in this plane. When uncertainty arises about the possibility of a fracture in the routine views, a custom-tailored tangential or en face view might resolve the situation. Figure 60-5 illustrates such a projection, obtained in the evaluation of the same patient. In this case, an oblique view better defines and localizes an obvious fracture. In other situations, such a view may make the diagnosis.

There are occasionally pitfalls encountered in evaluating the calvaria for fractures. Linear fractures must not only be distinguished from vascular grooves, sutures, and fissures but from the overlying radiolucency of air trapped in a scalp laceration. The double density frequently seen with depressed fractures can be simulated by the overlying radiodensity of a hair braid, by dressing materials, or by foreign objects in the hair or scalp. Don't hesitate to examine the patient for correlation or to request that he or she temporarily rearrange a hairstyle. An old fracture and the tracks of past neurosurgery may persist a long time. If previous skull radiographs aren't available for comparison, historical data and physical examination correlation regarding the site of a past or present injury will often provide the answer.

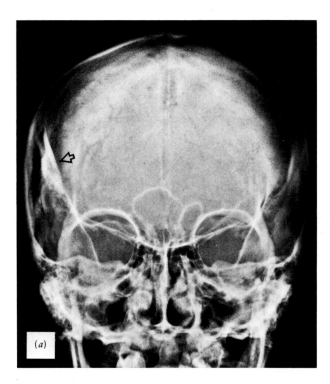

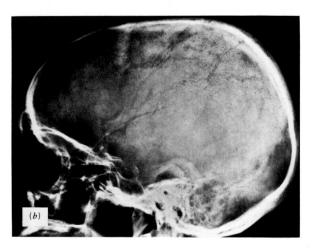

Figure 60-4. The radiographic skull series of a patient assaulted with a hammer. (*a*) frontal view, with a marked linear radiodensity with a vertical orientation visible in what appears to be the right frontotemporal region (arrow). (*b*) Lateral view, showing no increase in radiodensity at the fracture site.

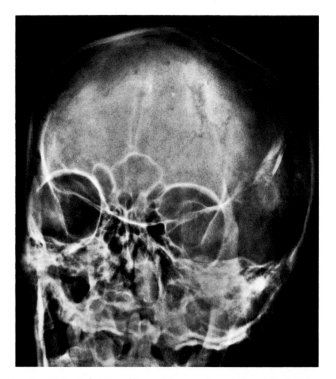

Figure 60-5. An oblique view of the same patient, confirming that the fracture does indeed lie in the temporoparietal region. You may have noted that the fracture now appears to be on the left in contradiction of Figure 60-4*a*. It is truly on the right, but the film is on the view box backward, a pitfall to avoid in the heat of the emergencies by carefully observing the right and left markers that must be placed on every radiograph.

Basilar Skull Fracture. Basilar skull fractures are often very difficult to visualize. When one is strongly suspected on clinical grounds, such as by the presence of otorrhea or rhinorrhea, care must be taken in the evaluation of the radiographs. The fracture itself may not be visible, but secondary signs such as an air-fluid level in the sphenoid sinus may aid in diagnosis (Fig. 60-6).

In Figure 60-6 the fracture itself is not visible but its sequellae are. Notice the perfectly straight, vertical, air/soft tissue density interface in the sphenoid sinus just anterior and inferior to the sella turcica. This is an air-fluid level resulting from a leak of cerebrospinal fluid through the fracture into the air-filled sphenoid sinus (Fig. 60-1*a*). Note that although the film is viewed as if the patient were erect, it was actually performed with the patient supine, accounting for the "vertical air-fluid interface seen in the lateral view.

Facial Fractures. Facial fractures are often complex and difficult to detect. Specialized views of the orbits, nasal bones, mandible, and temporomandibular joint area are frequently needed. In the absence of an obvious bony discontinuity, secondary signs such as an air radiolucency in the orbits from a fractured sinus or the presence of air-fluid levels in or opacification of a sinus secondary to a fracture may be seen.

Figure 60-7 is a Waters view of a patient who was struck in the left eye while engaging in fisticuffs. The patient was a combatant in a local bar brawl. She came in with left facial pain and swelling sufficient to limit opening the left eyelid. After aggressively opening her eye, the emergency room physician noted a limitation of upward gaze compared with the right eye.

Although no fracture can be identified in figure 60-7, note the soft tissue radiodensity in the superior aspect of

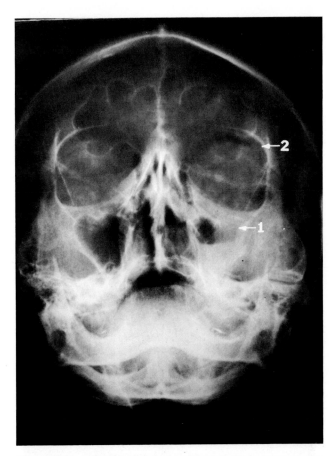

Figure 60-7. A Waters projection of the face after a direct blow to the left orbit, with soft tissue radiodensity adjacent to the roof of the maxillary antrum (arrow 1) and air in the orbital tissues caused by a fracture into the ethmoid air cells (arrow 2).

the left maxillary sinus, an air-fluid level in the sinus, and the air radiolucency in the superior aspect of the left orbit. These suggest a blow-out fracture of the floor of the orbit with entrapment of the orbital contents and hemorrhage into the maxillary sinus.

With a blow-out fracture, the force is transmitted from fist to fluid-filled globe to the thin orbital floor, fracturing it and entrapping the inferior extraocular muscles within the fracture. This results in the soft tissue radiodensity seen along the roof of the maxillary sinus. Hemorrhage from the fracture results in the air-fluid level in the sinus, and air escaping from the sinus has entered the orbit, as indicated by the gas radiodensity above the globe. So-called orbital emphysema should always suggest a fracture of either the orbital floor or the paper-thin medial wall of the orbit bordering the ethmoidal air cells, the lamina papyracea.

Keynotes

- *Skull films are of limited use in evaluating the patient for brain trauma. Most brain injuries and most fluid collections around the brain are not detectable on skull films.*

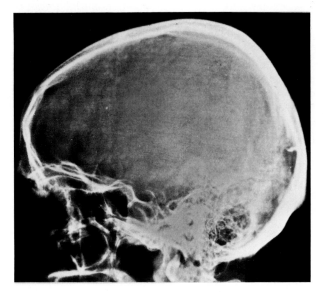

Figure 60-6. A lateral skull radiograph showing a basilar skull fracture.

- Tangential means viewed from an object's edge or profile.
- Fractures of the base of the skull may not be visible on radiographs; an indirect sign is an air-fluid level in the sphenoid sinus.
- A blow-out fracture of the floor of the orbit occurs when an injury suddenly increases the pressure within the orbit and this increase in pressure causes the orbital floor to fracture. Bone fragments may be so thin as to be not seen, but the protrusion of orbital contents through the floor may result in a soft tissue mass being seen in the superior portion of the maxillary sinus. A limitation of upward gaze is a common finding because the inferior rectus muscle becomes trapped among the fragments.

Neoplastic Disease

Skull radiography is less useful in the evaluation of intracranial neoplastic disease. Most often, only indirect evidence of a mass lesion is all that is encountered, unless, of course, the lesion directly involves the bony skull or facial structures. These indirect signs include evidence of increased intracranial pressure, midline shift, and pathological calcifications.

Increased Intracranial Pressure. Increased intracranial pressure may be of several etiologies, including mass lesions and edema resulting from trauma, neoplastic disease, or infectious processes. Increased intracranial pressure may also be related to congenital or acquired hydrocephalus. All will manifest similar bony changes that vary with the age of the patient and the severity of the problem. In the adult, erosion of the dorsum sellae is the most common sign of increased intracranial pressure.

Erosion of the Dorsum Sellae. Figure 60-8 is the lateral view of the sella turcica of a patient with a long history of

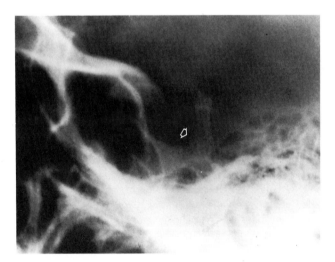

Figure 60-8. A coned-down lateral skull radiograph of a man newly admitted to the psychiatric service with a history of chronic "tension headaches." The radiograph, tailored to demonstrate the sella turcica to best advantage, reveals demineralization and erosion of the anterior cortex of the dorsum sellae (arrow), a sign of increased intracranial pressure.

increasing headaches who ultimately was sent for psychiatric evaluation. The psychiatric resident fortunately detected papilledema on the admission physical examination and ordered skull films and a CT scan. What does the skull film show? There is diminished cortical radiodensity of the dorsum sellae (compared with Fig. 60-1).

Subsequently, a CT scan demonstrated a neoplasm in the third ventricle blocking egress of CSF to the fourth ventricle. Sellar changes from sellar erosions secondary to an intra- or parasellar mass and those from the generalized bony demineralization of osteoporosis must be differentiated from the sellar changes of increased intracranial pressure.

Sutural Widening. In children, increased intracranial pressure may result in widening of the suture lines, which have not yet fused. Sellar changes in young children are less common. In the early teen years, there is some overlap with sutural widening or sellar changes occurring. Sutural widening may also be seen in cases of leukemia or metastatic neuroblastoma with metastases to the leptomeninges as well as in some metabolic disorders.

Pineal Shift. A tumor mass, secondary edema, or both together may cause a shift of the calcified pineal gland.

Tumor Calcification. Abnormal calcifications may also point to an intracranial mass. Tumors such as meningioma, craniopharyngioma, and oligodendroglioma may manifest calcification, the character and location of which may point to a likely diagnosis.

Mr. Carter had complained to his family doctor that he had been having recurrent headaches for some time. He had treated himself with aspirin and other patent remedies without success. Suspecting that this usually tranquil patient had more than a typical tension headache, the family physician ordered a skull series at the radiologist's office next door and scheduled the patient for a CT scan at the local hospital. He promptly received a call from the radiologist describing the skull films seen in Figure 60-9. What do you see?

These films depict the typical pattern of dense calcification seen in some meningiomas. The peripheral location (more cortical rather than in the deeper structures) also suggests this diagnosis, which was confirmed by the subsequent CT scan. The tumor was resected without complication.

Direct Effect on Adjacent Structures. Primary intracranial neoplasms may directly affect the adjacent bony structures. This may take the form of increased bony radiodensity, such as the sclerotic thickening of bone sometimes seen in portions of the skull adjacent to meningiomas (see Fig. 60-10). An area of bony destruction may be caused by an enlarging neoplasm as can occur with a sellar tumor or a neoplasm of the orbits or sinuses. An enlarging acoustic neuroma may widen the internal auditory canal. Views specially positioned to demonstrate the internal auditory canals may reveal a subtle asymmetry in the size of the

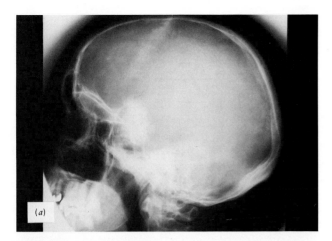

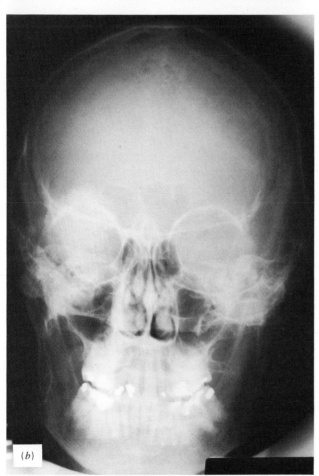

Figure 60-9. PA (a) and lateral (b) skull radiographs demonstrating a right sphenoid wing meningioma. A cluster of dense calcifications is present posterior to the right orbit.

canals suggesting the diagnosis. The canals can be well visualized by plain-film tomography but can also be evaluated by modern CT techniques. Magnetic resonance imaging is also quite useful in demonstrating acoustic neuromas directly.

Metastases. Metastases to the skull may be readily visualized as multiple areas of bony destruction (Fig. 60-11) or as areas of increased bony density.

Keynotes

- *Signs of increased intracranial pressure:*
  Adult: erosion of the dorsum sellae
  Child: spreading of the sutures
- *Primary intracranial neoplasms may be detected because of*
  a. *signs of increased intracranial pressure*
  b. *Shift of the normally midline calcified pineal gland*
  c. *Intratumor calcification in some tumors*
  d. *Reactive bone formation (with some meningiomas)*
  e. *Bone destruction (as of the internal auditory canal with acoustic neuromas)*
- *Metastases to the skull usually results in lytic destruction and less often in areas of increased bone density.*

Infectious Disease

Occasionally skull and facial radiographs may be helpful in the diagnosis of infectious disease.

Sinusitis. Views of the paranasal sinuses can be used to detect sinusitis when this is suspected clinically. Edematous, inflamed mucosa may be seen as a thickened soft tissue rim around the bony wall of the sinus and may impart a hazy appearance to what is normally a clear air-filled structure. In acute cases, air-fluid levels may be seen, indicating an obstruction to sinus drainage. Often, the swelling and retained fluid result in complete opacification of a sinus with soft tissue radiodensity. Long-term or particularly aggressive infections may lead to destruction of portions of the bony wall of a sinus.

Mrs. Milton had suffered several days with a "fever, stuffy nose, and tightness in her face" when she came to her internist for examination. Noting some tenderness in the area of her maxillary sinuses, he agreed with her diagnosis that her "sinuses were acting up." The Waters view of her sinus series is shown in Figure 60-12a. What do you see?

The view shows air-fluid levels and mucosal thickening in several sinuses, confirming their diagnosis of acute bilateral maxillary sinusitis. The frontal sinuses were also found to be involved.

Mastoiditis. Increased soft tissue radiodensity, dimished aeration, and sometimes bony destruction may be seen also in the mastoid air cells, indicating mastoiditis, although this condition has become less common since the advent of antibiotic therapy.

Other Infections. Excluding the sinus and mastoid examination, plain films are likely to be of little value in the work-up of intracranial infection. As already noted, a large abscess may occasionally produce secondary signs of a mass

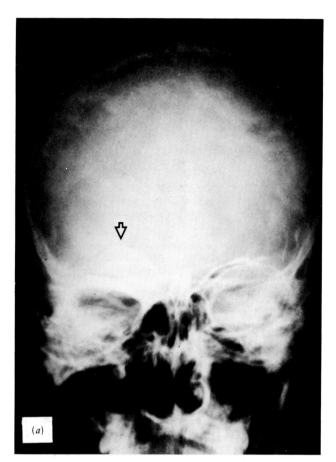 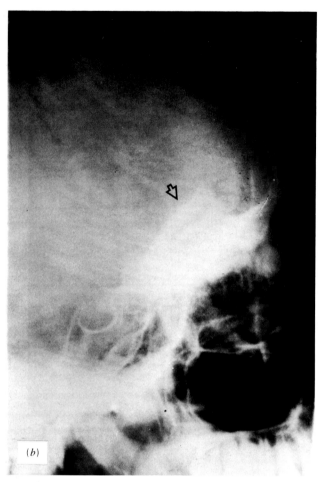

Figure 60-10. A second patient with a sphenoid wing meningioma. Although this patient's tumor has not calcified, it has invaded the sphenoid bone, inciting a sclerotic reaction. Here, thickening of the bone, with increased calcification, results in the increased radiodensity of the right sphenoid ridge as seen in the PA (a) and lateral (b) views (arrows). Compare the abnormal radiodensity on the right in *a* with the normal left side. Meningiomas can and do occur anywhere there are meninges, typical sites including the convexities, the parasagittal areas, the tentorium, and the olfactory groove.

effect. In pediatric patients, the detection of intracranial calcifications may support the diagnosis of prenatal infection. In cytomegalic inclusion disease, numerous small periventricular calcifications may be seen (Fig. 60-13).

In patients with toxoplasmosis or with old tuberculous granulomata, one or several small calcifications may also be seen. Osteomyelitis of the skull or facial bones may be diagnosed as an area of bony destruction. This is sometimes seen in the calvaria in patients after brain surgery or may be the result of an aggressive sinus infection.

Keynote

• *Sinusitis shows*

  a. *Thickened mucosa in the sinus*

  b. *Complete sinus opacification*

  c. *An air-fluid level in the sinus*

Endocrine and Metabolic Disorders

Endocrine and metabolic disorders may occasionally manifest changes visible on plain films. For example, in children multiple intrasutural bones may be seen in hypothyroidism and in several congenital dysplastic conditions, although these extra bones may also be seen in normal people.

Sellar enlargement may occur with growing pituitary tumors, some of which are hormone producers (Fig. 60-14a). The tumors may be large and grossly visible, with destruction of the floor of the sella and anterior clinoid processes. occasionally a very large lesion may erode into the underlying sphenoid sinus, where a soft tissue mass may be identified. More often, endocrine tumors are small and sellar erosion is focal, very subtle, and visible only faintly in detailed tomographic or CT sections of this area. This is frequently the case with diminutive but clinically important microadenomas of the pituitary gland.

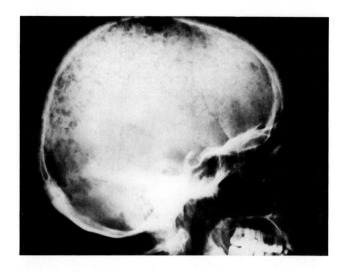

Figure 60-11. Lateral view from the skull series of a 36-year-old woman with bilateral inflammatory ductal carcinoma of the breast. This film was obtained approximately 6 months after diagnosis of the patient's malignancy. Although she underwent immediate bilateral mastectomies at the time of diagnosis, widespread metastases had already occurred. There are many small areas of osteolytic bony destruction.

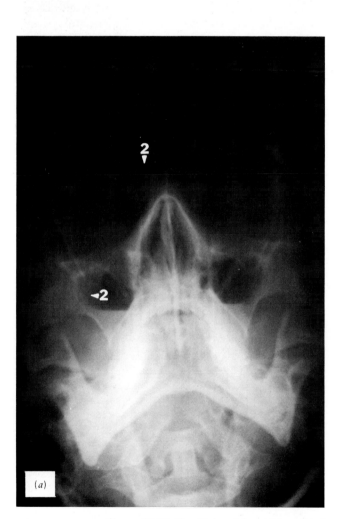

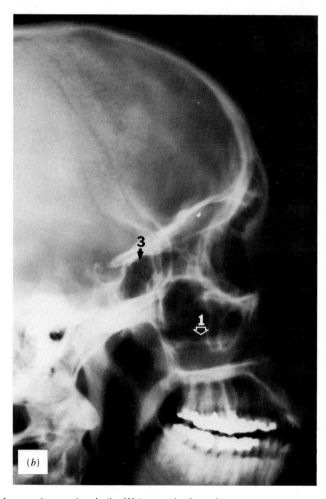

Figure 60-12. The Waters (a) and lateral (b) views from a sinus series. In the Waters projection, air-fluid levels compatible with acute sinusitis are easily seen in the maxillary sinuses. These fluid levels can also be seen in the lateral projection (arrow 1). Further inspection of the Waters view reveals swollen mucosa (arrow 2) in both the maxillary and frontal sinuses, also compatible with inflammation. The ethmoidal air-cells (best seen in the PA view in Fig. 60-1b) were normal in this patient, as was the sphenoidal sinus visible in b (arrow 3).

Changes in the cranial vault may also be seen in endocrine and metabolic abnormalities. Acromegaly may result in thickening of the calvaria and enlargement of the paranasal sinuses (Fig. 60-14b). The osteoporosis of hyperparathyroidism may, in contrast, lead to diminished radio- density in the calvaria, along with a punctate, patchy, salt-and-pepper appearance. The normally visible vascular grooves may become less distinct as bony radiodensity decreases.

Keynote

- *Large pituitary adenomas can cause sellar enlargement and erosions. Microadenomas may show only on tomographic sections or CT scans.*

Congenital, Developmental, and Dysplastic Disorders

Signs of congenital and developmental disorders are often readily visible on radiographs of the skull. These may be as simple as the premature closure of a suture, resulting in an abnormal cranial configuration, or they may be complex multicentric changes as is the case in many of the less common dysplastic syndromes.

Little Joyce's pediatrician had noticed on her routine well-baby visits that Joyce's skull was assuming an increasingly elongated configuration. With the possibility of synostosis of the sagittal suture in mind, the pediatrician requested the radiographic study in Figure 60-15. What does it show?

The films reveal the scaphocephalic (boatlike) configu-

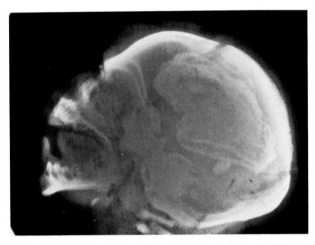

Figure 60-13. Lateral view of the skull of an infant with "failure to thrive." The periventricular calcifications seen with cytomegalovirus infection are grossly evident in this case, although they are usually not this pronounced. Here, the "boxing-glove" appearance outlining the ventricular system is striking.

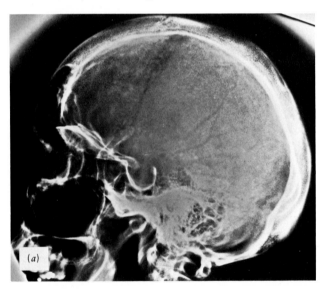

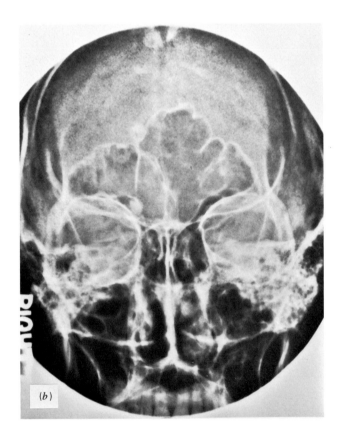

Figure 60-14. The skull series of a 40-year-old man who complained that he was constantly outgrowing his hats, gloves, and shoes. Succumbing to his wife's prodding, George finally saw his family physician, who quite cleverly requested these radiographs. Compare the two views (a and b) with the normal views in Fig. 60-1, particularly the lateral view. There are three key findings: (1) a large sella turcica, the result of a slowly enlarging pituitary neoplasm; (2) thickening of the calvarial bones, and (3) a large frontal sinus. The latter two findings are both secondary to continued growth of the flat bones of the calvaria responding to elevated growth hormone levels. The diagnosis was, of course, acromegaly.

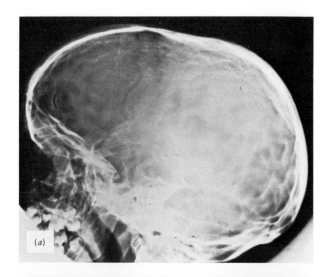

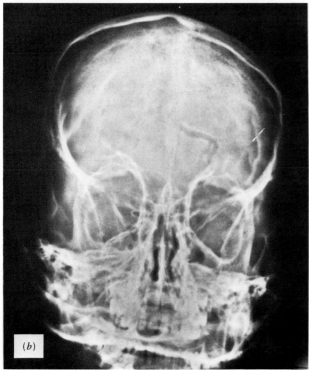

Figure 60-15. Premature closure of the sagittal suture in a young girl. As her brain grew, the skull was forced to enlarge solely from front to back as lateral growth was blocked by the early fusion of the sagittal suture. (a) Lateral view. (b) Frontal view.

ration the skull assumes when the normal lateral enlargement ceases with the early closure of a small portion of the sagittal suture. As the brain continues to grow normally, the cranial vault is thus forced to enlarge from front to back by growth at the normal coronal and lambdoidal sutures. Notice the active coronal suture in the lateral view, where normal sutural interdigitations are seen. Enlargement at this suture led to the elongated appearance of the

skull. In the frontal view, the fused sagittal suture is barely visible.

In studying these films, you've probably observed prominent convolutional markings of the cranial bones, which correspond to the gyri and sulci of the underlying brain. It would seem that these might be the result of increased intracranial pressure from the abnormal cranial growth, but they are actually within normal limits for a patient of this age.

Brain Growth and Skull Size. From the preceding discussion it is evident that growth of the calvaria is related to brain growth. Normal versus deficient brain growth may be roughly assessed by comparing the size of the cranial vault and its cross-sectional area to that of the face as seen in the lateral view of the skull. The normal newborn's cranial/facial ratio is approximately 4:1. A much lower ratio would suggest microcephaly, the result of diminished brain growth. This may be seen in prenatal viral infections such as cytomegalic inclusion disease. After reviewing Figure 60-13, would you agree? The normal adult ratio is roughly 1.5:1 or 2:1.

Dysplastic Conditions. Dysplastic conditions and other diseases affecting the bony calvaria and facial structures may be detected as changes in bone size and radiodensity.

Paget's Disease. Paget's disease, for example, may begin with a large area of bony destruction in the skull, termed *osteoporosis circumscripta,* and later develop the markedly increased bony radiodensity typically seen when this disorder affects the weight-bearing areas of the pelvis and hips. These changes of the disease are demonstrated in Figure 60-16.

Fibrous dysplasia may also affect the calvaria and face in various ways, sometimes as bubbly-appearing destructive lesions and at other times as markedly increased radiodensity limited to a solitary bone of the craniofacial region.

Vascular Diseases. Skull films are usually of little help in the diagnosis of vascular disease. Calcified atherosclerotic plaques may be seen in the major vessels at times but have no great diagnostic or prognostic value. Occasionally, the calcified wall of an intracranial aneurysm may be visible, as may punctate calcifications in the wall of an arteriovenous malformation.

Keynotes

- *Pagets disease is a disease of bone of unknown etiology in which there is destruciton and then replacement of bone. In this process, the shape of the bones involved is frequently changed.*

- *Fibrous dysplasia of bone is an uncommon disease in which abnormal deposits of fiber bone (an immature form of bone) are present. It results in deformity of the skeleton. In rare instances it is associated with accelerated sexual maturity.*

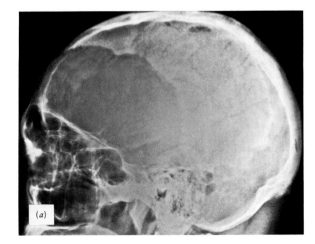

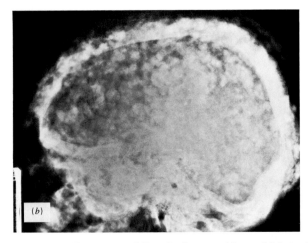

Figure 60-16. Two cases of Paget's disease of bone. (a) Lateral view demonstrating the osteolytic phase. Note the large, well-circumscribed area of destruction involving the frontal, parietal, and temporal regions of one side of the skull, resulting in diminished radiodensity. (*b*) Lateral view demonstrating the thick calvarial bones and "fluffy" increased radiodensity of the blastic phase of Paget's disease. Note the prominent vascular groove reflecting the increased blood flow to the skull.

SUMMARY

A systematic approach to viewing the skull film aids in the finding of abnormalities. The sutural lines demarcate the bones of the cranial vault. Widening of the sutures can be a sign of injury, increased intracranial pressure, or metastases. Premature fusion of the sutures can lead to skull deformity. Linear radiolucencies can be due to the arterial channels, venous channels, or skull fractures. Arterial channels branch and are less distinct than fractures. Venous channels often converge on larger areas of venous confluence called venous lakes.

If it has calcified, the pineal gland is a useful midline marker. Its shift from midline is a sign of brain swelling, mass, or focal brain atrophy. In most cases of brain injury, the skull films are normal. Fluid collections in and around the brain are best detected by CT. A skull fracture or pineal shift is seen in a minority of injured patients.

The signs of increased intracranial pressure include erosion of the dorsum sellae in the adult and spreading of the suture lines in the child. Primary intracranial neoplasms may result in the signs of increased intracranial pressure, a shift of the calcified pineal gland, intratumoral calcification (in some tumors), reactive bone formation (with some meningiomas), or bone destruction.

Large pituitary adenomas can cause sellar enlargement and erosion. Changes related to microadenomas, if any, may be visualized only on conventional or computed tomography. Areas of bone lysis and areas of bone deposition can be seen in metastatic disease of the skull, in Paget's disease of bone and in fibrous dysplasia.

REVIEW QUESTIONS

1. Describe the types of changes in the sutural bones that can occur with increased intracranial pressure or with leptomeningeal metastases.
2. What are venous lakes?
3. How would you differentiate a skull fracture from an arterial channel, from a diploic venous channel, and from a venous lake?
4. What types of processes can shift the calcified pineal gland?
5. How would you evaluate the patient with a head injury?
6. What is a blow-out fracture?
7. What are the signs of increased intracranial pressure?
8. What findings might be present on the skull films of a patient with a primary brain tumor?
9. What is the radiographic appearance of skull metastases?
10. What is Paget's disease of bone?

VOCABULARY

blow-out fracture	papilledema
depressed skull fracture	pituitary adenomas
diploic space	rhinorrhea
en face	scaphocephaly
falx	skull tables
fibrous dysplasia	spongiosa
microadenomas	Stenvers view
microcephaly	sutural lines
neuroradiology	synostosis
osteoporosis circumscripta	tangential
otorrhea	venous lakes
Paget's disease of bone	Waters view

61

CRANIAL COMPUTED TOMOGRAPHY

HARRY C. KNIPP

KEY CONCEPTS

Clinical

Cranial CT has become the primary imaging method in the evaluation of head trauma, neoplastic disease, cerebrovascular disease, hydrocephalus, and certain endocrine disorders. The patient with head trauma may have cerebral edema, intracerebral hemorrhage, or subdural or epidural hematomas. Patients who have sustained head trauma and have neurological symptoms (such as loss of consciousness, confusion, amnesia, etc.) or neurological signs (such as weakness , seizure, change in level of consciousness, etc.), and patients who for whatever reason are difficult to evaluate clinically should probably have cranial CT as part of their trauma evaluation.

CT is used in evaluating the patient with symptoms of a possible brain mass or suspected metastatic disease. It can be used both for the initial demonstration that a mass is present and to follow the effect of therapy

Cerebrovascular diseases include strokes, aneurysms, and arteriovenous malformations. Strokes are three types: embolic, thrombotic, and hemorrhagic. Embolic and thrombotic strokes may in part be treated with anticoagulation. Hemorrhagic strokes may worsen with anticoagulation. Prompt CT examination can demonstrate whether or not the stroke is hemorrhagic and can have a direct effect on the treatment method chosen.

Hydrocephalus can be due to obstruction of flow, decreased CSF resorption, or brain atrophy. The treatment of hydrocephalus from obstruction or decreased CSF resorption is an internal shunt drainage procedure. There is no specific treatment for cerebral atropy.

Radiological

Cranial CT examinations can be performed either with or without an intravenous contrast medium. Those obtained with contrast are called *enhanced scans*. Those obtained without intravenous contrast can be called *dry scans* or unenhanced scans. Unenhanced scans should be used in patients being evaluated for acute traumatic lesions and acute strokes. For most other conditions, a combination of dry and enhanced scans should be obtained.

Trauma can result in bleeding or cerebral edema. Bleeding can be recognized because new blood is radiodense compared with the brain and CSF, whereas older blood collections may be of the same radiodensity as brain and CSF. When the injury is not acute, both dry and enhanced scans should be obtained. Trauma can also result in cerebral edema. Cerebral edema decreases the radiodensity of the brain and, if sufficiently large, can compress the ventricles and sulci

Brain neoplasms may contain calcium and may be hypervascular. Dry scans are useful in looking for calcifications. Enhanced scans can demonstrate the degree of vascularity of the mass. In these patients both types of scans should be obtained.

The patient with a hemorrhagic stroke should not be given an anticoagulant. A dry CT scan will demonstrate blood as an area of whiteness, permitting identification of the hemorrhage.

The patient with obstructive hydrocephalus will, in general, demonstrate disproportional enlargement of only some of the ventricles. The patient with hydrocephalus caused by a problem with CSF resorption will usually have dilation of all the cerebral ventricles. The patient with cerebral atrophy will have enlargement of the ventricles and enlarged cortical sulci.

OBJECTIVES

When you complete this chapter you will be able to

1. Identify the presence of acute bleeding on selected CT scans.
2. Differentiate hemorrhagic and nonhemorrhagic strokes on selected CT scans.
3. List five changes that might be seen in the patient with head trauma.

4. Given a list of symptoms and signs, decide which trauma patient should have a cerebral CT.

5. Given a list of indications for cranial CT, decide which patient should have dry scans and which need both dry and enhanced scans. You should be able to explain your choice.

6. Identify masses on selected CT examinations.

7. Differentiate on selected CT scans obstructive hydrocephalus from cerebral atrophy.

In 1979 the Nobel Prize in Medicine was awarded to three men, none of whom were physicians. Their professions? Physics and engineering. Their achievements? The pioneering of what was rapidly to become the modern neuroradiologist's most basic tool: computed tomography. With its introduction in the mid-1970's, CT provided radiologists, neurosurgeons, and neurologists with a rapid, easily performed, and noninvasive means of examining the cranial contents and, what's more, provided heretofore unobtainable differentiation of the various soft tissue radiodensities present within the brain. For example, using sophisticated computer programming, the differences between gray and white matter, blood, and CSF become readily visible on the scan images, whereas with conventional x-ray techniques they would all have appeared as "water density."

The basic concepts of CT have been discussed in Chapter 4. In cranial CT, sections through the brain are usually obtained angled as shown in Figure 61-1. The initial positioning line is based on a line drawn from the outer canthus of the eye to the external auditory canal. Sections are obtained angled 15 ° to this line.

The sections obtained through the brain (Fig. 61-2) can differentiate different tissues and structures because of slight differences in radiodensity between them. As needed, the radiodensities can be assigned a numerical value that can be used to evaluate the nature of the tissue seen. The only specifically assigned number is that water is 0 Hounsfield units (HU). Other numbers are machine specific. Higher numbers are assigned to more radiodense tissues; for example bone is usually greater than 500HU.

Structures less radiodense than water have numbers less tha 0 HU; for example, air in the paranasal sinuses may be less than −500 HU.

Scans may be either enhanced or dry. An *enhanced CT scan* is one obtained after the injection of intravenous radiographic contrast material. A *dry scan* is one obtained without the prior injection of contrast. The injection of intravenous contrast medium will increase the radiodensity of the brain. This increased radiodensity may hide the presence of blood and, occasionally, of calcium. In general, scans obtained for acute trauma and suspected acute cerebrovascular accidents should not be enhanced because the presence of extravascular blood will affect treatment, and this blood might be concealed by the contrast. For most other conditions, scans should be obtained both dry and enhanced.

Any region receiving an abnormally increased amount of blood, such as a highly vascular tumor, the outer wall of an abscess, or an arteriovenous malformation, will enhance, aiding in its identification and accurate diagnosis. In addition to intravenous contrast, intrathecal contrast can be administered to outline the spinal canal, subarachnoid space, and cisterns.

The anatomy of the normal cranial CT is shown in Figure 61-2. These sections should be reviewed and then referred to as needed for comparison with later scans.

Keynotes

- *Tissue density numbers (approximate means values):*
  +500 HU bone
  +30 HU blood
  0 HU water, CSF
  −500 HU air

- *An enhanced scan is a scan performed with an intravenous or intrathecal contrast medium to "enhance," or add to, the image.*

- *A subacute or chronic abscess will usually be encased by a hypervascular zone of tissue, the abscess wall, or "rind."*

- *Intrathecal means within the coverings of the brain or spinal cord, within the subarachnoid space, or within the ventricular system.*

$\longrightarrow$

Figure 61-2. Normal cranial CT scan. (*a*) Enhanced scan: 1, orbit; 2, sphenoid sinus; 3, sella turcica; 4, basilar artery (with IV contrast); 5, pons; 6, 4th ventricle; 7, mastoid air cells in the petrous bone; 8, middle cranial fossa/temporal lobe; 9, posterior fossa/cerebellar hemisphere. (*b*) Dry scan: 1, frontal sinus; 2, orbital roof/sphenoid; bone; 3, olfactory groove/frontal lobe; 4, posterior clinoid processes; 5, pons; 6, middle fossa/temporal lobe; 7, posterior fossa/cerebellar hemisphere. (*c*) Enhanced scan: 1, frontal lobe; 2, middle cerebral artery (with IV contrast); 3, midbrain; 4, corpora quadrigemina; 5, vermis of cerebellum; 6, edge of tentorium; 7, occipital lobe. (*d*) Dry scan: 1, sylvian fissure; 2, third ventricle; 3, midbrain. (*e*) Enhanced scan: 1, frontal horn of lateral ventricle; 2, caudate nucleus; 3, third ventricle; 4, pineal gland. (*f*) Enhanced scan: 1, frontal horn of lateral ventricle; 2, septum pellucidum; 3, thalamus; 4, choroid plexus of lateral ventricle; 5, occipital horn of lateral ventricle. (*g*) Dry scan: 1, body of lateral ventricle; 2, parietal lobe; 3, falx. (*h*) Dry scan: 1, falx; 2, cortical gray matter; 3, white matter; 4, cortical gyri (light) and sulci (dark).

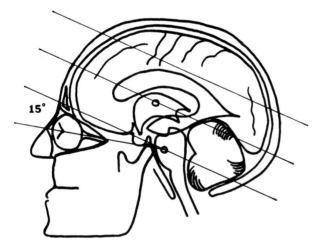

Figure 61-1. Schematic sagittal view of positioning usually used for cranial CT.

15°

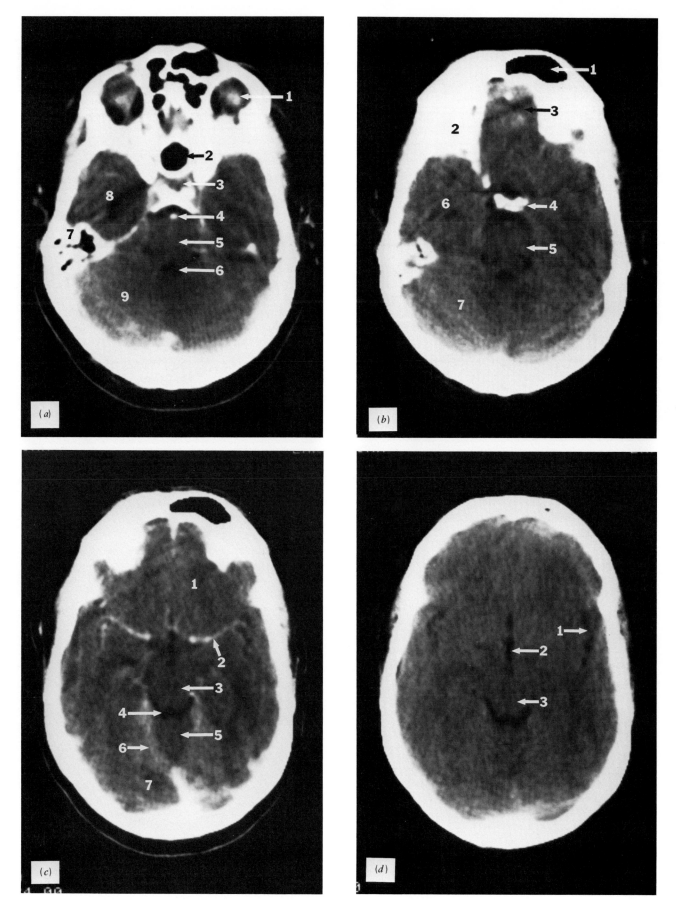

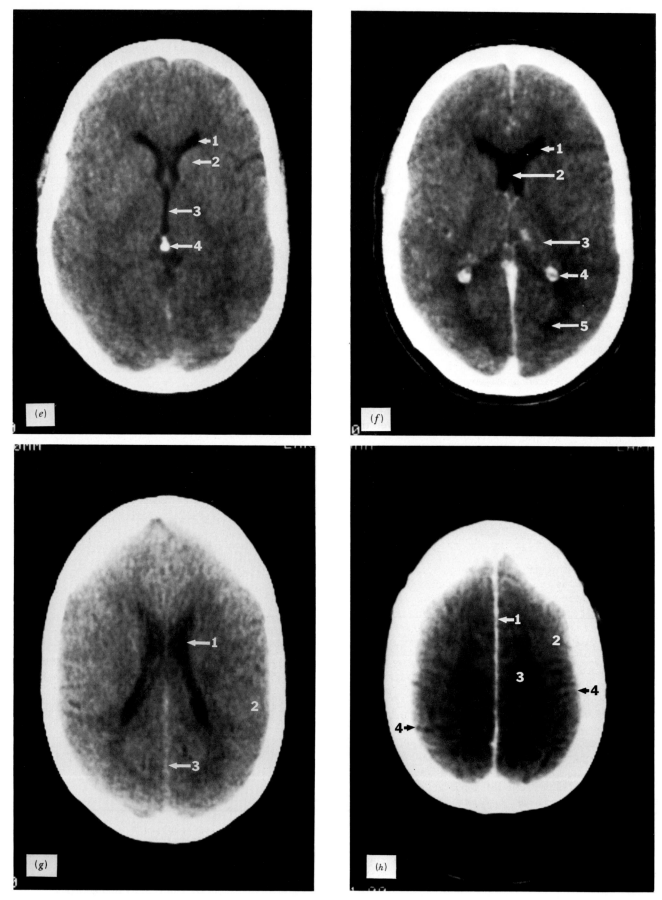

Figure 61-2. (Continued).

TRAUMA

Computed tomography has had a major impact on evaluation of head trauma. After a careful history and physical examination, a decision must be made on whether or not to obtain cranial CT. Who should have one? Any injured patient with neurological symptoms (i.e., loss of consciousness, confusion, amnesia, etc.) or neurological signs (weakness, seizure, change in level of consciousness, etc.) or any patient who cannot be evaluated accurately clinically because of belligerence, intoxication, inability to speak your language, or other reasons.

Doug B. was the unfortunate victim of a barroom brawl, in which, the police reported, he received a vicious beating with a heavy pipe. His emergency admission scans (Fig. 61-3) shortly before his death demonstrate a number of important findings in head trauma. What do you see? First, note the marked shift of the midline structures to the left. (Fig. 61-3b) This is the result of a mass effect caused by a subdural hematoma in the right temporoparietal region, which appears as a lenticular (lenslike) collection of medium-white density on the scan (no. 3 in Fig. 61-3b and c). Fresh blood, more radiodense than normal brain parenchyma, appears as a white area in the CT images.

Note also that swelling in the underlying brain also contributes to the shift. Cerebral edema, whatever the cause, appears as an area of darker density in the scan than normal brain tissue (Fig. 61-3c). It may be helpful to conceptualize that water-radiodensity edema fluid in the tissues "dilutes" the normal parenchymal radiodensity, making the computer's average density number in this area lower and thus making the image darker (further toward the black end of the cathode ray tube's gray scale).

Returning to the subdural hematoma, recall its concavo-convex lenticular shape. This is important because it helps the physician distinguish a subdural collection from an epidural hematoma, an altogether different lesion. The subdural hematoma assumes its classic shape because the loose dural connections in this space allow the blood, usually the result of venous bleeding, to spread easily over a wide area, conforming somewhat to the convexity of the brain and the concavity of the skull. The epidural bleed, often arterial, is more confined by the tight connections between the skull and dura. As the blood cannot spread laterally as freely as in the subdural space, the collection bulges inward under great pressure in a biconvex configuration.

The rounded areas of white seen in the right frontal area (no. 5 in Fig. 61-3b) and middle fossa (no. 4 in Fig. 61-3a) are intraparenchymal hematomas. What caused them? The clue to their origin is the location of the various lesions. The increased thickness of the soft tissues outside the skull in the left parietooccipital area represent swelling at the site of the impact. The blow to this area accelerated the soft, jellylike tissues of the brain in the direction of the force, causing them to impact against the jagged surfaces of the right orbital roof and petrous ridge; hence, the hematomas. This same accelerating force may have

sheared subdural veins on the right as well, resulting in the subdural collection noted initially. This type of injury is called a *contrecoup injury.* Injuries can result in bleeding into the subdural space, the epidural space, the brain, and the ventricular system.

Closed skull trauma also frequently results in cerebral edema. As in the example above, this may be localized to a particular area, or it may be generalized diffusely throughout the brain. In the latter case, the edema results in a slight diminution in the overall radiodensity of the brain, but more important, it narrows the ventricles and obliterates the normally visible cortical sulci.

Compare the scan of the patient in Figure 61-4 with the normal scan in Figure 61-2e and f. This patient has suffered a massive blow to the head, and though no bleeding can be seen on the CT image, she has developed increased intracranial pressure, the result of generalized cerebral edema. Notice how the swelling brain has encroached upon the normal ventricular spaces, making them appear slitlike, and how the cortical sulci have been effaced by the enlarging brain. Remember that these signs of cerebral edema may be seen with swelling of any etiology including infection, neoplastic disease, and stroke.

Keynotes

- *An emergency CT scan combined with a careful physical examination is the best method of evaluating the patient with head trauma. Who should have one? Any injured patient with neurological symptoms (loss of consciousness, confusion, amnesia, etc.) or neurological signs (weakness, seizure, change in level of consciousness, etc.).*

- *Midline shift can be demonstrated as shift*
  Of the third ventricle
  Of the lateral ventricles
  Of the calcified pineal gland
  Of the interventricular sulcus

- *Lenticular means lenslike either convexoconvex or concavoconvex.*

- *Cerebral edema results in focal swelling and appears on the scan as a darker area of decreased radiodensity; it may focally narrow and efface sulci and compress ventricular structures.*

- *In epidural hematoma, because the blood entering the epidural space is under arterial pressure, it expands rapidly, causing the rapid onset of severe cerebral symptoms. The subdural hematoma, filled under venous pressure, expands much more slowly, with symptoms often delayed in onset for days or weeks.*

- *A contrecoup injury is an injury to the brain occurring on the side of the brain opposite to the side of the blow.*

NEOPLASTIC DISEASE

Computed tomography has also made dramatic changes in the diagnosis and follow-up of intracranial neoplastic disease. Whereas physicians once relied upon the complexities of the patient's neurological examination to localize an intracranial lesion, CT can rapidly and accurately per-

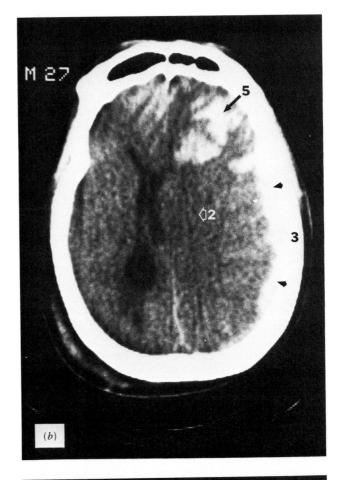

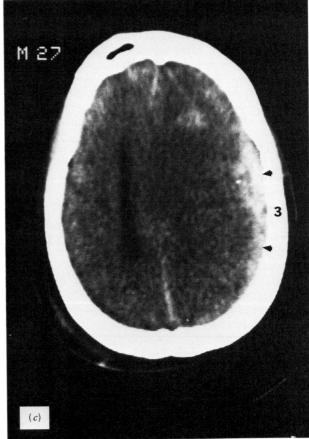

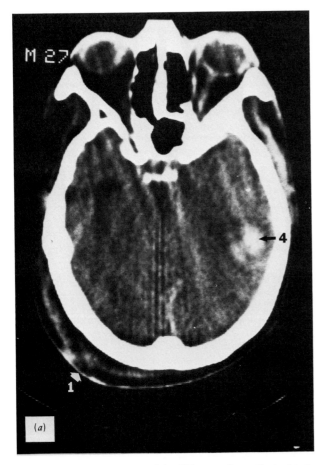

Figure 61-3. Three sections of the CT scan of a patient who received a massive blow from a lead pipe to the left parietooccipital area. The skull films demonstrated no fracture. (*a*) Temporal region. The white area 4 is an intracerebral hematoma. (*b*) Midventricular level. Both ventricles are shifted to the left (open arrow, 2). The lenticular region of whiteness (black arrows, 3) represents a subdural hematoma. The white region (black arrow, 5) is an intracerebral hematoma. (*c*) High ventricular level. The subdural hematoma (black arrows, 3) is again seen.

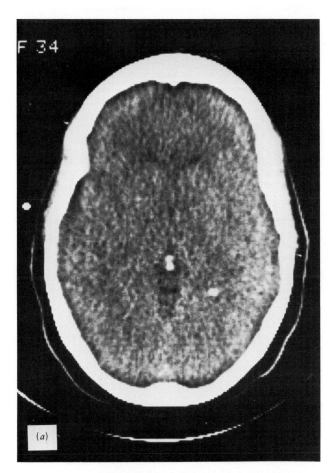 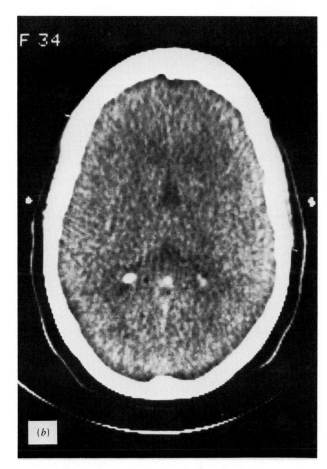

Figure 61-4. Adjacent sections from the midventricular level of a CT scan of a 34-year-old woman who developed diffuse intracranial swelling after a severe closed skull injury.

form this task as well as provide information on the tissue type involved.

Figure 61-5a is the unenhanced scan of a patient with headache. Note the slightly white lesion in the frontal region, which spreads the frontal horns of the lateral ventricles laterally. The tissue radiodensity numbers of this area measured approximately +175 HU. These numbers suggest some calcification within the lesion. The patient was subsequently injected with intravenous contrast material, and a second scan (Fig. 61-5b) was performed. The radiodensity numbers of the lesion were even higher after enhancement, and it appeared much brighter in the images. These findings suggest that the lesion is not only calcified but also very vascular. Putting the triad of a peripheral location, calcification, and increased vascularity together, you can predict the diagnosis of meningioma in this middle-aged female patient.

Figure 61-6 is the contrast-enhanced study of an unfortunate man who has been followed for a malignant brain tumor. He has undergone a partial resection, as evidenced by the craniotomy defect in the right parietal region, where the bone flap has been replaced (Fig. 61-6a). The large mass appears as irregular rings of increased radiodensity with low-radiodensity centers. These correspond respectively to the highly vascular rims of growing tumor and the necrotic central portions, which no longer have an adequate blood supply. Also note the low radiodensity (darker) areas surrounding the tumor. These represent edema in the adjacent portions of the normal brain displaced by the tumor mass. With the aid of CT, neurosurgeons can now follow their postoperative patients for tumor regrowth and spread and also evaluate postoperative complications such as infarction or infection.

Metastases

The early detection of metastatic disease may be of great value to the clinician in plotting the course of the future therapy. Radionuclide brain scanning can detect only the larger lesions, usually after the onset of related symptoms. The sensitivity of CT, particularly with intravenous contrast enhancement, allows diagnosis of intracranial metastases often long before they are sizable enough to result in detectable signs and symptoms. Figure 61-7 is the enhanced scan of a patient with oat cell carcinoma of the lung. Several early metastases are visible as small

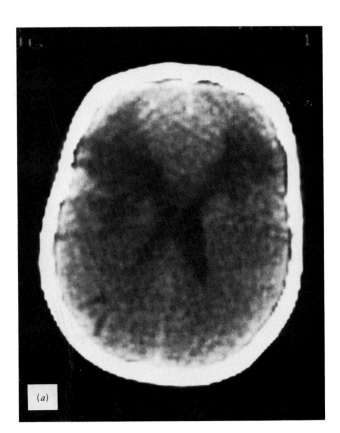

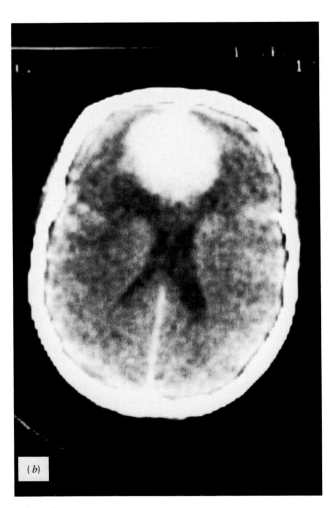

Figure 61-5. (*a*) Dry and (*b*) enhanced sections from scans of a woman with headaches and a slight change in behavior.

white areas of increased radiodensity, the result of increased vascularity in neoplastic tissue. These could not be visualized on the unenhanced images. After irradiation, a follow-up scan showed a decrease in the size of the lesions.

Figure 61-8 shows a metastasis in the brain of a patient with an adenocarcinoma. Note the larger ringlike appearance with a small central radiolucency indicating some necrosis. There is also radiolucent edema surrounding the lesion. The mass and the surrounding edema result in a midline shift to the left and obliterate the posterior horn of the right lateral ventricle.

Keynotes

• *If calcium has a tissue radiodensity number of +500 HU, how can a calcified lesion show a tissue radiodensity number of +175? Because the tissue is not totally calcified. The tissue radiodensities of calcified and noncalcified areas are volume-averaged, to yield a radiodensity of +175.*

• *Meningioma is a slowly growing, usually nonmetastasizing tumor originating from the layers of tissue covering the brain or spinal cord. Usually seen in young to middle-aged adults, meningiomas can recur locally after resection.*

CEREBROVASCULAR DISEASE

Stroke

The third major area where CT diagnosis has become a valuable asset is in the diagnosis of vascular disease. The diagnosis of stroke, primarily a clinical one before CT, has become a routine indication for head scanning. Figure 61-9 is the unenhanced scan of a patient with a right hemiparesis. You can easily see an area of decreased radiodensity (i.e., a blacker area) in the left parietal area. Such a low radiodensity in the distribution of a major vessel is the classical CT abnormality of a cerebrovascular acci-

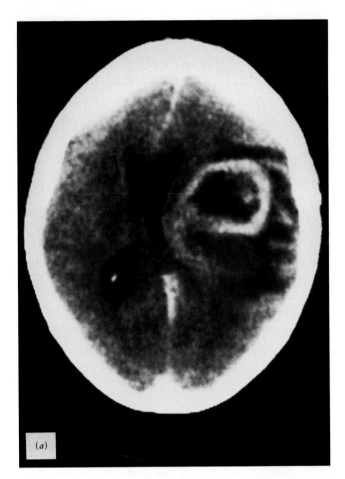
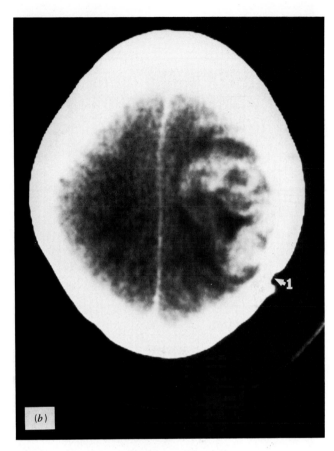

Figure 61-6. CT scan of a glioblastoma. (*a*) Midventricular level. (*b*) High-convexity section. The white arrow indicates the deformity resulting from a prior craniotomy with flap replacement.

dent, whatever the location. A faint low-radiodensity area usually first becomes visible 6–24 hours after the onset of symptoms, gradually decreasing in radiodensity and increasing in definition as several weeks pass. Occasionally some localized swelling may also be seen early in the course of the lesion, possibly with a slight displacement of the adjacent ventricle, focal flattening of cortical sulci, or both, as described in the discussion of edema.

Strokes can be of three types; embolic, thrombotic, and hemorrhagic. It is usually not possible to distinguish thrombotic from embolic lesions, but CT can diagnose hemorrhagic infarctions, which usually precludes clinical therapy with anticoagulants. Such infarcts appear as areas of increased radiodensity with some edema similar to the intracerebral hematomas.

Intravenous contrast enhancement is usually of little help in the diagnosis of stroke. Occasionally, a lesion may be detected slightly earlier with enhancement. Contrast radiodensity in an area of infarction may indicate luxury perfusion (increased blood flow at the margins of the infarction) with a breakdown in the blood-brain barrier.

Aneurysms

Aneurysms may also be visualized on dry scans if they are calcified or on enhanced images as bulges of major arteries. Many smaller aneurysms, however, are not seen. Computed tomography is better at demonstrating the bleed than at demonstrating the aneurysm. Blood can be seen in the subarachnoid space, ventricular system, and brain parenchyma. Figure 61-10 depicts such a case.

Arteriovenous Malformations

Subarachnoid hemorrhage may also result from bleeding from an arteriovenous malformation. These vascular lesions can be seen as enhancing masses because of their increased vascularity, but unlike tumors, they have no real mass effect or edema. Figure 61-11 is an enhanced scan demonstrating a right parietal arteriovenous malformation.

The serpentine shape of the large feeding and draining vessels seen here is often visible in such patients. The

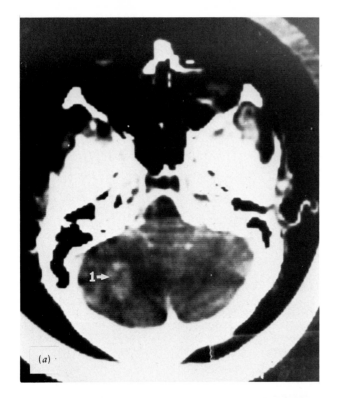

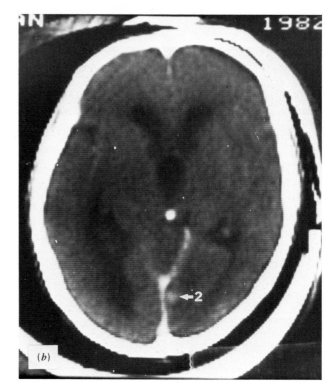

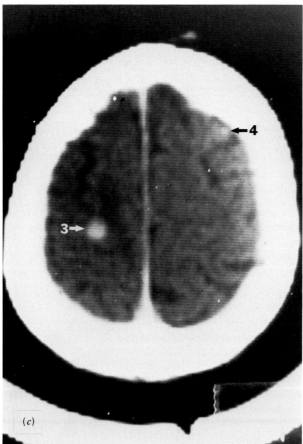

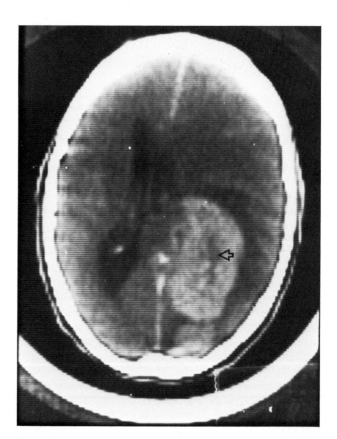

Figure 61-7. These three sections from the CT scan of a patient with metastatic oat cell cancer of the lung demonstrate four enhancing metastases (arrows) that could not be seen on the dry scans.

Figure 61-8. Enhanced cranial CT revealed a large ringlike lesion of the right parietooccipital area with a very vascular tumor mass, a small area of central necrosis (arrow), and surrounding edema.

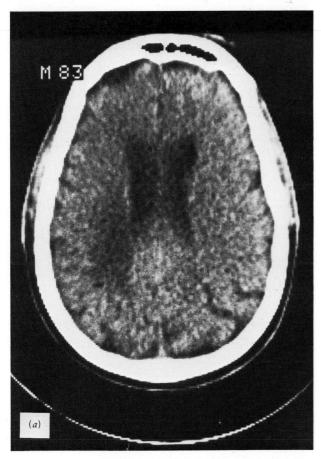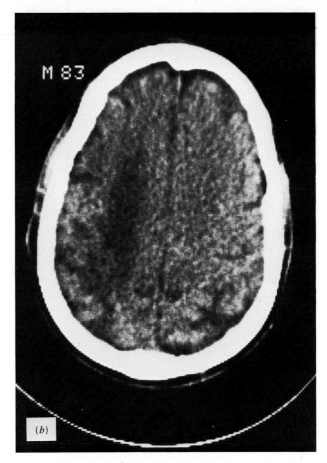

Figure 61-9. Two sections from the scan of an elderly man with right hemiparesis. Diminished radiodensity is readily seen in the left parietal region just lateral to the left lateral ventricle. The scan suggests a left middle cerebral artery infarction correlating perfectly with the clinical neurological examination. Notice how the cerebral gyri and sulci are more clearly seen in this 83-year-old man than in many of the younger patients' scans we have reviewed. Normal mild cerebral atrophic change results in decreased brain mass and thus the slightly more prominent sulci.

anomalous direct arterial-to-venous connection allows the shunting of great volumes of high-pressure arterial blood into the more distensible venous system, resulting in the dilated, tortuous veins. The arteries also gradually enlarge as more and more blood courses through this path of least resistance. These lesions may "grow" in this manner to great size and in doing so may deprive normal brain in adjacent areas of its vital blood supply. Usually these lesions develop gradually as the brain grows. They usually cause no mass effect unless bleeding occurs, forming a hematoma.

Keynotes

- Stroke *is a sudden onset of neurological disease with a vascular cause, usually the result of*

  a. *Embolization to an intracerebral vessel with infarction distally—the embolic stroke*

  b. *Thrombosis of an intracerebral vessel with infarction distally—the thrombotic stroke*

  c. *Nontraumatic intracerebral bleeding, usually in the basal ganglia of the brain and usually associated with systemic hypertension—the hemorrhagic stroke*

  d. *Bleeding from an aneurysm or arteriovenous malformation—the stroke with subarachnoid hemorrhage*

- *Decreased radiodensity in the distribution of a major cerebral vessel is the usual finding in the embolic or thrombotic stroke.*

- *Thrombotic and embolic strokes are frequently treated with anticoagulation, as this may decrease the size of the area of final brain injury. Anticoagulation should not usually be used in the treatment of hemorrhagic stroke because this therapy will often increase bleeding, enlarging the size of the area of brain damage.*

- *Luxury perfusion is an increase in blood flow at the margins of an area of infarction.*

- *An aneurysm is a dilated vessel. In the central nervous system the most common sites are at the*
  Posterior communicating artery origin
  Anterior communicating artery
  Middle cerebral artery at its point of division
  Basilar artery at the circle of Willis at the base of the brain

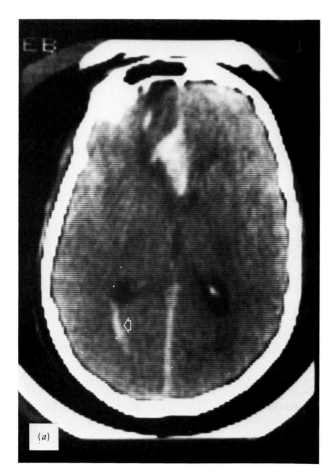
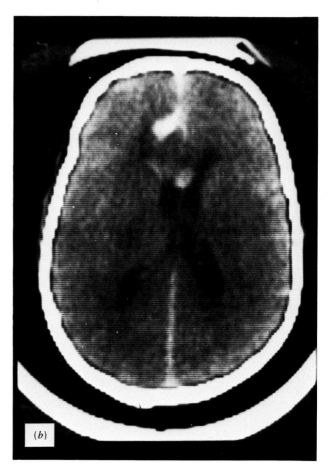

Figure 61-10. Two sections from the scan of a 36-year-old businessman who had complained to co-workers of a severe headache immediately before losing consciousness. A subarachnoid and intra-cerebral hemorrhage is evidenced by the white radiodensity of fresh blood in the left frontal region extending into the interventricular area and by the intraventricular bleeding. The white radiodensity in the posterior horn of the left lateral ventricle (a, arrow) is blood, heavier than CSF, which had fallen to the most dependent portion of the ventricle with the head in the routine scan position (cf. Fig. 61-2g). An anterior-communicating artery aneurysm was predicted based on the site of the bleeding and was confirmed by a subsequent angiogram. The aneurysm was clipped successfully and the patient recovered uneventfully.

• An arteriovenous malformation is an anomaly of development in which abnormal connections occur directly from artery to vein with no intervening capillary bed. Because they develop slowly as the brain itself is developing, they show no evidence of a mass or of edema surrounding them until they bleed.

HYDROCEPHALUS

Evaluation of hydrocephalus (enlarged CSF space in the brain) is another of the many areas in which CT has proven valuable. It is used in differentiating obstructive from communicating hydrocephalus and in following patients after various corrective CSF shunt procedures.

Obstructive Hydrocephalus

In obstructive hydrocephalus, there is a block to the egress of CSF from its point of production in the choroid plexus of the ventricular system, usually because of either a mass compressing or a stricture blocking the normal pathways of outflow. By pinpointing such a lesion or by assessing whether there is or is not ventricular dilation, the site of the obstruction can be diagnosed.

Figure 61-12 is the scan of a patient with congenital stenosis of the Sylvian aqueduct between the third and fourth ventricles. Notice that the lateral and third ventricles are grossly dilated, but the fourth ventricle remains normal in size, suggesting the point of obstruction.

Communicating Hydrocephalus

The patient in Figure 61-13 has communicating hydrocephalus. In this condition, there is usually normal egress of CSF from the ventricles, but a problem arises with the resorption of CSF at the arachnoid granulations high over the convexity of the cortex. All of this patient's ventricles,

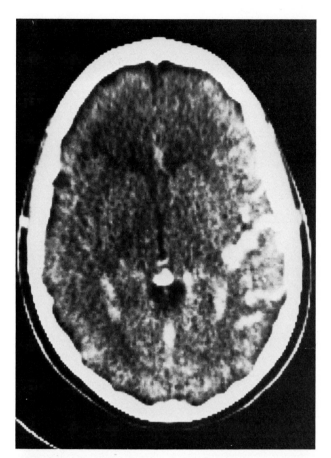

Figure 61-11. Section from the contrast-enhanced scan of a young woman with headache and left hemiparesis. Large, dilated serpentine blood vessels are visible in the right parietal region. No areas of diminished radiodensity are seen, indicating an absence of edema. The midline structures (e.g., the calcified pineal gland and third ventricle just anterior to it) are not displaced. These factors all support the diagnosis of arteriovenous malformation.

including the fourth, are enlarged. This information, added to the patient's history of meningitis in the past, suggests the diagnosis of communicating hydrocephalus. Scarring in the subarachnoid space limits the resorption of CSF; as CSF continues to be formed at a normal rate at the choroid plexus, hydrocephalus results. A subsequent shunt from the lateral ventricle to the abdominal peritoneal cavity helped to solve this patient's problem.

Cerebral Atrophy

A condition that also causes enlarged ventricles is the entirely different entity of cerebral atrophy. Before the introduction of CT, there was no imaging technique with which neurologists or psychiatrists could confirm this diagnosis. This condition is characterized by ventricular enlargement along with enlargement of the cortical sulci, which become wider and deeper as the brain atrophies. Computed tomography has provided a rapid, noninvasive test

that can demonstrate an overall decrease in brain mass and thus suggest generalized cerebral atrophy. Figure 61-14 demonstrates these findings well.

As the brain atrophies, its mass decreases, leaving all these CSF-filled spaces relatively large in appearance as they occupy the remaining intracranial space. The ventricular enlargement of atrophy can be differentiated from that of obstructive and communicating hydrocephalus by the diminished size of the cortical sulci in these latter conditions. In those cases, the grooves of the sulci are effaced as the brain is pushed outward by the increasing intraventricular pressure.

Keynotes

- *There are three conditions resulting in dilation of the ventricular system:*

  Obstructive hydrocephalus, in which there is obstruction to the outflow of CSF from the ventricular system

  Communicating hydrocephalus, in which there is decreased resorption of CSF over the brain convexity

  Cerebral atrophy, in which there is diffuse loss of brain tissue, resulting in large ventricles and large cortical surface sulci

- *Communicating hydrocephalus often occurs after an episode of meningitis or subarachnoid hemorrhage.*

ENDOCRINE DISORDERS

The work-up of endocrine disorders may include CT examination of the head for abnormalities of the hypothalamic-pituitary axis. Obviously, large, grossly evident tumors of the pituitary region may be seen. Enlargement of the sella turcica may also be identified. Even subtle pituitary lesions such as microadenomas may be detected, particularly with the use of intrathecal contrast agents and coronal scanning positions to better visualize the area of the sella turcica.

Figure 61-15a is the coronal scan of a young man with gynecomastia. Unlike the other scans in this section, it was performed with the head and scanner tilted in such a way as to section the patient's skull in the coronal plane (as if one were looking forward at the patient's face). The white radiodensity surrounding the basal structures of the brain is a water-soluble contrast material especially designed for intrathecal use. It was injected into the lumbar subarachnoid space, whence it flowed by gravity into the basilar CSF spaces of the brain known as *cisterns*.

Notice that there is a small, bony erosion of the sellar floor, best seen in Figure 61-15b, a magnified view of this area. The erosion was caused by the growth of a small pituitary tumor. Subsequently, a prolactin-secreting pituitary microadenoma was removed by transsphenoidal resection, resulting in rapid improvement in this patient's condition.

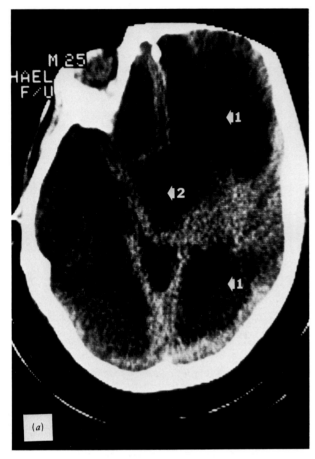

(a)

Figure 61-12. Two sections from the unenhanced scan of a 25-year-old man with long-standing hydrocephalus. (a) Massive enlargement of the lateral and third ventricles (arrows, 1 and 2 respectively). Only a thin residual layer of cerebral cortex can be seen peripherally in most areas. (b) A normal-sized fourth ventricle (arrow) is revealed, indicating that the level of obstruction is between the third and fourth ventricles, in other words, in the cerebral sylvian aqueduct. No mass lesions can be seen to account for the obstruction. A prior ventriculogram (a radiograph using water-soluble contrast material introduced into the ventricles, either by lumbar puncture or direct ventricular puncture) had demonstrated aqueductal stenosis.

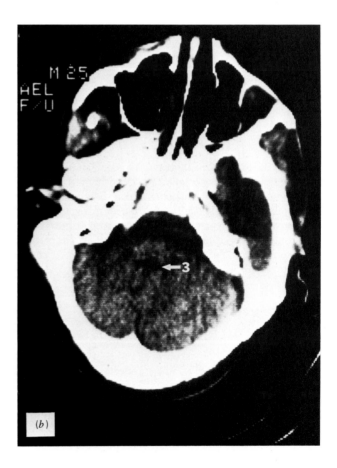

(b)

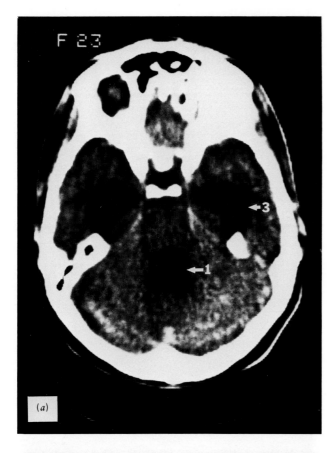

(a)

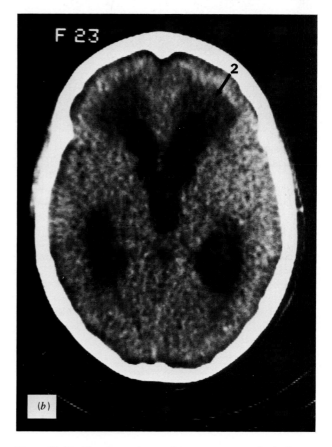

(b)

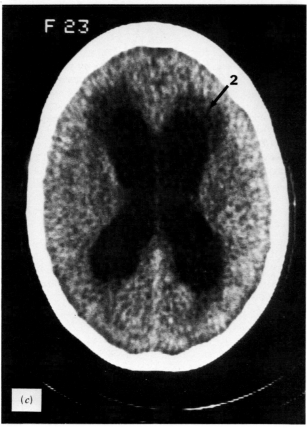

(c)

Figure 61-13. Unenhanced scan of a young woman who had recovered from a severe episode of meningitis several years previously. The marked dilatation of the entire ventricular system is easily seen. (a) The fourth ventricle (arrow, 1) is enlarged along with the third and lateral ventricles (arrow, 3), suggesting communicating hydrocephalus as opposed to the obstructive form (cf. Fig. 61-12). (b) and (c) Enlarged lateral ventricles. Note the areas of diminished radiodensity (arrow, 2) adjacent to the frontal horns. This is not edema but transependymal (i.e., across the ependymal lining of the ventricles) resorption of the excessive CSF (cf. Fig. 62-2 with normal CSF absorption).

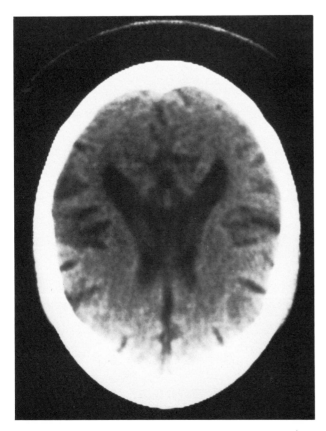

Figure 61-14. Single section from the unenhanced scan of a middle-aged woman with long-standing organic brain syndrome. Compare her scan with a normal section at this approximate level (fig. 61-2g). The prominent cortical sulci and interhemispheric fissure and the dilated lateral ventricles are readily seen in this patient with cerebral atrophy.

MRI OF THE BRAIN

Magnetic resonance images of the brain (see Chapter 5) compete with CT of the brain. As of this date, CT and MRI have both shown approximately the same percentage diagnostic yield with most brain processes, and because CT is substantially cheaper (1/2 to 1/3 the cost), it is preferred. For several processes, MRI has been shown much superior to CT and is therefore preferred for the evaluation of demyelinating diseases and small cranial nerve tumors. In the posterior fossa of the brain MRI is more sensitive for small lesions, but should probably be used only following a normal CT, since most posterior fossa lesions will be demonstrated on CT. Conversely, CT has been demonstrated more sensitive in the detection of meningiomas, and if a meningioma is suspected, CT is preferred (though the difference is probably not as great as initial clinical studies suggested; CT may offer only a slight advantage).

There is as yet, except for posterior fossa lesions, insufficient data to indicate whether or not a patient with a normal CT of the brain should have MRI and conversely, whether a patient with a normal MRI of the brain should have CT. Currently available studies indicate that for

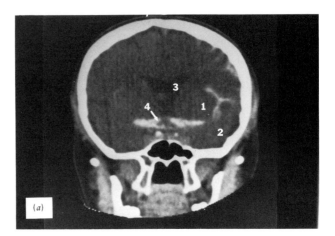

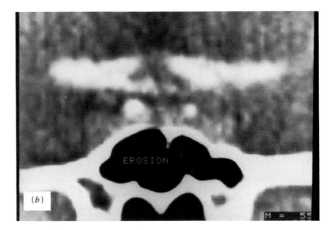

Figure 61-15. Coronal CT section from a scan of a young adult man suffering from gynecomastia with galactorrhea. Plain-film radiographs of the sella turcica were normal, demonstrating no sellar enlargement or erosion. Routine CT scans with intravenous contrast enhancement were also normal in appearance. This study is done in the coronal plane with intrathecal contrast material. (a) On the left, contrast material delineates the lateral sulcus, surrounding the insula (1) and the temporal lobe (2). The bodies of the lateral ventricles can be seen filled with CSF, which does not contain the contrast agent (3). The optic nerves (arrow, 4) are visible distal to the optic chiasm, outlined by the contrast agent, with the silhouette of the infundibulum in between. (b) Magnified view. A small erosion is visible in the floor of the sella turcica, just above the sphenoid sinus. Such a unilateral focal erosion can be seen with pituitary microadenomas, a diagnosis confirmed surgically.

most processes, CT and MRI have similar yields, but there are patients in whom CT has succeeded in finding abnormalities when MRI has failed, and vice versa.

SUMMARY

Cranial CT is one of the major advances in diagnostic studies in the last 15 years. Computed tomographic imaging of the brain permits the noninvasive evaluation of possible brain injury, tumor, metastasis, stroke, and subarachnoid hemorrhage and has greatly enhanced the ability of neurologists and neurosurgeons to evaluate and treat their patients safely.

The patient with a head injury may demonstrate intracerebral hematoma, sub- and epidural hematoma, and generalized or focal brain edema. In the acutely injured patient, areas of bleeding will appear as areas of increased radiodensity, whereas edema will appear as an area of decreased radiodensity. Generalized brain edema may decrease the size of the ventricles and sulci. In the subacute state, area of bleeding may be of the same radiodensity as the brain, and both dry and enhanced scans may be needed to demonstrate the abnormalities.

The CT images can demonstrate intracranial masses and the edema that surrounds them. Both primary and metastatic tumors can be identified.

A brain infarct shows on the CT scan as an area of decreased radiodensity, usually first visible 6–24 hours after the onset of symptoms. Thrombotic and embolic strokes cannot be distinguished. Hemorrhagic infarcts show as areas of increased radiodensity on the dry scan. Hemorrhage in an area of infarction is usually a contraindication for anticoagulation. Subarachnoid hemorrhage can be identified because of the increased radiodensity of the blood in the subarachnoid space.

There are three common forms of ventricular dilation: obstruction of CSF outflow (obstructive hydrocephalus); diminished CSF resorption (communicating hydrocephalus); and brain atrophy. Differential diagnosis is made by evaluating which ventricles are dilated (in obstructive hydrocephalus both lateral ventricles and the third ventricle are usually dilated; in communicating hydrocephalus and atrophy all ventricles are dilated) and by evaluating whether the brain sulci are enlarged (as in brain atrophy).

Some of the many diagnostic problems CT may help to resolve have been discussed briefly. Other areas of disease, including inflammatory conditions, demyelinating diseases, congenital disorders, extra-axial neoplasms, orbital/ocular lesions, and facial neoplasms, can also be evaluated by CT scanning, a technique less than a decade old but one of the major advances in modern medicine.

REVIEW QUESTIONS

1. Describe the axis of the usual brain slice viewed in CT.
2. What are the several effects of trauma to the brain that can be identified on CT scans? What is their appearance?
3. What is a contrecoup injury?
4. How would you differentiate an epidural from a subdural hematoma?
5. What is the clinical importance of the correct identification of an epidural hematoma?
6. What is the difference between an enhanced and a dry scan?
7. Describe the findings on CT of a brain tumor. How might the appearance of brain metastasis be different?
8. What are the four types of stroke? How do their CT appearances differ?
9. What are the three causes of ventricular dilation? How might they be differentiated by CT scanning?
10. Describe the role of CT scanning in the evaluation of endocrine disorders.

VOLCABULARY

arteriovenous malformation	hydrocephalus
cerebral atrophy	lenticular shape
cerebral edema	luxury perfusion
communicating hydrocephalus	meningioma
contrecoup injury	meningitis
dry scan	obstructive hydrocephalus
enhanced scan	prolactin
epidural hematoma	stroke
gynecomastia	subdural hematoma
hematoma	Sylvian aqueduct
hemiparesis	thecal space
hemorrhagic stroke	

SUGGESTIONS FOR FURTHER READING FOR CHAPTERS 61 AND 62

Ronald G. Quisling, Preston R. Lotz. *Correlative Neuroradiology: Intracranial Radiographic Analysis with Computed Tomography, Angiography, and Magnetic Resonance Imaging.* John Wiley & Sons: New York. 1985.

B. Felson, Ed. Primary brain tumors. *Seminars in Roentgenology,* **19** (1, 2), 1984.

62

NEUROANGIOGRAPHY

HARRY C. KNIPP

KEY CONCEPTS

Clinical

Neuroangiography is used for three main purposes: to guide the surgeon in the treatment of mass lesions and vascular lesions of the brain, to identify the sources of intracranial bleeding, and to evaluate brain ischemia to help identify a treatable lesion. In general, CT will precede angiography and will guide how the examination is performed. When ischemic disease is suspected, preliminary evaluation may also include carotid ultrasound and oculoplethysmography (pressure recordings from the eye).

Radiological

Depending on the clinical indications and the guidance provided by a preliminary CT examination or carotid ultrasound examination, angiograms of the external, internal, and common carotid arteries or the vertebral-basilar vascular system can be obtained. Subtraction techniques can be useful in removing the confusing shadows of overlying bony structures. Sometimes special oblique views are useful in better demonstrating the anatomic abnormalities encountered.

Mass lesions can demonstrate abnormal tumor vessels or may demonstrate a more diffuse vascular increase as a generalized blush within the tumor. Masses will also usually displace vessels. The displacement of vessels is an important guide to the location of the mass and to the neurosurgeon as he or she operates.

Vascular demonstration aids in the diagnosis and treatment of aneurysms and arteriovenous malformations and in the identification of possible treatable vascular causes of brain ischemia.

OBJECTIVES

When you complete this chapter you will be able to

1. List the main indications for neuroangiography.
2. Correctly identify on selected radiographs intracerebral masses, aneurysms, and arteriovenous malformations as well as plaques narrowing the internal carotid arteries.
3. Identify selected vascular shifts occurring from intracerebral mass lesions.
4. Give two common causes of subarachnoid hemorrhage.
5. Describe the method of evaluation of embolic stroke or transient ischemic attack.

The third major diagnostic modality used in neuroradiology is angiography. This technique involves radiography of the head and neck after opacification of the vasculature with water-soluble contrast material. Usually this is achieved by percutaneous catheterization of the major brachiocephalic arteries, most often via a femoral artery puncture site. Using fluoroscopic guidance, the angiographer can advance the catheter cephalad through the femoral and iliac arteries and the abdominal and thoracic portions of the aorta into the aortic arch, where he or she can selectively catheterize the carotid and vertebral arteries, injecting small doses of contrast material (the same water-soluble agents used for CT enhancement and IVU), while rapid-sequence radiographs of the head and neck are performed in various projections.

Figure 62-1 depicts selected films in the AP and lateral projections from the midarterial and venous phases of such an injection in the right internal carotid artery. The major vessels of the internal carotid circulation in their normal positions are well demonstrated.

Figures 62-2a and b are views of the arterial phase of a

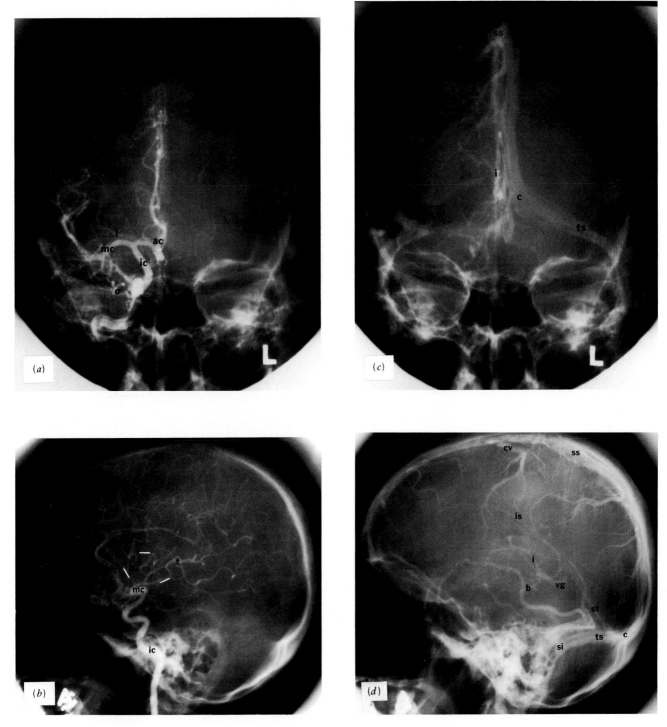

Figure 62-1. Arterial and venous phase films from a normal right internal carotid angiogram with major normal arterial and venous structures labeled. Remember to think in three dimensions when studying these films, comparing the frontal and lateral views to help sort out the many overlapping branches. (a) Frontal arterial-phase view; (b) lateral arterial-phase view; ic = internal carotid artery; ac = anterior cerebral artery; mc = middle cerebral artery; o = ophthalmic artery; l = lenticulostriate arteries; pc = pericallosal artery; p = parietal branches of the middle cerebral artery; t = temporal branches of the middle cerebral artery. The three small white lines in b help to define the sylvian triangle. (c) Frontal venous-phase view; (d) lateral venous-phase view; ss = superior sagittal sinus; is = inferior sagittal sinus; ts = transverse sinus; si = sigmoid sinus; st = straight sinus; c = confluence of sinuses; cv = a superficial cortical vein; vg = vein of Galen; i = internal cerebral vein; b = basal vein.

vertebral artery injection demonstrating the normal basilar, posterior fossa, and posterior cerebral circulation in the frontal and lateral projections. Occasionally, the bony structures of the cranial vault will obscure the opacified vessels, particularly the smaller ones such as the anterior inferior cerebellar artery, which is clearly seen in the frontal view but obscured by the petrous bone in the lateral one. Figure 62-2c demonstrates one technique for avoiding this problem: subtraction films. Here, a negative film of the skull is obtained before the vascular injection. It is used later to photographically subtract much of the bone radiodensity from the angiogram film, leaving a clearer negative image of the vessels.

You can see that angiography provides excellent visualization of the vascular anatomy. Unfortunately, the study is invasive, requiring violation of the major vessels by the catheter, and thus there is a possibility of the untoward secondary sequellae of thrombosis, embolization, and possible vascular damage. Although such events are uncommon, they do occur, and therefore the risk entailed by this examination must be weighted against the value of the information to be gained. Further, the test must be performed in a hospital environment under sterile conditions, with preoperative preparation and postprocedural observation usually requiring hospital admission and all the related expenses.

In this age of CT diagnosis, cerebral angiography is used primarily in three major areas:

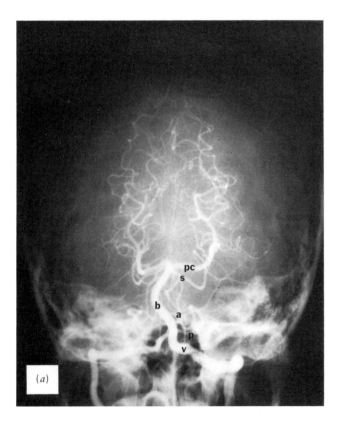

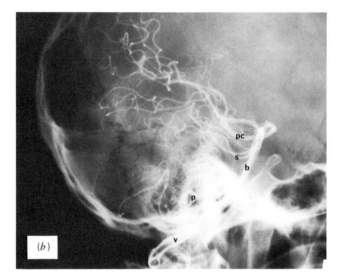

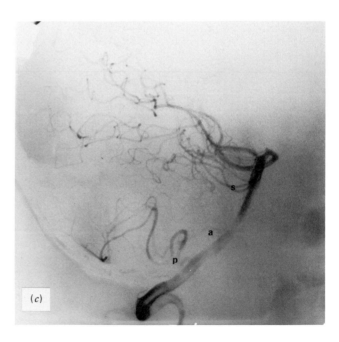

Figure 62-2. The normal anatomy of the vertebral-basilar arterial system. (a) Normal midarterial frontal view. (b) The comparable lateral projection, magnified by radiographic technique. The right and left vertebral arteries join to form the basilar artery, which then branches into the intracranial vessels to the right and left as labeled. (c) Subtraction image of b; v = vertebral artery; b = basilar artery; pc = posterior cerebral artery; s = superior cerebellar artery; a = anterior inferior cerebellar artery; p = posterior inferior cerebellar artery.

1. The preoperative evaluation of mass lesions for assessment of their vascularity and for the vascular anatomy of the surrounding area, so that the surgical route may be planned

2. The evaluation of atraumatic intracranial bleeding from such sources as aneurysms and arteriovenous malformations;

3. The work-up of cervicocranial embolic and vascular occlusive disease

MASS LESIONS

Before CT, angiography was the major modality with which intracranial masses were localized. By demonstrating abnormal tumor vasculature, many lesions became clearly visible. In the case of less vascular masses, the displacement of the surrounding vessels from their normal locations would usually closely localize a lesion. With CT, most lesions are already localized by the time of angiography, this study being used primarily to assist the surgeon in preoperative planning.

Mr. Clark's for example, has been diagnosed as having a right frontoparietal meningioma by an initial enhanced CT scan. His preoperative angiogram in Figure 62-3 shows that this is a vascular tumor. You can see the increased radiodensity of the lesion filled with contrast-laden blood in the arterial phase of the external carotid arteriogram shown in Figure 62-3a and b. These films also demonstrate that the primary vascular supply of this meningeal tumor is, as expected, from the meningeal branches of the external carotid artery. Typical areas of increased and decreased bone radiodensity are visible in Figure 62-3b at the tumor site (see Chapter 60).

In Figure 62-3c, involvement of the major cortical veins can be seen, allowing the surgeon to plot the least bloody course to the tumor. Figures 62-3d and e show frontal and lateral views of a right common carotid angiogram in the arterial phase. Notice the shift of the anterior cerebral arteries to the left of the midline in Figure 62-3d and the depressed position of the middle cerebral vessels in both films. These indicate the presence of a mass in the right frontoparietal cortex even before the blush of the contrast agent is seen in the many tumor capillaries (as shown in Figure 62-3a b).

Displacement of Vessels by a Mass

The displacement of vessels is one of the main findings of a mass. Figure 62-4 is a series of line drawings of simple but typical displacements of the normal vessels caused by lesions in various locations of the brain. Comparison of these with the normal vessels in Figure 62-1 should give you at least a basic concept of how masses were, and still are, localized by angiography.

Figure 62-4a is a schematic lateral view of a normal left internal carotid artery injection showing major branches of the anterior and middle cerebral arteries. It is included to demonstrate the actual positions (the numbered circles) of three individual masses. Their individual mass effects are not shown in this view, but arrows are included to indicate how each might affect adjacent vessels.

Figure 62-4c is a normal schematic frontal view of this left carotid injection showing the anterior and middle cerebral arteries.

Figure 62-4c demonstrates mass 1 in the left frontal region. It displaces the anterior loop of the left anterior cerebral artery smoothly to the right across the midline, including the frontopolar branch, which is also shown. The more posterior portion of the vessel, high near the schematic falx, is less affected and stays near midline. The left middle cerebral artery is not visibly affected because it is more posterior in position than this far frontal mass. This is a round shift of the anterior cerebral artery.

Figure 62-4d demonstrates mass 2, a left parietal parasagittal mass high in the coretex near the midline. Because the mass is more posterior, it has little effect on the anterior portion of the left anterior cerebral artery. Notice that the frontopolar branch (arrow) is unaffected here. But, as the anterior cerebral artery extends posteriorly (and thus higher in our frontal view), it shifts across the midline to the right as it nears the mass. Note, however, that it abruptly returns to the left under the edge of the relatively rigid falx. Because of this rigidity, the falx remains at midline. This is a *square shift* of the anterior cerebral artery. Again, the middle cerebral artery is not significantly affected because it is inferior and well lateral to the mass.

Figure 62-4e shows mass 3, a left temporal mass. The mass lies below and lateral to the middle cerebral artery and thus elevates and straightens the bend, or "knee," of the proximal middle cerebral artery and stretches the higher temporoparietal portion as well. The more proximal portions of the left anterior cerebral artery are shifted slightly to the right across the midline, but the frontopolar branch is less affected, and the high distal portions near the falx are involved minimally, if at all.

The vascular shifts depicted are admittedly schematic and simplified for clarity but do serve to demonstrate on a basic level how masses are evaluated angiographically. Although the availability of CT scanning has obviated the need for angiographic localization of lesions in nearly all cases, the principles of vascular displacement remain important in conceptualizing intracranial pathology.

Keynotes

- *Brain tumors displace cerebral vessels, aiding in tumor localization. Some brain tumors have increased tumor vascularity.*

- *Approximately one-half of all intracranial meningiomas are found over the convexities of the brain: laterally; parasagittally (i.e., high near the sagittal or superior longitudinal, venous sinus); or arising from the falx cerebri. Another 40% arise at the base of the brain, often in the olfactory groove or along the sphenoid wing.*

- *The shift of the anterior cerebral arteries can indicate by its shape the likely anteroposterior position of the tumor mass. A "round" shift indicates a frontal mass. A "square" shift indicates a parietal mass.*

CERVICAL AND INTRACRANIAL VASCULAR LESIONS

Cerebral Artery Aneurysms

Recall the patient shown in Figure 61-10, in whom bleeding from an anterior communicating-artery aneurysm resulted in subarachnoid and intraventricular hemorrhage. The work-up of patients with intracranial bleeding such as this is another major indication for arteriography. Figure 62-5 is a series of angiographic subtraction films of such an anterior communicating-artery aneurysm. Like the study of the patient in Figure 61-10, the CT scan of this patient also revealed subarachnoid hemorrhage.

The exact source of the hemorrhage could not be visualized by CT scan. After the patient was stabilized, the angiogram was performed, demonstrating the anterior communicating-artery aneurysm seen in Figure 62-5b, and c. Aside from diagnosing the probable source of the bleeding, the study aided the surgeons in several ways:

1. The size and position of the lesion indicated that it could be treated surgically and also aided in selecting the optimal route of surgical approach.
2. The configuration of the lesion suggested that its origin could be occluded with a special metal aneurysm clip.
3. By examining the other intracranial vessels, additional lesions were excluded, as multiple aneurysms are sometimes present.
4. Because subarachnoid blood is an irritant that can cause spasm of the adjacent arteries, resulting in distal ischemia, this possible complication was also excluded.

Postoperatively the patient did well. The follow-up skull film (Fig. 62-5d) reveals the metal aneurysm clip and a right craniotomy site with bone flap replaced.

Other common sites for aneurysms are at the trifurcation of the middle cerebral artery, where it divides into its frontal, temporal, and parietal branches, and at the origin of the posterior communicating artery. This vessel is visible in the lateral view (Fig. 62-5b arrow). The relatively wide caliber of its origin from the internal carotid artery is normal and does not represent an aneurysm.

Arteriovenous Malformations

Figure 62-6 demonstrates the angiogram of a patient with intracranial bleeding. This lesion is obviously a right parietal arteriovenous malformation. Notice the tangle of enlarged vessels as great volumes of high-pressure arterial blood from both the carotid and vertebralbasilar systems are shunted directly into the massively enlarged and tortuous draining veins. Three of the views depict *early-draining veins,* so named because the direct arterial connections of the malformation feed blood (and contrast material) to these veins before the normal cortical veins elsewhere are visualized. Imagine how these large, tortuous vessels would look in an enhanced CT scan image. Now review Figure 61-11, for it is the CT scan from the same patient.

Because of the location of this lesion, it could have blood supply from both the carotid and vertebralbasilar system. For this reason, a vertebralbasilar arteriogram was performed (Fig. 62-6d, e, and f), demonstrating both the vascular malformation and its early-draining veins. Angiography is used to help plan the surgical approach.

Keynotes

- *Once a CT scan identifies the presence of subarachnoid hemorrhage, an angiogram can be used to define its precise etiology. Angiography is useful in evaluating an intracerebral aneurysm*

  To define the best surgical approach

  To indentify the size of the neck of the aneurysm

  To identify possible additional aneurysms

  To evaluate the degree of vascular spasm present

- *An early-draining vein is a vein that fills before the normal cortical veins. It indicates blood flow through a lesion that is more rapid than normal. It aids in establishing a more precise diagnosis.*

Figure 62-3. Five films from an angiographic study of a patient with a right frontoparietal meningioma. (a) Frontal subtraction view, demonstrating a large tumor blush (arrow, 1) as the contrast agent enters the many capillaries of this vascular lesion. (b) Regular lateral view of a right external carotid artery injection. Because the meningeal vessels originate from the external carotid circulation, the external carotid was studied first. (Recall that the vessels and tumor will appear black with contrast material in the negative subtraction image [a] and more white in the regular film image [b].) The tumor's blush, or "stain" is evident in b, adjacent to an area of bony destruction (arrow, 2) caused by the enlarging tumor. (c) Lateral film from the venous phase of a right common carotid injection. The bony abnormalities are clear. Notice that the cortical veins in the area where the tumor blush was seen are displaced posteriorly (arrow, 3). They are obliterated in the area of bony erosion. (d and e) Earlier arterial-phase films from the right *common* carotid injection. Compare the frontal subtraction view (d) with a. The tumor blush is not as well shown by the common carotid injection, but this view does show that beneath the area of the blush, small vessels are "cupped" around the bottom of the mass (arrow, 4). The middle cerebral vessels are displaced downward (arrow, 5), and the anterior cerebral arteries are shifted across the midline to the left (arrow, 6). In the unsubstracted lateral view (e), the middle cerebral artery branches are displaced inferiorly (arrows, 7). Normally, these vessels form a rough triangular shape known as the *sylvian triangle* (outlined for comparison in the normal lateral view, Fig. 62-1b). In this case, it is flattened in appearance by the presence of the large tumor mass displacing the brain downward from above.

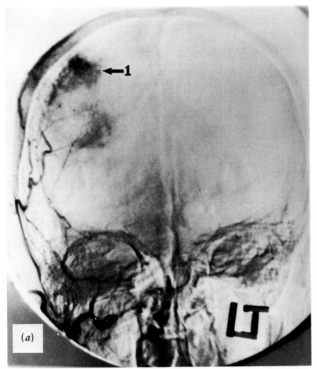

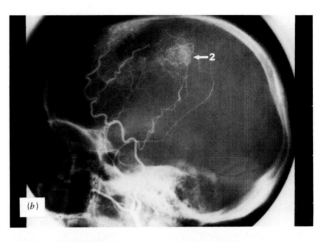

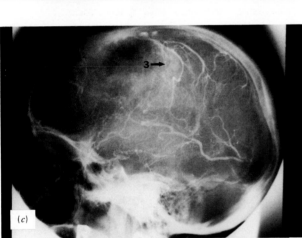

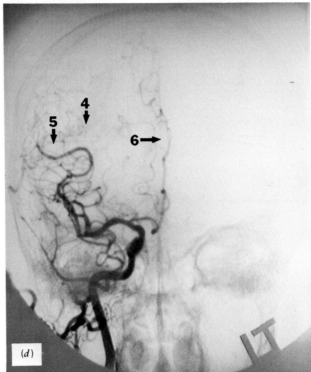

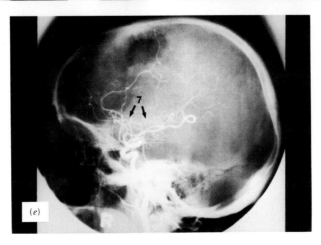

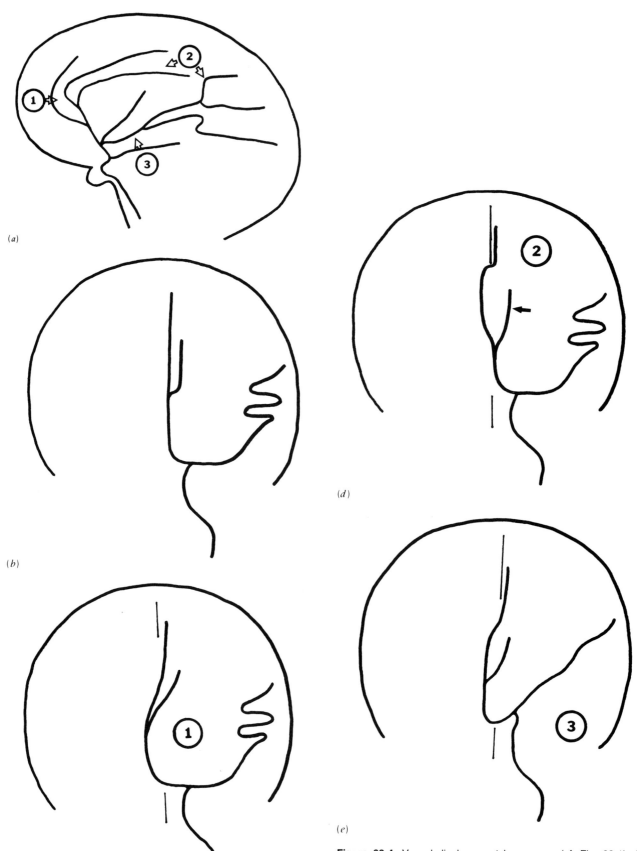

Figure 62-4. Vessel displacement by masses (cf. Fig. 62-1). (a) Normal lateral view of the internal carotid artery. (b) Normal frontal view of the internal carotid artery. (c) Left frontal mass. (d) Left parasagittal mass. (e) Left temporal mass.

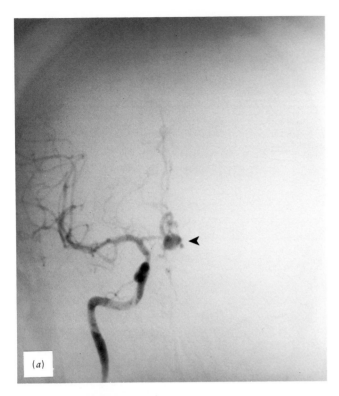

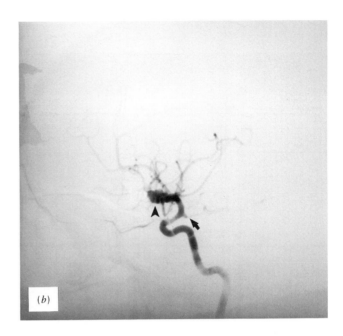

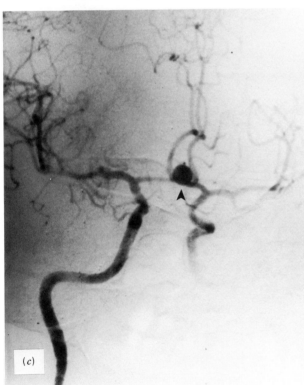

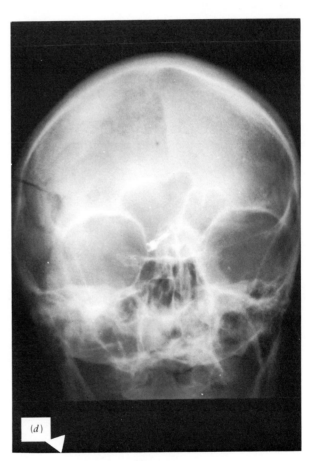

Figure 62-5. An anterior communicating-artery aneurysm (arrowheads) is demonstrated angiographically. Subtraction films of selected images from a right internal carotid artery injection are presented: (*a*) an AP view. (*b*) A lateral view. (*c*) A special oblique projection in which the lesion is viewed radiographically "through" the right orbit in order to avoid the overlapping of the adjacent vessels present in the other images. The balloonlike aneurysm is easily seen in all three images, with its location at the anterior communicating artery best demonstrated in *c*. (*d*) Postoperative skull film in the frontal view demonstrating the metallic clip used to occlude the origin, or "neck," of the aneurysm. A right-sided craniotomy site is visible with the bone flap replaced.

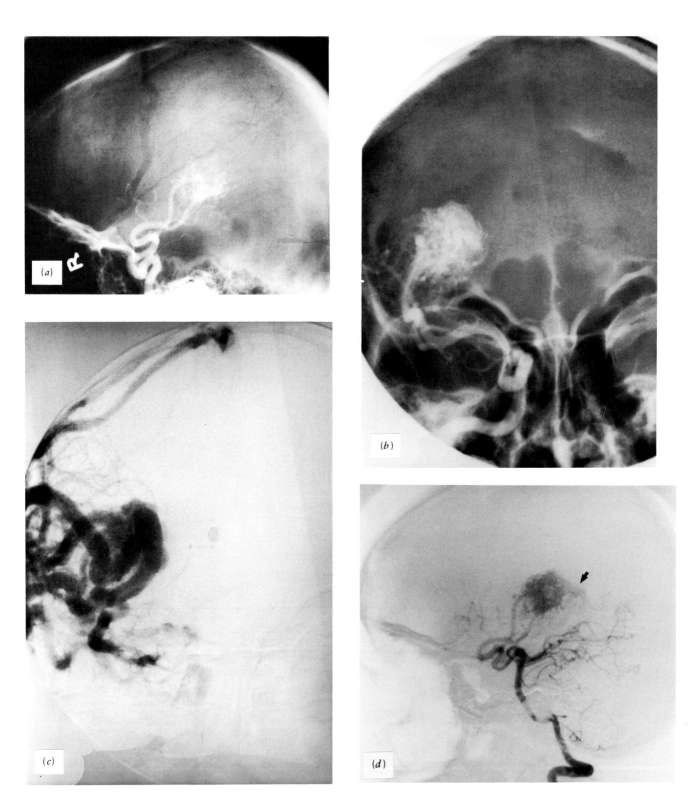

Figure 62-6. Right parietal arteriovenous malformation. On both *a* and *b* the vascular lesion can be easily seen. Note the relatively sparse filling of the normal intracerebral vessels. (*a*) Lateral view. (*b*) Frontal view. (*c*) Frontal subtraction view demonstrating the large, tortuous early-draining veins. (*d*) Lateral view, arterial phase. Early-draining veins are marked by an arrow. (*e*) Frontal view, arterial phase. (*f*) Frontal view, late arterial phase, demonstrating the early-draining veins. Subtraction views *d*, *e*, and *f* of a left vertebral artery injection demonstrate that the malformation also obtains a blood supply from the vertebral-basilar arterial system.

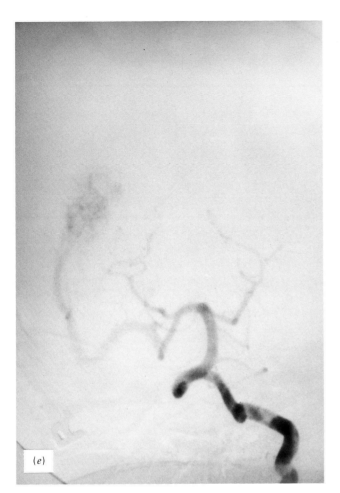

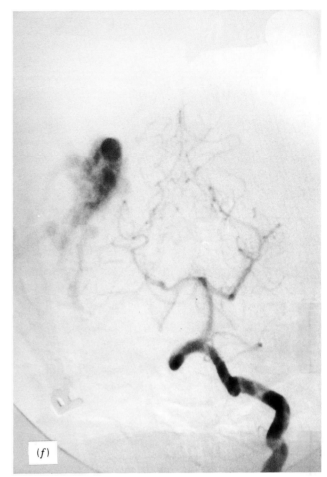

Figure 62-6. (Continued).

Strokes

Mr. Baker had suffered several "small strokes" without permanent sequellae when he was admitted to the vascular surgery service. His physical examination revealed a left carotid bruit, pointing to left carotid atherosclerosis as a possible etiology for the mild right hemiparesis he had suffered during his three prior transient ischemic attacks (TIAs).

Oculoplethysmography, a noninvasive test of gross carotid flow, also indicated a lesion of the left carotid system, but before endarterectomy could be performed, an angiogram (Fig. 62-7) was required to confirm and exactly localize the lesion. The images are frontal and lateral views of the right and left carotid arteries. Notice the smooth contours and absence of narrowing on the right and compare these to the marked narrowing of the lumen of the left internal carotid. The radiologist performing this study suspected an ulcerated atherosclerotic plaque along the posterior wall of the origin of the left internal carotid artery (Fig. 62-7c), a possible source for emboli, which may have caused the patient's problem. This was confirmed at surgery. Postoperatively, the patient ceased having TIAs.

Such evaluation of ischemic vascular disease is the third major indication for angiography. Typically, views of the aortic arch, cervical, and intracranial vessels are obtained so that lesions anywhere in the system, from major branch to small vessel, may be detected; this helps the surgeon to localize a repairable abnormality and to evaluate the potential improvement a patient may expect from a surgical procedure such as an endarterectomy or bypass.

With the advent of computer-enhanced radiographic techniques, similar images of the cervical arteries may be obtained after intravenous injection of contrast material, eliminating much of the risk and expense of conventional angiography. Such techniques, known as digital subtraction angiography, represent another major improvement in radiographic diagnosis. Basically, this technology involves digital computer subtraction of a preliminary fluoroscopic view of the area of interest from a second view obtained after intravenous bolus infusion of contrast material. The image remaining after subtraction is that of the blood vessels under study. Intra-arterial injections can also be performed with this technique.

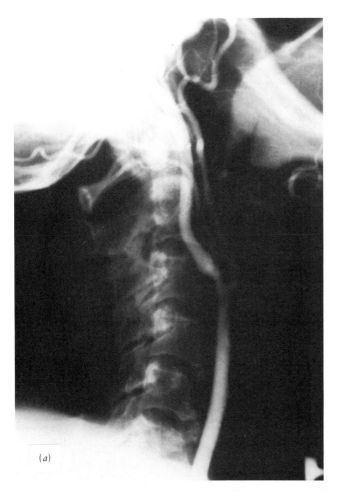
(a)

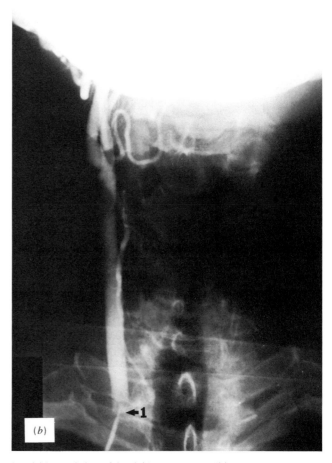
(b) ←1

Figure 62-7. Arteriogram of both common carotid arteries. (a) Lateral view of the right common carotid artery. (b) Frontal view of the right common carotid artery. (c) Lateral view of the left common carotid artery. (d) Frontal view of the left common carotid artery. Right common carotid artery lateral (a) and frontal (b) views demonstrate no abnormalities. The catheter tip (arrow, 1) can be seen in b. The vascular contours are smooth, and no narrowed areas are seen. The left common carotid artery lateral (c) and frontal (d) views both reveal marked narrowing at the origin of the left internal carotid artery (arrow, 2). The narrowing extends over a length of approximately 1 cm. Here, the lumen of the artery is approximately one-fourth of its normal diameter. Recall that if the radius of a circle is reduced, its area diminishes as the square of the radius. Thus, the narrowing of the circular cross-sectional area of the lumen of the artery at this point is considerably greater than the decrease in its diameter we can see radiographically. Blood flow through this point, therefore, is markedly altered. A small ulceration within an atherosclerotic plaque along the posterior aspect of the vessel may be present as shown by a small "beak" visible in c (arrow, 3).

Keynotes

- *Transient ischemic attacks are temporary episodes of cerebral dysfunction from a brief period of brain ischemia.*
- *Ulcerated atherosclerotic plaques in the carotid arteries probably predispose to embolic strokes.*
- *Computer-enhanced angiography is a technique that uses a computer to change image quality and to improve the diagnostic information on an angiographic study. It is currently called digital subtraction angiography or DSA, but it has broader applications than just subtraction, and a better term might be "computer-assisted radiographic imaging."*

SUMMARY

Neuroangiography is a technique in which the blood vessels of the neck and brain are filled with contrast medium so that they can be studied. Because this technique involves the placement of needles or catheters into arteries and the injection of contrast media, it is of some risk to the patient. Currently, neuroangiography is most often used to better define abnormalities already identified by CT to aid in their surgical treatment.

The angiographic work-up of tumors of the brain includes an evaluation of their degree of vascularity and an

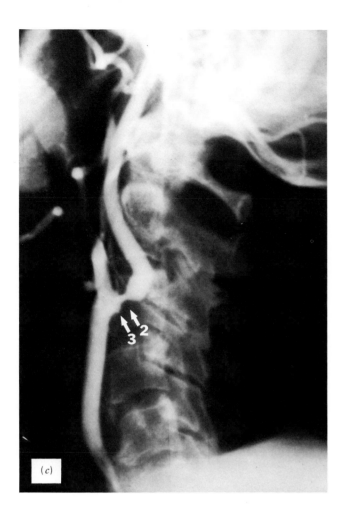

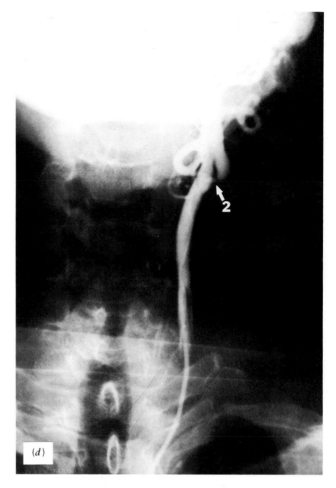

identification of their feeding vessels. Because tumors can displace the major cerebral vessels, the angiograms are studied to aid in choosing the surgical approach.

The patient with an embolic stroke or transient ischemic attack should have an evaluation made of the carotid arteries. Atherosclerotic changes resulting in luminal narrowing and ulceration can be identified with angiographic techniques. Often, these patients are screened initially with oculoplethysmography or Doppler and ultrasound imaging techniques, and those with positive studies are examined by angiography.

Subarachnoid hemorrhage can be identified as an area of increased radiodensity on CT scans. Once identified, an angiogram aids in the evaluation of the aneurysm or arteriovenous malformation that led to the hemorrhage. The presurgical evaluation of an aneurysm includes an evaluation of the vessel of origin of the aneurysm, an evaluation of the size of the neck of the aneurysm, and the identification of any other aneurysms. The evaluation of an arteriovenous malformation includes the identification of all vessels supplying the malformation.

REVIEW QUESTIONS

1. Describe the technique used in neuroangiography.

2. What is the role of angiography in the evaluation of a brain tumor?

3. What are the common causes of subarachnoid hemorrhage?

4. What does the surgeon need to know about a cerebral artery aneurysm?

5. What is an arteriovenous malformation?

6. What is the method of evaluating an embolic stroke or a transient ischemic attack?

VOCABULARY

arteriovenous malformation

digital subtraction angiography

early-draining vein

endarterectomy

oculoplethysmography

parasagittal

round shift

square shift

subarachnoid hemorrhage

transient ischemic attacks

SUGGESTIONS FOR FURTHER READING

For suggested reading see Chapter 61.

PART 7

CONTROLLING THE COST OF HEALTH CARE

Expenditures on health care in the United States now exceed 10% of the gross national product. Efforts to contain the cost of health care have so far focused mainly on high-cost areas: diagnostic testing, hospital admissions, and operations. Throughout this book recommendations on diagnostic imaging have included a concern for cost efficacy. Chapter 63 explains, in part, the economic basis of these choices and discusses some of the parameters affecting health care costs and their impact on the recommendations made for diagnostic testing.

63

COST CONTAINMENT

JOHN MEYERHOFF

KEY CONCEPTS

When U.S. expenditures for health care approached and then exceeded 10% of the gross national product, a general societal consensus was reached that, were costs not restrained, society would end up paying too much for health care and would be diverting too many of its resources away from other important needs. The response to this consensus was a major strengthening of the cost containment measures imposed on the medical care system.

Currently health care reimbursement can be on a fee-for-service basis in which a charge is generated for each service provided, a prepaid system in which care is provided for patients based on a monthly prepaid fee, via preferred provider systems in which a discounted fee-for-service payment is made, and via a prospective payment system in which a set payment is made for treatment of the patient's specific illness and in which the payment is the same no matter what the cost of providing the treatment.

Because the effect of eliminating a few high-cost procedures is great, emphasis in cost containment has initally been placed on the control of high-cost diagnostic tests, hospital admissions, and operations.

The key to reducing the cost of diagnostic testing is the carefully performed and evaluated clinical history and physical examination. Tests should be performed for specific purposes. For each test, the physician should consider whether the test is necessary, whether the test result will affect the patient's further evaluation or therapy, and whether there is a cheaper method of obtaining the same information.

The selection of the appropriate test should be based on a knowledge of its sensitivity, specificity, and cost, and this knowledge should be compared with the sensitivity, specificity, and cost of competing tests that might yield the same information. Unfortunately, for most diagnostic tests, this information is not available. Thus if you are not certain which test is best, consultation with the radiologist or knowledgeable specialist should be obtained.

The cost-efficient evaluation of the symptomatic patient will vary with the severity of illness and whether the patient is an outpatient or inpatient. Outpatient evaluation can usually proceed in a sequential fashion with each subsequent test based on the results of the preceding one. Because of the high cost of hospitalization, there may be less total expense with the hospitalized patient if test are clumped together, thus shortening the overall time needed for the patient's evaluation and thereby decreasing the duration of hospitalization.

OBJECTIVES

When you complete this chapter you will be able to

1. Describe the following practice systems and discuss the economic incentives and disincentives in each:
   a. Fee-for-service
   b. Prepaid group.
   c. Preferred provider organization
   d. Independent practice association
   e. Prospective payment system
2. Describe cost-efficient methods of evaluation in an outpatient and inpatient setting, explaining the differences between them.
3. List the three methods by which a hospital can decrease the costs of a hospital admission.
4. Define and differentiate "sensitivity" and "specificity."

The technology used in the practice of diagnostic imaging has changed dramatically in the past decade. Computed tomography scanners and MRI devices now produce images only imagined in the past. The amount and type of

583

information they produce has caused adjustments in the ways that patients' complaints are evaluated.

The cost of these machines and of the studies produced on them is high, and this with the other increasing costs of medial care has produced a countertrend of activity emphasizing cost containment. An assessment of costs should now be part of every decision about the care of a patient. With each decision you make, ask yourself, "Is what I am doing necessary? Is there a cheaper way to do the same thing?"

The elimination of a few high-cost procedures equals the effect of eliminating many inexpensive procedures. Thus the major initial focus of cost containment has been high-cost procedures—especially diagnostic imaging procedures, operations, and hospitalizations. Diagnostic imaging is one of the prime areas for cost cutting because of the high cost of many of the tests and the ability to generate significant savings if these tests are used appropriately

But cost containment in diagnostic imaging has to be viewed in a broader context. Medical care in the United States as a percentage of the GNP has steadily increased over the years, and as it approached and exceeded 10%, a general societal consensus crystallized (without any discussion of how much medical care there ought to be): too much was going toward medical care while society's other essential expenditures were restricted by the level of medical care expenditure. The federal government, state governments, and large and small employers, the payers for medical care, all have begun to adopt ways of reducing the costs of medical care. To understand the new cost containment methods and how they affect medicine in general and diagnostic imaging in particular, some definitions are needed.

Keynotes

- *An assessment of costs should now enter into every decision made about patient care.*
- *Ask yourself, "Is what I am doing necessary? Is there a cheaper way to do the same thing?"*
- *Appropriate controls on high-cost diagnostic imaging procedures, hospital admissions, and operations can help control the cost of health care.*
- *The cost of health care now exceeds 10% of GNP.*

REIMBURSEMENT SYSTEMS

Fee-for-service

Fee-for-service is the traditional medical reimbursement system. The patient sees the physician or has a radiological exam, and a fee is paid for this service. The fee may be paid by the patient or by an insurance company, but there is an one-to-one relationship between the service and the fee.

If you were responsible for managing employee benefits for a corporation that was interested in containing the cost of medical care, what would you think of this system and how would you react?

If you were a physician working in a FFS practice, what incentive is there for you to limit the cost of medical care?

Prepaid Group

The *prepaid group* (PPG) is the newer method of reimbursement as exemplified by health maintenance organizations (HMOs). There is a monthly fee prepaid on a per-patient basis to a primary care provider (or group), and all of the medical care required by the patient is provided without any additional cost. In the older HMO's all the physicians are employees of the group.

If you were a corporate executive trying to decide how to contain the cost of health care, how would you view an HMO system as a method of lowering your costs?

If you were a physician working for the HMO, what incentive is there for you to contain health care costs? What incentive is there for you not to order too few tests or provide too few services?

Preferred Provider Organization

The *preferred provider organization* (PPO) is a group of providers (physicians, hospitals, etc.) who have agreed to provide fee-for-service care at a discount to individuals who have signed up for the PPO. The provider gives the discount in the expectation of an increased number of patients, given that not all the providers in a community will be participating in the PPO. Because the additional cost (called the *marginal cost*) of providing one more unit of care is less than the average cost, the provider expects to make more money with more patients. Conversely, the provider may decide that not participating in the PPO will result in fewer patients coming to her or him and may decide to join the PPO to protect the size of her or his practice.

If you were the employee benefits manager at a corporation, how would you view the PPO as a method of containing costs?

If you were a physician, what incentives are there for you to join the PPO and what incentives are there in the PPO for you to contain costs?

Independent Practice Association

An *independent practice association* (IPA) is a group of providers (usually FFS physicians) who contract to provide prepaid care in their own offices. In many of the new HMO's the providers are not group employees but are working on a contract basis.

If you were the corporate employee benefits manager, what advantage does the IPA offer over the traditional HMO?

If you were an IPA physician, what incentives would you have to contain costs?

Prospective Reimbursement

The system currently used by the federal government in paying hospitals for Medicare patients is *prospective reimbursement*. Based on the type of illness that requires the patient to be hospitalized, the government will pay the hospital a fixed amount of money representing the average cost of taking care of similar patients in that part of the country. The classification system is based on payment for a diagnosis-related group (DRG), not on the actual charges generated by a specific patient. In a few states, all hospitalizations are reimbursed on a DRG basis regardless of who is paying.

What are the financial incentives to the hospital to contain costs under a prospective payment system?

Keynotes

- *In a Fee-for-service practice a fee is generated for each service provided.*
- *In a prepaid group practice a monthly fee is prepaid for each patient to cover all costs of health care.*
- *Health care providers include physicians, nurse practitioners, dentists, podiatrists, hospitals, clinics, and others.*
- *Preferred providers have agreed to provide fee-for-service care at a discount.*
- *Marginal cost is the cost of providing the next unit of service or product.*
- *An independent practice association is a group of providers who contract to provide prepaid care in their own offices.*
- *Prospective reimbursement is the payment of a set fee for covering all the costs of care.*
- *Diagnosis-related groups is a classification system based on grouping illnesses that have approximately the same costs associated with them.*

CORPORATE AND PROVIDER INCENTIVES TO CONTAIN COSTS AND PRESERVE QUALITY

Corporate benefits managers have two opposing incentives in choosing a health plan for their corporations' employees: the lowest cost possible for services and services that satisfy the employees and limit complaints about the plan. If benefits managers choose plans that employees will not accept, they can cause labor-management problems for their corporations. If they spend too much money on health plans they limit corporate resources for investment in other programs.

Those employees who already have a relationship with a physician are least likely to want to change plans. They would perfer a FFS plan unless their personal physician is a member of a PPO or IPA. Those without a personal physician will usually want a system that provides them with care that is convenient and personal. Depending on the specific systems available in a community, any of the above systems of physician reimbursement may be the preferred method of an employee benefits manager. An HMO or a PPO may or may not be the cheapest; it may provide a higher but known prospective cost. An HMO could provide good service or bad service to its members. It could be in an inconvenient location. It could have friendly or nasty personnel. Each of these factors enters into the decision.

What are the physician's economic incentives under each of the payment plans? With a FFS system, it would initially appear that the incentive is always to do more tests and have more visits from each patient; the more visits or more tests, the more earnings. In most FFS arrangements, however, insurance only covers 80% of the charge or less, so the patient always receives a bill for some of the costs of the service. In that situation, the physician whose bill to the patient is too high may lose that patient to a less costly alternative, even if it is another FFS physician. The pressure from HMOs and PPOs in an environment that competes for patients also serves to limit the charges of a FFS physician.

In addition, insurance companies and hospitals are beginning to keep track of how often each physician orders tests or office visits for common diagnoses. This allows them to develop profiles of high-cost and high-use physicians. In some states, hospitals and the companies that administer Medicare use these profiles to counsel those physicians rated high cost.

In the prepaid plans (the HMOs and IPAs), there are provider incentives to limit costs. In those where the physicians are employed by the group, each is usually paid a base salary and a year-end bonus based on any surplus or profit made by the group. If the group has a loss—that is, it provides more care during the fiscal year than the contract is paying for—then the providers often must make up some of the loss out of their salaries or work longer hours. Thus each individual physician has the economic incentive not to waste the monthly capitation fee on useless tests.

Before the era of intensive cost containment, most of the savings in PPG plans was generated by not hospitalizing patients and by providing care in less expensive settings. The savings were generated not by doing less in the outpatient setting than would have been done in a FFS system but by controlling the costs related to hospitalization. For a PPG to be able to offer less expensive care, the providers in the group must believe that less care in terms of frequency of visits, number of tests performed, and use of hospitals can provide equal or better care than the FFS arena.

To ensure that the PPG makes (and certainly does not lose) money, there must be someone watching how much money each physician is spending. This is particularly true in an IPA, where not every physician may really believe that less care may be good care. If a physician is ordering too many tests, putting too many people in the hospital, or seeing patients too often, the group administrator will suggest that he or she be more frugal. Similar controls exists in PPOs to make sure that a discounted fee for a procedure is not made up by doing more of the procedures when they are not indicated.

HOSPITAL INCENTIVES UNDER A PROSPECTIVE REIMBURSEMENT SYSTEM

If you were the hospital administrator managing a hospital under a prospective reimbursment system, what would you do to maximize profit? Under this system you receive payments for each patient admitted depending on the DRG that the patient is in. How would you attempt to control the use of diagnostic imaging procedures and limit other costs of the admission?

The hospital's incentives under a prospective payment system are three:

1. Shorten the length of stay.
2. Decrease the costs of each admission.
3. Eliminate services that cost more than is paid for them.

Reducing Length of Stay

Reducing the length of stay is important because the overhead costs (construction costs, heating, cleaning, etc.) of each bed in the hospital are fixed. If patients stay a shorter time, each bed can be used by more patients each year. By spreading the fixed costs of each bed over more patients, the cost per patient is decreased and, the increased admissions also result in more payments. If no additional admissions result, then decreasing the length of stay will mean fewer beds occupied at any time, so fewer beds have to be maintained, partially eliminating their cost.

Decreasing the Costs of Each Admission

The hospital can decrease its expenses by decreasing the nonfixed (or variable) costs of each admission. These nonfixed costs vary from patient to patient and range from big-ticket items like MRI examinations to small-ticket items like the adhesive bandage put on a venipuncture site. The hospital will attempt to reduce the cost of each item to the minimum.

Greater savings may be possible by not doing excessive numbers of laboratory or imaging tests, discouraging or forbidding the use of expensive drugs, and shifting diagnostic evaluations and follow-up care to outpatient or less expensive care facilities (such as nursing homes or home care services).

Eliminating Services That Are Not Reimbursed Adequately

If a service is not reimbursed adequately by the payers, then a decision must be made on whether it should be eliminated or whether it is so important to some other function of the hospital that it should be a loss leader.

SELECTION OF THE APPROPRIATE TESTS

Physicians who understand the medical care economic system know that cost containment is appropriate and essential in choosing diagnostic tests. Whether they work in FFS practices or for HMOs or have patients in both groups, they will find incentives for controlling the cost of health care in all systems. Working in this environment, physicians must select the tests they obtain and decide which patients really need hospitalization and which patients really need surgery. How are such determinations to be made?

Diagnostic Testing

Decisions on requesting diagnostic testing should be based on the knowledge gained from a careful history and physical examination. Most incorrect requests for tests come from an incomplete understanding of the patient's problem. Each test should be based on the need to make a decision about further evaluation or treatment. If no decision results from a test, the test is probably not needed to manage the patient. In deciding that a test is needed, the physician should have a knowledge of the test's specificity, sensitivity, and cost.

The *sensitivity* is how likely the test is to demonstrate the abnormality if the suspected disease is present. The *specificity* is how unlikely the normal patient is to have an abnormal result. A less expensive test may be justified, because it is less expensive, even if it is not as specific or as sensitive as a more expensive test. Conversely, an expensive test may be indicated because its increased sensitivity or specificity eliminates the need for several less expensive tests that are not as good.

It is unfortunate that for most diagnostic tests the true sensitivity and specificity, much less the relative sensitivity and specificity of competing tests, are unknown. A further complication is that in tests requiring special interpretive skills or special equipment, like most imaging examinations, a particular institution may have greater skill or better equipment in one area than another, which must be also considered in the choice of the appropriate test. For these reasons, the clinician should readily consult with the radiologist to obtain advice as to the best imaging test to request.

Keynotes

- *A careful analysis of a carefully obtained history and physical examination is the proper guide to the cost efficient selection of diagnostic tests.*
- *The sensitivity of a test is how likely the test is to demonstrate the abnormality if the suspected abnormality is present.*
- *The specificity is how unlikely the normal patient is to have an abnormal result.*

Screening Tests

For a test to be a good *screening test* for a particular disease, the test must be one that produces abnormal results in most of the patients with the disease (high sensitivity). Because the idea of screening is to pick up disease at a stage where treatment is still effective, it is important that the test give abnormal results early in the course of the disease. In addition, because excluding the presence of disease in a patient who has a false-positive test result is expensive and anxiety producing for the patient, it is desirable to have a test in which only a few normal people will have a positive test result (high specificity).

How well does the chest radiograph function as a screening device? To answer this question, you need the answer to the question: A screening device for what disease?

For COPD? For this disease, it is a poor screen. Its sensitivity is too low. Early COPD will not result in any changes on radiographs. With advanced disease, you may see some overinflation and flattening of the diaphragm, but if you have to use a chest radiograph to learn that your patient may have advanced emphysema, you didn't take a very good history.

For lung cancer or tuberculosis in asymptomatic individuals? For many years there were mobile x-ray vans that went to schools and job sites so that people could have chest radiographs done to screen for lung cancer and tuberculosis. This method of screening has been abandoned for several reasons. First, as the incidence of tuberculosis fell, the diagnostic yield of the examination decreased and therefore the cost per case found went up. Second, it was found that the populations that still had tuberculosis were not those that came to the mobile vans; they avoided them. The highest yield in screening for tuberculosis came from those arrested and sent to local jails.

Random screening for lung cancer with chest radiographs is usually not helpful because most of the patients found to have lung cancer have advanced cancer and can not be cured. While periodic screening of a set population with chest radiographs obtained every 6 months does find some curable cases, most of the patients found this way

still have metastatic cancer. In general, screening imaging examinations have proved of value only with screening mammography (Chapter 25).

Keynotes

- *A screening test ideally should be one that is of high sensitivity, high specificity, and low cost and that detects the disease sufficiently early in its course to result in effective treatment.*

Baseline Examinations

For years physicians have obtained chest radiographs, ECGs, and other tests as *baseline studies*. What does this mean? The assumption was that an asymptomatic person might have some chronic, but not pathologically significant, change on his or her chest radiograph or ECG. Later, if the person developed a cough, shortness of breath, or other pulmonary or cardiac symptom, the chronic change would not then be misinterpreted as a new finding leading to an expensive diagnostic work-up. When carefully considered, does this hypothesis really make sense?

First, it assumes that the abnormality would be one that could confuse the evaluation of the current symptom. Most of the abnormal findings in asymptomatic people (pleural thickening, small calcified granulomas, etc.) are not likely to cause symptoms.

Second, it assumes that the abnormality when first seen in an asymptomatic patient would not lead to a work-up yet would do so when the patient acquired some symptom. Actually, the work-up for almost all chest radiographic abnormalities is the same whether the patient is symptomatic or asymptomatic. It was also assumed that a "baseline" chest radiograph could help prevent an unneeded admission to the hospital by showing the physician caring for the patient that the suspicious change on the chest radiograph was in fact old and that the new symptoms did not require admission.

There is little evidence to support such uses of "baseline" examinations, and in general they should not be used. The main and important exception to this is the great usefulness of a baseline mammogram obtained at age 35. The lack of value in obtaining baseline studies does not apply, however, to the comparison of a preexisting examination result with a current study. If a patient with a suspected lung nodule has a previous chest radiograph, it is certainly worth comparing it with the current one to determine whether any change has occurred. The desirability of having an old study in a few select cases is not indication to obtain baseline examinations on everyone.

Keynote

- *A baseline study is one obtained so that a later change from this baseline will permit the earlier detection and treatment of disease.*

Cost-Efficient Evaluation of the Symptomatic Patient

The most cost-efficient methods of evaluating the symptomatic patient differ depending on whether the patient is an inpatient or an outpatient.

Outpatient Evaluation. The evaluation of the symptomatic outpatient should consist of a sequence of tests based on the presumptive diagnosis or diagnoses determined from the careful history and physical examination. Each selected test should be chosen to answer a specific question. Expensive tests should be sequential, with each subsequent more expensive test obtained in response to a positive or negative result of a previous test. Groups of tests should be obtained only when significant patient time or cost savings result.

Inpatient Evaluation. In a prospective reimbursement system in the hospital, remember that there are costs but no real charges. The hospital will be reimbursed only a fixed amount no matter how long the patient stays in the hospital or how many diagnostic tests are obtained. Because each day in the hospital costs money and each test costs money, it may be cheaper to obtain several tests on the same day to shorten the hospital stay, or if the tests are very expensive, to obtain them sequentially. The best system would be to discuss the clinical problem with the radiologist and allow the radiologist to manage the sequence of studies and the number of studies to be performed each day. With this method, once a definitive result is obtained, the remaining examinations can be canceled.

The alternate method is for the radiologist to have enough information about the patient so that if a specifically requested examination has not resulted in a diagnosis, the radiologist can proceed to the next stage of evaluation. In well-run radiology departments you will also find that all requests for imaging examinations are screened for appropriateness, and you should not be surprised to have the radiologist phone you, ask for more information, and then suggest a different or additional examination for your patient. This will occur particularly with the patients with difficult diagnostic problems.

Keynotes

- *The outpatient evaluation of the symptomatic patient should consist of a sequence of tests, each obtained in appropriate response to a previous normal or abnormal test result.*
- *The inpatient evaluation of the symptomatic patient may be less costly if diagnostic tests are clumped together so they are completed faster, thus shortening the hospital length of stay.*
- *Consultation with the radiologist or other specialist is an effective method of decreasing the cost of a diagnostic imaging evaluation.*

TWO ULTIMATE PRINCIPLES OF PHYSICIAN RESPONSIBILITY

This chapter may have seemed like a minicourse in economics, but some knowledge of the economics of our current health care system is necessary to understand the pressures that hospitals and physicians are working under. In this era of cost containment, two principles should guide our care of our patients:

1. Good care is always the best care and is often the most cost-efficent care. Patients want to know what is going on with them. They want a physician who listens to them and who talks to them and doesn't just order lots of tests.
2. We are our patients' advocates. Just because good care can sometimes be cheap care does not mean all cheap care is good care. Just because good care is sometimes expensive does not mean all expensive care is good care. If we see that our patients are being harmed by inadequate care as a result the new waves of cost containment, it is our responsibility to speak out. It is also our responsibility as physicians to monitor ourselves and our peers to ensure that we do not spend our patients' money just because it is there to spend.

SUMMARY

Expenditures for health care in the United States now exceeding 10% of GNP have led the payers for health care—the federal government, state governments, and small and large employers—to seek methods of controlling the cost of health care.

Current methods of payment for physician and hospital services include fee-for-service, prepaid group practice, preferred provider organizations, independent practice associations, and prospective payment plans. In each of these different systems, the incentives for controlling health care expenditures differ. In the FFS system the incentive is based on the need to limit the patient's co-payment for services and on competition from the HMOs and PPOs. In the HMOs the control is based on careful monitoring of the physicians' use of the HMOs' resources, sweetened by the provision of a bonus to the physician of funds unspent at the end of the year. Controls in PPOs are usually based on a monitoring of each physician's use of resources. Controls in an IPA may resemble those of an HMO or PPO, depending on the structure of the IPA.

Prospective reimbursement is currently used for Medicare payments to hospitals. The hospital receives a payment based on the DRG that the patient's diagnosis is in. This payment must cover all costs that result from the admission. If the hospital can keep its costs for the admission below the allowed amount, it makes a profit; if not, it has a loss for that patient.

The control of health care costs currently concentrates on the control of the most costly parts of health care: expensive diagnostic imaging tests, hospital admissions, and operations. The selection of appropriate tests should be based on a carefully performed history and physical examination. Each test should be selected to answer a question the answer to which would result in different management of the patient's problem. To evaluate which test should be performed, the test's sensitivity, specificity, and cost should be known and should be compared with the sensitivity, specificity, and cost of any competing test. Unfortunately, this information is unavailable for most of the tests used in diagnostic imaging. For this reason, consultation with the radiologist or a knowledgeable specialist may be helpful in difficult diagnostic problems.

In general, most screening tests using diagnostic imaging are not cost efficient. The main exception is mammography in screening for breast cancer. In most cases, the obtaining of baseline radiological examinations is not of value. Again, the main exception is mammography in screening for breast cancer.

Costs of diagnostic evaluation can be decreased by outpatient evaluation before admission with sequential testing. Because of the cost of hospitalization, clumping of tests in the hospitalized patient may be helpful in decreasing the total cost of the hospital admission.

REVIEW QUESTIONS

1. What is FFS practice, and what are its economic incentives and disincentives?
2. What is PPG practice, and what are its economic incentives and disincentives?
3. What is a PPO, and what are its economic incentives and disincentives?
4. What is an IPA, and what are its economic incentives and disincentives?
5. What is a prospective payment system, and what are its economic incentives and disincentives?
6. What is a DRG?
7. Major efforts at cost containment are directed at what three high-cost medical activities?
8. Define and differentiate "sensitivity" and "specificity."
9. Discuss the criteria that would make a screening test worthwhile economically.
10. Describe the function of baseline examinations.
11. How should the diagnostic evaluation of the symptomatic outpatient and the symptomatic inpatient differ?

VOCABULARY

baseline examination
cost containment
cost efficient
diagnosis-related group
fee-for-service
gross national product
health maintenance
  organization
independent practice
  association
length of stay
preferred provider
  organization
prepaid group
prospective payment system
prospective reimbursement
provider
screening test
sensitivity
specificity

SUGGESTIONS FOR FURTHER READING

Paul Starr. *The Social Transformation of American Medicine*. Basic Books,: New York. 1982.

Harold C. Fox, Jr., Ed. *Common Diagnostic Tests: Use and Interpretation*. American College of Physicians: Philadelphia. 1987.

INDEX